Orthopaedics

Questions and Answers

Preparatory Manual for Undergraduates

Second Edition

Orthopaedics
Questions and Answers
Preparatory Manual for Undergraduates

Sachin Upadhyay
MS (Ortho), FIJR BCBR GCP
Professor
Department of Orthopaedics
NSCB Medical College
Jabalpur, MP

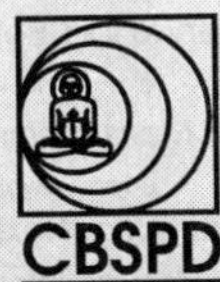

CBSPD

CBS Publishers & Distributors Pvt Ltd

New Delhi • Bengaluru • Chennai • Kochi • Kolkata • Lucknow • Mumbai
Hyderabad • Jharkhand • Nagpur • Patna • Pune • Uttarakhand

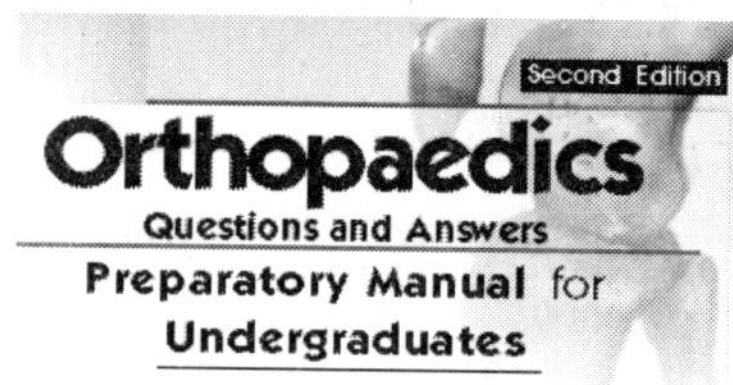

ISBN: 978-93-5466-614-8

Copyright © Author and Publisher

Second Edition: 2025

First Edition: 2013

Published by Satish Kumar Jain and produced by Varun Jain for

CBS Publishers & Distributors Pvt Ltd

4819/XI Prahlad Street, 24 Ansari Road, Daryaganj, New Delhi 110 002, India.
Ph: 011-23289259, 23266838   Website: www.cbspd.com
                                             e-mail: delhi@cbspd.com

Corporate Office: 204 FIE, Industrial Area, Patparganj, Delhi-110092
Ph: 011-4934 4934   Fax: 011-4934 4935   e-mail: publishing@cbspd.com; publicity@cbspd.com

Branches

- **Bengaluru:** Seema House 2975, 17th Cross, K.R. Road, Banasankari 2nd Stage, Bengaluru 560 070, Karnataka, India
  Ph: +91-80-26771678/79   Fax: +91-80-26771680   e-mail: bangalore@cbspd.com
- **Chennai:** 18/8B, Subbarayan Street, Shenoy Nagar, Chennai 600 030, Tamil Nadu
  Ph: +91-044-42032115, 26681266   e-mail: chennai@cbspd.com
- **Kochi:** 42/1325, 1326, Power House Road, Opp KSEB Power House, Ernakulam 682 018, Kochi, Kerala, India
  Ph: +91-484-4059061-65   Fax: +91-484-4059065   e-mail: kochi@cbspd.com
- **Kolkata:** 147, Hind Ceramics Compound, 1st Floor, Nilgunj Road, Belghoria, Kolkata 700 056, West Bengal, India
  Ph: +91-033-25633055, 033-25633056   e-mail: kolkata@cbspd.com
- **Lucknow:** Basement, Khushnuma Complex, 7-Meerabai Marg (behind Jawahar Bhawan), Lucknow 226 001, UP, India
  Ph: +91-522-400043, 9919002738   e-mail: tiwari.lucknow@cbspd.com
- **Mumbai:** PWD Shed, Gala no. 25/26, Ramchandra Bhatt Marg, Next to JJ Hospital Gate no. 2
  Opp. Union Bank of India, Noorbaug, Mumbai-400009, Maharashtra, India
  Ph: 022-60061880/89   e-mail: mumbai@cbspd.com

Representatives

• **Hyderabad**	0-9885175004	• **Jharkhand**	0-9811541605	• **Nagpur**	0-8692091830
• **Patna**	0-9334159340	• **Pune**	0-9664372571	• **Uttarakhand**	0-9716462459

Printed at: Mudrak, Noida, UP, India

__________ **to** __________

my parents
who are always loving and supporting me
and
my family
who have always been there for me, and have never doubted my dreams,
no matter how crazy they might be

Foreword

During university exams besides anxiety there is a lot of confusions in student's brain about the examination paper. What the question is actually asking? What are they expected to include in their answer? What matter will be relevant? And on the other side —The most common complaint from assessors is that the student did not answer the question appropriately and consequently they did not score well.

Ideally, students want textbook notes to supplement what they are learning in class. They will make the concrete base for any revision or further study they need to do. Proper revision is essential to learning to write effectively and is the most effective in improving the score on students' papers. Therefore, it is imperative to take notes effectively, making it easier for them to read and understand when they come back to revising the topic in the future.

A number of textbooks are available in the market with comprehensive relevant contents but lack sample answers and tips to score high during the university exams. No one can memorize page by page of contents. Keeping these facts, Dr Sachin Upadhyay has tried to condense the entire material into a succinct format, i.e. one which pulls all the important/relevant information and terminology out for them, avoiding any superfluous contents. He has tried to skim many textbooks and scientific journals and prepared notes (answers) on the most important contents. Being an eminent member in DNB exams panel and as a teacher I had always suggested Dr Sachin Upadhyay to write a book for undergraduate students, for I felt that a concise book concerning undergraduate's university exams is the need of the hour. I am happy that he has acted on my honest advice. The present *Orthopaedics Preparatory Manual for Undergraduates* though meant for the undergraduate students it has also become popular among postgraduates students pan India.

I remembered that Dr Upadhyay is one of the few Indians who has received word of Felicitation from Drs. Canale and Beaty the editor of *Campbell's Operative Orthopaedics* for his outstanding research on patella position in Indian population. Besides an eminent Researcher, innovator, author and skilled surgeon, Dr Upadhyay has unique style of teaching and writing which is popular among the students. The concise materials outlined in this book were not prepared overnight. They represent a hard and dedicated work of Dr. Upadhyay from the past few years of clinical work in the field of undergraduate academics. The second edition of the book provides a concise overview of orthopedic university theory exam in the form of questions and answer directed toward third- and fourth-year undergraduate students.

The best thing about *Orthopaedics Preparatory Manual for Undergraduates* is that it is provocative and expertly written. Simple writing, lucid language, crisp presentation, flow-charts; proper material headings and subheadings, important notes, inclusion of every possible question and clarity of the content make this book unique. The proper framing of questions in the form of short note and essay type format is also very good. Undoubtedly, the MCQs at the end are very useful for the university exam format. There is no doubt that this is a well-written informative book for the undergraduate and postgraduate students, and I have no hesitation to recommend this book to undergraduate and postgraduate students in medical universities for theory examinations.

It is my pleasure and honor to foreword this book which is dedicated to undergraduate and postgraduate students. I congratulate Dr Sachin Upadhyay on his prodigious efforts, and the very fact that the book is seeing its second edition is certainly a matter of great pride and honor for him. I wish him and the book all the best.

Prof. Dr. Javahir A Pachore
MS (Ortho), MCh (Ortho) (Liverpool), MNAMS (Ortho), D.Ortho, FCPS
ISHKS Founder President (2006–2008)
Director-Professor and Head
Department of Hip Replacement Surgery
Shalby Hospitals
Former Orthopaedics Consultant and Joint Replacement Surgeon
Bombay Hospital
Mumbai

Preface to the Second Edition

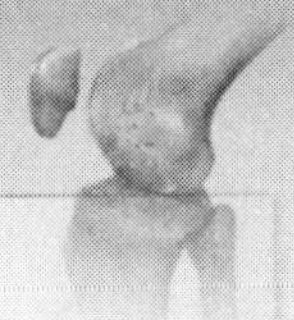

The second edition of *Orthopaedics: Preparatory Manual for Undergraduates* provides a concise overview of university question and answers directed toward prefinal and final undergraduate students. In response to our first-ever competitive text, we have updated and revised every chapter to reflect updated evidence-based material in this popular Preparatory manual which I believe gives better continuity. We have added few more questions and answers to every chapter in simple and lucid language supported by flowcharts and bullets points.

As in previous editions, I have kept the text in a standardized format as much as possible. The topics are presented from a straightforward practical point-of-view, with the content being condensed to its most salient features. As paying close attention to readers' feedback from previous edition, this edition has a well-organized index which helps the readers to save their precious time while searching for the topics.

Additionally, at the end of questions and answers, I have presented around 500 multiple-choice questions (MCQs) considered appropriate for medical students to be able to answer as per the new format from the medical universities. This section will help the students to score good marks as well as develop a strong foundation for the future NEET postgraduate exams.

Lots of standard textbooks/scientific journals have been referred before compiling this book. Still I would wholeheartedly accept fruitful suggestions/constructive criticism and comments offered by the readers for improvements in the pattern/text in its future editions.

At the end, I hope this book will meet all the requirements of the readers and come up to their expectations. This self-contained book would take the readers from a state of dilemmas and doubts to clarity and finally to their respective destinies.

If you need any kind of help regarding any questions or any special topic, you are most welcome to contact me via e-mail. I would try my level best to help you.

Sachin Upadhyay
e-mail: drsachinupadhyay@gmail.com

Preface to the First Edition

A large number of books on orthopaedics, both international and Indian, are available in the market. Many of these are voluminous and students find these somewhat hard to understand. The examination season is a difficult time – there seems to be so much of studying and revision to do on the top of your normal course, at times it seems that you will never get through it all. It is quite usual for students to experience the stress of revision during exam time as they have a huge syllabus to cover, but the worst thing that you can do is get so anxious that you spend more time worrying than revising. In this stressful environment if you have your own notes concerning the subjects you will finish your revision in no time as they play vital role during the last minute revisions. Preparing notes helps in better understanding of the topics that are given in the books. Currently no such book is available in the market, especially on orthopaedics, which helps you in exam revision stress. This book has been written keeping in mind the requirements of undergraduate students. This book will also help postgraduate students to refresh their basics of orthopaedics in their early phase. The text written will not only help the students to prepare for their exams but also helps them in retaining all important facts about the subject. Thus it maximizes productivity and results.

The overall objective of this comprehensive, self-contained book is to provide concise, consolidated yet authoritative/trustworthy coverage of the basics of orthopaedics. The book is divided into different sections which follows the general pattern of a textbook which includes general anatomy, trauma, diseases of joints, spine injuries, congenital anomalies, infections, skeletal tuberculosis, metabolic diseases, myopathy, regional orthopaedics, current facts about resuscitation, neurology, imaging, gait physiology, splints and instruments. Each of these sections includes series of *commonly asked questions* (*essays types* or *short note types*) *with appropriate* **answers**. The answers are point-wise, written *in lucid language and are very easy for students to follow*. In places of lengthy explanations I have incorporated a large number of *flow charts* at appropriate places for easy comprehension. While writing the chapters and compiling the questions, I have consulted syllabi of several universities to cover most of the topics prescribed for undergraduate medical students. The text provides an intelligent and comprehensive study.

A number of standard textbooks and scientific journals have been referred to before compiling this book. Still I would wholeheartedly accept fruitful suggestions, constructive criticism and comments offered by the readers for improvement in the presentation and text in its future editions.

In the end I hope this book will meet all the requirements of the readers and come up to their expectations. This self-contained book would take the readers from a state of dilemmas and doubts to clarity and finally to their respective destinations.

If you need any kind of help regarding any questions or any special topic, you are most welcome to contact me via e-mail. I would try my level best to help you.

Sachin Upadhyay
e-mail: drsachinupadhyay@gmail.com

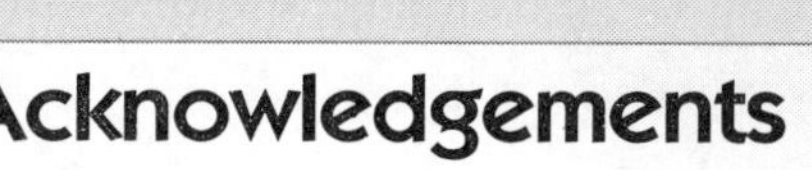

Acknowledgements

After almighty god, I would like to extend my heartiest gratitude to those who helped me in making this dream a living reality. These people have always encouraged and motivated me in all walks of life. They have acted as spur in the moments of doubts and dilemmas.

I am very thankful to all those who have made unforgettable contribution in collecting questions and giving their valuable advice, without their unselfish contributions this book would not have made it to your hands.

This book would not have been possible without the invaluable assistance, love and blessings of many of my teachers, colleagues, and friends. Special thanks go first and foremost to my mentors *Prof Javahir A Pachore, Prof HKT Raza* and *Prof HS Varma* for their efforts and time they have invested in helping me to improve my writing skills and strengthen my powers of arguments. For this and their excellent teaching I will always be deeply grateful to them.

My special thanks to all my teachers who have showered their blessings on me and shaped my career and made me competent to write a book of this nature. I respectfully bow and acknowledge their roles in my growth and understanding of what it means to have a body and to be present on this earth.

It is my privilege to express thanks to my young colleagues, without their continuing support and devotion this book would not have come to the fruition.

I want to thank all my students because all gave me inspiration to write this book. Each and every day that I listened to you guys talk (crazy at times), it further solidified the need to write this book.

I am grateful to *YN Arjuna* (Senior Vice-President—Publishing, Editorial and Publicity), *CBS Publishers & Distributors Private Limited, Delhi,* and their efficient and cordial staff for their valuable suggestions and all help in the production of this book.

I must express my deep reverence to my parents *late Smt Suman Upadhyay and late Shri Sharad Kumar Upadhyay* without whose encouragement and blessing it could not have been possible for me to complete the book.

Acknowledgements would be incomplete without my heartfelt thanks to those who have been with me throughout this long journey: my beloved wife Dr *Smita* and my darling angels *Juhi* and *Jahnavi*. Thanks for everything; thanks for being my inspiration and strength.

Sachin Upadhyay

Contents

1

Anatomy

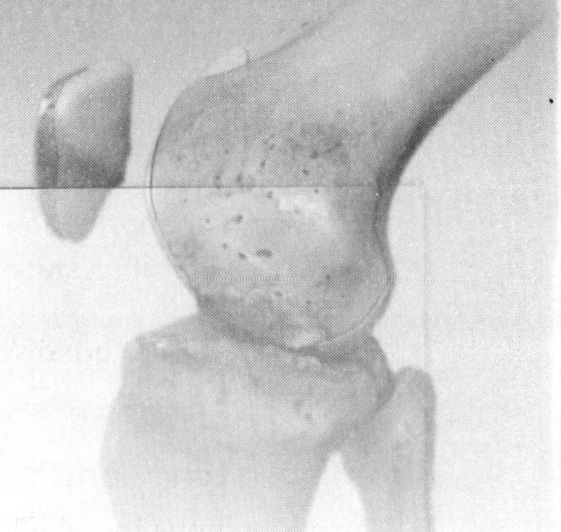

Q1. Discuss in brief the development of skeleton.

Human skeleton has 206 bones. The parent connective tissue is *mesenchyme*. In intrauterine life the mesenchymal tissue, differentiate into *bone, cartilage, fascia and muscles.*

Important Points:
- *Cartilage* first appears at 5th wk of intrauterine life.
- *Ossification* of fetus starts in 5–6th wk of intrauterine life.
- *Synovial tissue* is seen earliest in 12th wk of intrauterine life.
- *Bone* first appears at 7th wk of intrauterine life.
- *Somites* undergo division into three parts:
  - *Dermatomes*: forms the dermis of the skin
  - *Myotomes*: forms the skeletal muscle
  - *Sclerotome*: helps to form the vertebral column.
- Bones of the limbs, including the bones of the shoulder and pelvic girdles, are formed from mesenchyme of the *limb buds*. With the exception of the clavicle, they are all formed by enchondral ossification.
- *Limb buds* are outgrowth that arises from the side-wall of the embryo at the beginning of the second month of intrauterine life.
- *Forelimb buds* appears about the 26th day and the *hindlimb bud* about the 28th day.

Q2. Write in short ossification and growth pattern in bone.

Development and Ossification of Bones

Bones are first laid down as mesodermal (connective tissue) condensations. Conversion of mesodermal models into bone is called *intramembranous or mesenchymal ossification* and the bones are called *membrane (dermal) bones.*
- However, mesodermal stage may pass through cartilaginous stage by chondrification during 2nd month of intrauterine life.
- A conversion of cartilaginous model into bone is called *intracartilaginous or endochondral* ossification and such bones are called *cartilaginous bones.*
- Ossification takes place by centres of ossification.
- The centres of ossification may be *primary or secondary.*
- The *primary centres* appear before birth, usually during 8th week of intrauterine life; the *secondary centres* appear after birth, with a few exceptions.
- Many secondary centres appear during puberty.
- A primary centre forms *diaphysis,* and the secondary centres form *epiphyses.*

- Fusion of epiphysis with the diaphysis starts at puberty and is complete by the age of 25, after which no more bone growth can take place.
- The *law of ossification* states that 'secondary centres of ossification which appear first are last to unite".
- The end of a long bone where epiphysial fusion is delayed is the growing end of the bone.

Growth of a Long Bone

- A growing bone increases both in length and in thickness.
- Bone grows in *length* by multiplication of cells in the epiphysial plate of cartilage.
- Depending upon the distribution/arrangement of cells following zones are recognized:
- *Zone of resting cartilage (or resting zone)*: Cells are small and irregularly arranged.
- *Zone of proliferating cells*: the cells are larger and are undergoing repeated mitosis. During the process of multiplication, they come to lie in parallel columns, separated by bars of intercellular matrix.
- *Zone of calcification or calcified matrix*: the cell becomes still larger and the matrix becomes calcified.
- *Zone of ossification*: here the cartilage cells dead and the calcified matrix is replaced by bone.
- Bone grows in *thickness* by active multiplication of cells in the zone of proliferation.
- Bone grows by deposition of new bone on the surface and at the ends. This process of bone deposition of osteoblasts is called *appositional growth or surface accretion*. However, in order to maintain the shape the unwanted bone must be removed. This process of bone removal by osteoclasts is called remodelling. This is how marrow cavity increases in size.

Q3. What are osteoblast, osteocytes and osteoclast.

Bone is a dynamic tissue that is remodeled constantly throughout life where osteoblasts are responsible for bone formation (osteogenesis) and osteoclasts for its resorption.

Osteoblasts

- Theses are bone-forming cells.
- Osteoblasts synthesize and secrete the organic matrix
- Osteoblasts are specialized mesenchymal cells with a single, usually eccentric, nucleus; contain large volumes of synthetic organelles: endoplasmic reticulum and Golgi membranes.
- They lie on bone surfaces and undergo a process of maturation where genes like core-binding factor $\alpha 1$ (Cbfα1) and osterix (Osx) play a very important role.
- Recently it was found that Wnt/β-catenin pathway plays a part on osteoblast differentiation and proliferation.
- When active, they assume a round, oval, or polyhedral form and a seam of new osteoid separate them from mineralized matrix.
- When stimulated, osteoblasts form new bone organic matrix and participate in controlling mineralization of matrix.
- Osteoblasts also play vital role in regulation of bone resorption through receptor activator of nuclear factor-κB (RANK) ligand (RANKL), that links to its receptor, RANK, on the surface of preosteoblast cells, inducing their differentiation and fusion.

- Osteoblasts secrete a soluble decoy receptor (osteoprotegerin, OPG) that blocks RANK/RANKL interaction by binding to RANKL and, thus, prevents osteoclast differentiation and activation.

Osteocytes

- These cells are seen in mature bone.
- Osteocytes descend from osteoblasts (and during this, the cells lose a large part of their cell organelles).
- They are formed by the incorporation of osteoblasts into the bone matrix.
- Present in lacunae.
- Osteocytes remain in contact with each other and with cells on the bone surface via *gap junction-coupled* cell processes passing through the matrix via small channels, the canaliculi that connect the cell body-containing lacunae with each other and with the outside world.

Functions

- Osteocytes are actively involved in *bone turnover*.
- Through its large cell-matrix contact surface involved in *ion exchange*.
- Osteocytes are the mechanosensory cells of bone and play a pivotal role in functional adaptation of bone.
- Also, function as regulators of mineralization and as regulators of phosphate homeostasis

Osteoclast

- These cells are responsible for bone removal.
- These are multinucleated giant cells with acidophilic cytoplasm responsible for *bone resorption* derived from hematopoietic stem cells.
- Seen at the site of bone resorption.
- Formation of osteoclast requires the presence of *RANK ligand* and *M-CSF*.
- Morphology: Osteoclasts lie in resorption bays *"eaten out cavities"* called *Howship's lacunae*.
- Produce enzymes like acid phosphatase, collagenase, acid hydrolases and various glycolytic enzymes.
- Parathyroid hormone, 1,25-dihydroxyvitamin D3, TGT-alpha, and EGF act permissively in their formation whereas *calcitonin* inhibits its formation.

Q4. What is ossification and discuss in brief the ossification centers.

All bone is of *mesodermal origin*. The process of bone formation is called *ossification*.

Types of Ossification

Enchondral ossification

- In most part of the embryo, bone formation is preceded by the formation of cartilaginous model. This kind of bone formation is called *enchondral ossification*.
- Bones formed in this way are termed as *cartilage bones*.
- Example: *base of skull, trunk* and *limb bones*.

Intramembranous ossification

- If bone is laid down directly in fibrous membrane without the cartilaginous phase, this is called *intramembranous ossification*.

- Bones formed in this way are termed as *membrane bones*.
- Example: *Vault of skull, the mandible* and *the clavicle*.

Ossification Centers

An area where ossification starts is called *centre of ossification*.

Primary Center of Ossification

- Single or multiple
- Appear before birth b/w 6–8 wk of intrauterine life.
- When multiple, appear simultaneously.
- Diaphysis (shaft) of long bone develops from primary center.

Secondary Center of Ossification

- Multiple
- Appear after birth
- Epiphysis (ends) of long bone develops from secondary center.

Appearance of Important Ossification Centers

Bone	Time of appearance of ossification centers
Humerus head	Birth to 3 months
Scapula	First fetal week
Radial head	6 yr
Distal epiphyses of radius	1 yr
Lunate	4 yr
Scaphoid	5 yr
Olecranon	10 yr
Pisiform	12 yr
Distal epiphysis of femur	At birth (35–38 wk)
Capital epiphysis of femur	1 yr
Greater trochanter	3 yr
Lesser trochanter	11 yr
Upper tibial epiphysis	38 wk of intrauterine life
Talus	7th month
Calcaneum	5th month

Q5. Discuss the macroscopic and microscopic structure of bone.

Bone is a connective tissue, impregnated with calcium salts. The *inorganic* calcium salts (mainly calcium phosphate, partly calcium carbonate, and crystal of hydroxyapatite $Ca_{10}(PO_4)_6(OH)_2$ traces of other salts) make it hard and rigid, which can afford resistance to compressive forces of weight-bearing and impact forces of jumping. The *organic connective tissue* (collagen fibres) makes it tough and resilient (flexible), which can afford resistance to tensile forces.

Macroscopic structure

Macroscopically, the architecture of bone may be *compact* or *cancellous*.

Compact Bone

- It is dense in texture like ivory, but is extremely porous.
- It is best developed in the cortex of the long bones.
- This is an adaptation to bending and twisting forces (a combination of compression, tension and shear).

Cancellous Spongy or Trabecular Bone

- It is open in texture, and is made up of a meshwork of trabeculae (rods and plates) between which are marrow containing spaces.
- The trabecular mesh works are of three primary types, namely:
- Meshwork of rods
- Meshwork of rods and plates
- Meshwork compressive forces

Microscopically

The bone is of four types, namely lamellar (including both compact and cancellous), fibrous, dentine and cement.

- *Lamellar*: Most of the mature human bones, whether compact or cancellous, are composed of thin plates of bony tissue called lamellae.
- *Fibrous*: It is found in young fetal bones, but are common in reptiles and amphibia.
- *Dentine*
- *Cement* occurs in teeth.

Mineralized Bone

It could could be either:
- Woven bone (immature)
- Lamellar bone (mature)

Osteon

- The basic microscopic unit of bone is an 'osteon'.
- Haversian canals run through the entire length of the bone-carrying blood vessels.
- They are interlinked to each other through the Volkmann's canals.
- On a transverse section of the bone each of these Haversian canals is surrounded by a grouped of lacunae, which lodge an 'osteocytes'.
- The entire group of osteocytes link to each other and to the centrally located Haversian canal through cytoplasmic extensions that run through tiny channels called 'canaliculi'.

Q6. Discuss gross structure of an adult long bone.

Naked eye examination of the longitudinal and transverse sections of a long bone shows the following features:

Shaft

From without inwards it is composed of periosteum, cortex and medullary cavity.

Periosteum

- It is a thick fibrous membrane covering the surface of the bone.
- It is made up of an outer fibrous layer, and an inner cellular layer, which is osteogenic in nature.

- Periosteum is united to the underlying bone by Sharpey's fibres, and the union is particularly strong over the attachments of tendons and ligament.
- At the articular margin, the periosteum is continuous with the capsule of the joint.
- The abundant arteries nourish the outer part of the underlying cortex also.
- Periosteum has a rich nerve supply, which makes it the most sensitive part of the bone.

Cortex

It is made up of a compact bone, which gives it the desired strength to withstand all possible mechanical strains.

Medullary Cavity

- It is filled with red or yellow bone marrow.
- At birth, the marrow is red everywhere with widespread active hemopoiesis.
- As the age advances the red marrow at many places atrophies and is replaced by yellow, fatty marrow, with no power of hemopoiesis.
- Red marrow persists in the cancellous ends of long bones.
- In the llium, sternum, ribs, vertebrae and skull bones, the red marrow is found throughout life.

Articular End

The two ends of a long bone are made up of cancellous bone covered with hyaline cartilage (articular cartilage).

Q7. Discuss in brief the different part of a young bone.

Ans: A *typical long bone* ossifies in three parts, the two ends from secondary centres, and the intervening shaft from a primary centre.

Before ossification is complete, the following parts of the bone can be defined.

Epiphysis

- The tips and ends of a bone ossify from secondary centers are called epiphyses.
- Develop from secondary center
- Electropositive
- The epiphysis, which ossifies first, unites with the diaphysis last and epiphysis, which ossifies last fuses first (exception: distal end of fibula-ossifies first and fuse last).

These are of the following types:

Pressure Epiphysis

- It is articular and participates in transmission of the weight.
- Examples: Head of femur, lower end of radius, condyles of tibia, etc.

Traction Epiphysis

- It is also known as apophysis it is extra-articular and does not participate in the transmission of the weight.
- It always provides attachment to one or more tendons, which exert traction on the epiphysis.

- The pressure epiphyses ossify earlier than traction epiphyses.
- *Examples*: Trochanters of femur, tibial tuberosity tubercles of humerus, mastoid process, etc.

Atavistic Epiphysis

- It is phylogenetically an independent bone, which in man becomes fused to another bone.
- *Examples*: Coracoid process of scapula and os trigonum

Aberrant Epiphysis

- It is not always present.
- *Examples*: Epiphysis at the head of the first metacarpal and at the base of other metacarpal bones

Diaphysis

- It is the elongated shaft of a long bone between the two cartilaginous ends.
- Ossifies from a primary centre
- Contains marrow cavity
- Electropositive
- Site of muscle insertion

Metaphysis

- The ends of a diaphysis are metaphysis.
- Each metaphysis is the zone of active growth.
- Before epiphysial fusion, the metaphysis is richly supplied with blood through and arteries (*Circulus-Vasculosus of Hunter*) forming hair-pin bends.
- This is the commonest site of osteomyelitis in children because; the bacteria or emboli are easily trapped in the hair-pin bends, causing infraction.
- After the epiphysial fusion, vascular communications metaphysis contains no more end arteries, and is no longer subject to osteomyelitis.

Epiphysial Plate of Cartilage

- It separates epiphysis from metaphysis. Proliferation of cells in this cartilaginous plate is responsible for lengthwise growth of a long bone.
- After the epiphysial fusion, the bone can no longer grow in length. Both the epiphysial and metaphysial arteries nourish the growth cartilage.

Q8. Enumerate the functions of bone.

The first bone appears in the seventh embryonic week, it's the vertebra. The *clavicle* is the first bone in the skeleton to ossify.

Characteristics

- It is subject to disease and heals after a fracture.
- It has greater regenerative power than any other tissue of the body, except blood.
- It can mould itself according to changes in stress and strain it bears.
- It shows disuse atrophy and overuse hypertrophy.

Functions

- Bones give shape and support to the body, and resist all forms of stress.
- They provide surface for the attachment of muscles, tendons, ligaments, etc.
- They serve as levers for muscular actions.
- The skull, vertebral column and thoracic cage protect brain, spinal cord and thoracic viscera, respectively.
- Bone marrow manufactures blood cells.
- Bones store 97% of the body calcium and phosphorus.
- Bone marrow contains reticuloendothelial cells, which are phagocytic in nature and take part in immune responses of the body.
- The larger paranasal air sinuses affect the timber of the voice.

Q9. Discuss blood and nerve supply of bone.

BLOOD SUPPLY OF BONES

Long Bones

The blood supply of a long is derived from the following sources.

Nutrient Artery

- These enter the shaft through the nutrient foramen, run obliquely through the cortex, and divides into ascending and descending branches in the medullary cavity. Each branch divides into a number of small parallel channels, which terminate in the adult metaphysis by anastomosing with the epiphysial, metaphyseal, and periosteal arteries. The nutrient artery supplies medullary cavity, inner two-thirds of cortex and metaphysis.
- The nutrient foramen is directed away from the growing end of the bone; their directions are indicated by a jingle, *'To the elbow I go, from the knee' I flee.*
- The oblique direction of nutrient foramina opposite to the growing end of the bone is best explained by the growing-end hypothesis.
- Periosteal arteries are especially numerous beneath the muscular and ligamentous attachments. They ramify beneath the periosteum and enter the Volkmann's canals to supply the outer one-third of the cortex.

Epiphysial Arteries

These are derived from periarticular vascular arcades (circulus vasculosus) found on the non-articular bony surface.

Metaphyseal Arteries

- These are derived from the neighbouring systemic vessels.
- They reinforce the metaphyseal branches from the primary nutrient artery.
- In miniature long bones, the infection begins in the middle of the shaft rather than at the metaphysis because the nutrients artery breaks up into a plexus immediately upon reaching the medullary cavity.
- In the adults, however, the chances of infection are minimized because the nutrient artery is mostly replaced by the periosteal vessels.

Other Bones

- Short bones are supplied by numerous periosteal vessels, which enter their non-articular surfaces.

- In a vertebra, the body is supplied by anterior and posterior vessels, and the vertebral arch by large vessels entering the bases of transverse processes. Its marrow is drained by two large basivertebral veins.
- A rib is supplied by: (a) the nutrient artery, which enters it just beyond the tubercle, and (b) the periosteal arteries.

Veins

These are numerous and large in the cancellous, red marrow-bones (e.g. basivertebral veins). In the compact bone, they accompany arteries in the Volkmann's canals.

Lymphatics

- Present only in periosteum and haversian canal
- No lymphatics in bone marrow

Nerve Supply

- Nerves accompany the blood vessels. Most are sympathetic and vasomotor in function.
- Few are sensory which are distributed to the articular ends and periosteum of the long bones, to the vertebra, and to large flat bones.

Q.10 Discuss the classification of joints in brief.

Classification of Joints

Fibrous Joints (Synarthroses, Immovable)

- Sutures (in the skull)
- Syndesmoses
- Gomphoses

Cartilaginous Joints (Amphiarthroses Partially Movable)

- Synchondroses (hyaline cartilage)
- Symphyses (fibrocartilage)

Synovial joints (Diarthroses Freely Movable)

- Uniaxial
  - Ginglymus (hinge)
  - Trochoid (pivot)
- Biaxial
  - Condyloid
  - Saddle
- Triaxial
  - Ball and socket
  - Planar

Features and Examples

Fibrous Joints

This type of joint is held together by only a ligament.

Examples:
- *Sutures* in the sagittal and partial bones of skull
- Site where the teeth are held to their bony sockets (*Gomphoses*)
- Both the radio-ulnar and tibio-fibular joints (*Syndesmoses*)

Cartilaginous Joints

Cartilaginous (Synchondroses and Symphyses)
- These joints occur where the connection between the articulating bones is made up of cartilage.
- *Example*: Between vertebrae (intervertebral joint) in the spine and sacroiliac joint

Synchondroses are temporary joints, which are only present in children, up until the end of puberty.
Example: the epiphyseal plates in long bones

Symphysis joints are permanent cartilaginous joints.
Example: Pubic symphyses

Synovial Joints

Synovial (Diarthrosis):
- Synovial joints are by far the most common joint within the human body.
- They are highly movable and all have a synovial capsule (collagenous structure) surrounding the entire joint, a synovial membrane (the inner layer of the capsule) which secretes synovial fluid (a lubricating liquid) and cartilage known as hyaline cartilage which pads the ends of the articulating bones.
- There are 6 types of synovial joints which are classified by the shape of the joint and the movement available.
- Synovial joints are most evolved, and, therefore, most mobile type of joints.
- *Example*: Hip and knee joint, shoulder joint etc.

Q11. Discuss the characteristic features and different types of synovial joints with relevant examples.

Characteristic Features of a Synovial Joint

- *Hyaline (articular) cartilage* (occasionally *fibrocartilage* in certain membrane bones) covers the articular surfaces.
- *Articular cartilage* is avascular, non-nervous and elastic. Lubricated with synovial fluid, the cartilage provides slippery surfaces for free movements, like *'ice on ice'*.
- Between the articular surfaces there is a joint cavity filled with synovial fluid. An articular disc or meniscus divides the cavity partially or completely.
- An *articular capsule* encircling the joint, which is made up of a fibrous capsule lined by synovial membrane.
- Because of its rich nerve supply, the fibrous capsule is sensitive to stretches imposed by movements. This sets up appropriate reflexes to protect the joint from any sprain. This called the *'watch-dog'* action of the capsule.
- The *synovial membrane* lines whole of the interior of the joint, except for the articular surfaces covered by hyaline cartilage.
- The membrane secretes a slimy viscous fluid called the *synovial fluid*, which lubricates

the joint and nourishes the articular cartilage. The viscosity of fluid is due to hyaluronic acid secreted by cells of the synovial membrane.

- Varying degrees of movements are always permitted by the synovial joints.

Classification and Movements of Synovial Joints

S. no.	Type of joint	Movements
A.	Plane or gliding type	Gliding movement
B.	Uniaxial joints	
	a. Hinge jointb	Flexion and extension
	b. Pivot joint	Rotation only
C.	Biaxial joints	
	a. Condylar joint	Flexion and extension, and limited rotation
	b. Ellipsoid joint	Flexion, extension, abduction, adduction, and circumduction
D.	Multiaxial joints	
	a. Saddle joint	Flexion, and extension, abduction, adduction, and conjunct rotation
	b. Ball and socket joint	Flexion, extension, abduction, and adduction, circumduction, and rotation

Types of Synovial Joint

Plane Synovial Joints

- Articular surfaces are more or less flat (plane). They permit gliding movements (translations) in various directions
- *Examples:*
  - Intertarsal joints
  - Facet between superior and inferior articular process of vertebrae
  - Intercarpal joints
  - Jaw: Temporomandibular joint

Hinge Joints (Ginglymi)

- Articular surfaces are pulley-shaped. There are strong collateral ligaments.
- Movements are possible in one plane around a transverse axis.
- *Examples:*
  - Elbow joint
  - Ankle joint
  - Interphalangeal joints

Pivot (Trochoid) Joints

- Articular surfaces comprise a central bony pivot (peg) surrounded by an osteo-ligamentous ring. Movements are possible in one plane around a vertical axis
- Examples:
  - Median atlanto-axial joint
  - Superior and inferior radio-ulnar joints

Condylar (Bicondylar) Joints

- Articular surfaces include two distinct condyles (convex male surfaces) fitting into reciprocally concave female surfaces (which are also, sometimes, known as condyles, such as in tibia).

- These joints permit movements mainly in one plane around a transverse axis
- *Examples:*
  - Knee joint
  - Temporomandibular joints

Ellipsoid Joints

- Articular surfaces include an oval, convex, male surface fitting into an elliptical, concave female surface. Free movements are possible around the axes, flexion and extension around the transverse axis and abduction and adduction around the anteroposterior axis.
- Combination of movements produces circumduction.
- Typical rotation around a third (vertical) axis does not occur.
- *Examples:*
  - Wrist joint
  - Metacarpophalangeal joints
  - Atlanto-occipital joints

Saddle (Sellar) Joints

- Articular surfaces are reciprocally concavoconvex. Movements are similar to those permitted by an ellipsoid joint, with addition of some rotation (conjunct rotation) around a third axis, which, however, cannot occur independently.
- *Examples:*
  - First carpometacarpal joint
  - Sternoclavicular joint
  - Calcaneocuboid joint

Ball and Socket (Spheroidal) Joints

- Articular surfaces include a globular head (male surface) fitting into a cup-shaped socket (female surface). Movements occur around an indefinite number of axes, which have one common center. Flexion, extension, abduction, medial rotation, lateral rotation, and circumduction, all occur quite freely.
- *Examples:*
  - Shoulder joint
  - Hip joint
  - Talocalcaneonavicular joint

Classification of Fracture and Complications

Fracture is the breach in the continuity of bone or damage to the trabecular pattern, as a result of accidental implication of force with or without associated injuries.

Classification of Fractures

Based on Presence or Absence of Wound

Simple

When there is a fracture, but the overlying soft tissue and the skin is intact and there is no associated vital tissue damage.

Open

- When the fracture haematoma communicates with the exterior atmosphere, through an overlying wound in the skin and soft tissue.
- Evaluation and treatment depends on extent of soft tissue damage and level of wound contamination

The well-accepted classification of open fracture is as follows:

Gustilo's Classification of Compound Fractures

- *Type 1:* Clean wound of size <1 cm.
- *Type 2:* Lacerated wound >1 cm but without extensive soft tissue damage, skin flaps or avulsions.
- *Type 3A:* Extensive soft tissue lacerations/flaps, but maintain adequate soft tissue coverage of bone or they result from high-energy trauma regardless of the size of wound especially segmental/severely comminuted fractures.
- *Type 3B:* Extensive soft tissue damage with periosteal stripping and bony exposure, usually massively contaminated.
- *Type 3C:* Open fractures with an arterial injury that requires repair regardless of size of wound.

Based on the Extent of Fracture Line

Incomplete fractures: These fractures involves single cortex of the bone.

Complete fractures:

- These fractures involve the entire bone.
- Complete fracture could be undisplaced or displaced (muscles forces or gravity or improper handling)

OTA Classification, Based on Fracture Pattern

Linear: It could be transverse, spiral or oblique.

Comminuted:
- When bone breaks into multiple pieces as in crush injuries, commonly seen in run over accidents.
- Fracture with butterfly fragment is also included in this type.

Segmental: When the long bone breaks at two places, proximal and distal with a free-floating middle fragment.

Bone loss: This could be <50% or >50% of bone loss.

Miscellaneous or Atypical Type

Complicated fracture: When the fracture is associated with injury to vital tissue, viscera, vessels and nerves related to the bone, e.g. fracture of mid shaft humerus with radial nerve palsy, fracture pelvis with rupture of urethra.

Greenstick fracture: In a child, the bones are pliable and elastic, hence they bend under pressure, with or without a breach in the cortex. Greenstick fracture has intact periosteum on the concave side, where the bone buckles while the other cortex bends and breaks at the convex side

Torus fracture: Here both cortices are buckled, due to vertical compression, with intact periosteum, hence the fragments are undisplaced.

Stress or Fatigue Fracture

- Cyclic application of minor trauma over a prolonged period causing spontaneous partial or complete fracture in the long bones.
- *Most common site*: Metatarsal bones (2nd metatarsal seen in army recruits *(March fracture)*) followed by fibula and tibia, neck or subtrochanteric fracture of femur, pelvis, ulna and radius.
- Early diagnosis by Tc99 bone scans.
- *Examples*:
    - Runners fracture: Fracture lower third fibula
    - Jumping fracture: Fracture upper third fibula
    - March fracture: 2nd metatarsal
    - Ballet dancer's fracture: Mid shaft tibia (anterior cortex)

Pathological Fractures

- These fractures usually occur when invasive disease or destructive processes have compromised the normal integrity and strength of bone.
- The force required to bring about these fracture is trivial.
- Most common cause in children is a benign bone cyst
- Most common site (local lesion): Vertebral bodies and most common cause of local lesion is metastatic carcinoma
- Most common site (diffuse lesion): Thoracic or lumbar vertebrae and most common cause of diffuse lesion is senile osteoporosis

> **Q2. Discuss the mechanism of injury and an approach to diagnose a fracture and related injuries.**

Mechanism of Injury

- *Severe trauma*: Enough to cause a fracture (single or repeated).
- *Trivial injury:* As seen in pathological fracture.

Severe Trauma

Single Episode of Injury

Direct injuries: Always associated with (in adults) overlying soft tissue damage and the force passing through the soft tissue to the bone.
- ***Tapping force***: Transverse fracture shaft of long bones, depressed fracture of skull (Gutter fracture), fissure fracture of flat bones (scapula, pelvis fracture).
- ***Crushing injuries***: Comminuted fracture with extensive soft tissue damage. The damaging force passes through the skin and muscles down to the bone, crushing all the tissue along its path.
- ***Missile injuries***: Splintering fracture, seen in war, as bullet and blast injuries. This high energy force passes through the bone, blasting it into several pieces

Indirect injuries: The soft tissue escapes the line of force and hence is often undamaged.
- ***Twisting force***: Spiral fracture.
- ***Angulation force***: Transverse fracture without soft tissue damage
- ***Angulation + axial compression***: Fracture with butterfly piece.
- ***Angulation + axial compression + rotation***: Short oblique fracture

Vertical compression: Wedge/collapse as in vertebrae and calcaneum

Traction: Due to violent muscular contraction, it causes avulsion of bone, e.g. fracture patella (seen in epileptics and tetanus).

Repeated Episodes of Injury

Stress fracture: This is due to repeated, cyclic minor trauma over a long period of time, e.g. **March fracture** in military recruits.

Trivial Injury

Fracture occurs as a result of underlying pathology.
- ***Hereditary***: Osteogenesis imperfecta, brittle bone disease.
- ***Infection***: Osteomyelitis.
- ***Degenerative***: Osteoporosis.
- ***Metabolic***: Osteomalacia, hyperparathyroidism.
- ***Tumour***: Simple bone cyst in young and secondaries in old patients.

Diagnosis

- Careful history
- Thorough clinical examination
- Investigation

History

- Care should be taken to evaluate the fracture in view of the age, sex, occupation and previous history of fracture, mechanism of forces in injury, history of convulsions.
- Keep in mind the involvement of bladder, bowel habits and history of the drug allergies and addictions.

Clinical Examination

General

• Posture may be typical in cervical cord injury, fractures and dislocations, etc.

Lesion	Attitude
5th cervical segment	Immobile against the trunk and completely paralysis
6th cervical segment	Patient lies helplessly on the back with the arm "Hands up" position abducted and externally rotated and the forearm flexed and supinated
7th cervical segment	Arm is partially abducted and internally rotated with the forearm flexed and pronated paralysis of intrinsic muscle as hand will used to main en griffe
Posterior dislocation of hip	Flexion, adduction and internal rotation
Anterior dislocation of hip	Flexion, abduction and external rotation
Incomplete external rotation of lower limb	Intracapsular fracture neck femur

• Always keep in mind that the injured patient should be examined as a whole not just the injured part. The part should be well exposed for examination and compared with the normal.
• Always make it a point to examine head, eyes, ears, mouth, chest, its respiratory movements, abdomen, pelvis, the pelvic viscera and the functions of the spinal cord.
• Record the pulse, BP and respiration.

Whenever the patient comes to you, he may have three important complications.
Following trauma each may be fatal:
• Few hours: Shock
• Few days: Fat embolism
• Few weeks: Thromboembolism.

Local

Clinical features (important sign and symptoms):

• *Pain:* usually the first and most important symptom
• *Swelling:* it could be due to soft tissue damage or medullar bleeding or it may be reactionary haemorrhage. Swelling should be examined for size, shape, margins, consistency, tenderness, fixity to the underlying structures, fluctuations, transillumination, etc.
• *Deformity:* Certain classic deformities clinch the spot diagnosis just like seen in various fractures and dislocation.

Classic deformity	Probable diagnosis
Flat shoulder	Anterior dislocation of shoulder
S-shaped deformity of distal humerus	Supracondylar fracture of the humerus
Dinner fork deformity	Colles fracture
Mallet finger	Rupture of distal end of the index extensor
Flexion, adduction and internal rotation	Posterior dislocation of hip
Flexion, abduction and external rotation	Anterior dislocation of hip

- *Shortening*: A little amount of shortening is always expected in cases of fracture due to overlapping of fragment.
- *Tenderness*: It is important valuable sign of a fracture. Bony tenderness due to fracture is called local bony tenderness.
- *Bony irregularities*: On palpation there may be sharp elevation or a gap which is a definite sign of a fracture.
- *Crepitus*: It is a sensation of grating when fractured fragment are moved against each other. It adds nothing to the diagnosis but causes pain so it is always better to avoid it.
- *Abnormal mobility*: It is also a definite sign of fracture and it can be elicited by moving the one part against other.
- *Absence of transmitted movements*: When there is, breech in the continuity of the bone the transmitted movement will surely be absent.

Not to forget to examine:
- Bruising and blisters at fracture site.
- Examination of distal sensation and pulsation for neuromuscular damage.
- Always examine important related viscera, e.g. bladder, urethra in the pelvic injury and spinal cord in the vertebral injuries
- Range of movements and stability of relevant joints for intra-articular injuries.

Investigations

For Diagnosis and Subsequent Management

- *X-rays*:
    - It is an important diagnostic tool.
    - Full length of bone should be clearly visible in the skiagram.
    - Whenever writing a requisition for X-ray of an injured patient, following points must be kept in mind "Rule of 2".
    - *Two joints*, i.e. one above and one below the fracture should be included.
    - *Two view*, AP and lateral (if necessary oblique also especially in hand and foot injuries).
    - *Two occasions*, whenever in doubt as in stress fracture, scaphoid/greenstick fracture (repeat X-ray after an interval of 1–2 weeks).
    - *Two limbs*, in the epiphyseal injuries (for comparison with normal) especially in children.
- *CT scan*: It helps in detecting fracture of pelvis, skull, spine, joint, and loose intra-articular bodies.
- *MRI*: Besides fracture, it helps to assess the soft tissue injury, injury to ligaments or menisci and the status of the cord.
- *Myelography*: It helps to assess the continuity of the cord by the flow of the dye.
- *Nerve conduction study and electromyography*: These help to assess any neurological deficit.
- *Ultrasonography*: Fluid or joint effusion.
- *Doppler studies*: These help to assess vascular injuries or any vascular deficit.
- *Arthroscopy*: It helps to assess intra-articular injuries. It has both diagnostic and therapeutic significance.
- *Routine haematological* and serological evaluation to assess the status of health.
- *Urine routine* and microscopy.
- *Synovial fluid* for synovitis, haemarthrosis and arthritis.

Q3. Discuss in brief the management of fractures.

Management

Principles of Treatment

General

- Management of shock and haemorrhage, replace fluid and electrolytes, maintain input and output chart.
- Antibiotics, anti-inflammatory drugs, tetanus toxoid, etc.

Local

- Restoration of anatomy
- Care of the soft tissue
- Stabilization of bone
- Preservation of function

Aim

- Lower limbs: Maintenance of length
- Upper limbs: Recovery of function
- Correct alignment is on top priority than complete anatomical apposition.

Management of Simple Fracture

- Reduced and maintained in position for 6–12 weeks.
- Rehabilitation

Reduction

The fracture fragments are reduced by:
- Closed reduction under anaesthesia.
- Open reduction for:
    - Unstable fracture
    - Intra-articular fracture
    - Complicated fracture
    - Segmental fracture

Maintenance

Maintenance of reduction is achieved by:
- *External support*:
    - Plaster:
        - POP slabs
        - POP cast
        - A functional brace (permits movements while the fracture is still in cast)
    - Splint: Other than POP are Crammer wire splint, Thomas splint, Bohler-Braun splint etc.
    - Tractions: Skeletal or skin traction and can be employed as fixed, balanced or combined.
- *Internal fixation*:
    - Extramedullary fixation by plates and screws.
    - Intramedullary fixation by nails.

- *External fixators*: External fixation is for temporary stabilization of the fracture when there is :
    - Potentially contaminated wound.
    - Extensive soft tissue damage (Type III) to continue maintaining accurate reduction and stabilization of bone, till healing of fracture and soft tissue cover is achieved.

Rehabilitation

By means of physiotherapy and active and passive movements.

Management of Open Fractures

Principle of Management

- *First aid management (Airway, Bleeding, Circulation)*:
    - Clear airway and secure airway
    - Control of haemorrhage by firm compression bandage
    - Management of shock by adequate and appropriate fluid (crystalloid and colloid) and blood replacement.
    - Most of the deaths, which occur in the first few hours, are due to the mismanagement of shock and haemorrhage.
- *During transportation*: Take care during transport with cervical collar, other splints and support of injured part with maintenance of life support system.
- *Assessment of the patient*: Examine CNS, cardiothoracic function, abdomen, bladder, bowel status and always note down the vitals.
- *Supportive treatment*:
    - Broad spectrum antibiotics or nowadays using antibiotic impregnated PMMA (bone cement) beads
    - Anti-tetanus protection
    - Anti-gas-gangrene serum
    - Analgesics
- *Local (bone and soft tissue) management*:
    - Radical wound debridement to remove all dead and devitalized tissue.
    - Thorough wound debridement and excision of all necrotic debris is very essential to prevent infection.
    - Stabilization of bone (fracture fragment) by *external fixators* initially. These fixators helps:
        - Stabilize the fracture fragment
        - Allow daily wound inspection and dressing
        - Permit secondary procedure to close the wound like grafting or secondary suturing.
        - Allow soft tissue healing
        - Early mobiiization

Once the soft tissue status is healthy, the fixators can safely be changed to internal fixation like nailing.

Final Management of Wound

Primary closure if:
- The wound is clean
- Good circulation without neurovascular deficit.
- Wound age should be <6 hours.

Wound left open and delayed primary closure is preferable after few days if:
- Wound >6 hours
- Potentially contaminated

Delayed closure by autogenous graft using split thickness, rotational/cross leg flaps.
Secondary closure after 2 weeks by suture.

In cases where conditions are not, favorable for primary closure we have following alternative for secondary closure:
- Split thickness graft (SSG) over raw granulating tissue
- Full thickness graft over exposed bone, tendons
- Pedicle graft or flaps
- Suturing after 2–3 weeks
- Biological dressings
- Relaxing incisions to release the tension and mobilize the adjacent skin.
- **Delayed repair** of tendons/nerves.
- **Final stabilization** of bone by POP cast/internal fixation.

Q4. What are Lambotte's principles of surgical treatment of fractures?

Lambotte's principles of surgical treatment of fractures are:
- Anatomic reduction
- Stable internal fixation
- Preservation of blood supply
- Active mobilization

Q5. Enumerate the complications of fracture.

Complications of Fractures

General

Early
- Shock
- Haemorrhage
- Fat embolism
- Fracture fever

Late
- Thromboembolism
- Osteoporosis due to prolonged immobilization

Local

Immediate

Injury to important:
- Vessels (brachial artery injury in supracondylar fracture humerus)
- Nerves (radial nerve palsy in fracture shaft humerus, sciatic nerve palsy in posterior dislocation of hip)
- Viscera (bladder/urethral injury during pelvic fracture)

Infections such as:
- Pyogenic (osteomyelitis)
- Tetanus
- Gas gangrene

Late

Bone:
- Delayed union
- Malunion
- Nonunion
- Avascular Necrosis (e.g. head of femur in fracture neck)
- Growth Disturbance following epiphyseal injury in children
- Shortening

Soft tissues:
- Muscles:
    - Myositis ossificans following passive manipulation of an injured joint
    - Muscle adhesions leading to stiffness of joints.
- Tendons:
    - Adhesions
    - Rupture.

Vessels:
- Volkmann's ischaemia
- Contracture/atrophy due to compartmental syndrome

Nerves:
- Radial nerve palsy in fracture shaft humerus
- Sciatic nerve palsy in posterior dislocation of hip

Joints:
- Stiffness due to Sudeck's atrophy
- Instability due to ligament injuries.

Other: Malignancies following trauma, e.g. *osteoclastoma* and *osteogenic sarcoma* following injury to metaphyseal area.

Q6. Discuss the definition, classification, clinical features and diagnosis of Nonunion.

Definition

FDA panel defined nonunion as *"established when a minimum of 9 months has elapsed since injury and the fracture shows no visible progressive signs of healing for 3 months."* This criterion cannot be applied to every fracture as fracture neck femur or bone loss is day one nonunion.

So for all-purpose the nonunion is defined as "Nonunion is said to established when the biological activity of fracture healing has come to standstill both clinically and radiologically and further union cannot be achieved without external intervention such as surgery, electric stimulation, etc."

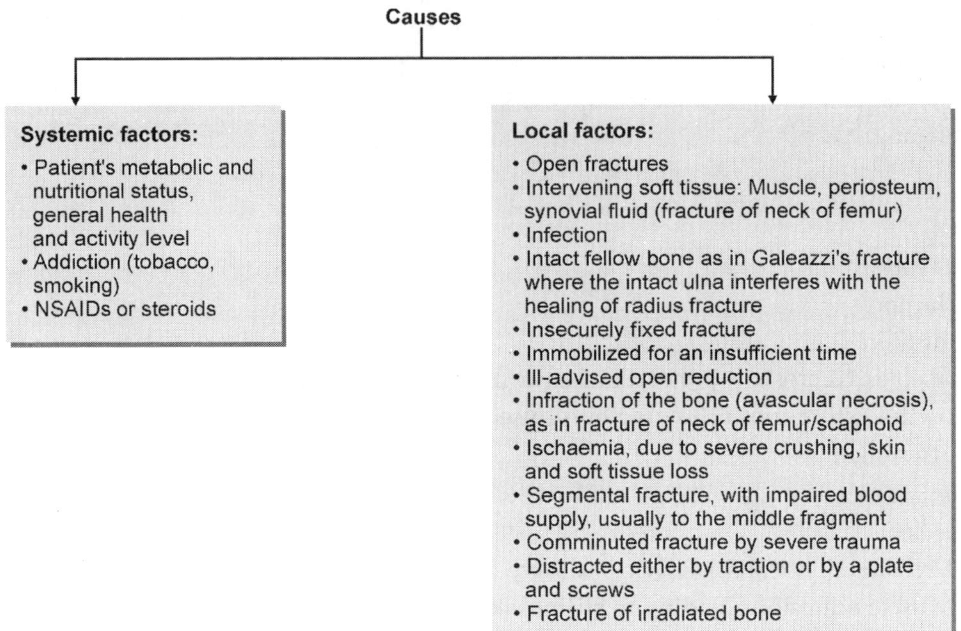

Classification

According to the Viability of the Ends of the Fragments

Judet and Judet, Müller, Weber and Cech, and others classified nonunions into two types:
- *Hypervascular (hypertrophic) nonunion or viable* is capable of biological reaction.
- *Avascular (atrophic) nonunions or inert*—are not capable of uniting without intervention

Hypervascular Nonunions

- The fracture fragment ends are capable of biological reaction.
- Shows increased uptake of *strontium-85*, which indicates a rich vascular supply in the ends of the fragments.

Hypervascular nonunions are subdivided as follows:
- *"Elephant foot" nonunions*:
  - Hypertrophic and rich in callus.
  - Result from insecure fixation, inadequate immobilization, or premature weight bearing in a reduced fracture with viable fragments.
- *"Horse hoof" nonunions*:
  - These are mildly hypertrophic and poor in callus.
  - Usually occur after a moderately unstable fixation with plate and screws.
  - Ends of the fragments show some callus, insufficient for union, and possibly a little sclerosis.
- *Oligotrophic nonunions*:
  - These are not hypertrophic, but are vascular
  - Callus is absent
  - They typically occur after major displacement of a fracture, internal fixation without accurate apposition of the fragments or distraction of the fragments.

Avascular (Atrophic) Nonunion or Inert

- The fracture ends are incapable of biological reaction.
- Shows decreased uptake of *strontium-85*, which indicates a poor vascular supply in the ends of the fragments.

Avascular nonunions are subdivided as follows:

- ***Torsion wedge nonunions:***
  - The characteristic feature is the presence of an intermediate fragment in which the blood supply is decreased or absent.
  - The intermediate fragment has healed to one main fragment, but not to the other.
  - Usually seen in tibial fractures treated by plate and screws.
- ***Comminuted nonunions:***
  - These are characterized by the presence of one or more intermediate fragments that are necrotic.
  - The skiagram shows absence of any sign of callus formation.
  - Typically, these nonunions result from the breakage of any plate (implant failure) used in stabilizing the acute fracture.
- ***Defect or gap nonunions:***
  - It is characterized by the loss of a fragment of the diaphysis of a bone.
  - Ends of the fragments are viable, but union across the defect is impossible.
  - In due course of time, the ends of the fragments become atrophic.
  - These nonunions occur after open fractures, sequestrectomy in osteomyelitis, and resection of tumors
- ***Atrophic nonunions*** :
  - The Intermediate fragment is replaced by a scar tissue that lacks osteogenic potential.
  - The ends of the fragments have become osteoporotic and atrophic.

According to the Bone Defect and Deformity

Paley et al. classified nonunions into two types:

Type A

- Nonunions with bone loss of less than 1 cm (type A).

Subdivided into:

- Type A1: Nonunions with a mobile deformity
- Type A2: Nonunion with a fixed deformity
  - Type A2-1, a stiff nonunion without deformity
  - Type A2-2, a stiff nonunion with a fixed deformity

Type B

- Nonunions with bone loss of more than 1 cm.

Subdivided into:

- Type B1: Nonunions with a bony defect B
- Type B2: loss of bone length
- Type B3: both.

Both of these classification systems can be modified further by the presence or absence of infection.

Clinical Features

- Usually there is history of trauma or head injury or multiple injuries.
- Painless abnormal mobility (most characteristic sign)
- Shortening
- Deformity
- Wasting of muscles
- Scar or sinuses
- Loss of function

Investigation

X-rays: Standard AP, lateral view and oblique views (to assess gap).

Radiological Features

- Persistence of fracture gap after adequate time
- Sclerosed margins of the fracture ends with surrounding osteoporosis.

Atrophic

- Conical bone ends.
- Medullary plug
- No signs of periosteal or endosteal callus formation.

Hypertrophic

Rounded elephant foot type of callus formation on both sides of fracture line, but fracture gap still persists.

Gap Nonunion

Loss of bone at fracture sites at the time of injury so that there is loss of contact between fracture ends.

Q7. Write in short the management of nonunion.

Treatment

Principle of Treatment

- It is an absolute indication for surgery.
- Excision of sclerosed and atrophic bone to create raw bleeding surface.
- Removal of medullary plug, to open up medullary vascular channels.
- Rigid cortical or medullary fixation in the proper alignment by DCP, intramedullary locked nail or Illizarov's fixator, compression at fracture site.
- Induce osteogenesis by bone grafting, bone marrow injection at fracture site, electrical stimulation by magnetic induction or by low-intensity ultrasound.
- Eradication of the infection (if this is the primary cause), removal of improper implant.
- Active mobilization to promote periosteal vascular inflow through muscles and to avoid stiff joints.
- Adequate skin and soft tissue cover.

Stabilization of Fragments (Rigid Fixation)

Adequate stabilization can be obtained by:
- Internal fixation, such as:
  - Plates and screws
  - Intramedullary nails (esp. interlocked nailing)
- External fixation such as:
  - Pin fixator
  - Ring fixator (Ilizarov): useful in nonunion associated with defects, shortening, and deformities
  - *Advantages*:
    - It can be used for temporary or definitive stabilization.
    - It is relatively noninvasive.
    - It does not disturb soft tissues surrounding the nonunion.
    - It correct deformity and provide stable fixation.

Choice of internal fixation depends on:
- Type of nonunion
- Condition of the soft tissues and bone
- Size and position of the bone fragments
- Size of the bony defect

Induce Osteogenesis

By Bone Grafting

- It is the most frequently used method of treatment of nonunions.
- Autogenous bone graft, allograft bone, or synthetic bone substitute used alone or in conjunction with internal fixation may help to stimulate bone formation.
- Different techniques includes:
  - *Onlay bone graft (Campbell)*: Used for nonunions of the shaft of any long bone
  - *Phemister technique*:
    - Type of onlay bone grafting for established nonunion.
    - Graft is placed subperiosteally across the fragments without mobilizing the fragments, i.e. bypassing the fracture.
    - *Advantage*: blood supply of the fragments and the normal impacting forces of the fracture were not disturbed
  - *Dual onlay graft (Boyd's)*:
    - Two cortical onlay grafts are kept opposite each other on the bone across the nonunion and are fixed with screws
    - They grip the fragments like a vise.
    - Any intervening space at the bone ends is packed up with cancellous chips.
    - It can also be used in nonunion of bones, which are thin and osteoporotic.
  - *Cancellous insert grafts (Nicolls):*
    - Bridging gaps in long bones with solid blocks of cancellous bone and fixing the fragments with compression plate and screws.
    - Useful in patients with defects less than 2.5 cm long.
  - *Massive sliding graft:*
    - Sliding graft about ½ the circumference of the bone and 10–15 cm long.

- ■ Useful for bridging bone defects especially nonunion of the tibia and femur
    Disadvantage: when a massive sliding graft fails, later grafting is difficult.
  - *Whole fibular transplants*: for bridging defects in the radius or ulna
  - *Vascularized free fibular graft*: useful in treatment of osteonecrosis of the femoral head to treat defects associated with tumor resections.
  - *Intramedullary fibular (peg graft) allografts*: using this technique of intramedullary grafting of the humerus with an allograft fibula and plating with a 4.5-mm compression plate give good result in treating nonunion humerus.

By Low-intensity Ultrasound

Theories: Several theories suggested that Ultrasound stimulation promotes bone healing. These are:

- It stimulates the genes involved in inflammation and bone regeneration.
- It increases blood flow through dilation of capillaries and enhancement of angiogenesis, increasing the flow of nutrients to the fracture site.
- It enhances the stimulation of chondrocyte, which leads to an increase in enchondral bone formation.

Current protocol: 20 minutes once a day

By Electrical and Electromagnetic Stimulation

Principle: When an optimal osteogenic potential of 20 μamp is delivered to the gap by inserting cathode electrodes a fibrous union can be converted to fibrocartilage, which then undergoes enchondral ossification.

Types of techniques: At least three electrical and electromagnetic methods are available for the treatment of non-unions. These are: (1) Invasive, (2) Semi-invasive, (3) Noninvasive

1. *Invasive*:
   - Electrodes are implanted
   - Titanium cathode is implanted within the fracture site
   - Platinum anode is placed in the soft tissue.
   - With the help of a generator, a constant current of 20 μamp is delivered.
   - Union is achieved in >90% of cases even in the presence of infection.
2. *Semi-invasive*:
   - Here the cathodes are inserted percutaneously under LA under X-ray control so that the tip of cathode comes to lie directly within the nonunion site and continuous small amount of direct current is delivered.
   - Main disadvantage is iatrogenic infection
3. *Noninvasive*: Weak electric currents in bone are induced by pulsing electromagnetic field (2 Gauses).

Q.8: Write in short about the management of an infected nonunion.

Infected nonunion is a very common and is difficult situation, because the problem is double fold.

Principle of Treatment

- First, it is necessary to eradicate the infection by drugs and local debridement of all the infective tissue from skin down to the bone and remove all devitalized tissue.
- The next step is to change or remove the implant (which is the most common cause) and to switch over to a suitable fixator for stabilization of the fracture.

- Finally, after control of infection, a well-planned procedure for bone grafting and fixation of fracture is done.

Methods

Conventional Treatment

Objective

- To convert an infected and draining nonunion into one that has not drained for several months
- To promote healing of the nonunion by bone grafting.

Steps

- *Radical debrima*: Wound is thoroughly saucerized and all foreign, devitalized, or infected materials are removed to provide a vascular bed.
- *Antibiotics*: Parenterally and locally after surgery.
- *Split-thickness skin graft (SSG)*: After 4–7 days of surgery, when a thin layer of granulation tissue has covered the wound SSG is applied.
- *Full-thickness pedicle skin graft*: 4–6 weeks after the wound has healed from the operation. Full-thickness pedicle skin graft is applied.
- *Bone grafting*: When the clinical signs of infection have subsided, the skin over the bone is good bone grafting must be considered.

Disadvantage of conventional treatment:

- It often requires 1 or more years to complete
- It usually results in stiffness of adjacent joints.

Active Treatment

Objective

- To obtain bony union early.
- To shorten the period of convalescence.
- To preserve motion in the adjacent joints.

Steps

- Restoration of bony continuity takes priority over treatment of infection.
- Expose the nonunion through the old scars and sinuses, decorticated subperiosteally
- All devitalized, necrotic and infected tissue should be removed.
- Fracture fragments are aligned and stabilized usually with external fixator.
- A suction drain is inserted
- Closed the wound as much as possible
- If necessary bone grafting is done.
- Once the non-union is healed split-thickness skin grafts are applied to remaining defect.

Other methods to induce soft tissue healing, union and eliminating:

Ilizarov

Indication: Infection associated with deformity, shortening, and segmental bone loss

Ilizarov frame allows multiple modes of treatment, including lengthening, compression, distraction, and bone transport besides improving the vascularity by corticotomy that is essential to eliminate infection and obtain union.

Huntington Method in Infected Tibial Nonunion

- Huntington describe centralization of the fibula and fixation of it to the tibia, i.e. Tibialization of the fibula (for massive tibial bone loss) or transposition of the ipsilateral fibula.
- Prerequisites: Intact fibula is required.
- *Disadvantage* includes prolonged immobilization and non-weight bearing is essential, segmental bone defect or short proximal or distal fragment are difficult to manage with this method.

Papineau (Open Bone Grafting)

Papineau et al. described an open bone grafting procedure for the treatment of infected nonunion and or chronic osteomyelitis.

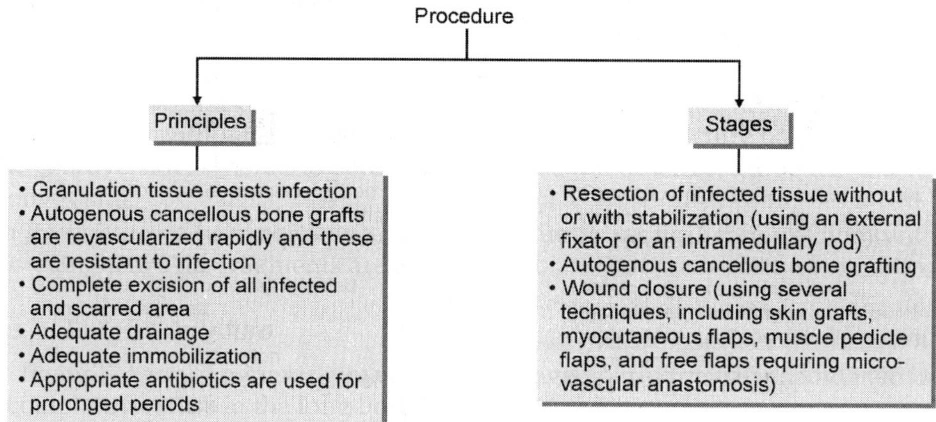

Soft-tissue Transfer

To fill a dead space left after radical debrima, soft tissue transfer may range from localized muscle pedicle flap to microvascular free tissue transfer.

Aim: Vascularized muscle flaps or graft by bringing in a blood supply improves the local biological environment that is significant for osseous and soft-tissue healing, in the host's defense mechanisms and for antibiotic delivery.

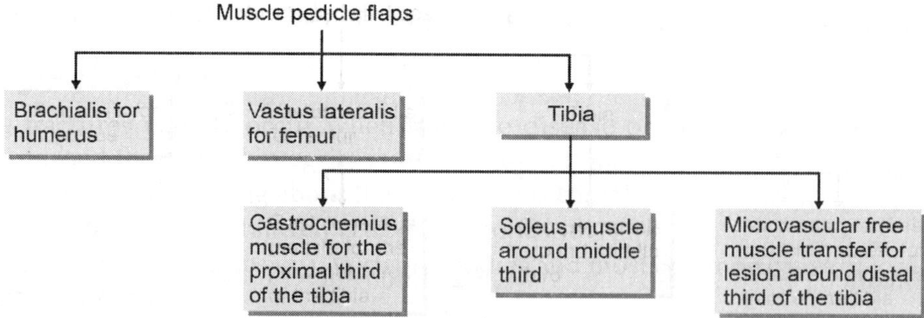

Polymethyl Methacrylate Antibiotic Beads

These can also be used to treat infected nonunion.

Aim: it is to deliver levels of antibiotics locally so that its concentration exceeds the minimal inhibitory concentrations.

Prerequisites:
- All infected, scarred and necrotic tissue should be excised adequately.
- All foreign material should be removed.

Antibiotic used:
- Thermostable and well-eluted antibiotic like aminoglycosides, penicillins, cephalosporins, and clindamycin.
- Vancomycin elutes much less effectively but it used most commonly in methacillin-resistant *S. aureus*.

Implantation:
- Short term: beads are removed within 10 days
- Long-term implantation: these beads may be left for 80 days

Q9. Write short note on fat embolism or post-traumatic distress syndrome.

It is *post-traumatic distress syndrome* seen within 48–72 hours of skeletal injury. It indicates the presence of fat globules (Olein in adults and palmitin and stearine in children) within lung parenchymatous tissue and peripheral circulation following a long bone fracture.

Fat Embolism

- Latent period: 12–24 hrs after fracture of major bones (femur, pelvis).
- Fat globules embolize in cerebral, white matter producing multiple petechial haemorrhages.
- Grey matter not involved.
- More frequent with closed fractures than open.
- Polytrauma and crush injuries.
- Following liposuction for cosmetic surgery.

Source of Fat

- Bone marrow (most common)
- From plasma by agglutination of chylomicrons which later acts as a embolus (less common)
- The free fatty acid directly destroys the penumocytes and causes ARDS.

Pathogenesis

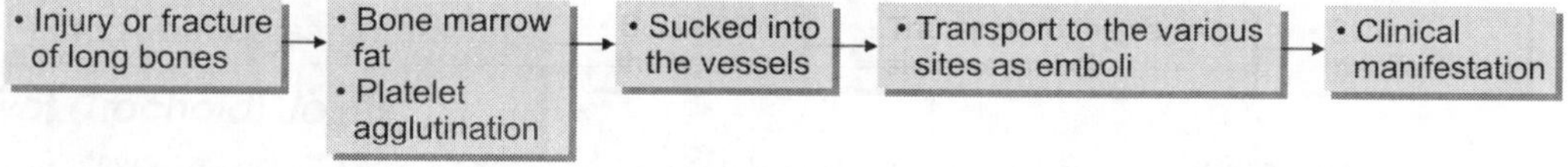

Clinical Features

- Depends on the organ involved, i.e. brain, lungs, heart, kidney, etc.
- The patient suddenly becomes:
  - Restless
  - Disoriented
  - Feverish
  - Dyspnoeic
  - Confusion

– Comatose
– Retention of urine
– Transient rash over neck and chest, might have conjunctival haemorrhage (subconjunctival rashes are pathognomonic)
– Hypertension with tachycardia(<140)
– Thrombocytopenia, petechial rashes and PaO_2 <60 mmHg constitute the triad of fat embolism

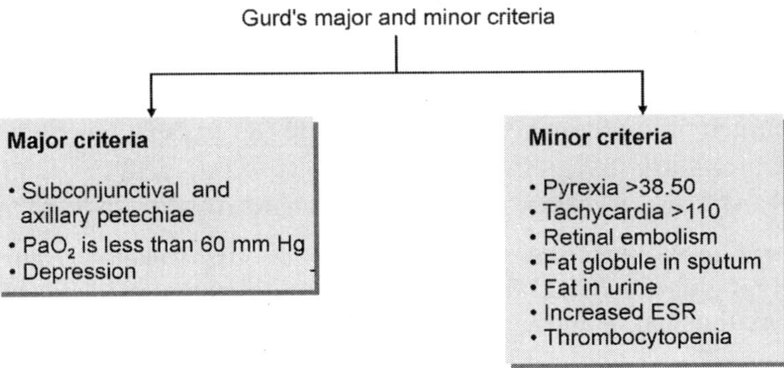

Investigations

- Lipuria: Earliest sign
- The sputum and urine contains fat globules.
- Sizzle test is positive (when platinum loop dipped in urine, it produces a sizzle when heated in a flame)
- X-ray chest, shows *snowstorm pattern* and bilateral infiltration of lungs.
- PaO_2 is always <60 mm (most important).
- ECG shows:
    - Prominent S wave in lead I
    - Prominent Q waves in lead II
    - ST depression and right axis strain
- Platelets counts <1.5 lakh.
- Fundoscopy may show characteristic findings.
- Anaemia, hypocalcemia may also occur
- MRI, CT scan helps to grade the severity.

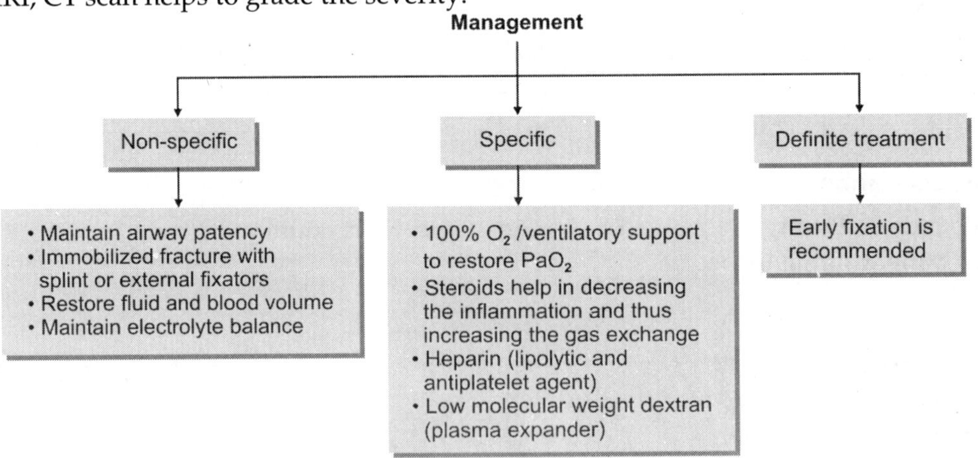

Q9. Describe the aetiology, clinical features, and management of compartmental syndrome.

Compartmental syndrome is a crippling complication of fracture due to impeded blood flow, increased compartmental pressure and progressive damage of all the tissues; skin, muscles, nerves and bone which are preventable to a great extent. Commonly involving the forearm/tibial compartment; first described by *Prof. Richard Volkmann, a German surgeon in 1881.*

Definition: *Mubarak* define compartment syndrome as "as an elevation of the interstitial pressure in a closed osseofascial compartment that results in microvascular compromise".

Compartment Involved

- Anterior compartments of the leg
- Deep posterior compartments of the leg
- Volar compartment of the forearm

Other Sites of Compartmental Syndrome

Buttock, thigh, shoulder, hand, foot, arm, and lumbar para-spinous muscles.

Classification

Depending on the cause of the increased pressure and the duration of symptoms it can be classified as *acute* or *chronic*

Stages

- I: Phase of ischemia
- II: Phase of contracture

Causes of Compartment Syndrome

Acute

- Fractures (Supracondylar fracture humerus, both bone forearm fracture, proximal tibial fracture)
- Soft-tissue trauma
- Arterial injury (Damage to the brachial artery following fracture supracondylar humerus, sometimes—posterior dislocation of elbow and fracture of radius/ulna, causing damage to forearm vessels)
- Occlusion of blood flow through the artery may be because of:
  - External pressure on the vessel due to:
    - Tight plaster bandage or wooden splints.
    - Grossly displaced fracture fragments.
  - Damage to the vessel wall by cut or contusion of artery/vein.
  - Occlusion of lumen due to:
    - Spasm
    - Thrombus
    - Intimal tear.
- Limb compression during altered consciousness
- Burns

- Intravenous fluid extravasation
- Anticoagulants.

Pathophysiology of Ischaemia

- Vessels, nerves (*most common nerve involved is Median nerve*) and muscles (*most common and earliest muscle involved is FDP and severely affected muscles are FDP and FPL*) are compressed resulting in increased pressure in tight osteofascial compartment due to oedema with no arterial inflow and poor venous return, slow tissue death, necrosis occurs, and this vicious cycles continues.
- This cycle of increasing muscle ischaemia was depicted by **Eaton and Green** as shown below:

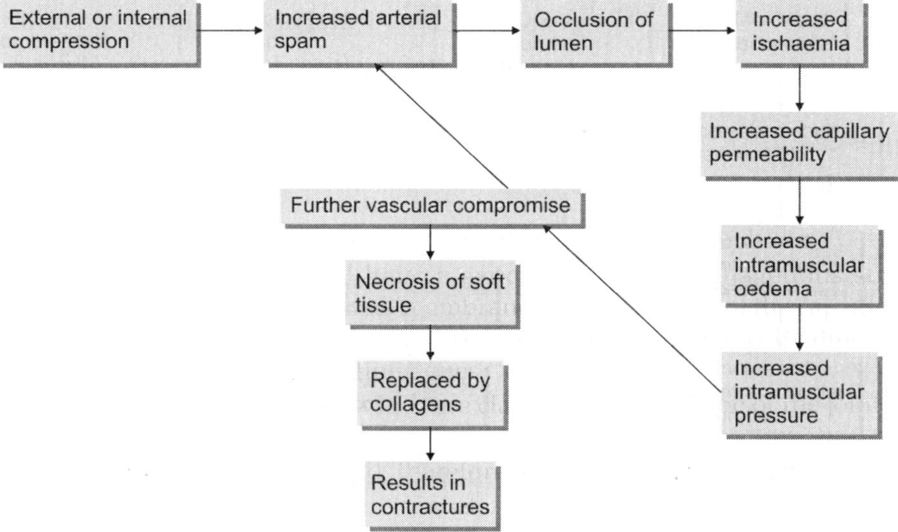

Clinical Features

Patient presents with following clinical features.

Five P's

Griffith's tetrad: Pain, Pallor, Pulselessness, Paresis.
- Pain in distal parts of forearm and hand, which is excruciating, unbearable and is the earliest symptom. Most important and earliest single sign is *Griffith's sign (passive stretching of the flexed finger causes severe pain).*
- Pallor of nail bed.
- Paresthesias, numbness and tingling.
- Pulselessness (absent radial/dorsalis pedis pulsations).
- Paralysis of the involved muscles, in late cases.

Principle of Management

To relieve the compression on the vascular channel and to restore the vascularity of the distal part at the earliest.

Treatment

Decompress

- Remove all external splintages and bandages immediately.
- Measuring of compartmental pressure: If no specialized instrument is available then it can be measured using intravenous tubing, a three-way stopcock, a syringe, and a mercury manometer, as described by Whitesides.
- If compartmental pressures are > 30 mmHg in the presence of clinical findings, immediate fasciotomy is indicated.
- Cool the limb by ice packs to reduce metabolic demands.
- If the fracture fragments are grossly displaced, do closed reduction under anaesthesia at the earliest.
- Watch for return of capillary circulation and the pulsation.

Repair

If within few hours circulation does not improve, Doppler study may show the type of arterial block, exploration of the damaged vessel, decompression and necessary repair should be done.

Phase of Contracture

VIC (Volkmann's Ischaemic Contracture)

It is the end result of prolonged ischaemia, causing irreversible damage to muscle and nerve.

Pathophysiology of Contracture

- Prolonged ischaemia leads to necrosis of muscles, nerves, atrophy of skin, bone and soft tissue.
- In due time necrosed muscles are replaced by fibrous tissue (bands) resulting into contracture.

Clinical Features

- Patient presents with a deformed hand, which is stiff, weak and numb.
- The extent of involvement may be mild, moderate or severe with extensive involvement of muscles, bones and nerves.

Deformity

- Fingers are flexed at interphalangeal joints due to contracture of flexor muscles of the forearm.
- This deformity increases with dorsiflexion and diminishes with flexion of wrist (Volkmann's sign); this is due to fibrotic flexor muscles

Other Changes

- *Joints*: Stiff and bones are atrophied and deformed.
- *Muscles*:
  - Loss of the power of grip.
  - Wasting of small muscles of hand/forearm.

- *Nerves*: Loss of sensation affecting the median and ulnar nerves.
- *Skin*: Skin becomes atrophic and so do nails and hair.

Tsuge Classification of Volkmann's Ischemic Contracture

Grading	Involvement of structures
Mild	• Involvement of flexor digitorum profundus and flexor pollicis longus
Moderate	• Involvement of flexor digitorum profundus and flexor pollicis longus
	• Involvement of superficial finger flexors
	• Involvement of wrist flexors
	• Involvement of thumb flexors
Severe	• All flexors
	• Few extensors
	• Neurological deficit (most common median nerve)
	• Joint contracture
	• Severe scarring of the skin
	• Deformity of bones

Treatment

Depending on the Extent of the Involvement

Mild

- Splinting
- Physiotherapy
- If there is involvement of single muscle then plan for its excision

Moderate

- Muscle sliding of the common flexors from the medial epicondyle (*MaxPage*).
- Excision of the dead fibrotic muscle
- Tendon transfers

Severe

- Excision of the scar
- Nerve grafting
- Proximal row carpectomy (Seddon's)
- Wrist arthrodesis in functional position

Q10. Write short note on: a. Malunion; b. Myositis ossificans; c. Gas gangrene; d. Avascular necrosis; e. Tetanus

a. Malunion

Definition

A *malunited fracture* is one that has healed with the fragments in a non-anatomical alignment.

Malunion Impairs Function Several Ways

- An abnormal or incongruent joint surface can cause irregular weight transfer and arthritis of the joint, especially in the lower extremities.

- Angulation or Rotation of the fragments can interfere with proper balance or gait in the lower extremities or proper positioning of the upper extremities
- Overriding of fragments or bone loss results in shortening.
- The movements of neighboring joints are restricted.

Causes

- Inaccurate reduction
- Ineffective immobilization during healing
- Commonly seen in closed treatment of fractures
- Malunion developing in patients with multiple injuries, fractures goes un-noticed as treatment of more life-threatening injuries takes precedence

Clinical Features

- Pain
- Deformity
- Stiffness
- Muscular wasting
- Shortening
- Loss of function
- Disability
- Restriction of movements at the joint

Investigation

- *X-rays*: Anteroposterior and lateral radiographs of the involved part including the joint above and below are of utmost important.
- *CT scan*: It is helpful to evaluate the potential for congruity of the joint (axial views) and the condition of the articular surface.

Treatment

In patients the fracture should be reduced as near to the acceptability criteria as possible
- *Factors determine the acceptability of fracture reduction:*
    - Alignment (most important)
    - Rotation
    - Restoration of normal length
    - Actual position of the fragments (least important)

Surgical Treatment

Indication

- To restore function
- Cosmetic reasons or appearance (relative)

Best time for surgery: 6–12 months after the fracture has occurred.

Type of Surgeries

- Corrective osteotomy or compensatory procedure may be necessary to restore function (e.g. Darrach's procedure in malunited fracture Colles)

- Ilizarov: simultaneous restoration of alignment, rotation, and length
- Sometimes pain may be the predominant symptom and may require fusion of a joint or arthrodesis.

b. Myositis Ossificans

Definition

It is a reactive condition where there is calcification and ossification of injured soft tissue usually in response to trauma (fracture or dislocation), most commonly in the flexor muscles of the upper arm, the quadriceps femoris, adductor muscles of the thigh, the gluteal muscles and the soft tissues of the hand resulting in stiff and painful joint.

Causes

- Most common cause: Repeated manipulations and massage of injuries around the joint.
- Most common area is around the *elbow joint*.

Types

- Traumatica: After injuries
- Progressiva: As a hereditary disease
- Heterotrophica: As in head injury

Pathogenesis

- Reactive
- History of trauma in 50% of cases

Gross Pathology

Location: Most commonly *(Muscle involvement)*:
- Flexor muscles of upper arm (especially brachialis anticus)
- Quadriceps femoris
- Adductor muscles of thigh (Prussian disease: Myositis of adductors in riders due to constant pressure of saddle)
- Gluteal muscles
- Soft tissues of hand

Histopathology

- Highly cellular stroma associated with:
    - Formation of new bone
    - Less commonly, cartilage
- *Early lesion*: Centrally placed areas may be difficult to distinguish from osteosarcoma due to extreme cellularity
- As process evolves, osteoid:
    - Appears in orderly pattern at periphery of mass
    - Subsequently matures into well-developed bone
- Maturation pattern *(Ackerman LV zonal phenomenon: Layer-wise differentiated activity in peripheral zones)*
    - Most important diagnostic feature

– It is characterized by:
  ■ Central cellular area
  ■ Intermediate zone of osteoid formation
  ■ Peripheral shell of highly organized bone

Ultrastructurally

Cells with features of myofibroblasts prominent.

Clinical Features

Acute Stage

• Pain
• Swelling
• Tenderness
• Painful restriction of movements

Late Stage

• No pain
• Bony lump is very well palpated
• Bony lump act as a mechanical block to the joint movements

Investigation

X-ray

Active stage: Hazy, translucent or cotton wool appearance with diffuse margins:
• In front (in the branchialis muscle)
• Behind (in triceps muscle)
• Sides (common flexor/extensor muscles) of elbow

Quiescent stage: Bony shadow with clear margins and visible trabecular pattern.

Treatment

Treatment is initially conservative, as some patients' calcifications will spontaneously be reabsorbed, and others will have minimal symptoms.

Active stage

• Ice can also be placed on the injured spot to relieve the pain
• Immobilization in a slab
• Avoid massage or any passive stretching,
• Anti-inflammatory drug like indomethacin.

Healed: Active mobilization of joint and surgical excision of the myositis mass after it has matured usually 6–12 months (with caution, as recurrence is frequent).

c. Gas Gangrene

Gas gangrene (also known as, *Clostridial myonecrosis* and *"Myonecrosis"*) is a deadly rapidly developing and spreading form of gangrene usually caused by *Clostridium perfringens* bacteria that produces gas tissues in gangrene. It is a medical emergency.

Offending organism

- Most commonly by a bacterium called *Clostridium perfringens*.
- Occasionally by Group A *Streptococcus. Staphylococcus aureus* and *Vibrio vulnificus* can cause similar infections.

Causes

- More than 50% of cases had history of trauma.
- Other cases occur spontaneously or in patients after operative procedures.

Predisposing Factors

- Trauma
- Open fractures
- Foreign bodies
- Frostbite
- Thermal or electrical burns
- Subcutaneous or intravenous injection of medications or illicit drugs
- Pressure sores
- Motor vehicle or roadside accidents

Postoperative

- Gastrointestinal tract surgery
- Genitourinary tract surgery
- Abortion
- Amputation
- Tourniquets, casts, bandages, or dressings applied too tightly

Spontaneous (or non-traumatic, idiopathic, or metastatic gas gangrene)

- It is usually a mixed infection caused by *C. septicum, C. perfringens, and C. novyi.*
- The gastrointestinal tract is the source of organisms.
- The organisms escape the bowel by translocation, enter the bloodstream, and seed distant sites where they can cause gas gangrene.
- Approximately 80% of patients without trauma have an overt or occult malignancy (hematologic malignancies and colorectal).

Pathophysiology

It is mainly the exotoxin produced by these organisms, which produce this disease.
Organism, which produce this disease:

- Alfa toxin (Lecithinase)—Haemolytic
- Collagenase is a proteinase and breaks down collagen, connective tissue elements of the muscle.
- Hyaluronidase beaks down hyaluronic acid
- Theta toxin-Haemolytic, necrotic
- Leucocidin kills the leucocytes.

Pathological events following Clostridium invasion:

- Clostridial invasion → Affects the involved muscle completely (origin to incretion) → Foul smelling muscle (origin to incretion) → Necrosis of the muscle

- Rapidly spreading edema of subcutaneous tissue and muscle with accumulation of gas.
- Collagens fibres become swollen, fragmented and get broken down.
- Blood vessels are damaged.
- Necrosis
- Ultimately, muscle becomes friable, soft and green to black.
- If septicaemia occurs, gas may produce in the other organ, notably the liver known as *'foaming liver'*.

Clinical Features

General: Vital signs—may indicate systemic toxicity and include:
- No or low-grade fever
- Tachycardia (relative tachycardia)
- Tachypnoea
- Hypotension
- Hypoxia

Local
- Pain in affected limb: Gas gangrene typically begins with the sudden appearance of pain in the region of the wound
- Edema bullae
- Erythema with purplish black discolouration
- Excruciating tenderness
- Brownish skin discolouration (bronzing, brawny) with bullae
- Profuse, "dish-watery," serous drainage from ruptured bullae
- Discharge—thin watery grayish and may have a peculiar, "mousy," sweet odor
- Minimal crepitant bullae
- Crepitus is always present due to gas in muscle and subcutaneous tissues.
- Crepitant tissue—May extend well beyond any skin discolouration, edema, or bleb formation
- Mental status—Paradoxically, may be depressed early during the disease course; sensorium then may clear as the disease progresses and the patient is near death.
- Profound shock and toxemia
- Finally death

Investigation

Laboratory Findings
- WBCs count may be normal or elevated.
- Elevated liver function test (LFTs) results may indicate progressive hepatic dysfunction.
- Elevated blood urea nitrogen (BUN) and creatinine may indicate azotemia, renal insufficiency, or renal failure.
- Myonecrosis may elevate serum aldolase, potassium, lactate dehydrogenase, and creatine phosphokinase levels (CPK).
- Profound anaemia may result from severe intravascular hemolysis.
- Arterial blood gas (ABG) analysis may reveal metabolic acidosis.
- Disseminated intravascular coagulation (DIC) may result from exotoxin release.
- Gram's stain of the wound discharge reveals gram-positive rods and an absence of

polymorphonuclear cells. Other organisms are also present in up to 75% of cases. This test is essential for rapid diagnosis.

- An assay for sialidases (neuraminidase) produced by clostridia also may be performed on serum and wound discharge. These tests provide rapid (<2 hours) confirmation of Gram's stain results.

Radiographs reveals: Fine gas bubbles within the soft tissues, dissecting into the intramuscular fascial planes and muscles.

CT scan: Intra-abdominal clostridial gas gangrene is evaluated usually with CT scanning, which demonstrates extraluminal gas.

Treatment

The most deciding factors in the successful treatment of gas gangrene are *early diagnosis and prompt treatment*.

Medical treatment

Resuscitative measures:
- Restore intravenous fluid volume
- Monitor urine output with an indwelling bladder catheter.
- Transfer to an ICU that has telemetry and pulse oximetry.
- Ensure that tetanus immunity is adequate.

Antibiotic:
- Inj. Penicillin 2 g (4 hourly)
- Mixed infections are common and antibiotic spectrum should include aminoglycosides, penicillinase-resistant penicillins, or vancomycin.
- For patients who are allergic to penicillin, alternatives include clindamycin, a third-generation cephalosporin, metronidazole, and chloramphenicol.

Passive immunization: Inj. Antigas gangrene serum (AGGS) 22500 IU, IM 4-6 hourly after AST.

Hyperbaric Oxygen

- Clostridia lack superoxide dismutase, making them incapable of surviving in the oxygen-rich environment created within a hyperbaric chamber. This inhibits Clostridial growth, exotoxin production (halts alpha toxin production), and exotoxin binding to host tissues.
- Hyperbaric oxygen therapy may also induce host polymorphonuclear cell function.
- Administer therapy 3 times a day for 2 days, then twice a day for several more days, until the disease process is well under control.
- The dose is usually 2.5 atmospheres absolute (ATA) oxygen for 120 minutes or 3 atmospheres absolute (ATA) oxygen for 90 minutes (1–2 hours) every 8–12 hours, for a total of 6–8 treatments. The pressure at sea level equals 1 ATA.

Complications include:
- Fire
- Seizures
- Decompression sickness
- Middle ear barotrauma
- Claustrophobia

Absolute contraindication: The presence of an untreated pneumothorax.

Surgical Treatment

- It represents a true surgical emergency.
- As soon as the diagnosis is established multiple longitudinal incision are given for decompression and drainage.
- It requires prompt aggressive and radical debridement of all devitalized or necrotic tissues.
- Extensive extremity involvement may require amputation.
- Because the disease process may continue to involve additional tissue, daily exploration and further debridement may be necessary.
- Wound exploration reveals gas, watery discharge, and necrotic muscle.
- If the patient survives, the wound is allowed to heal secondarily (by wound contraction and spontaneous re-epithelialization).

d. Avascular Necrosis

Avascular necrosis is death of bone from deficient vascular supply.

Causes of AVN

Idiopathic (most common).

Haemoglobinopathies

- Sickle cell disease
- Sickle Thalassemia

Traumatic

- Fracture neck femur (subcapital fractures are more prone for AVN and has worst prognosis)
- Dislocation of hip joint (>12 hours)
- SCFE

Infective

- Osteomyelitis
- Septic arthritis
- TB hip

Storage Disease

- Gaucher's disease
- Dysbaric osteonecrosis:
- Caison disease (due to N_2)

Malignancy

Haematological, e.g. leukemia, lymphoma.

Coagulation Disorders

- Familial thrombophilia
- Hypofibrinolysis

- Hypolipoproteinemia
- *Thrombocytopenic Purpura*

Others

- Pregnancy
- Alcohol
- Steroid
- Tobacco
- Perthes' disease
- Nephrotic syndrome
- Anaphylactic shock
- Renal transplant patients (16%)
- SLE
- Ionizing radiation

Common Sites of Avascular Necrosis

Site of avascular necrosis	Cause
Head of femur	Fracture neck of femur; posterior dislocation of the hip
Proximal pole of scaphoid	Fracture through the waist of the Scaphoid
Body of the talus	Fracture through neck of the talus
Lunate (entire bone)	Dislocation of lunate bone

Important Points

- In avascular necrosis of femoral head there is *first restriction of the internal rotation followed by abduction*
- On X-rays recognized 1–3 months after injury.
- Necrosed bone appears denser (sclerotic) due to its calcium being not absorbed, whereas surrounding normal bone shows osteoporosis due to hyperaemia.
- In advanced cases when the bone collapsed it appears on the x-rays as shrunken and crumbled bone.
- Investigation of choice is *MRI*

Treatment

- Early stages: Protective braces to prevent collapse
- Decompression (doubtful but helpful)
- Late stages: Hip: Total hip replacement; scaphoid: open reduction and Bone grafting

e. Tetanus

Tetanus results from infection with *Cl. tetani*, a mobile, spore-forming, anaerobic, gram-positive bacillus. The spores of *Cl. tetani* germinate and produce two exotoxin: *tetanolysin* (*a haemolysin; cardiotoxic*) and *tetanospasmin*, (*act on the brainstem and spinal cord;* responsible for the clinical manifestations of tetanus)

Mode of Transmission

Infection is acquired by contamination of wounds with tetanus spores.

Range of Injuries

- Open fractures
- Gangrenous limb
- Skin abrasion
- Puncture wound
- Unsterile surgeries
- Pin-prick
- Burns
- Human bites
- Animal bites and Stings
- Intrauterine deaths
- Bowel surgery
- Dental extractions
- Otitis media
- Chronic skin ulcers

Incubation Period

Usually 6–10 days.

Clinical Features

- Restless and headache
- Sore throat with dysphagia (early sign)
- Muscular rigidity
- Painful paroxysmal spasms of the voluntary muscles:
    - Masseters (trismus or lock- jaw)
    - Facial muscles (risus sardonicus)
    - Muscle of back and neck (opisthotonus)
    - Lower limbs and abdominal
- Periods of apnea resulting from spasm of the intercostal muscles and diaphragm
- Prone for fractures due to fall.

Prevention of Tetanus

Passive Immunization

- Provides temporary protection against tetanus.
- Human tetanus hyperimmunoglobulin.
- *Dose*: 250–500 IU
- Give protection up to 30 days
- Safe and no serum reaction
- If it is not available equine ATS should be used (dose: 1500 IU, S/C AST; causes sensitivity reaction)

Active and Passive Immunization

- Usually practiced in non-immune persons
- 1500 IU units of ATS or 250–500 IU units of human Ig in one arm and 0.5 ml of adsorbed tetanus toxoid into the other arm or in gluteal region.

- This should be followed 6-week later by another dose of 0.5 ml of tetanus toxoid, and a third dose 1year later.

Antibiotics

- Single IM injection of 1.2 mega units of long acting penicillin (benzathine penicillin)
- Patient who are sensitive to penicillin; give a 7-day course of erythromycin 500 mg 6 hourly.

Recommendations for Prevention of Tetanus in the Wound

- All wound Category I and II receive surgical toilet
- Category I: Wounds <6 hr old, clean, non-penetrating and with negligible tissue damage:

Immunity category	*Treatment*
Had a complete course of toxoid or a booster dose within 5 yr	Nothing more required
Had a complete course of toxoid or a booster dose >5 yr and <10yr	Toxoid 1 dose
Had a complete course of toxoid or a booster dose >10 yr	Toxoid 1 dose
Has not had a complete course of toxoid or immunity status is unknown	Toxoid complete course

- **Category II: Other wound:**

Immunity category	*Treatment*
Had a complete course of toxoid or a booster dose within 5 yrs	Nothing more required
Had a complete course of toxoid or a booster dose >5 yrs and <10yrs	Toxoid 1 dose
Had a complete course of toxoid or a booster dose >10 yrs	Toxoid 1 dose + Human Tet. Ig
Has not had a complete course of toxoid or immunity status is unknown	Toxoid complete course+ Human Tet. Ig

Treatment of Tetanus

Critical Care

- ICU admission
- Respiratory support (oxygen, ventilator)
- Tracheostomy if required
- Maintain strict isolation (as noise, light or any other sound may initiate painful spasms of muscles)
- Good nursing care

Drugs

- The goals of pharmacotherapy are to prevent complications and to reduce morbidity.
- Treat reflex muscle spasms, rigidity, tetanic seizures and infections.
- Antimicrobials: cover all likely pathogens; prevent any other infection
- Benzodiazepines: may act in the CNS to induce muscle relaxation. Administer diazepam IV, typically 10–40 mg every 1–8 hours. Vecuronium (by continuous infusion) or pancuronium (by intermittent injection) are adequate alternatives
- Sedative hypnotics, narcotics, inhalational anesthetics, neuromuscular blocking agents, and centrally acting muscle relaxants (e.g. intrathecal baclofen).

Surgical (if required): Meticulous management of wound (radical debrima plus thorough wound toilet).

> **Q11. Discuss in brief: a. List nerve and viscera prone for injury following fracture/ dislocation; b. Sudeck's Posttraumatic osteodystrophy**

a) Nerve and Visceral Injury Following Fracture

Injury to Nerves

Site of fracture /dislocation	*Most common injured nerve*
Shoulder dislocation	Axillary
Surgical neck humerus	Axillary
Distal humeral shaft fracture	Radial
Medial epicondyle fracture	Ulnar
Lateral condyle humerus	Tardy ulnar nerve palsy
Fracture neck of radius	Posterior interosseous nerve
Posterior dislocation of hip	Sciatic
Anterior dislocation of hip	Obturator
Both bones forearm	Ulnar
Both bone legs	Peroneal
Fracture neck fibula	Common peroneal (lateral peroneal)

Injury to Visceras

Fracture	*Visceral injury*
Fracture ribs	Laceration of lungs or pleura
Flail chest or stove in chest (double rib fracture)	Paradoxical respiration Traumatic wet lung Dead space ventilation Treatment: IPPV and rib traction
Fracture pelvis	Urinary bladder or urethral injury

b. Sudeck's Posttraumatic Osteodystrophy

- It is also known as Reflex sympathetic dystrophy.
- Causalgia and shoulder hand syndrome represent Sudeck's dystrophy.

Causes

- Most common cause in upper limbs: Colle's fracture
- Most common cause in lower limbs: Ankle injury

Pathology

- Due to disturbances of sympathetic nervous system
- Disuse decalcification due to prolonged immobilization.

Clinically characterized by:
- Symptoms appears 2 months after injury
- Pain
- Swelling
- Joint stiffness
- Osteoporosis
- Thickening of soft tissues
- Vascular stasis

Treatment

- Conservative treatment in form of active exercises of involved extremity.
- Some cases may required Stellate sympathectomy or peri-arterial sympathectomy

3

Epiphyseal Injuries, Fracture Healing, Bone Grafting and Substitute

Q1. What is a greenstick fracture?

Greenstick fracture occurs in resilient bones of children. It is an incomplete fracture and involves cortex on the convex side and concave half is only bent.
- In a child, the bones are pliable and elastic hence they bend under pressure, with or without a breach in the cortex.
- Green stick fracture has intact periosteum on the concave side, where the bone buckles while the other cortex bends and breaks at the convex side.

Q2. Discuss in brief types of epiphyses injury and their management.

Epiphyseal Injuries

These are fractures in children at the epiphysio-metaphyseal area, classified as shown below:

Salter-Harris Classification

Type I

- Complete separation of epiphysis from metaphysis without any X-ray evidence of a metaphyseal fragment attached to displaced epiphysis.
- Prognosis is usually excellent because of the preservation of the proliferative and reserve zones.

Type II

- Fracture plane travels transversely across the growth plate for a variable distance and then through the metaphysis producing a triangular-shaped fragment the *"Thurston-Holland"* sign.
- Periosteal hinge is intact on the side with the metaphyseal fragment.
- Prognosis is excellent, although complete or partial growth arrest may occur in cases of displaced fractures.

Type III

- Fracture plane passes along the growth plate and across the epiphysis (intra-articular), seen around the knee and elbow.
- Anatomic reduction and fixation without disturbing the physis are essential.
- Prognosis is guarded, because partial growth arrest and resultant deformity are common.

Type IV

- Fracture line is vertical passing across the epiphysis, growth plate and metaphysis (intra-articular).
- Anatomic reduction and fixation without disturbing the physis are essential.
- Prognosis is guarded, because partial growth arrest and resultant deformity are common.

Type V

- Compression or crush injury, destruction of growth plate, and growth disturbances.
- Prognosis is poor, because growth arrest and partial physeal closure are common.

Radiographs

- Comparison views of the opposite extremity may aid in diagnosing subtle deformities or a minimally displaced fracture.
- Skiagram must include orthogonal views of the involved bone as well as the joint proximal and distal to the suspected area of injury.
- CT scan: It helps in assessing the complicated intra-articular fractures in the older child.

Management

- CR and splint application: Type I and II injuries can be managed by closed reduction and maintain by splint in form of slab or cast.
- CR and percutaneous K wire fixation: If fracture is retained with splint then should be fixed with percutaneous K wires
- Intra-articular fractures, Salter-Harris types III and IV, require anatomic reduction (<1 to 2 mm of displacement both vertically and horizontally) to restore articular congruity.
- Indications for open reduction include:
    - Open fractures.
    - Displaced intra-articular fractures (Salter-Harris types III and IV).
    - Soft tissue interposition.
    - Fractures with vascular deficit.
    - Fractures with an associated compartment syndrome.
    - Unstable fractures.

Complications

- *Complete growth arrest*: It may result in limb length discrepancies necessitating the use of orthotics, prosthetics, or operative interventions including epiphysiodesis or limb lengthening.
- *Progressive angular or rotational deformities*: it is due to partial growth arrest or malunion. In cases of significant functional disabilities or cosmetic deformity, corrective osteotomy is required.
- *Overgrowth*: it is due to stimulation and hyperaemia due to physeal injury.

Q3. Discuss in brief the stages of fracture healing and outline the factor affecting it.

During the process of fracture repair, four basic types of new bone formation occur:
- Osteochondral ossification
- Intramembranous ossification

- Oppositional new bone formation
- Osteonal migration (*creeping substitution*):
  - The word *"creeping substitution"* coined by phemister.
  - It is the process of formation new bone on some surfaces and osteoclastic resorption on some other surfaces (acceptability of a graft).
  - It is a characteristic of autologous cancellous bone graft.

The type, amount, and location of bone formed can be influenced by:

- Fracture type
- Gap condition
- Fixation rigidity
- Loading
- Biological environment

Types of Fracture Healing

Primary

- It is seen when accurate anatomical reduction and firm/rigid fixation is done.
- Fracture heals without external callus formation
- The stage of cartilage formation is absent and direct endosteal bone formation occurs.
- There is no periosteal cuff of callus.
- Primary healing is radiologically invisible and much slower.
- Cutter head osteon indicates direct or primary bone healing.
- Calcium utilized in healing of a fracture comes from bloodstream.

Secondary

- Indirect or secondary bone healing characterized by *"re-generation torus"*.
- Healing occurs both by periosteal as well as endosteal callus.

Fracture Healing Time

Perkin's Rule of 6

	Healing time (in weeks)		
	Spiral fracture	*Transverse fracture*	*Consolidation time*
Upper limb	6	12	24
Lower limb	12	24	48

Stages of Fracture Healing (Classic Stages as Described by Hunter)

- Stage 1: Haematoma
- Stage 2: Granulation
- Stage 3: Soft callus
- Stage 4: Hard callus
- Stage 5: Remodelling
- Stage 6: Final healing

Stage of Haematoma (Inflammatory Phase)

- When a bone breaks, the gap is filled with blood from the ruptured periosteal and endosteal vessels.

- This blood distends to the soft tissues and clots to form a haematoma.
- This process takes about one to two days.
- Earliest change in healing is hyperemia, fibroblastic proliferation and inflammation.

Stage of Granulation Tissue

- The margins of the bone undergo aseptic necrosis.
- The soft tissues in the region undergo the usual changes of acute aseptic inflammation with vasodilatation and exudation of plasma and leucocytes.
- The clotted blood is invaded by fine capillaries and young connective tissue and is converted into granulation tissues in about two weeks.
- The multipotent cells can differentiate into fibroblast, chondroblast and osteoblast.

Stage of Soft Callus Formation (Chondrogenic Phase: Cartilage Formation with Subsequent Calcification)

- The granulation tissue matures into fibrocartilaginous mass, which subsequently is converted into spongy immature bone.
- First, a bridge of callus develops in the subperiosteal zone, this is called external callus.
- Subsequently, medullary callus formation starts, which is called the internal callus.
- Radially oriented callus: end of 4th week
- Longitudinally oriented callus: end of 8th week
- Maximum size of callus: 2–4 weeks
- First radiological sign of callus: 4–5 weeks

Stage of Hard Callus Formation (Osteogenic Phase: Cartilage Removal and Bone Formation)

Primary callus is removed by osteoclastic resorption, and the spongy bone is replaced by matured lamellar bone.

Stage of Remodelling

- The new formed bone starts arranging itself under stress and strain into sheets of new lamellae.
- The initially deformed bone undergoes the process of reorganization and contouring.
- The extra callus which is formed gradually gets absorbed.
- The fracture is clinically well united and takes about 3–6 months.

Stage of Final Healing

The original bone structure is restored and extra callus formation is completely reabsorbed. This takes about a year.

Factors Affecting the Fracture Healing

General/Systemic Factors

- Age: In children, quick healing is due to the high osteogenic potential, whereas it is, poor, in old age and debilitated persons.
- Activity level including:
  - General immobilization
  - Space flight

- Nutritional status: Protein, calorie and calcium are required for good callus formation.
- Hormonal factors:
  - Growth hormone
  - Corticosteroids (microvascular osteonecrosis)
  - Others (thyroid, estrogen, androgen, calcitonin, parathyroid hormone, prostaglandins)
- Diseases: diabetes, anaemia, neuropathies, tabes, tuberculosis, malignancies (they all decrease the rate of healing)
- Vitamin deficiencies: A, C, D, K
- Drugs: NSAIDs, anticoagulants, factor XIII, calcium channel blockers (verapamil), cytotoxins, diphosphonates, phenytoin (dilantin), sodium fluoride, tetracycline
- Other substances (nicotine, alcohol)
- Hyperoxia
- Systemic growth factors
- Environmental temperature
- Central nervous system trauma
- Addiction—especially to tobacco, smoking significantly increases the risk of nonunion

Local Factors

Factors independent of injury, treatment, or complications:
- Type of bone
- Abnormal bone
- Radiation necrosis
- Infection
- Tumors and other pathological conditions
- Denervation

Factors Depending on Injury

- Degree of local damage
- Open fracture
- Comminution of fracture
- Velocity of injury
- Low circulatory levels of vitamin K_1
- Extent of disruption of vascular supply to bone, its fragments (macrovascular osteonecrosis), or soft tissues; severity of injury
- Type and location of fracture (one or two bones, e.g. tibia and fibula or tibia alone)
- Loss of bone
- Soft-tissue interposition
- Local growth factors

Factors Depending on Treatment

- Extent of surgical trauma (blood supply, heat)
- Implant-induced altered blood flow
- Degree and kind of rigidity of internal or external fixation and the influence of timing
- Degree, duration, and direction of load-induced deformation of bone and soft tissues
- Extent of contact between fragments (gap, displacement, over-distraction).
- Factors stimulating posttraumatic osteogenesis (bone grafts, (BMP), electrical stimulation, surgical technique, intermittent venous stasis).

Factors Associated with Complications

- Infection
- Venous stasis
- Metal allergy (or corrosion)

Other Important Factors

- Status of soft tissue around; Soft tissue damage and infection leads to delayed healing.
- Compression/distraction can induce osteogenesis as stated by Wolff's law that "new bone is laid down along stress and compression lines".
- Status of the muscles acting across the joint, active mobilization and weight bearing encourages rapid healing and remodelling of fracture, by encouraging inflow of blood through the muscles and laying down of bone along stress lines.

Q4. Write short note on bone grafting.

Bone grafting is utilization of bone tissue live or preserved (bone bank) for a variety of indications:
- To provide osteogenic tissue in delayed union and nonunion.
- To fill up gap in areas of bone loss following trauma.
- To fill up cavities following curettage of tumours, defects in the bone.
- To provide stability and osteogenic potential in pseudoarthrosis.
- To bridge major defects and restoring continuity.
- Arthrodesis: to provide bone block to limit joint motion.

Sources

The grafts may be *cortical, cancellous, or both.*
- Cancellous bone grafting: Posterior or anterior iliac crest
- Cortical bone graft: Tibia (junction of upper and middle third), fibula
- Cortico-cancellous graft: Ribs

Functions

- Immobilization/support: Dense cortical graft
- Osteogenesis: Cancellous bone
- Replacement: For extensive loss of a long bone

Types

Autograft

- These are grafts taken from the patient himself
- The usual sites of harvesting are:
    - Cortico cancellous: Iliac crest
    - Cortical: Fibula and ribs
    - Unicortical: Upper tibia
- Disadvantages
    - Morbidity of graft harvesting (pain, cosmetic defect, fatigue fracture, heterotopic bone formation)
    - Limited bone availability
    - Risk of pathological fracture

Allografts (Homografts)

- These are taken from other person's like relatives or fresh corpse.
- The bone is deep-frozen, stored in antiseptic solution, boiled and autoclaved.
- Advantages
  - Ready availability in various shapes and sizes
  - Avoidance of donor site morbidity
- The disadvantage of using this is:
  - Slow incorporation
  - The possibility of rejection
  - The risk of disease transmission (viral infection), although extremely small, is greater, however, with fresh frozen grafts

Xenografts (Heterografts)

- These are obtained from non-human animal cells tissue or organ.
- Advantages:
  - Abundant source
  - Favorable clinical performance
  - Ease of use
- Disadvantages:
  - Significant risk of transmission of diseases
  - Rejection (greater immune response)
  - Risk of transmission of Bovine spongiform encephalopathy

In general *(types based on technique and application)*:

Graft	Indication/application
Autograft	Bone of patient himself
Allograft (homograft)	One person to another, of same species
Isograft	Between genetically identical (twins)
Xenograft (heterograft)	From one person of one species to a person of another species, e.g. calf bone to human
Orthotopic	Positioning of graft in an appropriate site, e.g. bone in a bed of bone
Heterotopic	Positioning of graft in inappropriate site, e.g. bone in a bed of muscle
Slabgraft	From cortical bone, e.g. tibia
Silver or strip graft	From spongy cancellous bone, e.g. iliac bone
Chip graft	From cancellous bone
Vascularized graft	Taken with its vascular supply (artery and vein). Common sources: fibula, iliac crest. Maximum osteogenic potential
Inlay graft	A gutter is prepared on bone across the fracture and graft is fixed with a screw
Onlay graft	By removing the periosteum and little bit of cortex a bed for the graft is prepared, then graft fixed with screws across the fracture
Double onlay graft	Used for nonunion near joints
Peg or IM graft	Graft is introduce in intramedullary cavity, e.g. peg grafts (fibula) in non-union fracture shaft humerus or ICFN
Nicolls graft	Cancellous bone graft (block) plus plating/screws (usually for gap non-union <2.5 cm)
Phemister graft	Onlay strips of cancellous boneBypass the fracture site (need not disturb non-union site)
Prophylactic bone graft	Used in open fractures between 6–12 weeks to prevent delayed or non-union

Q5. Write short note on bone substitutes.

Bone substitutes are variety of natural and synthetic materials, such as polymers, ceramics, and composites and factor-based and cell-based techniques that can be used for filling bone defects in place of auto- and Allografts.

Types of Bone Graft Substitutes

Laurencin et al. classification of bone graft substitutes:

Type	Description	Examples
Allograft-based	Allograft bone used alone or in combination with other materials	Allogro Dynagraft Opteform Grafton
Cell-based	Use cells to generate new tissue either alone or seeded onto a support matrix	Mesenchymal stem cells (marrow)
Factor-based	Natural and recombinant growth factors used alone or in combination with other materials	TGF-β BMP-7—(OP)-1 BMP-2—Infuse PDGF + TGF-β + autograft Symphony FGF
Ceramic-based	Includes calcium phosphate, calcium sulfate, and bioactive glass used alone or in combination	Osteograft Norian STS Proosteon Osteostet
Polymer-based	Degradable and non-degradable polymers used alone and in combination with other materials	Cortoss OPLA Immix

Assessment of Polytrauma Patient and Resuscitation

Q1. Discuss an approach to manage a Polytrauma patient.

The initial evaluation of a seriously injured/polytrauma patient is a challenging task, and mandates rapid assessment of the injuries and institution of life-preserving therapy since every minute can make the difference between life and death. It is a multidisciplinary approach and requires dedicated trauma team.

Definition of a Polytrauma Patient

The polytrauma patient is defined as follows:
- Injury severity score >18
- Hemodynamic instability
- Coagulopathy
- Closed head injury
- Pulmonary injury
- Abdominal injury

Golden Hour

In World War I which took place in 1918, there was a real appreciation of the time factor between wounding and adequate shock treatment. If the patient was treated within one hour, the mortality was 10%. This increased markedly with time, so that after eight hours, the mortality rate was 75%. This data was subsequently used by R Adams Cowley in his "Golden hour" concept.

Rapid transport of the severely injured patient to a trauma center is essential for appropriate assessment and treatment. The patient chance of survival diminishes rapidly after 1 hour, with a threefold increase in mortality for every 30 minutes.

Early Trauma Deaths Result

- Failed oxygenation of the vital organs
- Massive central nervous system injury or
- Both the above factors

Objective of Evaluation

The objectives of the initial evaluation of the trauma patient are:
- To stabilize the trauma patient.
- To identify life-threatening injuries and to initiate adequate supportive therapy.

- To efficiently and rapidly organize either definitive therapy or transfer to a facility that provides definitive therapy.

Initial Assessment

The initial evaluation follows the protocol of:
- Primary survey
- Resuscitation
- Secondary survey
- Definitive treatment or transfer to an appropriate trauma centre for definitive care.

Primary Survey

The steps of the primary survey are encapsulated in the mnemonic *ABCDE:*
- **A:** Airway maintenance with cervical spine protection (Protection of the spine and spinal cord is an important management principle)
- **B:** Breathing and ventilation
- **C:** Circulation with haemorrhage control
- **D:** Disability: Neurologic status
- **E:** Exposure/environment control: Completely undress the patient, but prevent hypothermia

Airway Maintenance with Cervical Spine Protection

- Airway is the first priority.
- It should be assessed first to ascertain patency.
- The rapid assessment for signs of airway obstruction should include inspection for foreign bodies and facial, mandibular, or tracheal/laryngeal fractures that may result in airway obstruction.
- Measures to establish a patent airway should be instituted while protecting the cervical spine.
- The patients head and neck should not be hyper-extended, hyperflexed or rotated to establish and maintain the airway.
- Protection of the patient's spinal cord with appropriate immobilization devices (Philadelphia collar) should be accomplished and maintained.
- If immobilization devices must be removed temporarily, one member of the trauma team should stabilize the head and neck with manual in-line immobilization.

Breathing and Ventilation

- Ventilation requires adequate function of the lungs, chest wall, and diaphragm and each of these must be examined and evaluated rapidly.
- The patient's chest should be exposed to adequately assess chest wall excursion
- Auscultation: to assure gas flow in the lungs.
- Percussion: it may demonstrate the presence of air or blood in the chest.
- Visual inspection and palpation may detect injuries to the chest wall that may compromise ventilation.
- Injuries that may acutely impair ventilation include:
  - Tension pneuomothorax
  - Flail chest with pulmonary contusion

– Massive haemothorax
– Open pneumothorax

Circulation with Haemorrhage Control

- Haemorrhage is the predominant cause of post-injury deaths that are preventable by rapid treatment in the hospital setting.
- Haemorrhage into the thoracic or abdominal cavities, into soft tissue surrounding a major long bone fracture, into the retroperitoneal space from a pelvic fracture or penetrating torso injury are major sources of occult blood loss.
- Hypotension following injury should be considered to be hypovolemic in origin until proved otherwise.
- The elements of clinical observation that yield important information within seconds are:
  - Level of consciousness
  - Skin colour
  - Pulse
- Rapid, external blood loss is managed by direct manual pressure on the wound.
- Pneumatic splinting devices may also help control haemorrhage.
- Tourniquets should not be used (except in unusual circumstances such as traumatic amputation of an extremity) because they crush tissues and cause distal ischaemia.

Disability (Neurologic Evaluation)

- This establishes the patient's level of consciousness, as well as the pupillary size and reaction.
- A simple mnemonic to describe the level of consciousness is the AVPU method.
  - A: Alert
  - V: Responds to vocal stimuli
  - P: Responds only to painful stimuli
  - U: Unresponsive to all stimuli
- The Glasgow Coma Scale (GCS) is a more detailed neurologic evaluation that also is quick, simple, and predictive of patient outcome.
- *Glasgow coma scale* useful in determining the level of consciousness by measuring three behavioral responses: *eye opening (E), best verbal response (V), and best motor response (M).*

Coma scale	C score	Coma scale	C score
Eyes Open (E)		Incomprehensible words	2
Spontaneous	4	None	1
To sound	3	**Best Motor Response (M)**	
To pain	2	Obeys commands	6
Never	1	Localizes pain	5
Best Verbal Response (V)		Flexion withdrawal	4
Oriented	5	Abnormal	3
Confused conversation	4	Extension	2
Inappropriate words	3	None	1

GCS = E+M+V (range, 3–15)

Patients should be sent to a trauma center if:

- Glasgow coma scale of <13
- Systolic blood pressure of <90
- Respiratory rate of >29 or <10/min

Exposure/Environmental Control

- The final step in the primary survey includes patient exposure and control of the immediate environment.
- The patient should be completely undressed, to facilitate thorough examination and assessment.
- After the assessment is completed, it is important to cover the patient with warm blankets or an external warming device to prevent hypothermia.
- Intravenous fluids should be warmed before infusion, and a warm environment (room temperature) should be maintained.

Resuscitation

Control of Airway

- The airway should be protected and secured when the potential for airway compromise exists.
- A nasopharyngeal airway may initially establish and maintain airway patency in the conscious patient.
- If the patient is unconscious and has no gag reflex, an oro-pharyngeal airway may be helpful temporarily.
- Definitive control of the airway should be accomplished with continuous protection of the cervical spine.
- A surgical airway should be performed if oral or nasal intubation is contraindicated or cannot be accomplished.
- Every injured patient should receive supplemental oxygen to achieve optimal oxygenation..

Control of Bleeding

- Control bleeding by direct pressure or operative intervention.
- Traction with Thomas splints or extremity splints to limit haemorrhage from unstable fractures.

Establishing IV Line and Insertion of an Indwelling Bladder Catheter

- When establishing the intravenous lines, blood should be drawn for type and cross-match and for baseline haematologic studies.
- Monitoring of urine output is a sensitive indicator of the volume status of the patient and reflects renal perfusion.

IV Fluids Therapy

- Intravenous fluid therapy should be initiated with a balanced salt solution.
- Ringer's lactate solution is preferred as the initial crystalloid solution and should be administered rapidly.
- Such bolus intravenous therapy may require the administration of 2–3 liters of solution to achieve an appropriate response in the adult patient.
- All intravenous solutions should be warmed.

Administration of Group Specific Blood

- If the patient remains unresponsive to bolus intravenous therapy, type-specific blood may be administered.

- Type O negative blood is used for life-threatening exsanguinations.
- If blood loss continues, it should be controlled by operative intervention.

Drugs

- The shock state associated with trauma is usually hypovolemic in origin.
- Hypovolemic shock should not be treated by vasopressors, steroids, or sodium bicarbonate, or by continued crystalloid/blood infusion.

Final Assessment

The endpoints of resuscitation are:
- Normal vital signs
- Absence of blood loss
- Adequate urine output (0.5–1.0 cc/kg/hour)
- No evidence of end organ dysfunction

Adjuncts to Primary Survey and Resuscitation

- ECG monitoring
- X-rays and diagnostic studies:
  - X-rays should be used judiciously and should not delay patient resuscitation.
  - Lateral cervical spine: Must see all seven vertebrae and the top of T1
    - Swimmers view or CT scan if needed.
    - A rigid cervical collar must be maintained until adequate views or a CT scan can be obtained.
  - Anteroposterior (AP) chest
  - AP pelvis
  - Lateral thoracolumbar spine (if possible)
  - Possibly a CT of the head, cervical spine (if not cleared by plain radiographs), thorax, abdomen, or pelvis with or without contrast as dictated by the injury pattern
- Urinary output: Transurethral bladder catheterization is contraindicated in patients in whom urethral transection is suspected
- Monitoring:
  - Ventilatory rate and arterial blood gases
  - Pulse oximetry measures the oxygen saturation of Hb colourimetrically.
  - Blood pressure

Secondary Survey

- The secondary survey begins only when the patient is demonstrating normalization of vital functions
- It includes head-to-toe evaluation of the trauma patient, i.e. a complete history and physical examination, including a reassessment of all vital signs
- Complete neurologic examination is performed, including a GCS score determination, if not done during the primary survey.
- During this evaluation, indicated X-rays are obtained.
- Specific radiological evaluations and laboratory studies are also obtained at this time.

During primary survey and resuscitation phase's information (Table on next page) to indicate the need for transfer of the patient to another facility.

Revised Trauma Score

- The Revised Trauma Score is a physiological scoring system, with high inter-rater reliability and demonstrated accuracy in predicting death.
- It is scored from the first set of data obtained on the patient
- It consists of *Glasgow coma scale (GCS), systolic blood pressure (SBP) and respiratory rate (RR).*

Glasgow coma scale (GCS)	Systolic blood pressure (SBP)	Respiratory rate (RR)	Score
13–15	>89	10–29	4
9–12	76–89	>29	3
6–8	50–75	6–9	2
4–5	1–49	1–5	1
3	0	0	0

- RTS = 0.9368 GCS + 0.7326 SBP + 0.2908 RR
- RTS <4; patient should be treated in a trauma centre

Patient Transfer for Definitive Care

- Once the decision to transfer is made, referring doctor-to-receiving doctor communication is essential.
- Once the patient is stabilized hemodynamically definitive treatment as per injury should be instituted.

Decision to Operate

Early operative intervention is indicated for:
- Femur or pelvic fractures, which carry high risk of pulmonary complications (e.g. fat embolus syndrome, ARDS).
- Active or impending compartment syndrome (most commonly associated with tibia or forearm fractures)
- Open fractures
- Vascular disruption/compromise
- Unstable cervical or thoracolumbar spine injuries
- Patients with fractures of the femoral neck, talar neck, or other bones in which fracture has a high risk of osteonecrosis

> **Q2. Write short notes on: a. Abbreviated injury scale (AIS); b. Injury severity score (ISS); c. Basic life support (BLS); d. *Cardiopulmonary resuscitation* (CPR)**

a. Abbreviated Injury Scale (AIS)

- The abbreviated injury scale (AIS) is an anatomical scoring system first introduced in 1969.
- Injuries are ranked on a scale of 1–6, with 1 being minor, 5 severe, and 6 non-survivable injury.
- This represents the 'threat to life' associated with an injury.

Injury	AIS score
1	Minor
2	Moderate
3	Serious
4	Severe
5	Critical
6	Unsurvivable

b. Injury Severity Score (ISS)

- The injury severity score (ISS) is an anatomical scoring system that provides an overall score for patients with multiple injuries.
- Each injury is assigned an abbreviated injury scale (AIS) score and is allocated to one of six body regions (head, face, chest, abdomen, extremities (including pelvis), and external).
- Only the highest AIS score in each body region is used.
- The three most severely injured body regions have their score squared and added together to produce the ISS score

Region	Injury description	AIS	Square top three
Head and neck	Cerebral contusion	3	9
Face	No injury	0	
Chest	Flail chest	4	16
Abdomen	Minor contusion of liver complex rupture spleen	2 5	25
Extremity	Fractured femur	3	
External	No Injury	0	
		Injury severity score	50

- The ISS score takes values from 0 to 75. If an injury is assigned an AIS of 6 (Unsurvivable injury), the ISS score is automatically assigned to 75

C. Basic Life Support (BLS)

BLS (*or basic life support*) refers to maintaining an airway and supporting breathing and the circulation.

Elements

- Initial assessment
- Airway maintenance
- Expired air
- Ventilation (rescue breathing; mouth-to-mouth ventilation)
- Chest compression

When all are combined the term cardiopulmonary resuscitation (CPR) is used.

Purpose

It is to maintain adequate ventilation and circulation until a means can be obtained to reverse the underlying cause of the arrest

d. CPR

CPR (or cardiopulmonary resuscitation) is a combination of rescue breathing (mouth-to-mouth resuscitation) and chest compressions. It is more effective when done early. It can restore heart function.

It is done in:
- Any life threatening condition
- Unconsciousness/non-breathing person
- Cardiac arrest
- Ventricular fibrillation
- Also for near-drowning/asphyxiation/trauma cases

Call

- Ensure safety of rescuer and victim
- Check responsiveness
- Check the victim and see if he responds:
- Gently shake his shoulders and ask loudly: "Are you OK?"
- If he does not respond:
- Phone 108 or emergency number
- Get Automatic External Defibrillator or send second rescuer (if available) to do this

Blow

- Open airway, check breathing.
- Look, listen and feel for no more than 10 seconds
- If not breathing normally, pinch nose and cover the mouth with yours and blow until you see the chest rise.
- Give 2 breaths.
- Each breath should take 1 second.
- If no response, check pulse:
    - Do you definitely feel pulse within 10 seconds?
- If definite pulse present
- Give 1 breath every 5–6 seconds.
- Recheck pulse every 2 minutes.

Pump

If no pulse present:
- Give cycles of 30 compressions (push hard and fast (100/min; faster than once per second) and release completely) and 2 breaths until AED/defibrillator arrives, ALS providers take over, or victim starts to move.
- Elbow should be straight and place the other hand over the first while pumping
- Push the chest 3–4 cm

Number of Persons Doing CPR

- Continue with 30 pumps and 2 breaths (30:2) until help arrives
- This ratio is the same for one-person and two-person CPR.
- In two-person CPR, the person pumping the chest stops while the other gives mouth-to-mouth breathing.

The five major changes in the 2005 emergency cardiovascular care guidelines:
- Emphasis on and recommendation to improve delivery of effective chest compressions.
- A single compression to ventilation ratio (30:2) for all single rescuers for all victims (except neonates)
- Recommendation that each rescue breath be given over 1 second and should produce a visible chest rise.
- A new recommendation that single shock, followed by immediate CPR, be used to attempt defibrillation for ventricular fibrillation cardiac arrests. Rhythm checks should be performed every 2 minutes.
- Endorsement of the 2003 ILCOR recommendation for use of AED's in children 1–8 years old (and older) Use a child dose-reduction system if available.

Q3. Write in short: a. Triage; b; Concept of damage control orthopaedics (DCO)

a. Triage

Triage is the sorting of patients based on the need for treatment and the available resources to provide that treatment. Treatment is rendered based on the ABC priorities (airway with cervical spine protection, breathing and circulation with haemorrhage control).

Objective

To prioritize patients with a high likelihood of early clinical deterioration.

A triage of trauma patients considers:
- Vital signs
- Prehospital clinical course
- Mechanism of injury
- Patients age
- Comorbid conditions.

Findings that lead to an accelerated work up include:
- Multiple injuries
- Extremes of age
- Evidence of severe neurologic injury
- Unstable vital signs
- Preexisting cardiac or pulmonary disease
- *Multiple casualties:* The number of patients and the severity of their injuries do not exceed the ability of the facility to render care. In this situation, patients with life-threatening problems and those sustaining multiple system injuries are treated first.
- *Mass casualties:* The number of patients and the severity of their injuries exceed the capability of the facility and staff. In this situation those patients with the greatest chance of survival with the least expenditure of time, equipment, supplies and personnel are managed first.
- In *mass casualties' events*, the triage process is very complex. After initial assessment the injured are placed into a specific category based on the probability of survivorship and severity of injury.

The following categories of injured have been accepted.

Priority 1: Immediate (Red)

- Patients with critical injury, requiring minimal treatment time and resources, and after being treated have good prognosis for survival.
- *Case: Massive haemorrhage that can be controlled with a simple procedure.*

Priority 2: Delayed (Yellow)

- Patients with significant injury the care of which can be delayed without risk of significant subsequent morbidity
- *Case: Isolated major long bone fracture.*

Priority 3: Minimal, Non-urgent (Green)

- Patients, also known as walking wounded, with injuries that can wait for treatment.
- *Case: Small bones fractures, abrasions, lacerations, sprains.*

Priority 4: Expectant (Black)

- Patients with injuries so severe that chance of survival is minimal
- *Case: Massive head injuries, third degree burns with 95% body coverage.*

b. Concept of Damage Control Orthopaedics (DCO)

The concept of *damage control orthopaedics (DCO)* originally concerned the provisional immobilisation of long bone fractures—mainly the femur (in recent years also includes: *pelvis fractures, spine fractures and upper limb injuries*)—in the severely traumatized patient (STP) in order to minimise the traumatic effects of non-lifesaving surgical procedures, termed the *"second hit"* effect.

Example: **DCO** emphasizes the stabilization and control of the injury, often with use of spanning external fixation, rather than immediate fracture fixation.

Purpose

- Doing *"as little as possible"* (*Temporary fixation*) but *"sufficient"* to save the patient's life
- Avoid major bleeding and pathological inflammatory response, termed as *"second hit"* effect
- Delay definitive fracture fixation (*usually 6 to 8 days after the first procedure*) until a time when the general condition of the patient is optimized

Physiology

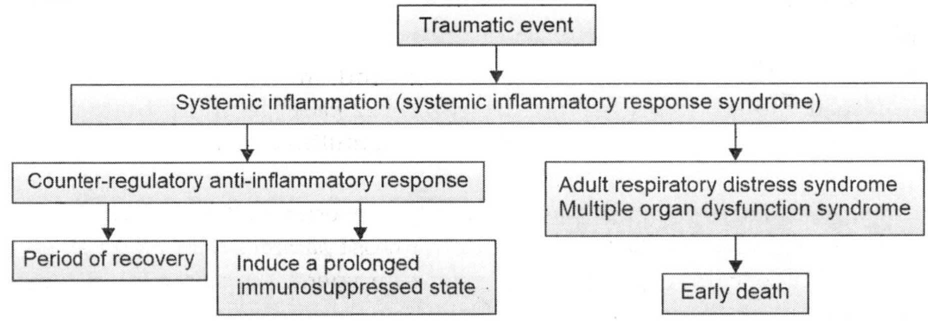

Key Players (in the Host Response)

- Cytokines, leukocytes, the endothelium, and subsequent leukocyte-endothelial cell interactions
- Reactive oxygen species, eicosanoids, and microcirculatory disturbances

5

Open Fracture: Classification and Management

Definition

When the fracture haematoma communicates with the exterior atmosphere, through an overlying wound in the skin and soft tissue.

Soft tissue injuries in an open fracture may have following consequences:

- Contamination of the fracture and wound by exposure to the external environment.
- Stripping, crushing, and devascularization results not only in soft tissue compromise but also there is increased susceptibility to infection.
- Destruction or loss of the soft tissue envelope may result in derangement of process of fracture and healing loss of function from muscle, tendon, nerve, vascular, ligament, or skin damage.

Classification

The well-accepted classification of open fracture is as follows:

Gustilo's Classification of Compound Fractures

Type	Wound	Contamination	Status of soft tissue	Bone injury
I	<1 cm	Clean	Minimal	Simple, comminution minimal
II	Lacerated wound >1 cm	Moderate	Moderate damage No extensive soft tissue damage, skin flaps or avulsions	Moderate comminution
IIIa	Usually >10 cm long	High	Extensive soft tissue lacerations/flaps, but maintain adequate soft tissue coverage of bone	Soft tissue coverage of bone is possible Segmental/severely Comminuted fractures
IIIb	Usually >10 cm long	High	Extensive soft tissue damage with periosteal stripping and bony exposure	Bone coverage is poor. Moderate-to-severe comminution
IIIc	Irrespective of size	High	Open fractures with an arterial injury that requires repair regardless of size of wound or arterial injury with very severe loss ofcoverage	Bone coverage is poor. Moderate-to-severe comminution

Tscherne Classification of Open Fractures

This takes into account wound size, level of contamination, and fracture mechanism.

- **Grade I:** Small puncture wound without associated contusion, minimal bacterial contamination, low-energy trauma
- **Grade II:** Small lacerated wound, skin and soft tissue contusions, moderate bacterial contamination, variable mechanisms of injury
- **Grade III:** Large laceration with heavy bacterial contamination, extensive soft tissue damage, with frequent associated arterial or neural injury
- **Grade IV:** Incomplete or complete amputation with variable prognosis based on location of and nature of injury (e.g. cleanly amputated middle phalanx versus crushed leg at the proximal femoral level)

Management

Aim

- To convert contaminated wound into clean wound so that it can be closed later and thus help in converting an open fracture into close fracture.
- To establish sound union in acceptable alignment
- To prevent clostridial and other pyogenic infections

Principle of Management

I. First Aid Management (Airway, Bleeding, Circulation)

- Clear airway and secure airway
- Control of haemorrhage by firm compression bandage
- Management of shock by adequate and appropriate fluid (crystalloid and colloid) and blood replacement.
- Most of the deaths, which occur in the first few hours, are due to the mismanagement of shock and haemorrhage.

II. During Transportation

Take care during transport with cervical collar, other splints and support of injured part with maintenance of life support system.

III. Assessment of the Patient

Examine CNS, cardiothoracic function, abdomen, bladder, bowel status and always note down the vitals.

IV. Supportive Treatment

- Broad-spectrum antibiotics or nowadays using antibiotic impregnated PMMA (bone cement) beads
- Anti-tetanus protection
- Anti-gas-gangrene serum
- Analgesics

V. Local (Bone and Soft Tissue) Management

- Radical wound debridement to remove all dead and devitalized tissue.
- Thorough wound debridement and excision of all necrotic debris is very essential to prevent infection.

Stabilization of bone or fracture fragment by *external fixators* initially. These fixators helps to:
- Stabilize the fracture fragment
- Allow daily wound inspection and dressing
- Permit secondary procedure to close the wound like grafting or secondary suturing.
- Allow soft tissue healing
- Early mobilization

Once the soft tissue status is healthy and infection is controlled, the fixators can safely be changed to internal fixation like intramedullary nailing

VI. Final Management of Wound

Primary closure if:
- The wound is clean
- Good circulation without neurovascular deficit
- Wound age should be <6 hours.

Wound left open and delayed primary closure is preferable after few days If:
- Wound > 6 hours
- Potentially contaminated

Delayed closure by:
Autogenous graft using split thickness, rotational/cross leg flaps.

Secondary closure after 2 weeks by:
Suture: In cases where conditions are unfavorable for primary closure, we have following alternative for secondary closure:
- Split thickness graft (SSG) over raw granulating tissue
- Full thickness graft over exposed bone, tendons
- Pedicle graft or flaps
- Suturing after 2–3 weeks
- Biological dressings
- Relaxing incisions to release the tension and mobilize the adjacent skin.

VII. Delayed Repair of Tendons/Nerves

VIII. Final Stabilization of Bone by POP Cast/Internal Fixation

> **Q2. Write short note on: a. Mangled extremity score (MESS); b. Injury severity score for Gustilo Type IIIA and IIIB open tibial fractures (Ganga injury severity score)**

a. Mangled Extremity Score

- Mangled extremity severity score (MESS) designed to predict the injury patterns that would best be treated by early amputation.
- It is based on a four-group system:
    - Skeletal and soft-tissue injuries
    - Shock
    - Ischaemia
    - Age

Mangled Extremity Severity Score (MESS) Score

Type	*Characteristics*	*Injuries*	*Points*
Skeletal/Soft-tissue Group			
1.	Low energy	Stab wounds, simple closed fractures, small-caliber gunshot wounds	1
2.	Medium energy	Open or multiple-level fractures, dislocations, moderate crush injuries	2
3.	High energy	Shotgun blast (close range), high-velocity gunshot wounds	3
4.	Massive crush	Logging, railroad, oil rig accidents	4
Shock Group			
1.	Normotensive hemodynamics	Blood pressure stable in field and in operating room (Systolic blood pressure always >90 mm Hg)	0
2.	Transiently hypo-tensive	Blood pressure unstable in field but responsive to intra-venous fluids	1
3.	Prolonged hypo-tensive	Systolic blood pressure <90 mm Hg in field and respon-sive to intravenous fluid only in operating room	2
Ischemia Group			
1.	None	Pulsatile limb without signs of ischaemia	0*
2.	Mild	Diminished pulses without signs of ischaemia	1*
3.	Moderate	No pulse by Doppler, sluggish capillary refill, pares-thesia, diminished motor activity	2*
4.	Advanced	Pulseless, cool, paralyzed and numb without capillary refill	3*
Age Group			
1.	<30 years		0
2.	30–50 years		1
3.	>50 years		2

* If ischaemia time >6 hours, add 2 points

- Limbs with scores of 7–12 ultimately required amputation, whereas limbs with scores of 3–6 were viable

b. Injury Severity Score for Gustilo Type IIIA and IIIB Open Tibial Fractures (Ganga Injury Severity Score): For Predicting Salvage and Outcome

More recently, *Rajasekaran et al.* proposed a new scoring system for Gustilo type IIIA and IIIB open fractures of the tibia that evaluated skin coverage, skeletal structures, tendon and nerve injury, and comorbid conditions to assess the possibilities of limb salvage.

Characteristics	*Points*
Covering structures: Skin and fascia	
Wound without skin loss:	
• Not over the fracture site	1
• Exposing the fracture site	2
Wound with skin loss	
• Not over the fracture	3
• Over the fracture	4
Circumferential wound with skin loss	5

(Contd.)

Characteristics	Points
Skeletal structures: Bone and joints	
Transverse or oblique fracture or butterfly fragment <50% circumference	1
Large butterfly fragment >50% circumference	2
Comminution or segmental fractures without bone loss	3
Bone loss <4 cm	4
Bone loss >4 cm	5
Functional tissues: Musculotendinous and nerve units	
Partial injury to musculotendinous unit	1
Complete but repairable injury to musculotendinous units	2
Irreparable injury to musculotendinous units, partial loss of a compartment, or complete injury to posterior tibial nerve	3
Loss of one compartment of musculotendinous units	4
Loss of two or more compartments or subtotal amputation	5
Comorbid conditions: Add 2 points for each condition present:	
• Injury leading to debridement interval >12 hours	
• Sewage or organic contamination or farmyard injuries	
• Age >65 years	
Drug-dependent diabetes mellitus or cardiorespirator diseases leading to increased anesthetic risk	
Polytrauma involving chest or abdomen with injury severity score >25 or fat embolism	
Hypotension with systolic blood pressure <90 mm Hg at presentation	
Another major injury to the same limb or compartment syndrome	

A score of ≥14: Indicator for amputation

6

Traumatology (Upper and Lower)

ACROMIOCLAVICULAR AND STERNOCLAVICULAR INJURIES

Q1. Write short note on acromioclavicular and sternoclavicular injuries.

I. Acromioclavicular Injuries

Incidence:

- Most common in the 2nd decade of life, associated with road traffic accidents, assault and contact athletic activities.
- Male preponderance.

Mechanism of Injury

Direct

- Most common mechanism
- Resulting from a fall onto the shoulder with the arm adducted, driving the acromion inferior and medial.

Indirect

- Less common
- Fall onto an outstretched hand.

Associated Fractures and Injuries

- Fractures: clavicle, acromion process, and coracoid process
- Pneumothorax or pulmonary contusion

Clinical Features

- Classic anatomic feature is a downward sagging of the shoulder and arm.
- Injured limb is supported by holding the elbow with contralateral hand.
- Obvious prominence at the outer end of clavicle is characteristic.
- Pain
- Swelling
- Tenderness
- Apparent step off deformity at the joint (step sign is diagnostic)
- Sometime there may be tenting of the skin overlying the distal clavicle.
- Painful restriction of shoulder motion.

Radiographic Evaluation

- True AP, scapular-Y, and axillary views
- Stress radiographs: Weights (10–15 pound) are strapped around the wrists, and an AP radiograph is taken of both shoulders to compare acromioclavicular and coracoclavicular distances.

Classification

- Type I: Sprain of the AC ligament.
- Type II: AC joint disruption with ligament tear; coracoclavicular ligament sprained.
- Type III: Acromioclavicular and coracoclavicular ligaments torn with AC joint dislocation.
- Type IV: Type III + Distal clavicle displaced posteriorly into or through the trapezius muscle.
- Type V: Type IV + Distal clavicle grossly and severely displaced superiorly
- Type VI: Acromio-clavicular joint is dislocated, with the clavicle displaced inferior to the acromion or the coracoid process.

Treatment

Type I

- Rest for 7–10 days
- Ice packs, and sling immobilization.
- Avoid full activity until painless
- After 2 weeks full range of motion.

Type II

- Sling immobilization for 1–2 weeks
- Gentle range of motion started as soon as pain subsides.
- Avoid heavy activity for 6 weeks.

Type III

Non-operative treatment comprises of sling, early range of motion, strengthening, and acceptance of deformity indicated in:

- Inactive, non-laboring
- Recreational athletic patients especially for the non-dominant arm

Operative stabilization indicated in:

- Younger, more active patients with gross displacement
- Laborers who use their upper extremity above the horizontal plane may benefit from.

Types IV, V and VI

Open reduction, internal fixation, surgical repair of the coracoclavicular ligaments and reconstruction.

Complication

- Coracoclavicular ossification
- Osteolysis of distal clavicle: Associated with chronic dull ache and weakness
- AC joint arthritis

II. Sternoclavicular Joint Injuries

Incidence:
- Rare injury
- Accounts for 3% of total 1,603 shoulder girdle dislocations (according to Cave et al.)

Mechanism of Injury

Direct

- Direct blow over the anteromedial aspect pushes the clavicle posteriorly into the mediastinum to produce posterior dislocation.
- This may occur:
  – Athlete falls on another athlete lying in supine position
  – When an individual is run over by a vehicle
  – When an individual is pressed against a wall by a vehicle.

Indirect

Blow from the anterolateral or posterolateral direction produces anterior or posterior SC dislocation especially seen during the football game.

Clinical Features

- Patient characteristically presents supporting the injured limb across the trunk with the contralateral, uninjured arm.
- Pain
- Swelling
- Tenderness
- Medial clavicle prominence depending upon the degree and direction of the impact.
- Painful restriction of shoulder motion
- Proper and through assessment of neurovascular status

Radiographic Evaluation

- AP chest radiographs typically demonstrate asymmetry of the clavicles
- Hobbs view: 90° cephalocaudal lateral view. In anterior dislocation the clavicle project above the interclavicular line, while in posterior dislocation the clavicle project below the interclavicular line.
- Serendipity view: This 40° cephalic tilt view is aimed at the manubrium.
- CT scan: Best technique for evaluation of SC joint injuries. CT is able to distinguish medial fractures from dislocation as well as delineate minor subluxations that would otherwise be missed.

Classification

Anatomic

- Anterior dislocation (most common)
- Posterior dislocation

Aetiological

- Atraumatic
- Sprain or subluxation

- Mild: Joint stable, ligamentous integrity maintained
- Moderate: Subluxation, with partial ligamentous disruption
- Severe: Unstable joint, with complete ligamentous compromise
- Acute dislocation
- Recurrent dislocation: Rare
- Unreduced dislocation

Treatment

Mild Sprain

- Ice for the first 24 hours
- Sling immobilization for 3–4 days
- Gradual return to normal activities as tolerated.

Moderate Sprain or Subluxation

- Ice for the first 24 hours
- Clavicle strap, sling and swathe, or figure-of-8 bandage for 1 week followed by sling immobilization for 4–6 weeks.

Severe Sprain or Dislocation

Anterior dislocation:
- Treat conservatively
- Closed reduction and maintain it with sling or reverse figure-8-bandage for 4–6 weeks.

Posterior dislocation:
- Closed or open reduction after rule out any neurovascular injury.
- Immobilized with clavicle strap, sling and swathe, or figure-of-8 bandage is used for 4–6 weeks.

Operative Management

- Fixation of the medial clavicle to the sternum using fascia lata, subclavius tendon, or suture
- Osteotomy of the medial clavicle.
- Resection of the medial clavicle.

Complication

- Poor cosmesis
- Complications are more common with the posterior dislocation. These includes the following:
    - Subclavian artery compression
    - Carotid artery compression
    - Voice changes
    - Severe pneumothorax
    - Laceration of the superior vena cava
    - Venous congestion in the neck
    - Oesophageal rupture
    - Thoracic outlet syndrome

CLAVICLE FRACTURE

Q.1: Discuss the clinical feature and management of clavicle fracture.

Fracture clavicle is one of the most common bony injuries, rarely requires open reduction. It is the most common bone fracture in body as well as in baby. It derives its name from the Latin word *'clavicula' (little key)* because the bone rotates along its axis like a key during abduction.

Anatomy

- It is the only long bone in body that lies horizontally.
- It has no medullary cavity.
- Doubly curved bone connects the arm (upper limb) to the body (trunk).
- Clavicle is the first bone to ossify.
- Only long bone ossifies from a membrane (intramembranous ossification).
- Ossified from two primary centers.

Commonest Site

Junction of two curves, i.e. lateral one-third and medial two-thirds.

Displacement of Fragment (Deforming Forces)

Lateral fragment is pulled:
- Down by the weight of limb.
- Medially by the pull of pectoral major muscle.

Medial fragment: It is pulled up by sternomastoid muscle.

Mechanism of Injury

- Falls onto the affected shoulder account for most (87%) of clavicular fractures.
- Direct blow to the shoulder by stick or boxing (7%).
- Fall on the outstretched hand (6%).
- Pulling out the fetus during the breech presentation (shoulder dystocia).
- In spite of the fact that this bone is subcutaneous throughout its length, compound fracture is very uncommon because skin overlying is freely mobile.

Clinical Features

- Patients typically present with splinting of the injured extremity, with the arm adducted across the chest and supported by the contralateral hand.
- Painful lump involving the clavicle after trauma
- Palpable bony crepitus
- Inability to move the upper limb, especially in neonates (pseudoparalysis).
- Always examine the pulsation and the sensations to rule out the possibility of underlying subclavian vessel and brachial plexus injury.
- If the patient has surgical emphysema then the apical zone of lung has been damaged.

Radiographs

- Standard anteroposterior radiographs is usually sufficient to confirm the fracture.
- Apical oblique view: to assess the undisplaced fracture especially in children.

- CT scan: In proximal third fractures, to differentiate sternoclavicular dislocation from epiphyseal injury, or distal third fractures, to assess any articular involvement.

Classification

Allman

Group I

- Fracture of the middle one-third (80%)
- Most common fracture in both children and adults
- Proximal and distal fragments are secured by muscular and ligamentous attachments.

Group II

- Fracture of the lateral or distal third (15%)
- This is subdivided according to the location of the coracoclavicular ligaments relative to the fracture:

  Type I:
  - Minimal displacement: Interligamentous fracture between the conoid and trapezoid or between the AC and coracoclavicular ligaments
  - In these fractures, ligaments still intact.

  Type II:
  - Displaced secondary to a fracture medial to the coracoclavicular ligaments
  - There is higher incidence of nonunion
  - IIA: Conoid and trapezoid attached to the distal segment
  - IIB: Conoid torn, trapezoid attached to the distal segment

  Type III:
  - Fracture of the articular surface of the acromioclavicular joint
  - No ligamentous injury
  - It may be confused with first-degree AC joint separation

Group III

- Fracture of the medial or proximal third (5%).
- Minimal displacement occurs if the costoclavicular ligaments intact.
- It may represent epiphyseal injury in children and teenagers.
- Subgroups include:
  - **Type I:** Minimal displacement
  - **Type II:** Displaced
  - **Type III:** Intra-articular
  - **Type IV:** Epiphyseal separation
  - **Type V:** Comminuted

Treatment

Nonoperative

Majority of clavicle fractures can be treated conservatively with some form of immobilization.

Goals of immobilization or principles of treatment:
- To counter the deforming forces as mentioned above.
- Support the shoulder girdle

- Raising the lateral fragment in an upward, outward, and backward direction.
- Depress the medial fragment.
- Maintain some degree of fracture reduction.
- So, the shoulder should be immobilized or braced up and back.

Duration of immobilization
- Usually for 4–6 weeks.
- During this period, active range of motion of the elbow, wrist, and hand should be encouraged.

Neonates and infants

- Reassurance of the parents
- Triangular sling with arm to chest bandage, for a few days.

Adults

Simple fracture:
- Figure of '8' bandage with good axillary cotton padding for 3–4 weeks, with cuff and collar sling.
- Meck's clavicle brace.

Other

Billington yoke method: POP over well-padded figure of "8" dressing.

Open fracture

Fixation with K-wires or with contoured cortical plates and screws, if necessary with bone grafting.

Operative

Require open reduction and internal fixation in the following situations:
- Open fractures
- Cosmetic problems
- Nonunion
- Neurovascular involvement (subclavian vessel and medial cord of brachial plexus (ulnar nerve))
- Fracture of the lateral end near the acromioclavicular joint in an adult.
- Interposition of soft tissue between the fragments.
- Floating shoulder.

Complications

Bone

- Malunion (most common) (unavoidable, lump) but remodeling occurs later.
- Nonunion (rare) is seen in comminuted fracture.
- Posttraumatic arthritis

Nerve

- Damage to the medial cord of the brachial plexus.
- Entrapment of the middle branch of the supraclavicular nerve in the callus causing paresthesia over the pectoral region.

Vessels

Damage to the subclavian vessel (patient may bleed to death on the spot).

Lungs

Emphysema due to pulmonary injury involving the apical lobe.

SCAPULA

Q.1: Write short note on scapular fractures.

Incidence

- Comparatively less common injury
- Represents only 3–5% of all shoulder fractures and 0.5–1% of all fractures.
- Average age of patients with fracture of the scapula is 35–45 years.

Mechanism of Injury

Direct injury

- Significant trauma as in road traffic accidents.
- Direct blow or fall (scapula body fracture)
- Direct blow to the point of the shoulder (acromion, coracoid fracture)

Indirect injury

Axial loading on the outstretched arm

Other

- Glenoid fracture may occur during shoulder dislocation.
- Muscles or ligaments may cause an avulsion fracture.

Associated Injuries

35–98% of scapula fractures occur in the presence of comorbid injuries including:
- Ipsilateral injuries: Fractured ribs, clavicle, sternum, shoulder trauma.
- Injuries to neurovascular structures: Brachial plexus injuries, vascular avulsions.
- Pneumothorax
- Pulmonary contusion
- Spine injuries
- Others: Skull fracture, blunt abdominal trauma, pelvic fracture, and lower extremity injuries.

Clinical Features

- Injured extremity supported by the contralateral hand in an adducted position.
- Pain
- Swelling
- Tenderness
- Rule out associated injuries mentioned above
- Thoroughly assess the neurovascular status.

- *Comolli sign*: is triangular swelling of the posterior thorax overlying the scapula and is indicative of hematoma resulting in increased compartment pressures.

Radiographic Evaluation

X-rays

- True AP view
- Axillary view
- Scapular-Y view
- Chest radiograph (in view of injuries to thoracic structures)

CT scan

It may be helpful in characterizing intra-articular glenoid fractures.

Classification

Anatomic Classification (Zdravkovic and Damholt):

- Type I: Scapular body
- Type II: Apophyseal fractures, including the acromion and coracoid
- Type III: Fractures of the superolateral angle, including the scapular neck and glenoid

Intra-articular Glenoid Fractures (Ideberg Classification)

- **Type I:** Avulsion fracture of the anterior margin
- **Type IIA:** Transverse fracture through the glenoid fossa exiting inferiorly
- **Type IIB:** Oblique fracture through the glenoid fossa exiting inferiorly
- **Type III:** Oblique fracture through the glenoid exiting superiorly and often associated with an acromioclavicular joint injury
- **Type IV:** Transverse fracture exiting through the medial border of the scapula
- **Type V:** Combination of a type II and type IV pattern
- **Type VI:** Comminuted glenoid fracture.

Treatment

Open reduction with or without internal fixation rarely is required for fractures of the scapula.

Nonoperative

Most fractures can be treated conservatively just by:
- Supporting the upper extremity in a sling
- Rest
- Strapping
- Instituting early active shoulder motion.

Operative

Indications: Though controversial, it includes:
- Displaced intra-articular glenoid fractures involving >25% of the articular surface.
- Scapular neck fractures with >40° angulation or 1 cm medial translation.
- Floating shoulder: Scapular neck fractures with associated displaced clavicle fracture.

- Fractures of the acromion that impinge on the subacromial space.
- Fractures of the coracoid process that result in a functional acromioclavicular separation (>10 mm).
- Comminuted fractures of the scapular spine.

Specific Condition

Significantly displaced fractures of the acromion and lateral scapular spine with retraction of the fragment and encroachment on the subacromial space:

- ORIF using Kirschner wires or plate and screws

Fractures of the coracoid with acromio-clavicular separation:

- ORIF of the coracoid with a screw or heavy suture and repair of the acromioclavicular ligament

Glenoid Rim Fractures

- Involves 1/4 of the articulating surface: primary ORIF
- Small glenoid rim fractures: Conservative measures.

Complication

- Associated injuries: as mentioned above.
- Malunion
- Nonunion (rare)
- Suprascapular nerve injury

GLENOHUMERAL DISLOCATION

Q1. Discuss in brief the clinical features and management of anterior shoulder dislocation.

Shoulder joint is the most commonly dislocated major joint of the body, accounting for up to 45% of dislocations. Over 95% of shoulder dislocation cases are anterior. It is caused by combination of *abduction, extension, and external rotation forces.*

Mechanism of Injury

- Trauma is the most common cause.
- Indirect trauma (most common): Indirect trauma when the shoulder is in *abduction, extension, and external rotation.*
- Direct impact to the posterior shoulder.

Clinical Features

- Patient comes with arm abducted and externally rotated, forearm and elbow supported by other hand.
- Round contour of the deltoid is lost (flat shoulder or squaring of shoulder) with positive Hamilton's ruler test.
- Head palpable below clavicle in abnormal position.
- The glenoid area appears hollow.
- Diminished length of the arm.

- Examine the sensation over insertion of the deltoid, to rule out the injury to axillary nerve.
- Integrity of musculocutaneous nerve can be assessed by the presence of sensation on the anterolateral forearm
- Due to spasm of muscles around the shoulder, all the movements are painfully restricted.

Clinical Tests

Hamilton's Ruler Test

- In *normal shoulder*, straight ruler cannot touch the acromion above and the lateral epicondyle below, simultaneously because of shoulder contour due to deltoid bulge.
- If *there is dislocation* of the head of humerus, the deltoid becomes flat, loss of round shoulder contour.
- Now a ruler kept on the lateral side of the arm, will touch the acromion above and the lateral epicondyle below at the same time.

Positive Duga's Sign

Inability to keep the elbow adducted in front of abdomen and palm touching the opposite shoulder (Internal rotation).

Calloways

- *Normally*, girth from the axillary base to shoulder top is symmetrical and same on both sides.
- Measure girth of affected shoulder and compare to unaffected side.
- Increased girth indicates dislocation

Bryants Sign

- Look for lowering of axillary fold.
- In anterior dislocation esp. subcoracoid, the anterior axillary fold looks elongated and seems to be at low level.

Radiographic Evaluation

- Anteroposterior (AP), scapular-Y, and axillary views of the shoulder to see the type of the dislocation and to rule out associated fractures.
- Special views: West point axillary, Hill-Sachs view, Stryker notch view, etc.
- Hill-Sachs view: AP radiograph is taken, keeping the shoulder in maximal internal rotation to visualize a posterolateral defect.
- CT scan: Used to assess humeral head or glenoid impression fractures, loose bodies, and anterior labral bony injuries (bony Bankart lesion).
- Arthrography: Single- or double-contrast, to evaluate rotator cuff pathologic processes.
- MRI: to identify rotator cuff, capsular, and glenoid labral (Bankart lesion) pathologic processes.

Types

It could be *subcoracoid (commonest), subglenoid, subclavicular,* and, very rarely, *intra-thoracic.* The subtypes denote position of the dislocated head.

Management

Nonoperative

Reduction: *Done under GA.*

Various Techniques

Kocher's Technique
- Counter traction given by the assistant who pulls through well-padded axillary sling.
- The surgeon pulls and manipulates in 4 steps—*TEAM*
    - **T:** Traction in the line of the deformity with the elbow flexed.
    - **E:** External rotation.
    - **A:** Adduction so that the tip of the elbow comes in front of the abdomen.
    - **M:** Medial rotation, so that palm touches the opposite shoulder (Duga's position).

Hippocrates' Method

The traction with gentle internal and external rotation is applied with forearm extended and the surgeon pulling against the pressure of the foot in the axilla (it is now obsolete and dangerous).

Stimson's Method

- If patient is unfit for the anaesthesia then the patient is kept prone and appropriate traction (Gentle, manual traction or 5 lb of weight is applied to the wrist,) is applied in forearm with the forearm hanging down.
- This is more so for the post dislocation of the shoulder.

Milch Technique

With the patient supine and the upper extremity abducted and externally rotated, thumb pressure is applied by the surgeon to push the humeral head into place.

Maintenance: Arm is strapped to the chest with the elbow in front of the umbilicus and the palm touching the opposite shoulder (Duga's position) for 3 weeks.

Rehabilitation: Start gentle active movements of the shoulder and build up the power of the rotator cuff after 3–4 weeks.

Operative

Indications for surgery include:
- Soft tissue interposition
- Displaced greater tuberosity fracture
- Glenoid rim fracture >5 mm in size
- Selective repair in the acute period (e.g. in young athletes)

Surgical options for stabilization include:
- Repair of the anterior labrum
- Capsular shift
- Capsulorrhaphy
- Repair of muscle or tendon transfers, and bony transfers

Complications

Bone

Associated fracture, greater tuberosity, and surgical neck of humerus.

Joint

- Recurrent dislocation (most common)
- Old unreduced dislocation
- Stiff shoulder

Tendon

Rupture of the supraspinatus.

Muscle

Rotator cuff injury.

Nerve

Brachial plexus, axillary nerve injury.

Q2. Write short note on Posterior dislocation shoulder joint.

It is a relatively uncommon injury. Posterior dislocations are occasionally due to *electrocution or seizure* and may be caused by *strength imbalance* of the rotator cuff muscles.

Mechanism of Injury

Indirect Trauma (Most Common)

- The shoulder typically is in the position of adduction, flexion, and internal rotation.
- Electric shock or convulsive mechanisms may produce posterior dislocations.

Direct Trauma

This occurs from force application to the anterior shoulder, resulting in posterior translation of the humeral head.

Clinical Features

- Affected upper extremity is held in the "classical sling position" of shoulder internal rotation and adduction.
- Deformity is less severe than in anterior dislocation.
- Palpable mass posterior to the shoulder
- Flattening of the anterior shoulder, and coracoid prominence may be observed

Radiographs

- AP, scapular-Y, and axillary views.
- A Velpeau axillary views (see earlier), if the patient is unable to position the shoulder for a standard axillary view.
- Signs suggestive of a posterior glenohumeral dislocation on a standard AP view of the shoulder, include:
  - Absence of the overlapping of normal elliptic of the humeral head on the glenoid.
  - Vacant glenoid sign: glenoid appears partially vacant (space between anterior rim and humeral head >6 mm).

- Trough sign: Impaction fracture of the anterior humeral head caused by the posterior rim of glenoid (reverse Hill-Sachs lesion).
- Loss of profile of neck of humerus: The humerus is in full internal rotation.
- CT scans: Assessing the percentage of the humeral head involved with an impaction fracture.

Types

- Subacromial (98%)
- Subglenoid (very rare)
- Subspinous (very rare)

Treatment

Nonoperative

Reduction
- Done under GA
- With the patient supine, traction applied to the adducted arm in the line of deformity with gentle lifting of the humeral head into the glenoid fossa.

Maintenance: 3–6 weeks of immobilization in a sling if shoulder is stable or if it is unstable or subluxates, it should immobilizes in shoulder spica with amount of external rotation, which is determined by the position of stability.

Rehabilitation: Once the duration of immobilization is complete, an aggressive external and internal rotator strengthening started.

Operative

Indications for surgery
- Lesser tuberosity fracture
- Large posterior glenoid fragment
- Irreducible dislocation or an impaction fracture on the posterior glenoid preventing reduction.
- Open dislocation.
- An anteromedial humeral impaction fracture (reverse Hill- Sachs lesion):
  - 20–40% humeral head involvement: Transfer the lesser tuberosity with attached subscapularis into the defect (modified McLaughlin procedure).
  - >40% humeral head involvement: Hemiarthroplasty with neutral version of the prosthesis.

Surgical options
- Open reduction
- Plication of infraspinatus muscle/tendon (reverse Putti-Platt procedure)
- Transfer of long head of the biceps tendon to the posterior glenoid margin (Boyd-Sisk procedure)
- Humeral and glenoid osteotomies
- Capsulorrhaphy

Complication

- Recurrent dislocation
- Associated fractures of the posterior glenoid rim, humeral shaft, lesser and greater tuberosities, and humeral head.
- Neurovascular deficit: Much less common than anterior dislocation of shoulder.

Q3. Discuss inferior dislocation of shoulder.

It is the least common among three occurring in less than 1% of all cases. This condition is termed as Luxatio erecta because the arm appears to be permanently held upward or behind the head. This rare injury is more common in elderly individuals.

Mechanism of Injury

It is caused by a *hyperabduction of the arm* that forces the humeral head against the acromion.

Clinical Features

- Patient present with a typical attitude of an upper limb in fixed abduction with the hand raised and inability to bring the elbow back to the body.
- Head is palpable on the lateral chest wall and axilla.
- Thorough neurologic and vascular examination must be performed as it often results in injury to great vessels and brachial plexus.

Radiographs

AP radiograph is usually diagnostic, with inferior dislocation of the humeral head and superior direction of the humeral shaft along the glenoid margin.

Management

Nonoperative

- Reduction done under general anesthesia.
- Traction-counter traction maneuvers.
- Axial traction applied in line with the humeral position (superolaterally), with a gradual decrease in shoulder abduction.
- Counter-traction should be applied with a sheet around the patient, in line with, but opposite to the traction vector.

Post Reduction

- The arm should be immobilized in a sling for 3–6 weeks.
- Older individuals may be immobilized for shorter periods to minimize stiffness of shoulder joint.

Operative

Indication: Soft tissue (inferior capsule and soft tissue envelop) interposition that prevents closed reduction.
Procedure: Open reduction and repair of all damaged structures.

Complication

- Rotator cuff tear
- Fracture of acromion with or without inferior glenoid fossa and with or without fracture of the greater tuberosity
- Neurovascular injury

Q4. Discuss pathology, clinical features and management of recurrent dislocation shoulder.

It occurs as a result of the damage to anterior part of the capsule and rotator cuff or detachment of the glenoid labrum *(Bankart lesion)*. Sometimes, defect in the posterosuperior quadrant of the head of humerus *(Hill-Sachs lesion)*. Even trivial injury or abduction and external rotation of the shoulder causes recurrent dislocations.

Pathological Anatomy

No single pathological lesion is responsible for recurrent subluxation or dislocation. Few important pathology have been cited and considered to be the *"essential" lesion* in recurrent dislocations.

Hill-Sachs Lesion

- *Hill-Sachs lesion* is a defect in the *posterolateral aspect of the humeral head.*
- This is due to the impaction of humeral head against the sharp rim of the glenoid at the time of dislocation.
- If these lesions involve >20% of the glenoid, they can result in recurrent instability

Bankart's Lesion

- During acute anterior dislocation humeral head is forced anteriorly out of the glenoid cavity and tears not only the fibrocartilaginous labrum from almost the entire anterior ½ of the rim of the glenoid cavity, but also the anterior capsule and periosteum from the anterior surface of the neck of the scapula
- This traumatic detachment of the glenoid labrum is called the *Bankart's lesion.*
- *Bankart's lesion* is the most commonly found pathological lesion in recurrent subluxation or dislocation of the shoulder joint.

Other Relative Lesions

- Excessive laxity of the shoulder capsule.
- Erosion of the anterior glenoid rim.
- Stretching of the anterior capsule and subscapularis tendon.
- Fraying and degeneration of the glenoid labrum.

Clinical Features

- History of previous episode of traumatic dislocation.
- Wasting of deltoid and other muscles.

Clinical Test

Sulcus Test

- This test is done with the arm in 0° and 45° of abduction.
- It is done by pulling distally on the extremity and observing for a sulcus or dimple between the humeral head and the acromion that does not reduce with 45° external rotation.
- This indicates laxity of the inferior glenohumeral ligament complex and of laxity at the rotator interval.

Positive Apprehension Test

Abduction and external rotation movement causes pain and insecure feeling. The patient becomes anxious and resists the maneuver.

Relocation Test for Evaluating Instability

It comprises of dislocation and relocation of the humeral head in the glenohumeral joint by manual pressure.

Radiographic Evaluation

- Diagnosis often is made by history and physical examination.
- Anteroposterior and axillary lateral views of the shoulder.
- If radiographs view are inconclusive then, special views (West point or Rokous view, and the Stryker notch view), gadolinium-enhanced MRI, or CT arthrography can be used.
- Gadolinium-enhanced MRI gives the best view of capsular or labral damage.

Treatment

Conservative

Develop the power of the muscles of rotator cuff by physiotherapy.

Surgical

Bankart's operation:
- Suturing of the detached labrum glenoidale to margins of glenoid cavity by sutures/ staples.
- Subscapularis and shoulder capsule are opened vertically.
- Lateral leaf of the capsule is reattached to the anterior glenoid rim.
- A medial leaf of the capsule is imbricated, and the subscapularis is approximated.

Putti Platt's Operation

Double breasting of the capsule and subscapularis tendon in front of the shoulder joint.

Bristow's Operation

- Especially for athletes (anterior bone block).
- Coracoid with its attachment is reposed in front of anterior rim of glenoid margin.

Maclaughlin's Procedure

Dividing the subscapularis tendon close to its insertion to the lesser tuberosity and transplanted or suturing it into the defect using bone drill holes.

Eden-Hybinette Procedure

Small bone block is applied to the anterior rim of the glenoid either intra- or extra-articularly.

PROXIMAL HUMERAL FRACTURE

Q1. Discuss the proximal humeral fracture under headings of classification, clinical features and management?

These fractures of the shoulder are common injuries and occur in all age groups.

Mechanism of Injury

Indirect injury

- Most common
- Fall on to outstretched upper extremity from a standing height.
- Especially in older, osteoporotic woman.

Direct injury

- High-energy trauma, such as a road-side accident.
- Usually seen in young patients

Classification

Most commonly used classification system is that of *Neer's four-segment classification.*

Four-part Anatomy of the Proximal Humerus

- The four different parts are *greater* and *lesser tuberosities*, humeral head, and proximal humeral shaft.
- A part is defined as displaced if more than 1 cm of fracture displacement or >45° of angulation.

Fracture types
- One-part fractures: No displacement of fragments regardless of number of fracture lines.
- Two-part fractures:
    - Anatomic neck
    - Surgical neck
    - Greater tuberosity
    - Lesser tuberosity
- Three-part fractures:
    - Surgical neck with greater tuberosity
    - Surgical neck with lesser tuberosity
- Four-part fractures
    - Osteonecrosis is most likely after displaced four-part fractures, as there is highest likelihood of disrupting the major blood supply to the proximal humerus.
- Fracture dislocation
- Articular surface fracture.

Clinical Features

- Patients typically present with the injured limb held closely to the chest by the contralateral hand
- Pain
- Swelling
- Tenderness
- Painful restriction of movements
- Axillary nerve function is assessed by the presence of sensation on the lateral aspect of the proximal arm overlying the deltoid *(the classical regiment badge sign)*

Radiographic Evaluation

- X-rays: Important views:
  - AP view of the shoulder in the plane of the scapula
  - Lateral view of the scapula (Y view)
  - Supine axillary view
- CT scan: If displacement is unclear on radiographs, an axial CT scan with 2-mm sections is indicated.
- MRI: May be used to assess rotator cuff integrity.

Treatment

Minimally Displaced Fractures

- These comprises the vast majority (86%)
- Sling immobilization
- Radiographic follow-up to detect loss of fracture reduction.
- Early shoulder motion may be started at 7–10 days if the patient has a stable or impacted fracture.
- Physical therapy regimen with pendulum exercises is started initially followed by passive range-of-motion exercises.
- At 6 weeks, active range-of-motion exercises are encouraged.
- Resistive exercises are instituted at 12 weeks.

Two-part fracture

Anatomic neck fractures:
- Rare and difficult to treat by closed reduction and are associated with a high incidence of osteonecrosis.
- In younger patients: Open reduction and internal fixation (ORIF)
- In elderly patients: Prosthesis (e.g. shoulder hemiarthroplasty)

Surgical neck fractures: In case of reducible fracture with good quality bone:
- Closed reduction and fixation with percutaneously threaded pins.
- Problems associated with multiple pin fixation include:
  - axillary nerve injury
  - Loosening of pin
  - pin migration
  - Inability to move the arm

Irreducible fractures (usually interposed soft tissue), widely displaced fractures, fractures with comminution or with osteopenic bone:

ORIF with:
- Threaded pins
- Intramedullary nails with or without a supplemental tension band
- Locking compression plate and screws

For extremely osteopenic patients:
- *Banco et al.* described a *"parachute"* technique, comprises *valgus impaction osteotomy and tension-band fixation incorporating transosseous sutures.*

Greater tuberosity fractures

Undisplaced fracture: Managed conservatively

Displacement > 5–10 mm:
- Open reduction and internal fixation with or without rotator cuff repair; otherwise, they may develop nonunion and subacromial impingement.
- Usually these fractures are stabilized with *trans-osseous sutures* or occasionally with screws in larger fragments

Fracture associated with anterior dislocation: Closed reduction and be managed non-operatively.

Lesser tuberosity fractures:
- Usually managed closed unless displaced fragment (>1 cm) blocks internal rotation
- One must rule out posterior dislocation associated with isolated fracture of lesser tuberosity.

Three-part Fractures

- Closed reduction and maintenance of reduction are often difficult as these fractures are unstable due to opposing muscle forces.
- Displaced fractures require operative fixation

Younger individuals:
- ORIF (LCP)
- stripping is kept to a minimum to avoid further damage to the humeral head blood supply.

Older patients: Usually primary prosthetic replacement (hemiarthroplasty).

Four-part Fracture

In young, active patients: Open reduction and LC plate fixation

In the elderly: Primary prosthetic replacement of the humeral head (hemiarthroplasty) is the procedure of choice.

Fracture-dislocations

Two-part fracture-dislocations
- Treated closed after shoulder reduction unless the fracture fragments remain displaced.
- If there is significant displacement then ORIF may be necessary

Three- and four-part fracture-dislocations:
- *In younger individuals*: ORIF is used.
- *In the elderly*: hemiarthroplasty.

Complications

Vascular Injury

Axillary artery is the most common site (proximal to anterior circumflex artery).

Neural Injury

- Brachial plexus injury:
- Axillary nerve injury: This is particularly vulnerable with anterior fracture-dislocation
- Complete axillary nerve injuries that do not improve within 2–3 months may require electromyographic evaluation and exploration.

Chest Injury

- Intrathoracic dislocation may occur with surgical neck fracture-dislocations.
- Pneumothorax
- Hemothorax

Myositis Ossificans

Due to:
- Chronic unreduced fracture-dislocations
- Multiple attempts at closed reduction.

Shoulder Stiffness

It may be minimized with an aggressive physical therapy regimen and sometimes requires open lysis of adhesions for refractory cases.

Osteonecrosis

A high rate of anatomic neck fractures followed by four-part fractures and three-part proximal humeral fractures.

Nonunion

- Common in displaced two-part surgical neck fractures with soft tissue interposition.
- Other causes include:
  - Excessive traction
  - Significant fracture displacement
  - Systemic or other general disease
  - Poor bone quality or stock
  - Inadequate fixation or immobilization
  - Infection.

It is treated:
- ORIF with or without bone graft
- Prosthetic replacement.

Malunion: Common:
- After inadequate closed reduction
- Failed ORIF.

Q2. Write in short surgical neck humerus.

Fracture—Neck of Humerus

- *In children*: Due to fall on outstretched hand, pathological (due to bone cyst).
- *In old age*: Due to the osteoporosis or secondaries

Clinical Features

- Contussion/ecchymosis
- Pain
- Swelling
- Tenderness

- Bony crepitations
- Loss of transmitted movements
- All movements are painful and restricted, extensive bruising and ecchymosis over arm, especially in old patients.

Treatment

Children and old age: Undisplaced and impacted fracture is immobilized in a *triangular sling*.

Adults:

- *In displaced fractures*: Reduction under GA and immobilization in 'U slab' with arm to chest bandage for 3 weeks.
- *For irreducible fracture*: Open reduction and internal fixation by K-wire or T-plate

Complication

- Most common nerve injured is *axillary*.
- Post-traumatic arthritis.

HUMERAL SHAFT FRACTURE

Q1. Discuss mechanism of injury, clinical features and management of fracture shaft humerus.

Fracture shaft humerus accounts roughly 3% of all fractures; most cases can be managed conservatively.

Mechanism of Injury

- *Direct (most common mode)*: Direct trauma to the arm from a blow or road-side accident results in transverse or comminuted fractures.
- *Indirect*: A fall on an outstretched arm results in oblique or spiral fractures, especially in elderly patients.

Displacement

- Proximal fragment is abducted by deltoid
- Overriding of fragments due to contraction of the biceps and the triceps.

Clinical Features

- Pain
- Swelling
- Deformity of arm
- Bony crepitus
- Loss of transmitted movements
- Shortening
- All movements restricted by pain.
- Always examine distal pulsations and sensations especially radial nerve in mid shaft fracture (may cause wrist drop).

Radiographic Evaluation

Standard AP and lateral view with the shoulder and elbow joints.

Classification

For descriptive purpose:
- Open or closed.
- Location: proximal 1/3rd, middle 1/3rd, distal 1/3rd.
- Degree: nondisplaced, displaced.
- Direction and character: Transverse, spiral, oblique, segmental, comminuted.
- Articular extension.

Treatment

Nonoperative

- Most humeral shaft fractures (>90%) will heal with conservative management.
- Acceptable limit: 20° of anterior angulation, 30° of varus angulation, and up to 3 cm of bayonet apposition are acceptable and will not compromise function or appearance.
- *In neonates*: Arm to chest bandage.
- *In adults*:
  - Hanging 'U' cast (weight of limb and plaster acts as reducing forces) with thoraco-brachial immobilization (Velpeau dressing).
  - Functional bracing: This utilizes hydrostatic soft tissue compression to effect and maintain fracture alignment while allowing motion of adjacent joints. It is typically applied 1–2 weeks after injury, after the patient has been placed in a hanging arm cast or U cast and swelling has subsided.

Operative

Open reduction and internal fixation for irreducible and unstable fracture.

Goal: Reestablish length, alignment, and rotation with stable fixation.

Indication for operative treatment:
- Polytrauma
- Failed conservative procedure
- Nonunion
- Pathologic fracture
- Associated vascular injury
- Floating elbow
- Progressive radial nerve palsy following fracture manipulation (controversial)
- Segmental fracture
- Intra-articular extension
- Bilateral humeral fractures
- Open fracture
- Neurologic loss following penetrating trauma

Children: Rush nail fixation.

Adults:
- *Plate osteosynthesis* (Cortical fixation by plates and screws): 4.5 mm DCP with fixation of 8–10 cortices proximal and distal to the fracture is used.

- *Intramedullary nail* by 'V' nails, flexible nails and interlocked nails. Either types of nails can be inserted through antegrade or retrograde techniques.

  Indications:
  - Segmental fractures
  - Humerus fractures in extremely osteopenic bone.
  - Pathologic humerus fractures
- *External fixators* is done whenever there is extensive soft tissue damage and risk of contamination

  Indications:
  - Infected nonunions.
  - Burn patients with fractures.
  - Open fractures with extensive soft tissue damage.

Complications

Bone

- Delayed union
- Nonunion due to muscle entrapment or soft tissue interposition (may necessitate open reduction and internal fixation with bone grafting)
- Malunion

Joint

Shoulder and elbow stiffness.

Nerve

- Radial nerve injury (wrist drop).
- Delayed surgical exploration should be done after 3–4 months if there is no evidence of recovery by EMG or NCV studies.

Vessel

Injury to brachial artery (VIC).

> **Q2. What is the treatment algorithm for radial nerve palsy associated with humeral shaft fracture?**

Radial nerve palsy was most frequent with fractures of the middle and middle-distal humeral shaft and often seen with transverse and spiral fractures than with oblique or comminuted fractures.

Important point to be remembered before dealing with such cases:
- In most of the cases, radial nerve injury is neurapraxic in nature that show spontaneous recovery.
- Nerve palsies that occur with a closed fracture usually recover without treatment.
- If an open fracture of the humeral shaft results in radial nerve palsy, the nerve should be explored at the time of the irrigation and debridement of the wound.
- If it is found intact, only watchful waiting is required while the fracture heals.
- Early exploration is required if evidence suggests that the radial nerve is impaled on a bone fragment or is caught between the fragments.

- Complete transection of the radial nerve usually occurs in association with open fractures, requires nerve repair or grafting.

Shao et al. developed an algorithm for the treatment of radial nerve palsy associated with humeral shaft fractures.

Case 1

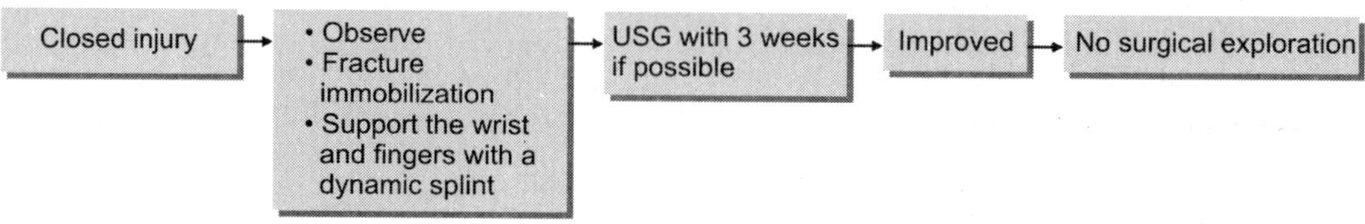

Case 2

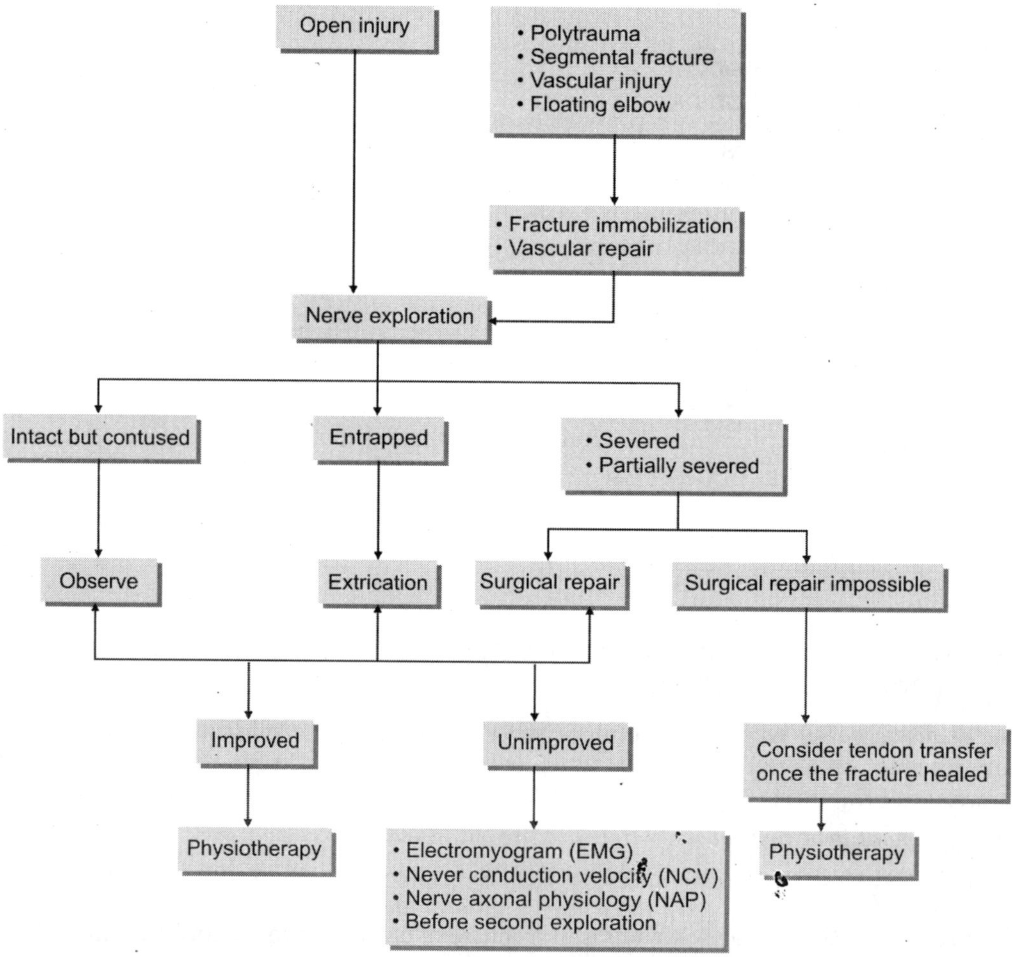

Q3. What is Holstein-Lewis fracture?

It is distal 1/3rd fracture of humerus shaft, which may entrap or lacerate the radial nerve as it passes through the lateral intermuscular septum. It usually results in radial nerve palsy.

DISTAL HUMERAL FRACTURE

Q1. Write in brief the ossification centre of ossification of elbow joint:

With the exception of the capitellum, ossification centers appear ~2 years earlier in girls compared with boys.

The following is a mnemonic for the appearance of the ossification centers around the elbow: "Cat and Rat Meet aT Olive Lake".

- *Cat*: **C**apitellum: 6 months to 2 years; includes the lateral crista of the trochlea
- *Rat*: **R**adial head: 4 years
- *Meet:* **M**edial epicondyle: 6–7 years
- *aT* : **T**rochlea: 8 years
- *Olive:* **O**lecranon: 8–10 years
- *Lake* : **L**ateral epicondyle: 12 years.

Q2. Discuss the mechanism of injury, classification, clinical features and management of supracondylar fracture humerus.

Most common and most serious fracture in childhood as it is often associated with complication. It is the fracture occurring through the supracondylar zone (metaphysis) of humerus. If any child comes with injury and swelling around the elbow, always think of this fracture unless or until proved otherwise.

Incidence

- Comprise 55–75% of all elbow fractures.
- Peak incidence is from 5–8 years, after which dislocations are more frequent.
- Male-to-female ratio is 3:2.

Mechanism of Injury

- Extension type: Hyperextension with or without varus/valgus force during fall onto an outstretched hand
- Flexion type: Fall on point of flexed elbow.

Types

According to the position of the distal fragment in relation to the proximal fragment the fracture may be:

Extension/Posterior Type

- Most common type (95%)
- Fall on outstretched hand with elbow extended and forearm pronated.
- The distal fragment carrying the elbow with it gets displaced *posteriorly, laterally, shifted proximally and gets pronated*

Flexion/Anterior Type

- Less common type (5%).
- Mechanism of injury fall on point of flexed elbow.
- Distal fragment with elbow displaced *proximally, anteriorly, laterally and supinated.*

Clinical Features

- Pain
- Gross swelling
- Tenderness
- Deformity (S-shaped deformity of the distal humerus) following injury.
- Relationship of three bony prominences of elbow maintained.
- Shortening of the arm length
- All movements painfully restricted.
- Palpable bony crepitus (should not be elicited for fear of damaging the vital neurovascular structures)
- *Pucker* or *Dimple sign*: spikes of the proximal fragment pears the brachialis muscle and tethering the skin, clinically visible as dimpling on the anterior aspect of the distal arm.
- Always examine the distal pulsations as well as sensations and make a note of it, after comparing it with the other side.

Radiographic Evaluation

To see the type of fracture, displacement and to rule out associated injury.

Few Important Point to be Remembered

- AP view: Remember normal carrying angle is about 10°.
- Lateral view: Anterior inclination of condyle about 45° in relation to the shaft humerus.
- Normal epiphysis should not be confused with the fracture line.
- If in doubt always, compare the X-rays with that of the uninjured elbow.
- Gross displacement of distal fragment is invariably seen. At times X-ray may show no fracture line on 1st day, but a positive fat pad sign is indicative of hairline fracture without displacement.

Radiological parameters to be assessed on AP view

- *Baumann's angle*: on AP view, angle between the line through physis of lateral condyle and the Line perpendicular to midline diaphysis of humeral shaft.
  - Normal: 64–81°
  - >81° suggestive of varus alignment
- *Metaphyseal-diaphyseal angle*: On AP view, angle between the transverse line through metaphysis at its widest point, and longitudinal line through axis of diaphysis
  - Normal angle is 90°.
  - Angle >90° indicates varus angulation.
  - Angle <90° indicates valgus angulation.

Radiological Parameters to be Assessed on Lateral View

- *Anterior spike*: Implies rotation rather than posterior displacement.
- *Crescent sign*: Normal lucent gap of elbow joint is missing and a crescent-shaped shadow due to overlap of the capitulum over the olecranon is visualized. It implies tilt medially or laterally.
- *Teardrop sign*: It is disturbed in supracondylar fracture. Normally, it is a radiographic shadow constituted by the posterior margin of the coronoid fossa anteriorly, the anterior margin of the olecranon fossa posteriorly, and the superior margin of the capitellar ossification center inferiorly.

- *Anterior humeral line*: In case of posterior displacement of the distal fragment in supracondylar fracture, this line passes through anterior third. Normally when extended distally, this line should intersect the middle third of the capitellar ossification center.
- *Posterior (olecranon) fat pad sign*: Normally it is not seen as the deep olecranon fossa completely contains the posterior fat pad. In cases of moderate to large effusions due to trauma or infection, distension of capsule leads to posterior displacement, resulting in a high specificity of the posterior fat pad sign as a radiolucent gap for intra-articular disorders (a fracture is present >70% of the time when the posterior fat pad is seen).

Classification

Extension variety; classified further into the following:

Gartland Classification

This is based on the degree of displacement.
- Type I: Non-displaced
- Type II: Displaced with intact posterior cortex; may be angulated or rotated
- Type III: Complete displacement with no cortical contact; posteromedial (a) or postero-lateral (b).

Management

Principles of Treatment

- To restore accurate anatomical reduction
- Early good range of elbow movement
- Emergency care of the injured vessels.

Hairline Fracture and Fracture with Minimal Displacement

Posterior above elbow slab with cuff and collar sling for 21 days.

Displaced Fracture without Neurovascular Deficit

- Closed reduction under anaesthesia, with a posterior above elbow POP slab in more than 90° flexion at elbow with compatible radial pulse and nail bed circulation for 3 weeks.
- When the elbow is flexed beyond 90°, the triceps provides a posterior splinting effect and stabilizes the fracture.
- Fracture is stabilized. Two lateral pins can be inserted which must be divergent, one engaging the lateral column and other the medial column or the reduction is fixed with cross K wires which gives a better configuration and stability.

Open or comminuted fracture or displaced fracture with massive edema and blisters:

- Skeletal traction: Olecranon pin traction
- Skin traction: Dunlop traction
- Advantages:
  - Easy to apply
  - Provide sustained traction
  - Give time for soft tissue healing
  - Facilitate dependent drainage

Irreducible Simple Fracture or Closed Reduction is Unsatisfactory or Failed or Fracture with Vascular Injury

Open reduction by posterior exposure with K-wire fixation.

Complicated Fracture Management of Vascular Injury

Elevation, ice pack and if necessary exploration of vessel and repair.

Q3. Discuss the complication of supracondylar fracture humerus.

The complication of supracondylar fractures can be summarized into:
- Early complication
- Late complication

Early Complication

Neurological Compromise

- Usually a neurapraxic injury
- Reported to occur in 3–22% of cases of supracondylar fracture
- Order of nerve involvement in decreasing frequency: *Anterior interosseous nerve (most common) > Median nerve > Radial nerve > ulnar nerve (mc in flexion type of fracture)*
- Most are *neurapraxias* requiring no treatment.
- Surgical exploration is required if nerve function has not returned within 6–8 weeks of reduction.

Vascular Injury

- Injury to the brachial artery occurs in 10% of cases of supracondylar fractures.
- Type of injury: It could be spasm, tear or complete transection.
- Often the circulation is returns to normal after the fracture has been reduced and fixed with percutaneous pinning.
- Means of evaluating circulation after reduction: *Signs of capillary refill and pulse, Doppler measurements or a pulse oximeter.*
- Surgical exploration of the brachial artery may be required: if circulation does not return to normal (with the elbow flexed to <45°) within about 5 minutes.
- Complete transection: Requires segmental resection and reverse vein graft.

Compartment Syndrome (Volkmann's Ischaemia)

- Rare but dreaded and serious complication of supracondylar fracture.
- Cause: hypoxic damage caused by interruption of the circulation to the muscles (anterior compartment) especially to flexor digitorum profundus (most common) and flexor pollicis longus.

Clinical Sign of Compartment Syndrome

- *5Ps:*
  - Pain on passive stretch (stretch pain: earliest sign)
  - Pallor
  - Pulselessness
  - Paraesthesia
  - Palsy

- Most important and earliest single sign is *Griffith's sign* (passive stretching of the flexed finger causes severe pain).

Principle of Management

To relieve the compression on the vascular channel and to restore the vascularity of the distal part at the earliest.

Decompress

- Remove all external Splintage and bandages immediately.
- Cool the limb by ice packs to reduce metabolic demands.
- Fasciotomy (*standard Henry approach*) is indicated to release the compartment pressure.

General indications for fasciotomy are:
- Clinical signs such as demonstrable motor or sensory loss
- Compartment pressures > 35 mm Hg (slit or wick catheter technique) or > 40 mm Hg (needle technique)
- Interrupted arterial circulation to the extremity for > 4 hours.
- If the fracture fragments are grossly displaced, do closed reduction under anaesthesia at the earliest.
- Watch for return of capillary circulation and the pulsation.

Repair

If within few hours circulation does not improve, Doppler study may show the type of arterial block, exploration of the damaged vessel, decompression and necessary repair should be done.

Late Complication

Malunion

Malunion in:
- Anteroposterior plane: causing limitation of flexion/extension.
- Mediolateral plane: This can be of two types:
    - Cubitus varus showing gunstock deformity
    - Cubitus valgus showing increased carrying angle.

Angular Deformity (Varus > Valgus) or Cubitus Varus or Gunstock Deformity

- Cubitus varus is the most common angular deformity.
- Three static components of cubitus varus deformity are: Posterior displacement, horizontal rotation and coronal tilt
- Cause (most common) for cubitus varus: Medial displacement and rotation of the distal fragment.
- It is a cosmetic problem, and there is no functional impairment.
- Requires corrective osteotomy (after skeletal maturity): There are osteotomies:
    - A medial opening wedge osteotomy (King and Secor) with a bone graft
    - An oblique osteotomy with derotation
    - A lateral closing wedge osteotomy (French and modified French).
- The occurrence of angular deformity is decreased with percutaneous pinning compared with reduction and casting alone.

Myositis Ossificans Traumatica

Rare and is usually seen after vigorous manipulation/massage.

Loss of mobility: Greater than 5-degree loss of elbow motion occurs; secondary to poor reduction or soft tissue contracture.

Volkmann's Ischemic Contracture (VIC)

It is the end result of prolonged ischaemia, causing irreversible damage to muscle and nerve.

Pathophysiology of Contracture

- Prolonged ischaemia leads to necrosis of muscles, nerves, atrophy of skin, bone and soft tissue.
- In due time necrosed muscles are replaced by fibrous tissue (bands) resulting into contracture.

Clinical Features

- Patient presents with a deformed hand, which is stiff, weak and numb.
- The extent of involvement may be mild, moderate or severe with extensive involvement of muscles, bones and nerves.

Deformity

- Fingers are flexed at interphalangeal joints due to contracture of flexor muscles of the forearm.
- This deformity increases with dorsiflexion and diminishes with flexion of wrist (Volkmann's sign); this is due to fibrotic flexor muscles

Other Changes

- *Joints*: Stiff and bones are atrophied and deformed.
- *Muscles*:
  - Loss of the power of grip.
  - Wasting of small muscles of hand/forearm.
- *Nerves*: Loss of sensation affecting the median and ulnar nerves.
- *Skin*: Skin becomes atrophic and so do nails and hair.

Tsuge Classification of Volkmann's Ischemic Contracture

Grading	Involvement of structures
Mild	• Involvement of flexor digitorum profundus and flexor pollicis longus
Moderate	• Involvement of flexor digitorum profundus and flexor pollicis longus
	• Involvement of superficial finger flexors
	• Involvement of wrist flexors
	• Involvement of thumb flexors
Severe	• All flexors
	• Few extensors
	• Neurological deficit (most common median nerve)
	• Joint contracture
	• Severe scarring of the skin
	• Deformity of bones

Treatment

Depending on the extent of the involvement:

- *Mild*:
  - Splinting
  - Physiotherapy
  - If there is involvement of single muscle then plan for its excision
- *Moderate*:
  - Muscle sliding of the common flexors from the medial epicondyle (*MaxPage*).
  - Excision of the dead fibrotic muscle
  - Tendon transfers
- *Severe:*
  - Excision of the scar
  - Nerve grafting
  - Proximal row carpectomy (Seddon's)
  - Wrist arthrodesis in functional position

Q4. Short note on: a. Fracture lateral condyle and its management; b. Fracture medial condyle and its management

a. Fracture Lateral Condyle

Incidence

- Most common distal humeral epiphyseal fracture.
- These are more common than fractures of the medial epicondyle or the medial condyle.
- Occurs at approximately age 6 years.

Mechanism of Injury

Two theories:

- "Pull off": due to a varus stress exerted on the extended elbow, there occurs avulsion injury by the common extensor origin.
- "Push off": A fall onto an extended upper extremity results in axial load, which is transmitted through the forearm.

Clinical Features

- Pain
- Swelling
- Tenderness to palpation
- Sometimes crepitus may be elicited during supination-pronation movements.
- Painful range of motion
- Pain on resisted wrist extension

Radiographic Evaluation

- AP, lateral, and oblique views of the elbow.
- Varus stress views may accentuate displacement of the fracture.

Classification

Milch

- Type I:
  - Rare (less common)
  - Fracture line courses medially to the trochlea through and into the capitellar-trochlear groove.
  - It is a true Salter-Harris type IV fracture.
  - Elbow is frequently stable because the trochlea is intact.
- Type II:
  - More common
  - Fracture line extends into the area of the trochlea
  - It represents a Salter-Harris type II fracture
  - The elbow is unstable because of the ability of the distal fragment and the forearm to angulate and translate into a lateral position.

Jakob's Classification:
- Stage I: Fracture undisplaced (<2 mm) with an intact articular surface
- Stage II: Fracture with moderate displacement (>2 mm)
- Stage III: Complete displacement and rotation with elbow instability.

Treatment

Nonoperative

- Jakob type I fracture.
- Immobilized in long posterior splint or above elbow POP cast in neutral position with elbow flexed in 90° for 3–4 weeks.
- Physiotherapy

Operative

- Open reduction and internal fixation is required for unstable Jakobs stage II and stage III fractures (60%).
- The fracture fragments are fixed with two crossed, smooth Kirschner wires that diverge in the metaphysis.
- Postoperatively the elbow is immobilized in above elbow splint at 60–90° of flexion with the forearm in neutral rotation.
- After 3–4 weeks, the pin and the splint are removed.
- Active range-of-motion exercises are encouraged.

If treatment is delayed (>3 weeks) or in late presenting cases: Closed treatment should be preferred, regardless of displacement, as there is high incidence of osteonecrosis of the condylar fragment.

Complication

Nonunion

- Due to pull of extensors and poor metaphyseal circulation of the lateral condylar fragment
- Often seen in patients treated conservatively.
- Results in cubitus valgus necessitating anterior transposition of ulnar nerve for tardy ulnar nerve palsy.

Angulation Deformity
- Cubitus valgus occurs more frequently than varus due to lateral physeal arrest.
- Resulting in tardy ulnar nerve palsy.
- Tardy ulnar nerve is treated by anterior transposition of the nerve.

Neurological Compromise
Tardy ulnar nerve palsy managed by anterior transposition of the nerve.

Osteonecrosis

- Osteonecrosis of the capitellum occurs with *"fishtail" deformity* (deepening of the trochlear groove) with a persistent gap between the ossification centre of the lateral and medial physis.
- It is usually iatrogenic especially when the surgery is delayed

Lateral condylar overgrowth with spur formation:
- During surgery or at the time of injury an ossified periosteal flap raised from the distal fragment resulting in lateral prominence due to bone formation.
- Cubitus pseudovarus
- Cosmetic problem.

b. Medial Condyle Fracture

Incidence

- These fractures are least common injuries of the elbow In adults and children.
- These are Salter-Harris type IV fractures.

Mechanism of Injury

- Direct: Trauma or blow to the point of the elbow, such as a fall onto a flexed elbow.
- Indirect: An avulsion injury due to fall onto an outstretched hand with valgus strain on the elbow

Clinical Features

- Pain
- Swelling
- Tenderness to palpation
- Sometimes crepitus may be elicited during supination-pronation movements.
- Painful range of motion
- Pain on resisted wrist flexion
- Assess neurological deficit (ulnar nerve).

Radiographic Evaluation

- AP, lateral, and oblique views of the elbow
- Stress views helps to differentiated the epicondylar (valgus laxity) from condylar fractures (both valgus and varus laxity).

Classification

Milch
- Type I:
  - More common type

– Fracture line traversing through the apex of the trochlea
– It is Salter-Harris type II
- Type II:
    – Less common
    – Fracture line through capitulo-trochlear groove
    – It is Salter-Harris type IV.

Kilfoyle Classification

- Stage I: A greenstick or impacted fracture
- Stage II: Fracture line complete with minimal displacement
- Stage III: Complete displacement with rotation of fragment from pull of flexor mass

Treatment

Nonoperative

- Kilfoyle type I fracture.
- Immobilized in long posterior splint or above elbow POP cast in neutral position with elbow flexed in 90° for 3–4 weeks.
- Physiotherapy

Minimally displaced fracture:
- Close reduction done with the elbow extended and the forearm pronated in order to relieve tension on the flexor origin
- Immobilized in a posterior splint or above elbow cast.

Operative

Unstable reduction: Fixed with two parallel metaphyseal percutaneous pins.

Irreducible fracture or Kilfoyle type II and III fracture:
- Open reduction an internal fixation.
- The fracture fragments are fixed with two parallel, smooth Kirschner wires that extend to the metaphysis.
- Postoperatively the elbow is immobilized in above elbow splint at 60—90° of flexion with the forearm in neutral rotation.
- After 3–4 weeks, the pin and the splint are removed.
- Active range-of-motion exercises are encouraged.

If treatment is delayed (>3 weeks) or in late presenting cases: Closed treatment should be preferred, regardless of displacement, as there is high incidence of osteonecrosis of the condylar fragment.

Complication

- Nonunion
- Angular deformity (usually varus)
- Ulnar neuropathy
- Osteonecrosis.

Q5. Discuss the classification, clinical features and management of inter-condylar fractures of humerus.

Incidence

- Most common type of distal humeral fracture
- Articular comminution is common in these injuries

Displacement of Fracture

Unopposed muscles pull at the lateral (extensor mass) and medial (flexor mass) epicondyles, which rotate the articular surfaces.

Mechanism of Injury

Due to longitudinal forces directed toward the elbow flexed >90°

Clinical Features

- Elbow is in 90° of flexion with the forearm pronated
- Pain
- Gross swelling
- Tenderness
- Intercondylar distance is increased
- Three-point relationship is disturbed
- Crepitus
- Severe painful restriction of the elbow motion
- Neurological assessment should be carefully done.

Radiological Evaluation

- Standard AP and lateral views of elbow
- CT scan to delineate the fracture pattern

Classification

Mehne and Matta Classification

- A: High T
- B: Low T
- C: Y-type
- D: H-type
- E: Medial Lambda
- F: Lateral Lambda

Riesborough and Radin Classification

- Type I: Undisplaced condylar fracture of the elbow
- Type II: Displaced but not rotated T-condylar fracture
- Type III: Displaced and rotated T-condylar fracture
- Type IV: Displaced, rotated, and comminuted condylar fracture

OTA Classification

- A: extra-articular
- B: partially articular
- C: completely articular (T or Y)

Treatment

Nonoperative

Indication:
- Undisplaced fractures
- Elderly patients with displaced fractures
- Severe osteopenia

- "Bag of bone" or gross comminution
- Medically unfit or patients with significant comorbid conditions

Nonoperative measures:
- Cast immobilization
- Olecranon pin traction
- Cuff and sling with extreme flexion especially in cases of "bag of bones."

Operative Treatment

Open reduction and internal fixation

Goal:
- Anatomical restoration of the joint surface
- Stable internal fixation
- Early motion

Indication

Displaced reconstructible fracture.

Preferred approach: Posterior approach with an olecranon osteotomy (Chevron)

Methods of fixation:
- Interfragmentary screws
- Dual plate fixation:
    - Pre-contoured or 3.5 mm compression plates are preferable to 1/3rd tubular and 3.5-mm reconstruction plates
    - One plate medially and another plate placed postero-laterally, 90° from the medial plate
- Total elbow arthroplasty or TER (semi-constrained): in markedly comminuted fractures and with fractures in severely osteopenic bone.

Postoperative Treatment

- Elbow is immobilized in extension (long-term immobilization should be avoided).
- Drain is removed 2 days after surgery
- Range of motion is begun 3 days after surgery.
- No bracing is used.

Complication

- Post-traumatic arthritis
- Implant failure
- Heterotopic bone formation
- Neurologic injury: Ulnar nerve is most commonly injured especially during surgical exposure

Q.6: Write short note on: a. Trochlea fracture; b. Capitellum fracture

a. Trochlea Fracture

Incidence

- It is also known as *Laugier fracture*.
- Extremely rare
- Associated with elbow dislocation

Mechanism of Injury

Tangential shearing force during an elbow dislocation.

Treatment

Undisplaced Fractures

- Immobilized in posterior splint for 3 weeks
- After 3 weeks, remove the splint and encourage-of-motion exercises.

Displaced Fractures

- ORIF with K-wire or screw fixation.
- Fragments not amenable to internal fixation should be excised.

Complications

- Post-traumatic arthritis
- Restricted range of motion (result from malunion)

b. Capitellum Fracture

Incidence

- Accounts for <1% of all elbow fractures.
- Always intra-articular.

Mechanism of Injury

- A fall onto an outstretched hand with the elbow in varying degrees of flexion
- Resulting force is transmitted through the radial head to the capitellum.
- Fracture occurs secondary to shearing force.
- Sometimes associated with radial head fractures.

Clinical Features

- Pain
- Swelling
- Tenderness over the lateral aspect of the elbow
- Haemarthrosis (joint effusion)
- Anterior displacement of the articular fragment into the coronoid or radial fossae may cause block to flexion.
- Posterior displacement limits the extension.
- Painful restriction of elbow movements.

Radiographic Evaluation

True lateral view of elbow. Presence of Mckay's "Double arc sign" is characteristic.

Classification

- Type I: *Hahn-Steinthal fragment*: large osseous component of capitellum
- Type II: *Kocher-Lorenz fragment*: articular cartilage with minimal subchondral bone attached: "uncapping of the condyle"
- Type III: Markedly comminuted

Treatment

Nonoperative

- Undisplaced fractures.
- Splinting in a posterior splint for 3 weeks followed by active range of elbow motion.

Operative

Open reduction and internal fixation:
- Indicated in displaced fracture
- ORIF with screws placed from a posterior to anterior direction or headless screws placed from anterior to posterior

Excision

- Indicated for severely comminuted type I fractures and most type II fractures.
- It is relatively contraindicated in the presence of associated elbow fractures as it results in elbow instability.

Complication

- Posttraumatic arthritis
- Osteonecrosis
- Cubitus valgus (usually after excision of the fragment) may be associated with tardy ulnar nerve palsy.

ELBOW DISLOCATION

Q1. Discuss the types, clinical features and management of dislocation of elbow.

- Elbow is the second most common joint dislocated in adults.
- ~ 20% of dislocations are associated with fractures.

Anatomy

- Elbow joint is a modified hinge joint.
- The three separate articulations are:
  - Ulno-humeral (hinge).
  - Radio-humeral (rotation).
  - Proximal radio-ulnar (rotation).
- Structures impart stability to joint are: Joint congruity, ligamentous structures and opposing action/tension of extensors and flexors.

Mechanism of Injury

- This is due to fall on outstretched hand or on the elbow (most common).
- Posterior dislocation is a combination of valgus stress, elbow hyperextension, arm abduction, and forearm supination.
- Anterior dislocation is due to direct force that strikes the posterior forearm when the elbow is in a flexed position.

Types

Depending on the position of the olecranon and head of radius:
- Anterior
- Posterior (most common)

It may be isolated or part of complex injury with associated fracture of olecranon, coronoid process, head/neck of radius or side-swipe injury.

Clinical Features

- The most common is posterior dislocation and is diagnosed by obvious posterior prominence of olecranon elbow flexed at 130°, with severe pain, spasm and immobility.
- The three bony point's relationship is reversed.
- There is often associated median nerve palsy. Always look for damage to ulnar and median nerve.
- Anterior dislocation is often associated with fracture olecranon.

Associated Injuries

- Associated fractures most often involve the radial head and/or coronoid process of the ulna.
- Acute neurovascular injuries are uncommon; the ulnar nerve and anterior interosseous branches of the median nerve are most commonly involved.
- With an open dislocation, there may be risk of injury to the brachial artery.

Radiographs

Standard anteroposterior and lateral radiographs of the elbow joint to assess the dislocation and other associated injuries.

Classifications

Based on the direction of displacement of the ulna relative to the humerus:
- Posterior
- Posterolateral
- Posteromedial
- Lateral
- Medial
- Anterior

Management

Nonoperative

Acute Episode

- Closed reduction under GA by gentle traction in the line of deformity and gradual flexion of elbow, beyond 90°.
- Neurovascular status should be reassessed, followed by evaluation of stability of elbow joint during full range of elbow motion.
- Post-reduction radiographs should be advised.
- POP post-slab for three weeks and followed by active physiotherapy.

Operative

Indications:
- Unstable reduction
- Unreduced dislocation
- Late presenting cases
- Associated injuries

Unstable reduction: Cross pinning of the joint.

Unreduced dislocation or late presenting cases:
- Unreduced dislocation may require *Open Reduction and V-Y Lengthening of Triceps Muscles* by post approach.
- Hotchkiss reported good results in unreduced dislocations treated by *hinged external fixation* to maintain joint reduction, to enhance muscle-tendon and stretching to permit motion.
- Unreduced dislocation for longer than 3 months will require some type of *elbow arthroplasty or arthrodesis*.

Other associated injuries: Fixation of associated fracture of ulna and dislocation.

Complications

- *Bones*: Associated fractures are olecranon, coronoid, supracondylar humerus and head of radius.
- *Joint*:
  - Unreduced dislocation
  - Stiff elbow
- *Muscle*: Myositis ossificans due to repeated manipulation and massage by bone -setters or quacks.
- *Vessel*:
  - Damage to brachial artery leading to VIC.
  - Compartment pressure monitoring and Serial neurovascular examinations may be necessary
- *Nerve*: Damage to median and ulnar nerve.

Q2. What is terrible triad of Hotchkiss?

It is triad of *posterior dislocation of elbow, radial head fracture and coronoid fracture*.

OLECRANON

Q1. Discuss the clinical features, classification and management of olecranon fracture.

Olecranon fracture may be:
- Isolated
- Part of complex injury: Fracture olecranon with anterior dislocation of elbow side-swipe injury (associated fracture of ulna and humerus).

Types

- Avulsion
- Transverse
- Comminuted

Mechanism of Injury

- Injury to elbow due to fall or blow to a flexed elbow.
- A fall onto the outstretched upper extremity accompanied by a sudden contraction of the triceps typically results in a oblique or transverse fracture.
- Epileptic seizures.

Clinical Features

- Patients present with the injured extremity supported by the contralateral hand with the elbow in relative flexion.
- Pain
- Boggy swelling over posterior side of elbow, palpable gap in the posterior border of olecranon
- Effusion
- Three bony points of elbow are disturbed.
- Inability to extend the elbow.

X-ray

- Standard anteroposterior and true lateral radiographs of the elbow joint.
- To see the type of fracture and decide appropriate treatment.
- To rule out associated injuries.
- Always keep in mind—'Patella cubitae' (where developmentally two separate centers of ossification are present) and may be mistaken for fracture in a child. In such situation, it is always advisable to take X-rays of the other uninjured elbow.

Classification

Schatzker Classification

Based on fracture pattern:
- Transverse
- Transverse-impacted
- Oblique
- Comminuted fractures with associated injuries
- Oblique-distal
- Fracture-dislocation

Colton Classification

- Nondisplaced fractures (<2 mm)
- Displaced fractures (avulsion fractures)
- Oblique and transverse fractures
- Comminuted fractures
- Fracture dislocation

Principles of Treatment

- Accurate Reduction.
- Restoration of the articular surface.
- To provide a stable elbow with good range of motion and power of extension.

- Early Mobilization.
- Prevention of complications

Treatment

Conservative

Indicated in:
- Nondisplaced fractures
- Displaced fractures in poorly functioning elderly.

Method of immobilization:
- Immobilization in a long arm cast with the elbow in 45–90° of flexion.
- Posterior slab or orthosis with gradual initiation of range of motion after 5–7 days.

Follow-up radiographs: It should be done within 5–7 days after treatment to rule out any fracture displacement.

Operative Treatment

Indicated in:
- Displaced fracture (>2 mm)
- Disruption of the extensor mechanism.

Operative treatments commonly used are:
- Open reduction and fixation with a figure-of-eight wire loop.
- Medullary fixation.
- Combination of intramedullary K-wires or screw and tension bands.
- Contoured plate and screws.
- Excision of the proximal fragment.

Choice of method depends on:
- Nature and location of the fracture.
- Amount of comminution.
- Age of the patient.

Avulsion fracture:
- Excision of fragments with triceps repair.
- Immobilize by posterior slab in 45° extension for 3 weeks followed by gentle active elbow movements.

Transverse fracture:
- Tension band wiring with intramedullary K-wires or cancellous olecranon screw fixation (6.5 mm AO cancellous screw).
- A posterior slab is applied with the elbow at 90°.
- At 7–10 days, gentle active and active-assisted motions are started, once the wound is healing satisfactorily.
- The elbow is supported between exercise periods with a removable splint.
- Usually support can be discontinued by 4 weeks postoperatively.

Principal of tension band wiring: It counteracts the tensile forces and converts them to compressive forces.

Comminuted fracture or comminution with bone loss:
- Contoured plates and screws provide rigid fixation
- Plate is applied most easily on the posterior surface
- Unicortical screws are used near the articular surface

Contoured plate and screws indicted in:
- Comminuted olecranon fractures
- Monteggia fractures
- Olecranon fracture-dislocations

Excision of the proximal fragment with triceps repair: Excision of as much as 50% of olecranon is sufficiently effective in treating comminuted fractures.

Method of choice in the following circumstances:
- In severely comminuted fractures in which open reduction and internal fixation are not technically possible
- In non-articular fractures
- After failed ORIF
- In nonunions
- In type III open fractures
- If local soft-tissue conditions are precarious, and the subcutaneous location of the internal fixation implant might create a problem.

Contraindication

Contraindicated in:
- Fracture-dislocations of the elbow
- Fractures of the radial head

  In these cases, excision results in compromised elbow stability

Complications

- Implant symptoms occur in 22–80% of patients.
- Require implant removal.
- Implant failure
- Infection pin migration occurs in 15%.
- Ulnar neuritis
- Heterotopic ossification
- Nonunion
- Decreased range of motion: This may complicate up to 50% of cases, particularly loss of elbow extension, although most patients note little if any functional limitation.

RADIAL HEAD

Q1. Discuss in brief the relevant anatomy, clinical feature and management of radial head and neck fracture.

Radial Head and Neck Fracture

- Epiphyseal injuries of childhood—Type II.
- Fracture in adults with or without displacement.

Anatomy

- The radial head articulates with capitellum.
- The radial head and capitellum are reciprocally curved.

- Transmission of Force across the radiocapitellar articulation occurs at all angles of elbow flexion and is greatest in fully extended elbow.
- Accurate anatomic positioning in the lesser sigmoid notch is essential for full rotation of the head of the radius.
- Though there is controversy, radial head plays a role in valgus stability of the elbow.

Mechanisms of Injuries

- Fall on the outstretched hand.
- It is associated with injury to the ligamentous structures of the elbow.

Types

- Chisel split (type I)
- Marginal (type II)
- Comminuted (type III)

Clinical Features

- Fullness of radial fossa, lateral to the triceps insertion.
- Swollen painful elbow.
- Limitation of forearm movements
- Palpable bony crepitus
- Tenderness present as thumb is pressed over the head of radius when forearm is rotated.

X-ray

- Standard anteroposterior (AP) and lateral radiographs of elbow in full pronation/ supination to the see the head all over, type of fracture and extent of displacement.
- Sometime CT scan may be required, especially in cases of gross comminution or fragment displacement for further fracture definition before preoperative planning.

Classification (Mason)

- Type I: Non-displaced fractures
- Type II: Marginal fractures with displacement (depression, impaction, angulation, segmental)
- Type III: Comminuted fractures involving the entire head
- Type IV: Associated with dislocation of the elbow (Johnston)

Treatment

Treatment varies with the type of fracture and age of patient.

Goal

- Correction of any mechanical block to forearm rotation
- Early and full range of elbow and forearm motion
- Stability of the elbow joint and forearm

Children

- Reduction of the displaced epiphysis (head of radius) open or closed and if necessary, fixed it with K-wire.

- Excision of radial head should never be advised in children because it is a growing end, as growth occurs the radius is liable to ride up toward the humerus with consequent disturbance of its relationship to the ulna, the inferior radioulnar joint subluxates and rotation become limited.

Adults

Conservative management:
- Especially for type I fracture.
- Most isolated fractures of the radial head can be treated conservatively.
- Symptomatic management comprises of a sling and early range of motion 24–48 hours after injury as pain subsides.
- Aspiration of the radiocapitellar joint has been advised by some authors for pain relief.

Posterior slab for 3 weeks if:
- Chisel split or type I fracture
- Undisplaced marginal fracture of head and fracture neck with tilt <15°.

Operative indications

The following fractures require operation:
- Fractures with gross comminution.
- Fractures of the margin involving >1/3rd of the articular surface, particularly if the fracture involves the radioulnar joint.
- Fractures with loose bony fragments in the elbow joint.
- Fractures of the neck with angulation that interfere with rotation.

Open reduction and internal fixation: Uncomminuted isolated or minimally comminuted fractures can be treated by *ORIF with mini AO screws, Herbert screws, or Acutrak screw.*

Excision of head (excised just proximal to the annular ligament) if:
- Comminuted fracture
- Displaced fracture head and neck in adults.
- If the radial head fracture is technically irreparable.

Postoperative treatment

- Posterior plaster slab at 90°.
- At about 1 week, the slab is removed, and the arm is supported in a sling.
- Active and active-assisted exercises advised.
- Discontinue the sling at about 3 weeks
- Gradually increasing the exercises as tolerated.

Excision and Prosthetic Replacement
- Indicated in Mason type III fractures with associated instability and Mason type IV fracture-dislocations.
- The rationale for use is to prevent proximal migration of the radius.
- Metallic (titanium, vitallium) radial head implants are superior to silicon implants.

Complications

- *Joint stiffness*:
  - *Radioulnar:* Limitation of supination and pronation.
  - *Radiohumeral:* Limitation of flexion and extension.

- Myositis ossificans around the head of radius and stiff elbow.
- Proximal migration of radius with subluxation of wrist, following excision of head of radius, hence, it is always better to wait for a few days to allow the interosseous ligament to recover and then do excision.
- Reflex sympathetic dystrophy very rarely following surgical interventions.
- Injury to posterior interosseous nerve.

RADIUS AND ULNA

Q1. Discuss the clinical features and management of fracture shaft radius and ulna.

Anatomy

Types

- Children: Greenstick fracture.
- Adults: Transverse, spiral, displaced, comminuted, segmental.
- Single bone.
- Both bones.
- Fracture of one bone with dislocation of proximal/distal radioulnar joint.

Mechanism of Injury

Fall on outstretched hand, direct blow, crushing injury.

Clinical Features

- Swelling
- Deformity
- Shortening
- Painful restriction of all movements,
- Palpable crepitus.
- Always examine the distal pulsation and sensation.

X-ray

Full length of radius and ulna, including the elbow and wrist joint AP and lateral view.

Principles of Treatment

- To restore accurate anatomical alignment of both bones and joints.
- Maintenance of interosseous space.
- Full range of hand and forearm movements with adequate power

Treatment

Children with greenstick fracture

Correction of the deformity under anaesthesia and AE POP cast for 6 weeks.

Always note while treating a fracture radius, in AE POP Cast.

- *Fracture of upper third*: The proximal fragment is supinated due to the strong supinators; hence *immobilize the forearm in full supination* so that the two fragments are well aligned.

- *In lower third*: As there are strong pronators, *immobilize in pronation.*
- *In middle third*: As there is balance between the supinators and the pronators, *mid-prone position* should be kept for immobilization in AE POP cast.

  In any case, when the forearm is in the cast, active movements of the shoulder and the fingers should be encouraged to avoid stiffness.

Adults

Even in spite of good position, the chances of displacement are there, hence open reduction and internal fixation is always best.

Simple

Intramedullary nailing: *Intramedullary square nail or interlocking nail* for distal one-third ulna and proximal two-thirds radius (narrow medullary canal).

Indications for intramedullary nailing of forearm fractures are:
- Segmental fractures
- Poor skin conditions (e.g. burns)
- Selected nonunions or failed compression platings
- Multiple injuries
- Diaphyseal fractures in osteopenic patients
- Selected type I and type II diaphyseal fractures (non-reamed nails are used)
- Massive compound injuries for which non-reamed ulnar nails can be used as an internal splint to maintain forearm length while soft-tissue loss is treated

Contraindication for intramedullary nailing:
- Active infection
- Medullary canal smaller than 3 mm
- Open physis

Plating: *Plating (3.5-mm AO dynamic compression plate)* with screws is best for, upper third of ulna and lower third of radius (wide marrow cavity). It provides rigid fixation and can withstand rotational distortion.

Principles of plating: Principles of plate fixation:
- Restore ulnar and radial length to prevent subluxation of either the superior or the inferior radioulnar joint.
- Restore rotational alignment.
- Restore radial bow that is essential for rotational function of the forearm.

Open fractures: External fixators (JESS).

Complications

Bone

- Delayed union.
- *Nonunion:* Due to soft tissue entrapment or bone loss.
- *Malunion:*
  - Angulatory.
  - Rotational
  - Cross union: Union through the interosseous space between radius and ulna.

Joint

Stiffness of hand and fingers.

Vessels

VIC, compartmental syndrome.

Muscle

Myositis.

Tendons

Entrapment of the tendons in between the fracture fragments.

Q2. Discuss briefly the Monteggia fracture-dislocation.

First described by Monteggia as fracture of the upper third ulna and dislocation of head of radius in 1814.

Mechanism of Injury

- Direct blow in front or behind the upper third, fall on outstretched hand with forearm pronated.
  As per Bado classification the various mechanism results in Monteggia fracture and dislocation
  - **Type I:** Forced pronation of the forearm
  - **Type II:** Axial loading of the forearm with a flexed elbow
  - **Type III:** Forced abduction of the elbow
  - **Type IV:** Type I mechanism in which the radial shaft additionally fails

Clinical Features

- Deformity of proximal ulna.
- Head of radius palpable in abnormal position (anterior, posterior, lateral).
- Movements of elbow and forearm restricted, painful with shortening of forearm.
- Neurovascular examination is necessary, as there may be risk of nerve injury, especially to the radial or posterior interosseous nerve, especially with type II Bado fractures.

X-ray

- Full-length forearm with elbow (AP and lateral view).
- To avoid missing of diagnosis of radial head dislocation on X-rays, Maclaughlin's line is usually employed. The radial head must always line up with the capitellum on all lateral radiographs, no matter in what position the elbow is placed and this line is Maclaughlin's line.

Classification

Bado Classification of Monteggia Fractures

- Type I: Anterior dislocation of the radial head with fracture of ulnar diaphysis at any level with anterior angulation (most common type)
- Type II: Posterior/posterolateral dislocation of the radial head with fracture of ulnar diaphysis with posterior angulation

- Type III: Lateral/anterolateral dislocation of the radial head with fracture of ulnar metaphysis
- Type IV: Anterior dislocation of the radial head with fractures of both radius (below the bicipital tuberosity) and ulna within proximal third at the same level

Treatment

These fracture-dislocation usually can be treated conservatively in children, but routinely requires open reduction in adults

Anterior type which is the most common:
- In pediatric population, close reduction under anaesthesia— immobilization in A/E slab with forearm fully supinated with 90° flexion at the elbow.
- In adult rigid fixation of the fracture of the ulna with 3.5 mm DCP, closed reduction of the radial head, and immobilization of the elbow for 6 weeks in a position of flexion above 90° with the forearm supinated.
- If closed reduction fails then open reduction of head of radius and DCP fixation of ulna should be done.

In old unreduced dislocation: Excision of head of radius and realignment of ulna and fixation by dynamic compression plate should be done and is supplemented by cancellous bone grafts if required.

After-treatment

- At 2 weeks: POP slab and suture are removed and usually a long-arm cast is applied.
- At 4 weeks, the cast is removed, and the extremity is supported with a collar and cuff sling, maintaining the elbow at 110–120°.
- Gentle pronation and supination motions started.
- After 6 weeks extension permitted.

Complications

Bone

- Malunion
- Nonunion of ulna
- Persistence of the dislocation of head of radius.
- Traumatic ossification around head of radius.

Joint

- Stiffness
- Loss of flexion/extension at elbow, supination/pronation of forearm.

Q3. Write short note on Galeazzi fracture-dislocation.

Fracture of the lower third radius with dislocation of the distal radio-ulnar joint. Campbell called Galeazzi or Piedmont fractures "the fracture of necessity" because it requires open reduction and internal fixation to achieve a good result.

Mechanism of Injury

- Direct trauma
- Indirect trauma, such as a fall onto an outstretched hand

Deforming forces includes:
- *Weight* of hand
- *Pronators:* causes pronation, dorsal and volar displacement.
- *Brachioradialis:* causes proximal displacement and shortening.
- *Thumb extensors and abductors:* shortening and relaxation of the radial collateral ligament causes displacement despite adequate immobilization.

Clinical Features

- Wrist pain or forearm pain that is exacerbated by stressing of the inferior radioulnar joint in addition to the radial shaft fracture.
- Deformity of the forearm in the lower third and subluxation of inferior radioulnar joint so that the two styloid processes come to lie in the same plane.
- There is bony crepitus and loss of transmitted movements of the radius.

X-ray

- AP and lateral radiograph of forearm, elbow, and wrist joint.
- To see the type of fracture and decide the line of treatment.

Radiographic signs suggesting inferior radio-ulnar joint injury are:
- Fracture base of the ulnar styloid process.
- Increased distal radio-ulnar joint space on AP X-ray.
- Subluxation of ulna on lateral X-ray.
- >5 mm of radial shortening.

Treatment

- Conservative treatment is associated with a higher failure rate.
- Open reduction of the radial shaft fracture through standard anterior Henry approach and internal fixation with a 3.5 mm AO dynamic compression plate is the treatment of choice in adults.
- Rigid anatomical fixation generally reduces the inferior radioulnar joint dislocation.
- If this joint is still unstable, it should be temporarily transfixed with a single 'K' wire with the forearm in full supination.

After treatment

Depends upon the status of distal radioulnar joint:
- If joint is stable: Early motion is recommended.
- If joint is unstable: Immobilize the forearm in supination for 4–6 weeks in a long arm splint or cast.
- Transfixing Distal radioulnar joint pins, if needed, are removed at 6–8 weeks

Complications

Bone

- Nonunion of the radius
- Malunion leading to loss of supination pronation of forearm.
- Radioulnar synostosis (uncommon)

Joint

Persistence of subluxation of inferior radioulnar joint.

DISTAL RADIUS

Q1. Discuss clinical features and management of Colles' fracture.

Abraham Colles describe this fracture in 1814. This is the most common of all fractures after the age of 40, invariably associated with osteoporosis.

Definition

Fracture of lower end of the radius, within an inch of the distal articulating surface with subluxation of inferior radioulnar joint with or without fracture of ulnar styloid.

Mechanism of injury

Fall on outstretched hands with the wrist in dorsiflexion (most common).

Clinical Features

- Commonest fracture in elderly patients and women due to osteoporosis.
- Pain
- Wrist is swollen with ecchymosis
- Dinner fork deformity
- Tenderness
- Loss of all movements of wrist and hand.
- Both the styloid come to lie at the same level due to impaction and proximal shift of the fracture end of the radius (normally radial styloid is lower than ulnar).
- Neurovascular assessment should be done, with particular attention to median nerve function

X-ray

Standard AP and lateral view of wrist joint

Normal anatomy of the wrist joint:
- Radial angulation—23°
- Radial length—12 mm
- Palmar angulation—11–12°

X-ray is done: To see the displacement and the associated fracture.

Classical displacements (six deformities) of the distal fragment are:
- *Impaction*
- *Dorsal tilt and shift*
- *Lateral tilt and shift*
- *Supination.*

   Additional findings may be, fracture ulnar styloid, subluxation of inferior radioulnar joint.

Classification

Frykman Classification of Colles' Fractures
This is based on the pattern of intra-articular involvement.

Fracture	*Distal ulna*	
	Absent	*Present*
Extra-articular	I	II
Intra-articular involving radiocarpal joint	III	IV
Intra-articular involving distal radioulnar joint (DRUJ)	V	VI
Intra-articular involving radiocarpal and DRUJ	VII	VIII

Management

Aim

- Restore fully functional hand and forearm
- Restore full range of movement
- No deformity

Nonoperative

Indications:
- Undisplaced or minimally displaced fractures.
- Displaced fractures with a stable fracture pattern

Closed reduction and cast application:
- Closed reduction *(traction, counter traction and manipulation)* under general anesthesia.
- Well-moulded and padded below elbow POP cast or colles cast in ~*10–15° palmar flexion* and ~*20° ulnar deviation* (*Cotton-Loder position*) extending upto the proximal palmar crease for 4–6 weeks.
- The cast should leave the metacarpophalangeal joints free.
- Completed cast must allow free movement of the elbow joint and metacarpophalangeal joint.
- Extreme flexion of wrist should be avoided, because it increases the risk of carpal canal pressure (and thus median nerve compression) as well as digital stiffness.
- Check radiographs during follow-up period to assess any significant displacement.

Operative

Indications:
- High-energy injury
- Secondary loss of reduction
- Articular comminution
- Metaphyseal comminution or bone loss
- Loss of volar buttress with displacement
- Distal radioulnar joint incongruity

Unstable fractures

- Percutaneous K-wire fixation (Closed reduction followed by percutaneous pinning of the distal radius through the radial styloid) or Kapandji pinning.
- JESS distractor (Ligamentotaxis is used to restore radial length and radial inclination,)
- AO distractor
- Buttress plating (Ellis plating, if associated with Barton's variety)

Indication for external fixators
- Open fracture
- Comminuted fractures with dorsal angulation of 25°
- Radial shortening of more than 10 mm
- Marked comminution with intra-articular fragments
- Loss of reduction after closed treatment
- Bilateral Colles' fractures

***Malunited fracture** with painful limitation of wrist movement and pronation/supination:*
- Corrective Osteotomy *(Fernandez (dorsal wedge osteotomy), Campbell (lateral wedge osteotomy)*, fixation and grafting
- *Darrach's excision* of distal ulna.

Complication

The most important complication is *stiffness of wrist, fingers and malunion. Finger stiffness* is the commonest complication while *nonunion* is least common.

Bone

- Malunion of radius
- Nonunion of ulnar styloid
- Subluxation of inferior radioulnar joint

Joint

- *Sudeck's atrophy* (this is *painful reflex sympathetic osteodystrophy* and presents as extremely painful and swollen hand and stiff fingers. X-ray shows *patchy osteoporosis* around the wrist). This is treated by physiotherapy and exercises.
- Shoulder hand syndrome, the hand and shoulder is stiff after the injury due to immobilization.
- Post-traumatic osteoarthritis

Tendon

Rupture of extensor pollices longus after a few weeks, due to friction at fracture site, near the Lister's tubercle.

Nerve

Carpal tunnel syndrome due to median nerve entrapment at the wrist.

Q2. Discuss in brief other fractures of distal end radius.

Fractures of distal end radius include:
- Smith fracture
- Barton fracture
- Fracture of radial styloid process
- Epiphyseal Injuries

Smith Fracture

- It is described by Smith.
- It is reverse Colles.

- It is caused by fall on the dorsum of the flexed wrist with the forearm fixed in supination.
- It differs from the Colles' fracture in that is ventral displacement of the distal fragment and is associated with ventral tilt, which is also known as *"Garden-spade deformity"*
- Treatment consists of manipulation and immobilization in an above-elbow POP cast with the wrist dorsiflexed and forearm supinated.
- It is a notoriously unstable fracture, which frequently requires ORIF because of difficulty in maintaining adequate closed reduction.
- ORIF can be done with ELLIS buttress plate fixation.

Barton Fracture

- Barton describes it in 1838.
  - Anterior marginal type—volar Barton fracture
  - Posterior marginal type—dorsal Barton fracture
- It is caused by fall on a dorsiflexed wrist with the forearm fixed in pronation.
- It is a intra-articular marginal fracture of the radius with subluxation of the wrist and inferior radioulnar joints.
- The carpus and the hand are displaced forwards with large marginal fragment with the fracture extending into the wrist joint.
- The treatment is similar to that of Smith's fracture discussed earlier.

Fracture of Radial Styloid Process

- Chauffeur's fracture, Back-fire fracture, and Hutchinson fracture.
- It is an avulsion fracture with extrinsic ligaments remaining attached to the styloid fragment.
- It is caused by compression of the scaphoid against styloid with the wrist in dorsiflexion and ulnar deviation.
- The injury is caused by forced radial deviation of the wrist and may occur after a fall or when the starting handle kicks back—so called the *Chauffeur's fracture.*
- It is often associated with intercarpal ligamentous injuries.
- *Treatment*:
  - Minimal displacement: immobilization of the wrist in plaster cast (Colles' cast) for 6 weeks
  - If not managed in cast: ORIF.

Epiphyseal Injuries

- Occurs in older children whose lower radial epiphysis as not yet fused.
- Caused by fall on an outstretched hand.
- Separation is adjacent to the epiphyseal disc (not through it)
- The line of cleavage is on the metaphyseal side of the epiphyseal plate so the cartilage cells are undamaged.
- Physeal fractures are mostly *Salter Harris type 1 or type 2* with the epiphysis tilted backwards and radially.
- Type V injuries are unusual and are diagnosed in retrospect when premature epiphyseal fusion occurs.
- Metaphyseal injures may appear as mere buckling of the cortex, greenstick fractures or complete fractures with displacement and shortening

- They can be missed easily however can be visualized when the appropriate views are available.
- Treatment:
  - Physeal fractures are reduced under anesthesia by pressure over the distal fragment.
  - The arm is immobilized with the wrist slightly *flexed and ulnar deviated* and the elbow at 90°.
  - The cast is retained for 4 weeks.
  - These fractures very rarely interfere with growth.
  - Even if reduction is nor perfect, further growth and remodelling prevents any deformity.

WRIST AND HAND

Q1. Write in brief the clinical features and management of scaphoid fracture.

Fracture of the scaphoid bone is the most common fracture of the carpus and account for about 50–80% of carpal injuries. Delay in the diagnosis and treatment of scaphoid fracture may alter the prognosis for union.

Incidence

- Most common carpal bone fracture.
- Age: it is most common in young men though it has been reported in individuals ranging from 10 to 70 years old.

Mechanism of Injury

This is due to fall on the outstretched palm, resulting in severe hyperextension and slight radial deviation of the wrist joint.

Anatomy and Blood Supply

- The precarious blood supply of the scaphoid predisposes fracture of this carpal bone to AVN, delayed union or nonunion, disability of the wrist joint.
- As scaphoid articulates with the distal radius and with four of the seven carpal bones any alteration of its articular surface due to fracture, subluxation or dislocation results in severe secondary changes

Blood supply

- 67% of scaphoid bones have: arterial foramina throughout the length
- 13% have: blood supply predominantly in the distal third
- 20% have most of the arterial foramina in the waist area
- No more than a single foramen near the proximal one-third of bone

This shows that fractures at proximal third results in osteonecrosis in 35% of cases. Due to inadequate blood supply these fracture take longer to heal and usually have higher rates of nonunion.

Clinical Features

- Pain, swelling and tenderness in the anatomical snuff box
- Loss of grip
- Wrist movements are painful.

Clinical Tests

- *Scaphoid lift test*: Reproduction of pain with dorsal-volar shifting of the scaphoid.
- *Watson test*: Painful dorsal scaphoid displacement while moving wrist from ulnar to radial deviation with compression of the tuberosity.

Radiographic Evaluation

- PA and lateral views of the hand/wrist
- *Oblique views*: 45° supination and pronation
- Clinched fist view
- Scaphoid view: ulnar deviation/wrist extension
- Plain radiographs may be falsely negative in 35–75% of cases

Even if the X-ray is negative and the patient has tenderness in the anatomical snuff-box, he is treated as fracture scaphoid. Immobilize the wrist in a cast or splint for 2 weeks and obtain follow-up radiographs.

Triple Phase Bone Scan

- Should be positive within 24 hours and always positive within 48 hours.
- Dynamic flow images are most reliable in acute fractures of the scaphoid.
- Useful in shortening the duration of immobilization without fracture and also decreasing complication rate in case of fracture unrecognized by plain films.

CT (in the Sagittal Plane of the Scaphoid)

- Best for surgical planning and accurate assessment of fracture, displacement, angulation
- Greater sensitivity and specificity than bone scan.

MRI

- MRI, especially with gadolinium enhancement, also is useful in assessing the vascularity of a fractured scaphoid
- The gold standard investigation
- Sensitivity: 100%; hence allows early exclusion of occult fracture.
- Accurately detects presence of other occult fractures about the wrist.

Classifications

Based on location or Anatomical classification (Weissman and Sledge):
- Waist: 66–70%
- Transverse: 45–48%
- Tuberosity: 17–20%
- Horizontal oblique: 13–14%
- Distal pole: 10–12%
- Vertical oblique: 8–9%
- Proximal pole: 5–7%

Based on displacement (Cooney, Dobyns and Linschield)
- Stable: undisplaced fractures
- Unstable: displacement with:
    - >1 mm step-off on AP and oblique view

- Scapholunate angulation is >45° in the lateral view
- Lunocapitate angulation is >15°

Based on fracture pattern (Russe)
- Horizontal oblique (distal third, middle third and proximal third)
- Transverse
- Vertical oblique

Treatment

Conservative Management

Indications for conservative treatment
- Nondisplaced distal third fracture
- Tuberosity fractures

Nondisplaced, Stable Scaphoid Fractures

Scaphoid cast: For 6 weeks:
- Started just below the elbow proximally to the base of the thumbnail (incorporating the proximal phalanx of thumb) and the proximal palmar crease distally.
- Wrist in slight radial deviation and in dorsi flexion.
- Hand in glass holding position.
- Thumb is maintained in a functional position
- Fingers are free to move from the metacarpophalangeal joints distally

   Review after 6 weeks and if evidence of delayed union is seen, one more cast for another 6 weeks.

Operative Treatment

Indications for surgery:
- >1 mm step-off on AP and oblique view
- Scapholunate angulation is >45° in the lateral view
- Luno-capitate angulation is >15°
- Nonunion
- "Humpback" deformity

Techniques

- *Open techniques (ORIF with screw or K wires)* are needed for nonunions and fractures with gross displacement. *Closed techniques (CRIF)* are best suited for acute fractures with minimal displacement.
- Most involve the insertion of screws commonly used are the *AO screw, the Acutrak screw, and the Herbert-Whipple screw.*
- *Postoperative immobilization consists of a long arm thumb spica cast for 6 weeks.*

Advantages of the Herbert Screw

- Reduces the time of external immobilization
- Provides relatively strong internal fixation
- Produces compression at the fracture site.
- The headless screw remains below the bone surface, removal usually is unnecessary.

Complications

Bone

- Delayed union
- Nonunion (treated by Herbert screw fixation with bone grafting)
- Avascular necrosis of the proximal pole (the vascular supply of scaphoid is distal to proximal, hence fracture waist of scaphoid causes AVN of the proximal pole

Joint

- Osteoarthritis of the wrist and intercarpal joints causing loss of power of grip.
- If associated with unbearable pain, then it is managed by arthodesis of wrist or proximal row carpectomy.

Q2. Write short note on Bennett's fracture.

Bennett's fracture is an *intra-articular fracture* through the base of the first metacarpal in which the shaft is laterally dislocated by the unopposed pull of the abductor pollicis longus.

Displacement: Displacement of Bennett fractures is due to unopposed pull primarily by the abductor pollicis longus and the adductor pollicis resulting in *flexion, supination, and proximal migration.*

Clinical Features

- Pain
- Swelling
- Tenderness at the base of the carpometacarpal joint
- Weakness of pinch and of grip
- Painful movements

Radiographic Evaluation

Standard AP and lateral view of hand.

Treatment

Conservative

- CR is obtained with longitudinal traction with abduction and pronation of the thumb and pressure on the base of the metacarpal
- Reduction by traction is easy, but is difficult to maintain first metacarpal shaft is displaced by divergent pull of muscles.
- B/E spica POP cast with incorporation of thumb.

Operative

- Closed percutaneous pinning (described by Wagner) is the most preferred technique.
- Check the reduction pon by radiographs.
- Apply a forearm cast or BE thumb spica, holding the wrist in extension and the thumb in abduction; the thumb interphalangeal joint is keep free.
- If the reduction is unsatisfactorily then open reduction and internal fixation by K-wire done.

Complication

- Malunion with persistent subluxation (treated by corrective osteotomy)
- Degenerative arthritis (managed by arthrodesis or arthroplasty)

Q3. What is Rolando fracture?

It is an *intra-articular 'Y-shaped' comminuted* fracture involving the base of the thumb metacarpal that usually not results in diaphyseal displacement as in a Bennett fracture. It was first, described by Rolando.

Treatment

- Aim: Because of the likelihood of post-traumatic arthritis after these fractures, accurate reduction is of paramount important
- Closed or open reduction and internal fixation by any of the following devices:
  - Use of small K-wires
  - Plate fixation with a mini-fragment T-plate if the articular fragments are of sufficient size.
  - Combination of tension band wiring and an external fixator.
- For severely comminuted fractures: combines external fixation, limited internal fixation, and bone grafting.

Q4. What is reverse Bennet fracture or ulnar bennet fracture?

It is an intra-articular fracture of base of 5th metacarpal bone. It is inherently unstable because the distal fragment is pulled by flexor carpi ulnaris.

Q5. Write short note on Gamekeeper's thumb.

An injury to the ulnar collateral ligament of the thumb metacarpophalangeal joint results in *Gamekeepers thumb*. Complete tear of ulnar collateral ligament with interposition of adductor pollicis constitutes *Stener lesion*.

Aetiology and Mechanism of Injury

- It is common during snow skiing accidents.
- It also occurs on fall on outstretched hand.
- Forceful palmar and radial abduction of the thumb results in *Gamekeepers thumb*.

Associated Injuries

Avulsion fractures, dorsal capsular tears and volar plate tears of the interphalangeal joint of the thumb.

Clinical Features

- Pain
- Tenderness over the ulnar aspect of interphalangeal joint.
- Sometimes on palpation there is a lump representing the torn ulnar collateral ligament, displaced by adductor pollicis.
- Painful movements.

Radiographic Evaluation

- AP view: $\leq$2 mm displaced fracture signifies a complete tear without Stener lesion.
- Stress AP view: To assess partial or complete tear.

Treatment

- Incomplete tear: Thumb spica usually for 4–6 weeks.
- Complete tear: repair of the ligament and older injuries requires palmaris longus graft, extensor pollicis brevis or a strip of fascia.

Q6. Write in brief the management of the metacarpal and phalangeal fractures.

Metacarpal Fracture

- *Undisplaced*: Dorsal slab, finger cot, ball and bandage.
- *Displaced*: ORIF with K-wires or fixators or mini-plate and screws.

Phalanx Fracture

- *Undisplaced*: Buddy strap two fingers together (injured + normal), finger splint/ball and bandage.
- *Displaced*: ORIF K-wire, with JESS frame for compound fracture.

Q7. Write in brief about baseball or mallet finger deformity.

Mallet finger is due to avulsion of the extensor tendon at the base of the distal phalanx causing inability to extend the distal phalanx, which in due course ends up with a flexion deformity of the terminal phalanx. Although closed injuries are more common, open injuries caused by crush abrasions and lacerations also occur.

Mechanism of Injury

- Forceful blow to the tip of the finger causing sudden flexion.
- Hyperextension injury with fracture of the dorsal lip of the distal phalanx.

Classification

- Type 1: Closed or blunt trauma with loss of tendon continuity with or without a small avulsion fracture (most common)
- Type 2: Laceration at or proximal to the distal interphalangeal joint with loss of tendon continuity
- Type 3: Deep abrasion with loss of skin, subcutaneous cover, and tendon substance
- Type 4:
    - 4A—transphyseal fracture in children (Seymore fractures)
    - 4B—hyperflexion injury with fracture of articular surface of ~20–50%
    - 4C—hyperextension injury with fracture of the articular surface >50% with early or late volar subluxation of the distal phalanx.

Treatment

- Type I:
    - Continuous DIP extension splinting with a molded polythene (Stack) or aluminum or frog splint for 6–8 weeks

- The splint keeps the proximal interphalangeal joints in flexion and the distal joint in hyperextension so as to repose the avulsed tendon along with its bony insertion in the distal phalanx.
- Type II:
  - Closed reduction after through wound debridement
  - Repair of the extensor tendon, using a roll stitch with K-wire fixation of the distal interphalangeal joint in full extension.
  - Splint and K-wire are removed at 6 weeks, and range-of-motion exercises are begun.
- Type III: Require soft-tissue coverage and pinning of the DIP joint and possible primary arthrodesis
- Type 4A: CR and splinting of the DIP joint in neutral or slight extension for 4 weeks
- Type 4B and 4C:
  - If Joint congruity is maintained then splinting only.
  - If joint is subluxates then open reduction using a pullout wire and transarticular K-wire in extension.
  - Splint and K-wire are removed at 6 weeks, and range-of-motion exercises are begun.

Q8. Write short note on trigger finger.

Tenosynovitis involving long flexor of thumb or finger causing locking of finger in flexion due to entrapment of the nodular tendonitis within its sheath. The term "triggering" is used because when the finger unlocks, it pops back suddenly and abruptly, as if releasing a trigger on a gun.

Aetiology

- Idiopathic
- It is often seen in diabetics.
- Stenosing tenosynovitis following trauma or unaccustomed activity.
- Rheumatoid tenosynovitis
- Middle-aged women are frequently the victim.
- Most commonly affected finger is the middle or ring finger.

Pathoanatomy

- Flexor tendon may become trapped at the portal of entry to its sheath; on forced extension, it passes the constriction with a snap i.e. *"triggering effect"*.
- Narrowing and thickening of the sheath, with occasional formation of a ganglion cyst.
- An intra-tendinous nodule may be palpated proximal to the first annular pulley opposite the head of the metacarpal or metacarpophalangeal joint.

Clinical Features

- It is characterized by snapping or locking of the involved finger flexor tendon, associated with dysfunction and pain.
- Extension of the involved finger is difficult and unequal so that the initial effort by the patient is insufficient to produce any extension and with further effort, it suddenly straightens with a snap.
- Sometimes patient has to straighten it passively.

Treatment

- *Early cases*: local steroid injection into the sheath of the tendon.
- *Refractory cases*: excision of the synovial sheath around the nodular tendonitis.
- Recent study shows: Most cost-effective treatment is *two trials of local corticosteroid injection, followed by open release of the first annular pulley.*
- In cases with *rheumatoid arthritis* the fibrous pulley must be preserved otherwise, its damage may result in ulnar deviation of the digits.

TENDON INJURIES

Q1. What are flexor tendon zones and pulleys?

Verdan divide the flexor surface into following five zones:
- Zone I—extends from just distal to the insertion of the sublimis tendon to the site of insertion of the profundus tendon.
- Zone II (critical area of pulleys)—is in the critical area of pulleys *(Bunnell's "no man's land")* between the distal palmar crease and the insertion of the sublimis tendon.
- Zone III—comprises the area of the lumbrical origin between the distal margin of the transverse carpal ligament and the beginning of the critical area of pulleys or first anulus.
- Zone IV—the zone covered by the transverse carpal ligament.
- Zone V—the zone proximal to the transverse carpal ligament and includes the forearm.

Importance of Zones

Zone II is the *"no man's land"* as this is the critical area of pulleys and primary repairs at this level usually fail because of adhesions in the area of the pulleys.

Pulleys

- There are fibrous pulleys namely A1 to A5. These fibrous pulleys hold the flexor tendons to the phalanges and prevent bowstringing during movements.
- A1, 3 and 5 are attached to the palmar plate near each joint.
- A2 and A4 have a crucial tethering effects and must always be preserved or reconstructed otherwise the tendon will bowstring and results in flexion deformity of the finger.

Extensor Tendon Zones

- Zone I is at the level of the DIP joint
- Zone II is the area over the middle phalanx
- Zone III is the area of the PIP joint.
- Zone IV includes the area over the proximal phalanx
- Zone V includes the area at the MCP joint

Q2. What are the principles of management of hand injuries and the discuss treatment of flexor tendon injury

Mechanism of injury

Crush, blast, mutilating injuries.

Principles of Management

- Thorough irrigation done, debride all devitalized tissue and salvage remaining parts, and give broad-spectrum antibiotics.

- Stabilize in functional position by K-wires or JESS frame.
- Mobilize uninjured joints.
- Prevent infection.
- Promote primary healing by primary/secondary skin cover.
- Repair of tendons and nerves.
- Restores function of pinch, grasp and grip.

Flexor Tendon Injury

Examination

- If the wound is distal to the wrist, the injured finger should be stabilized to obtain specific joint movements.
- With the PIP joint stabilized, the *flexor digitorum profundus* is presumed severed if the DIP joint cannot be actively flexed.
- If the *flexor superficialis* is injured, the DIP joint hyperflexes, and the PIP joint assumes an extended position.
- If neither the proximal nor the distal interphalangeal joint can be actively flexed with the metacarpophalangeal joint stabilized, both flexor tendons probably are severed.
- In the thumb if the *flexor pollicis longus* is severed, flexion at the interphalangeal joint is absent.

Purpose of Tendon Suturing

- To approximate the ends of a tendon
- To fasten one end of a tendon to adjoining tendons or to bone and to hold this position during the process of healing

Characteristics of an Ideal Tendon Repair

- Easy placement of sutures in the tendon
- Secure suture knots
- Smooth juncture of tendon ends
- Minimal gapping at the tendon repair site
- Minimal interference with tendon vascularity
- Adequate strength throughout healing to permit application of early motion stress to the tendon

Suture Material

- Braided polyethylene and braided stainless steel wire were most suitable mechanically.
- Braided polyester was intermediate
- Monofilament sutures of nylon and polypropylene are least satisfactory
- 3-0 suture may be useful to repair tendons in the forearm, palm, and larger digits, whereas a 4-0 suture may handle better in smaller digits.

Suture Configurations

Keeping aim of achieving strongest intratendinous suture arrangement to allow early passive and active motion, there are varieties of suture configurations at the repair site.

Group	Suture configurations
I	Simple sutures suture pull is parallel to the tendon collagen bundles
II	Bunnell suturestress is transmitted directly across the juncture by the suture material
III	Pulvertaft technique (fish-mouth weave) sutures are placed perpendicular to the tendon collagen bundles and the applied stress

Techniques for End-to-end Flexor Tendon Repair

- Bunnell
- Kessler grasping stitch
- Kessler-Tajima stitch
- Double loop
- Mason-Allen (Chicago) stitch
- Interlock stitch
- Tsuge stitch
- Bevel technique
- 4, 6 and 8-stranded repair

Types of Tendon Repair

Primary Repair

- It is done within the first 12 hours of injury.
- It can be extended to within 24 hours of injury in rare situations.
- *Delayed primary repair* is one that is done within 24 hours to approximately 10 days

Indications:

- Clean wound with tendon injury
- Clean wound with tendon injury combined with a neurovascular bundle injury
- Clean wound with a fracture if it can be fixed and stabilized satisfactorily

Secondary Repair

- If flexor tendons cannot be repaired within the first 10–14 days (delayed primary repair), the repair is considered to be secondary.
- Tendon repairs done between 10 days and 4 weeks as early secondary repairs
- Repairs done after 4 weeks as late secondary repairs.

Indication:

- Wound contamination
- Crushing or avulsing injuries
- Soft-tissue loss
- Multiple comminuted fractures
- Lack of available surgical skill
- Severe neurovascular injury
- Severe joint injury
- Skin loss requiring a coverage procedure, such as skin grafting or flap coverage.

Before going for secondary repair, certain requirements must be met:

- Wound erythema and swelling should be minimal
- Skin coverage must be adequate

- Tissues through which the tendon is expected to glide must be relatively free of scar
- Alignment of bones must be satisfactory, and any fractures must be healed or fixed securely.
- Joints must have a useful range of passive motion.
- Sensation in the involved digit must be undamaged or restored, or it should be possible to repair damaged nerves directly or with nerve grafts at the time of tendon repair.

After 1 month: Depend upon the status of scarring, disturbance of tendon sheath and joint mobility:

Tendon grafting (in order of preference Palmaris longus, Plantaris, long extensors of toes)

- In the absence of extensive scarring and destruction of the tendon sheath, traditional single-stage flexor tendon grafting can be done.
- In the presence of extensive disturbance of the flexor sheath and pulleys, joint contractures, and nerve injury, two-stage tendon grafting should be considered.

Tendon Transfer

Indication:
- Late presentation
- Previous measures fails.

In this procedure a normal functioning, which fulfill all the criteria of tendon transfer is used to replace the damaged tendon.

Postoperative Treatment

- After primary flexor tendon repair or flexor tendon graft, wrist and hand are immobilized in dorsal plaster splint.
- The wrist usually is in 20–30° of flexion with the metacarpophalangeal joints in approximately 50–70° of flexion and interphalangeal joints left in the neutral position
- Affected finger is held in flexion by elastic band or rubber band attached at wrist level and at fingernail by wire through nail or glued-on garment hook.
- Rubber or elastic band should allow full extension of the proximal interphalangeal joint against the traction of the band.
- Beginning on the first day after surgery, active extension exercises within the limitations of the splint are encouraged that decreases the adhesion at the repair site and enhances tendon repair.
- After 3 weeks: the dorsal splint is removed, and a wrist -band with a hook for the rubber band is used for an additional 3 weeks.
- At 6 to 8 weeks: Wrist band splint is discontinued, and dynamic extension splinting is used to prevent contractures of the proximal interphalangeal joint.
- At 8 to 10 weeks, strengthening exercises are permitted
- At 10 to 12 weeks, the patient progresses to using the hand normally after the repair.

Q3. Write short note on extensor tendon injury.

Extensors of hand are less commonly injured as compared to the flexors tendon so it is not described here in detail.

Important facts about extensor tendon injury

- From the lateral side to the medial side of the extensor retinaculum, the compartments contain the following numbers of tendons: two, two, one, five, one, and one.
  - The first compartment contains the *extensor pollicis brevis and the abductor pollicis longus*
  - The second, the *extensors carpi radialis longus and brevis*
  - The third, the *extensor pollicis longus*
  - The fourth, the four tendons of the *extensor digitorum communis plus the extensor indicis proprius*
  - The fifth, the *extensor digiti quinti*
  - The sixth, the *extensor carpi ulnaris*
- An extensor tendon is presumed to be severed between the PIP and DIP joints when active extension of the distal interphalangeal joint is lost.
- If the long extensors are severed, extension of the MCP joint is not possible.
- Extensors tendons are also divided into different zones but unlike in flexors tendons, these can be primarily repaired (any of the technique) at almost any level if the injury is clean cut.
- In presence of wound contamination secondary repair should be considered.

HIP DISLOCATION

Q1. Discuss the clinical features and management of posterior dislocation of hip.

Posterior dislocation of the hip occurs much more frequent than anterior hip dislocations.

Mechanism of Injury

Longitudinally directed force applied to the flexed knee *(e.g. dashboard injury)* with the hip in varying degrees of flexion

Clinical Features

- History of trauma
- Attitude: Flexion, adduction and internal rotation at hip *(classic appearance)*.
- True shortening of the thigh is present.
- Femur head palpable in gluteal area.
- All movements are painful and restricted due to muscle spasm.
- Trochanter shifted proximally (change in Bryant's triangle).
- In dislocation of hip, the femoral artery pulsations are feeble due to lack of posterior bony support, i.e. vascular sign of Narath (positive).
- Assess the distal neurovascular deficit (if any)

Radiographic Evaluation

- AP view of the pelvis
- Lateral view of the injured hip joint
- Judet view (oblique 45°) to assess:
  - Presence of osteochondral fragments
  - Integrity of the acetabulum
  - Congruence of the joint spaces

- CT scan: If closed reduction is not possible and planning for an open reduction:
  - To detect the presence of intra-articular fragments
  - To rule out associated femoral head and acetabular fractures

Management

Hip dislocation is a medical emergency and demands immediate intervention/reduction (closed or open).

Closed Reduction under GA

The preferred method is to perform a closed reduction under general anesthesia by one of the following maneuvers.

Reduction Maneuvers

Gravity Method of Stimson

Position: Patient is laid prone on a table or couch with both lower limbs hanging off the end.

Maneuvers
- Assistant stabilizes the pelvis
- Involved hip and knee are flexed 90°
- The surgeon holds the leg just distal to the flexed knee and applies an anteriorly directed force on the proximal calf.
- Gentle internal and external rotation of the hip may assist the reduction.

Allis Maneuver

Position: Patient is laid supine on a table, couch, or floor.

Maneuvers
- Assistant stabilizes the pelvis
- Surgeon applies traction in the direct line of the deformity followed by flexion of the hip to 90° while continuing traction.
- Rotations of the hip are performed until reduction is achieved.

Bigelow Maneuver

Position: Patient is laid supine on a table, couch, or floor.

Maneuvers:
- Assistant stabilizes the pelvis
- Longitudinal traction is applied in the direction of the patient's deformity
- continuing traction, flex the adducted and internally rotated hip to 90° or more
- Femoral head is reduced into the acetabulum by the combination of abduction, external rotation, and extension of the hip.

East Baltimore Lift

Position: Patient is laid supine on a table or couch.
Maneuvers
- Surgeon and an assistant stand on either side of patient.
- Patient's injured leg is flexed so that the hip and knee are at 90°.

- Both surgeons an assistant's arm passes under the proximal calf of the patient and rests on the each others shoulder
- Surgeon's other hand grips the patient's ankle
- Second assistant stabilizes the pelvis
- The surgeon and his assistant squat slightly with knees bent and straighten up together to apply traction to the hip
- The surgeon rotates the leg at the ankle.

Open Reduction

Indications

- Dislocation failed to reduce by closed means.
- Old and neglected dislocation (presented late)
- Non-concentric reduction.
- Fracture of the femoral head or acetabulum requiring excision or open reduction and internal fixation.
- Ipsilateral femoral neck fracture.

Approach:
- Posterior approach (Kocher-Langenbeck)
- Anterior (Smith-Peterson) approach for isolated femoral head fractures.

After treatment: The reduction achieved is maintained by above knee skin traction or skeletal traction through the upper tibial pin for 3 weeks and avoid weight bearing for further 3 weeks.

Complications

Bone

Associated fractures of:
- Posterior lip of acetabulum, a large piece requires open reduction and screw fixation for a stable hip reduction
- Head and neck femur
- Upper third shaft of femur
- Avulsion of greater trochanter
- Avascular necrosis of the head of femur.

Joint

Unreduced dislocation, early secondary osteoarthritis.

Muscle

Myositis ossificans or heterotopic ossification around the hip joint.

Nerve

Sciatic nerve palsy.

Others

- Recurrent dislocation
- Thromboembolism

Q2. Discuss the clinical features and management of anterior dislocation of hip.

Anterior dislocations of the hip are uncommon and constitute only 12% of traumatic hip dislocations.

Mechanism of Injury

It occur with the hip externally rotated and abducted

Clinical Features

- History of trauma
- Attitude: Flexion, abduction and externally rotated leg with lengthening of thigh.
- Head palpable in the femoral triangle
- All movements are painful and restricted due to muscle spasm.
- Trochanter shifted proximally (change in Bryant's triangle).
- Assess the distal neurovascular deficit (if any).

Radiographic Evaluation

- AP view of the pelvis
- Lateral view of the injured hip joint
- Judet view (oblique 45°) to assess:
  - Presence of osteochondral fragments
  - Integrity of the acetabulum
  - Congruence of the joint spaces
- CT scan: If closed reduction is not possible and planning for an open reduction:
  - To detect the presence of intra-articular fragments
  - To rule out associated femoral head and acetabular fractures

Classification

These are classified according to the position assumed by the femoral head:
- Pubic
- Obturator
- Perineal

Management

Closed Reduction under GA

- These can be reduced easily in most of the cases without surgery.
- Appropriate traction is applied longitudinally on the thigh and applying lateral force on the proximal thigh while levered the femoral head toward the acetabulum

Open Reduction

Indications:
- Dislocation failed to reduce by closed means.
- Old and neglected dislocation (presented late)
- Nonconcentric reduction

- Fracture of the femoral head or acetabulum requiring excision or open reduction and internal fixation.
- Soft tissue interposition (rectus femoris, Ilio-psoas muscles and the torn hip capsule)
- "Buttonhole" entrapment of the femoral head by the capsule

Approach: Anterior (Smith-Peterson) approach

After-treatment and complication: Already discussed above.

Q3. Write short note on central fracture dislocation.

In these cases, head bursts through the floor of acetabulum and moves into the pelvis.

Clinical Features

- Pain down the course of obturator nerve
- Greater trochanter is less prominent
- Medial displacement of trochanter
- Shortening
- Abduction and external rotation
- Gross limitation of abduction and rotational movements
- Rectal examination: feels femoral head in pelvis

Management

This is best treated by *lateral traction* through a hook screw passed into the head and neck of femur.

Complications

- Obturator nerve injury
- Traumatic arthritis
- Myositis ossificans
- Avascular necrosis

FEMORAL HEAD

Q1. Discuss the classification and management of fracture head femur.

Fracture head femur is usually associated with dislocation of hip joint.

Mechanism of Injury

High velocity trauma.

Clinical Features

- Pain
- Swelling
- Tenderness
- Deformity (associated with posterior (most common) or anterior dislocation of hip)
- Painful range of motion
- Careful assessment of neurovascular status

- May be associated with ipsilateral femur shaft fracture, knee ligamentous injuries or acetabular fracture

Radiographic Evaluation

- AP and Judet (45° oblique) views of the pelvis
- *CT scan*:
  - To evaluate the reduction of the femoral head fracture
  - To rule out the presence of intra-articular fragments
  - To evaluate associated acetabular fractures.

Classification

Pipkin Classification

- Type I: Hip dislocation with fracture of the femoral head inferior or caudad to the fovea capitis femoris
- Type II: Hip dislocation with fracture of the femoral head superior or cephalad to the fovea capitis femoris
- Type III: Type I or II injury associated with fracture of the femoral neck
- Type IV: Type I, II or III injury associated with fracture of the acetabulum

Brumback Classification

- Type 1: Posterior hip dislocation with fracture of femoral head involving inferomedial (non-weight bearing) portion of femoral head
- Type 1A: With minimal or no fracture of acetabular rim and stable hip joint after reduction
- Type 1B: With significant acetabular fracture and hip joint instability
- Type 2, posterior hip dislocation with fracture of femoral head involving superomedial (weight bearing portion) portion of femoral head
- Type 2A: With minimal or no fracture of acetabular rim and stable hip joint after reduction
- Type 2B: With significant acetabular fracture and hip joint instability
- Type 3: Dislocation of hip (any direction) with femoral neck fracture
- Type 3A: Without fracture of femoral head
- Type 3B: With fracture of femoral head
- Type 4: Anterior dislocation of hip with fracture of femoral head
- Type 4A: Indentation type, depression of superolateral surface of femoral head
- Type 4B: Indentation type, depression of superolateral surface of femoral head
- Type 5: Central fracture-dislocation of hip with femoral head fracture

Management

Pipkin Type I and II

- Closed reduction
- If closed reduction is impossible or if the reduction is not concentric:
  - Open reduction and internal fixation with small subarticular screws
  - Open reduction with excision of small fragments

Pipkin type III

- *In younger patients*: Open reduction and internal fixation of the femoral neck fracture, followed by internal fixation of the femoral head and use of some type of vascularized graft
- *In older individuals*: Hemiarthroplasty is usually recommended.

Pipkin Type IV

Open reduction and reconstruction of the acetabulum is usually recommended

Complication

- Osteonecrosis
- Secondary osteoarthritis

FEMORAL NECK FRACTURES

Q1. Write in brief the blood supply of proximal femur.

The blood supply to the femoral head after femoral neck fracture is precarious and therefore there is increased incidence of osteonecrosis following fracture. Crock described the blood supply to the proximal end of the femur, dividing it into three major groups:
- An extracapsular arterial ring located at the base of the femoral neck
- Ascending cervical branches of the arterial ring on the surface of the femoral neck
- Arteries of the ligamentum teres.

Vascular Supply

- Base of the femoral neck: Anteriorly by the *ascending branch of the lateral femoral circumflex artery* and posteriorly by the *medial femoral circumflex artery* forms an *extracapsular ring*.
- Extracapsular ring gives off the *ascending cervical branches* that pierce the hip capsule becoming the *retinacular arteries* coursing along the femoral neck. Most supplying the femoral head are posterosuperior in location.
- These *retinacular arteries* form a *subsynovial intracapsular arterial ring* at the base of the femoral head. They unite to form the *lateral epiphyseal arteries* as they enter the femoral head.
- The *lateral epiphyseal arteries (most important)* that arise from the posterosuperior ascending cervical branches supply the majority of the femoral head (supplying the lateral weight bearing portion of the femoral head.).
- The *artery of the ligamentum teres*, usually a branch of the obturator is limited to the area around the fovea capitis. It offers a small supplemental contribution to the femoral head.

Q2. Discuss the classification, clinical features and management of fractures neck femur.

80% occur in women, and the incidence in younger patients is very low and is associated mainly with high-energy trauma.

Mechanism of Injury

- Low-energy trauma
  - Most common in older patients
  - A fall onto the greater trochanter (valgus impaction) or
  - Forced external rotation of the lower extremity
- High-energy trauma: Younger and older patients (such as motor-vehicle accident or fall from a height)

Clinical Features

- Usually seen in the old patients, if he slips in bathroom or after a very trivial injury falls to the floor and is unable to stand up or bear weight on the injured limb.
- Children and adults: There is always history of major trauma/trivial in pathological fracture (bone cyst).
- Limb shortened slightly and externally rotated by 45°.
- Inability to raise the leg against the resistance.
- Tenderness over mid-inguinal point.
- Bitrochanteric compression test positive.
- Trendelenburg sign and pump handle test is positive (in old fracture)
- Supratrochanteric shift seen in Bryant's triangle
- Nelaton's line and Shoemaker's line deviates as compared to the normal side.
- Painful restriction of range of motion.

Radiographic Evaluation

- An anteroposterior (AP) view of the pelvis.
- An internal rotation (15°) view of the injured hip to further clarify the fracture pattern.

Classification

Anatomic Location

- Subcapital
- Transcervical
- Basicervical

Pauwel's Classification

Based on the angle of fracture from the horizontal.
- Type I: 30°
- Type II: 50°
- Type III: 70°

Garden's Classification

Based on the degree of valgus displacement:
- Type I: Incomplete/valgus impacted; head tilted in a posterolateral direction
- Type II: Complete and nondisplaced on AP and lateral views
- Type III: Complete with partial displacement (the two fragments remain in contact with each other); trabecular pattern of the femoral head does not line up with that of the acetabulum
- Type IV: Completely displaced; trabecular pattern of the head assumes a parallel orientation with that of the acetabulum (femoral head realign themselves with the trabeculae within the acetabulum)

AO Classification System

- Type B1: Subcapital with no or minimal displacement:
  - Type B1.1: Fractures may be impacted in valgus of 15° or more
  - Type B1.2: Impacted in valgus of less than 15°
  - Type B1.3: Non-impacted

- Type B2: Transcervical
    - Type B2.1: Basicervical
    - Type B2.2: Midcervical with adduction
    - Type B2.3: Midcervical with shear
- Type B3: Displaced subcapital fractures (worst prognosis)
    - Type B3.1: Moderately displaced in varus and external rotation
    - Type B3.2: Moderately displaced with vertical translation and external rotation
    - Type B3.3: Markedly displaced

Management

Manipulation and closed reduction of femoral neck fractures.

Method

Whitman:
- Involves traction on the limb in extension
- Position: Patient supine on the fracture table
- With the extremity externally rotated, it is abducted approximately 20°
- Finally internal rotation of the externally rotated and abducted limb.

Leadbetter
- Manipulation with the hip in flexion
- Affected limb is flexed at the hip to 90°, and the thigh is slightly internally rotated
- Traction is applied in line with the femur
- Limb is circumducted into abduction, maintaining the internal rotation; the limb is brought down to table level in extension

Clinical Evaluation

Heel-Palm test: The patient's heel is placed in the palm of the surgeon's outstretched hand. If reduction is achieved, the limb does not externally rotate spontaneously.

Assessment of Reduction

Garden proposed an index for acceptable reduction using the trabecular pattern alignment on AP and lateral X-rays.

AP View

- The angle formed by the central axis of the medial trabecular system in the head fragment and the medial cortex of the femoral shaft should not be <160° and >180°
- <160° denotes an unacceptable varus reduction
- >180° indicates severe valgus (*increase the risk of osteonecrosis and degenerative changes*)

Lateral View

On the lateral view, Garden's alignment index should be within 20° of the normal 180° straight line along the neck.

Management

Goals
- To minimize patient discomfort
- To restore hip function
- To allow rapid mobilization by obtaining anatomic reduction and stable internal fixation or prosthetic replacement.

Children

- Undisplaced and impacted injury requires hip spica for 6 weeks.
- Displaced (save the head), closed reduction under general anaesthesia and fix the neck by *Austin Moore's pins or Knowle's pins or cannulated cancellous screws.*

Adult

Fresh case: Reduction and fixation by:

- Knowle's pin
- Dynamic hip screw (especially Basicervical type)
- Cannulated cancellous screw

Old case: Up to 3 months:

- McMurray's osteotomy with hip spica for 8 weeks, valgus subtrochanteric osteotomy and fixation with a plate.
- Vascularized muscle pedicle bone grafting with fixation of fracture neck (Meyer's quadratus femoris graft), Sartorius graft.

Old age (>65 years): Partial hip replacement (hemiarthroplasty)

- If 2 cm calcar is present, Austin Moore's prosthesis is used.
- If no calcar then Thomson's prosthesis, and use bone cement if necessary.

Early OA changes of hip then

- Bipolar prosthesis (incidence of protrusio acetabuli than in unipolar prosthesis) is required.
- These prosthesis may be augmented by using bone cement if the patient is osteoporotic

In women with sedentary house living

- Excision arthroplasty in which the head of femur is removed.
- This causes shortening and instability but provides a good range of painless mobility.
- The procedure may combine with pelvic support osteotomy

Fracture neck with AVN or severe OA changes of hip joint then: Total hip replacement is required.

In general, the treatment for displaced Intracapsular fracture neck femur

Physiological age (yr)	*Functional Status*	*Treatment*
<65	Community ambulator	Close reduction and internal fixation Open reduction and internal fixation if necessary
65–75	Community ambulator	Close reduction and internal fixation Cemented bipolar arthroplasty (if closed reduction unsuccessful)
>75	Community ambulator	Cemented bipolar arthroplasty
>75	Minimal household ambulator	Cemented unipolar arthroplasty
>75	Household ambulator; extremely ill	Percutaneous CRIF (± local anesthesia with sedation)
NA (not applicable)	Preexistent arthritis	Total hip replacement
NA (not applicable)	Nonambulator	CRIF or nonoperative if extremely ill

After-treatment: Stress should be made on the maintenance of the quadriceps and gluteal power by exercises for good recovery after surgery.

Complications

Nonunion

Causes

- Synovial fluid bathing the fracture washed away the haematoma and thus interfere with the healing process.
- No periosteal layer, all healing must be endosteal.
- Angiogenic-inhibiting factors in synovial fluid inhibit the healing process.
- Precarious blood supply to the femoral head.
- It leads to absorption of neck, unstable gait and shortening.

Treatment

If there is no sign suggesting of osteonecrosis or AVN:
- Open reduction, osteosynthesis and muscle pedicle graft (*Meyers procedure*)
- Osteosynthesis by: Cannulated cancellous screw or screw with fibular strut graft or dynamic hip screw.
- Osteotomy
- Displacement osteotomy (McMurray), made just proximal to the lesser trochanter (Based on biomechanical principle)
- Angulation osteotomy (Schanz), made through or just distal to the lesser trochanter.
- Mechanical advantages: Line of weight bearing is shifted medially, and shearing force is decreased because the fracture surface has become more horizontal.
- If there are signs suggesting of AVN:
  - Hemiarthroplasty (if acetabular surface is normal)
  - Total hip replacement (if acetabular surface also shows arthritic changes)

Avascular Necrosis of Head

It leads to painful motion.

Treatment

- *Early stage*: Decompression
- *Late stages*:
  - Hemiarthroplasty (if acetabular surface is normal)
  - Total hip replacement (if acetabular surface also shows arthritic changes)

Q3. What are indications, advantages and disadvantages of hemiarthroplasty?

Indications for Hemiarthroplasty

- Comminuted, displaced femoral neck fracture in the elderly
- Pathologic fracture
- Implant failure several weeks after operation
- Malignancy
- Old/neglected, undiagnosed fractures of the femoral neck
- Fracture of the neck of the femur with complete dislocation of the femoral head
- Poor medical condition (patient who probably cannot withstand two operations)
- Poorer ambulatory status before fracture
- Neurologic condition (dementia, ataxia, hemiplegia, parkinsonism)

Advantages over Open Reduction and Internal Fixation

- It may allow immediate full weight bearing.
- It eliminates nonunion, osteonecrosis, failure of fixation as complication of fracture neck femur.
- It reduces the incidence of reoperation compared with internal fixation.

Disadvantages

- It is a more extensive procedure with greater blood loss.
- Risk of acetabular erosion exists in active individuals.

Contraindications

- Active sepsis
- Active young person
- Preexisting acetabular disease (e.g. rheumatoid arthritis)

Q4. What is arthroplasty? Enumerate the indication of total hip replacement.

Arthroplasty is defined as the surgical replacement of a joint with artificially produced material. *Total arthroplasty* (TA) refers to the replacement of all joint surfaces concerned, while *partial replacement* (PR) involves the replacement of only one or some of the surfaces but not the entire joint. *Hip and knee joints* are the most frequently replaced.

Most Common Reason for Arthroplasty

Destruction of articular surface from wear of the cartilage lining due to degenerative diseases such as osteoarthritis, fractures and other changes in bone and connective tissue structures.

Aim

To restore the function of a joint.

Indications

- Symptomatic osteoarthritis (most common)
- Peri-articular fractures, such as femoral neck fractures
- Chronic inflammatory rheumatic diseases
- Femoral head necrosis (osteonecrosis)
- Ankylosing spondylitis

INTERTROCHANTERIC FRACTURES

Q1. Discuss the classification, clinical features and management of intertrochanteric fracture or extracapsular fracture neck femur.

Mechanism of Injury

- High-energy injury such as a motor vehicle accident or fall from a height in younger individuals.
- 90% of intertrochanteric fractures in the elderly result from a simple fall.
- Direct impact to the greater trochanteric area in most of the cases.

Clinical Features

- Fall or severe trauma involving the trochanteric area.
- Pathological fracture as seen in:
    - Children: Osteogenesis imperfecta.
    - Young adults: Osteoclastoma, bone cyst, fibrous dysplasia.
    - Old age: Secondaries.

Examination

- Massive swelling of upper third of thigh and femoral triangle
- Shortening
- Leg externally completely rotated
- Bitrochanteric compression and trochanteric pressure: Painful
- Widening of the trochanter
- Shift in Bryant's triangle.
- Pain and bony crepitus with lack of transmitted movements
- Painful restriction of movements

Radiographic Evaluation

To know the type and the extent of the fracture and associated injuries.
- Anteroposterior (AP) view of the pelvis
- An internal rotation view of the injured hip may be helpful to clarify the fracture pattern further.
- For nondisplaced or occult fractures: Technetium bone scan or preferably magnetic resonance imaging may be of clinical utility in delineating these fractures that are not apparent on plain radiographs.

Classification

Boyd and Griffin

To decide the type of fixation they classified fractures into four types:
- Type 1: Fractures that extend along the intertrochanteric line from the greater to the lesser trochanter
- Type 2: Comminuted fractures, the main fracture being along the intertrochanteric line, but with multiple fractures in the cortex
- Type 3: Fractures that are basically subtrochanteric with at least one fracture passing across the proximal end of the shaft just distal to or at the lesser trochanter associated with Varying degrees of comminution
- Type 4: Fractures of the trochanteric region and the proximal shaft, with fracture in at least two planes, one of which usually is the sagittal plane.

Mechanical

Depending on the geometry of fracture line.
- Stable: The abductors and adductors create force of compression at the fracture line.
- Unstable: The adductors pull the distal fragment medially, while the gluteal abductors pull and rotate the proximal fragment laterally

Evans Classification

Based on the division of fractures into stable and unstable groups (pre- and post-reduction stability):

- Type I fracture, the fracture line extends upward and outward from the lesser trochanter.
- Type II, reverse obliquity fracture, the major fracture line extends outward and downward from the lesser trochanter (tendency toward medial displacement of the femoral shaft because of the pull of the adductor muscles)

AO Classification of Trochanteric Fractures

- Group A1: Simple two-part fracture
- Group A2: Fracture extends over two or more levels of medial cortex
- Group A3: Fracture extends through lateral cortex of femur.

Kyle classification

- Type I: Undisplaced, stable
- Type II: Displaced into varus with a small lesser trochanteric fragment
- Type III: Displaced into varus with posteromedial comminution, greater trochanter fracture; unstable
- Type IV: Type III+ subtrochanteric extension; unstable

Treatment

Nonoperative

Indications

- Medical unfit patient
- Demented patient with mild hip pain
- Patients with brief life expectancies
- Techniques:
  In children: Reduction under anaesthesia and hip spica for 6–12 weeks
  In adults:
  - Fixed traction in Thomas splint
  - Sliding balanced skeletal traction for 6–12 weeks
- Closed methods of treatment of intertrochanteric fractures have largely been abandoned due to increased risks and complications of prolonged recumbency, including:
  - Poor pulmonary toilet
  - Atelectasis
  - Venous stasis or DVT
  - Pressure ulceration/bed sore

Operative

Goal

- Strong, stable fixation of the fracture fragments
- Early mobilization

Fixation depends on:

- Bone quality
- Fracture pattern/geometry
- Fracture reduction
- Implant design
- Implant placement

Rigid internal fixation of intertrochanteric fractures with early mobilization.

Internal fixation by: Sliding compression hip screw devices (DHS: Dynamic compression screw):
- Most commonly used device for both stable and unstable fracture patterns.
- Richard's screw and barrel plate fixation
- It is available in plate angles from 130 to 150°
- Permits controlled impaction at the fracture site

Technical aspects of screw insertion are:
- Placement within 1 cm of subchondral bone to provide secure fixation
- Central position in the femoral head
- Baumgartner's tip-apex distance (TAD) is used to determine lag screw position within the femoral head. It is expressed in millimeters, is the sum of the distances from the tip of the lag screw to the apex of the femoral head on both the AP and lateral radiographic views (after controlling for radiographic magnification) .The sum should be <25 mm to minimize the risk of lag screw cutout.

Biaxial compression plate fixation: Medoff sliding plate indicated especially in intertrochanteric fractures with a significant subtrochanteric component

Fixation with intramedullary devices: Closed reduction and internal fixation by intramedullary hip screw

If there is subtrochanteric extension:
- Gamma nail
- Interlocking intramedullary nails inserted in the Recon mode
- Trochanteric femoral nail
- Intertrochanteric nail (small PFN)

If fracture of neck, trochanter associated with shaft femur fracture: Reconstruction nail.

Advantage
- Limited fracture exposure
- Decreased blood loss
- Less tissue damage
- Less operating time
- These implants are subjected to a lower bending moment
- Step ahead in treating unstable fractures, especially fractures with reverse obliquity and subtrochanteric extension

Disadvantage
- Femoral fractures at the tip of the device or through the distal locking screws especially in cases with Gamma nail, short PFN.
- Require more fluoroscopic exposure

Other Implants
Provide rigid fixation not controlled impaction as in DHS:
- McLaughlin nails plate fixation and early mobilization
- 95°-blade plate fixation
- Cobrahood plate fixation for comminuted fracture

Prosthetic Replacement

Indicated in:
- Patient where open reduction and internal fixation have failed.
- Unsuitable candidates for repeat internal fixation.
- Primary bipolar arthroplasty for comminuted, unstable intertrochanteric fractures.
- Occasionally in:
  - Patient with an intertrochanteric nonunion
  - Failure of fixation when the head is damaged or the bone is poor
  - Salvage of failed fixation of intertrochanteric fracture

Type of prosthesis: Calcar replacement hemiarthroplasty is indicated because of loss of most of the femoral neck and the lesser trochanter.

Disadvantages include:
- Morbidity associated with extensive surgical procedure
- Internal fixation problems with greater trochanteric reattachment
- Postoperative prosthetic dislocation

After treatment:
- The patients is mobilized the first day after surgery.
- With stable fixation early full weight bearing is allowed.
- Full weight bearing is permitted as tolerated.

Intertrochanteric osteotomy: *Dimon and Hughston Osteotomy* for restoration of medial continuity indicated for internal fixation of three-part and four-part intertrochanteric fractures (comminuted).

Complication

- Malunion:
  - Shortening
  - External rotation deformity
  - Coxa vara (reduction of neck shaft angle) causing difficulty in walking
- Nonunion (rare, occurring in <2% of patients)
- Implant failure
- Lag screw-side-plate separation
- Lag screw migration into the pelvis
- Laceration of the superficial femoral artery by a displaced lesser trochanter fragment.

SUBTROCHANTERIC FRACTURE

Q1. Discuss the classification and management of subtrochanteric fractures.

A subtrochanteric femur fracture is a fracture between the lesser trochanter and a point 5 cm distal to the lesser trochanter. These fractures account for 10–34% of all hip fractures.

Mechanism of Injury

- Bimodal age distribution
- Different mechanisms of injury
- Older patients typically sustain low-velocity trauma
- In younger patients these fractures commonly result from high-energy trauma (motor vehicle accidents, gunshot wounds, or falls from a height) and are associated with other fractures and injuries
- Pathologic fracture (17–35% of all subtrochanteric fractures)

Clinical Features

- Pain
- Swelling of the proximal thigh
- Tenderness over the proximal region
- Deformity
- Unable to bear weight and walk
- Hip motions are painfully restricted
- Any neurovascular deficit should be carefully examined

Radiographic Evaluation

An anteroposterior (AP) view of the pelvis and AP and lateral views of the hip and femur

Classification

Fielding

Based on the *location of the primary fracture line* in relation to the lesser trochanter:
- Type I: At the level of the lesser trochanter
- Type II: <2.5 cm below the lesser trochanter
- Type III: 2.5–5 cm below the lesser trochanter

Seinsheimer

Based on the *number of fragments* and *the location* and *configuration* of the fracture lines:
- Type I: Nondisplaced fracture or any fracture with <2 mm of displacement of the fracture fragments, regardless of pattern
- Type II: Two-part fractures
  - IIA: Two-part transverse femoral fracture
  - IIB: Two-part spiral fracture with the lesser trochanter attached to the proximal fragment
  - IIC: Two-part spiral fracture with the lesser trochanter attached to the distal fragment (reverse obliquity pattern)
- Type III: Three-part fractures
  - IIIA: Three-part spiral fracture in which the lesser trochanter is part of the third fragment, which has an inferior spike of cortex of varying length
  - IIIB: Three-part spiral fracture of the proximal third of the femur, with the third part a butterfly fragment
- Type IV: Comminuted fracture with four or more fragments
- Type V: Subtrochanteric-intertrochanteric fracture, including any subtrochanteric fracture with extension through the greater trochanter.

Russell and Taylor

Based on lesser trochanteric continuity and fracture extension posteriorly on the greater trochanter involving the piriformis fossa, the major two variables influencing treatment:
- Type I: Fractures with an intact piriformis fossa in which:
  - IA: The lesser trochanter is attached to the proximal fragment.
  - IB: The lesser trochanter is detached from the proximal fragment.
- Type II: Fractures that extend into the piriformis fossa and:
  - IIA: a stable medial construct (posteromedial cortex).
  - IIB: comminution of the piriformis fossa and lesser trochanter, associated with varying degrees of femoral shaft comminution.

Treatment

Nonoperative

It involves skeletal traction in the 90/90° position followed by spica casting or cast bracing.

Indications

- Elderly individuals who are not operative candidates.
- Children.

Disadvantages

- Increased morbidity and mortality in adults
- Nonunion
- Delayed union
- Malunion with varus angulation
- Rotational deformity
- Shortening.

Operative

- Indicated in most subtrochanteric fractures
- Closed reduction and internal fixation with intramedullary nails
- Open reduction and internal fixation with plates and screw (sliding hip screw, cobra hood plate or 95° fixed angle device).

Implants

Interlocking Nail

- First-generation (centromedullary) nails are indicated for subtrochanteric fractures with both trochanters intact.
- Second-generation cephalomedullary (i.e. reconstruction or Recon nail, gamma nail, PFN) nails are indicated for fractures with loss of the posteromedial cortex and also for fractures extending into the piriformis fossae.

Precautions

- With use of an intramedullary nail, one must monitor for the nail exiting posteriorly out of the proximal fragment.
- One must also monitor for the common mal-alignment of varus and flexion of the proximal fragment.

After treatment

- Allowed partial weight bearing with crutches the day after surgery.
- Progressive weight bearing as per radiographic evidence of callus formation

Advantages

- Retained blood supply to bone fragments
- Less operative blood loss
- Less disruption of the fracture environment
- Minimally invasive
- Less postoperative complications

Disadvantage

Late femoral fracture at the tip of the device especially with short intramedullary nail (gamma nails).

Cobrahood Plating

- Designed by Dr. HKT Raza (based on the trabeculae system of the proximal femur).
- Well -moulded broad DCP (Cobrahood) provide static stable fixation.
- It can be used in every configuration of subtrochanteric fractures.
- Used extensively in our institution besides closed intramedullary nailing.

95° Fixed Angle device

Fractures involving both trochanters

Sliding Hip Screw

Subtrochanteric fractures with intertrochanteric extension

In general: Treatment recommendations based on Russell-Taylor classification of subtrochanteric fractures.

Grade	Fracture pattern	Type of implant used
IA	Piriformis fossa and lesser trochanter intact	Standard interlocking intramedullary nail or cobrahood plating
IB	Piriformis fossa intact, lesser trochanter fractured	Reconstruction intramedullary nail or cobra-hood plating
IIA	Piriformis fossa fractured, lesser trochanter intact	Hip screw or reconstruction Intramedullary nail or cobrahood plating
IIB	Piriformis fossa and lesser trochanter fractured	Hip screw with bone graft or reconstruction Intramedullary nail or cobrahood plating

Complication

- Implant failure
- Non-union
- Malunion (Coxa varus)

FEMORAL SHAFT

Q1. Discuss the classification and management of fracture shaft femur.

Ans: *Fracture shaft femur* is among the most common fractures encountered in day-to-day practice. Fractures of the femoral shaft may be associated with multiple system injuries

Mechanism of Injury

- In neonates, during labour of breech presentation
- In children, due to the epilepsy and often fall from tree tops
- High-energy trauma (mc), usually in adults
- Pathologic fractures, especially in the elderly due to secondaries and osteoporosis.

Clinical Features

- History of trauma
- Gross swelling

- Deformity
- Leg is externally rotated
- Shortening
- Tenderness
- Bony crepitus
- Abnormal mobility of the thigh
- Loss of transmitted movements
- Unable to bear weight
- Painful range of motion
- Carefully assess the distal pulsations and sensations to rule out any complications.

Radiographic Evaluation

- AP and lateral view of femur, hip and knee
- AP view of pelvis

Classification
Descriptive

- Open or closed
- Location:
  - Proximal one-third
  - Middle one-third
  - Distal one-third
  - Isthmal
  - Infraisthmal
  - Supracondylar
- Pattern:
  - Spiral
  - Oblique
  - Transverse
  - Comminuted, segmental, or butterfly fragment
- Angulation or rotational deformity
- Displacement:
  - Shortening
  - Translation

Winquist and Hansen Classification

Based on fracture comminution:
- Type I: Minimal or no comminution
- Type II: Cortices of both fragments at least 50% intact
- Type III: 50–100% cortical comminution
- Type VI: Circumferential comminution with no cortical contact

Management

- Transportation of the patient with the injured leg bandaged to the healthy lower limb with a wooden plank or in Thomas splint (if available).

- Up to 1.5 L of the blood can be extravasated into the thigh and hence the patient may come in shock.
- Blood and fluid replacement and management of shock,
- Once the patient is stabilized, examine carefully to rule out other injuries of the head, chest, abdomen and the pelvis.

Principles of Treatment

- Restoration of alignment, length and rotation
- Preservation of the blood supply to aid union and prevent infection
- Rehabilitation of the extremity and the patient

Factors Influencing the Method of Treatment

- Type and location of the fracture
- Degree of comminution
- Age of the patient
- Patient's social and economic demands
- Infrastructure (availability of implants and image intensifier)

Treatment

Children

- *1–3 years*: Gallow's traction in wooden frame for three weeks
- *3–10 years*:
    - Reduction under anaesthesia and hip spica for 6 weeks
    - Flexible enders nail/Rush nail/DCP for unstable fracture

Adults

Conservative: For soft tissue injury and compound fracture
- External fixation or skeletal traction in Thomas splint with Perkin's attachment for knee flexion

Operative: Interlocking intramedullary nailing (IM) currently is considered to be the treatment of choice for most femoral shaft fractures

In short: Various operative options available are chosen depending on the fracture site and its geometry.
- Intramedullary 'K' nailing, upper one-third and additional bone grafting in comminuted fracture
- Interlocked nail for comminuted, segmental fractures and early mobilization
- DC Plating for middle and lower third
- Cobrahood plate/blade plate fixation for subtrochanteric fractures
- Ilizarov fixation for difficult comminuted fractures

Implants Used for Internal Fixation

Intramedullary (IM) nailing:
Interlocking nailing: Closed interlocking nailing is the treatment of choice in majority of fractures.
- Advantages
    - Minimally invasive
    - Maintaining both the fracture hematoma and the attached periosteum

- Early functional use of the extremity
- Restoration of length and alignment with comminuted fractures
- Rapid and high union (>95%)
- Low fefracture rates
- Low infection rates

Open Intramedullary Nailing

- Indication:
  - Old neglected fracture
  - Soft tissue interposition
  - Non-availability of image intensifier
- Disadvantage:
  - Skin scars
  - Fracture hematoma is evacuated
  - Infection rate is increased
  - Rate of union is decreased
  - Increased morbidity
- Techniques:
  - Antegrade (piriformis fossa)
  - Retrograde
    - Relative indication for retrograde nailing:
    - Obese patients(difficult to obtain an antegrade entry portal)
    - Ipsilateral femoral neck and shaft fractures (to allow the use of separate fixation devices for the shaft and neck fractures)
    - Floating knee injuries to allow fixation of the femoral and tibial fractures through the same anterior longitudinal incision
    - Multiple trauma patients to decrease operative time by not using a fracture table.

After treatment
- Touchdown weight bearing is permitted on the first postoperative day.
- Hip and knee range of motion is encouraged.
- Start straight leg raising exercises.
- Start hip abduction exercises after wound healing.
- Weight bearing is progressed as there is radiographic evidence of callus formation.

External Fixation

Indication
- Open femoral shaft fractures
- Severely injured patient (temporary devise)
- Severe soft tissue contamination
- Ipsilateral vascular injury

Configuration
- Six-pin uniplanar or multiplaner frame is used laterally
- Ring fixation with thin wires in a multiplanar configuration

Disadvantage
- Pin track infection
- Knee stiffness

- Angular malunion
- Femoral shortening

Plate and Screw

- 4.5 mm broad DCP with approximately eight cortical screws on either side of a transverse fracture
- Open or a submuscular technique can be used
- Provide anatomical reduction and interfragmentary compression
- Preserves the endosteal blood supply

Disadvantages
- Extensive approach (soft tissue and periosteum stripping)
- Blood loss
- High risk of infection
- Cortex underlying the plate is devitalized
- Load-bearing device therefore increased incidence of implant failure
- Early weight bearing and unprotected ambulation usually are not possible

After treatment
- Patient is allowed to sit on the day of the surgery (as tolerated)
- Drain removed after 48 hours
- Encouraged active quadriceps exercises
- Partial weight bearing after 1 month
- Weight bearing is progressed as fracture union evident radiographically.

Special Conditions

- *Subtrochanteric fracture*: Already discussed.
- *Fracture of the femoral shaft with dislocation of the hip*: Reduction of hip dislocation and than femoral shaft fracture could be treated in traction or internal fixation.
- *Fracture of the femoral shaft with a femoral head prosthesis*: Open reduction and internal fixation using compression plating (depending upon the type of fracture).
- *Fracture of the femoral shaft and neck*: Closed or open reduction of the femoral neck, provisional screw fixation, and static locked reconstruction nailing using two proximal and two distal locking screws.

Complication

General

The rule of two:
- Within 2 hours: Shock.
- Within 2 days: Fat embolism.
- Within 2 weeks: Thromboembolism.

Local

- Bone:
  - Delayed union
  - Malunion
  - Nonunion

  – Associated fractures of pelvis, neck of femur, patella especially in dash-board injuries.
* Joint:
  – Posterior dislocation of hip
  – Stiffness of the knee joint due to quadriceps adhesion
* *Nerve*: Sciatic nerve palsy in injuries of the upper third.
* *Vessels*: Damage to the femoral artery in compound mid-shaft fracture with penetrating injuries.
* *Muscle*: Quadriceps wasting and myositis ossificans.
* *Infection*: Osteomyelitis in compound fracture and after operations at times.

DISTAL FEMUR

Q1. Discuss the classification and management of fracture distal femur.

These fractures account for about 7% of all femur fractures. The incidence is highest in women >75 years and in adolescent boys and men 15–24 years old. Fractures often are unstable, comminuted, and some times regaining full knee motion and function may be difficult.

Mechanism of Injury

* Severe axial load with a varus, valgus, or rotational force results majority of the fractures.
* In young adults: High velocity trauma (motor vehicle collision or fall from a height)
* In the elderly: Trivial trauma (minor slip or fall onto a flexed knee).

Deforming Forces

These are muscular attachments cause characteristic displacement patterns:
* Gastrocnemius: Flexes the distal fragment, causing posterior angulation and displacement.
* Quadriceps and hamstrings: Exert proximal traction, resulting in shortening of the lower extremity.

Clinical Features

* Pain
* Swelling
* Haemarthrosis
* Deformity in the lower thigh and knee
* Unable to bear weight
* Painful range of motion
* Careful assessment of neurovascular status
* In polytrauma patients assessment of ipsilateral hip, knee, leg, and ankle is essential

Radiographic Evaluation

* Careful radiographic evaluation, including AP, lateral, tangential patellar, and tunnel views, is necessary
* CT scan: Helpful especially in cases where anteroposterior and lateral radiographs appear normal

Classification

Müller Classification

It is based on the location and pattern of the fracture:
- Type A fractures: Involve the distal shaft only with varying degrees of comminution.
- Type B fractures: Condylar fractures
- Type B1: Sagittal split of the lateral condyle
- Type B2: Sagittal split of the medial condyle
- Type B3: Coronal plane fracture (Hoffa's fracture)
- Type C: T-condylar and Y-condylar fractures
- Type C1: Fractures have no comminution
- Type C2: Fractures have a comminuted shaft fracture with two principal articular fragments
- Type C3: Fractures have intra-articular comminution.

Descriptive Classification

- Open or closed
- *Location*:
  - Supracondylar
  - Intercondylar
  - Condylar
- *Pattern*:
  - Spiral
  - Oblique
  - Transverse
- Articular involvement
- Comminuted, segmental, or butterfly fragment
- Angulation or rotational deformity
- Displacement
  - Shortening
  - Translation

Management

Nonoperative

Indications:
- Medically unfit patient
- Undisplaced or incomplete fractures
- Impacted stable fractures in elderly patients
- Severe osteopenia
- Advanced underlying medical conditions

Stable undisplaced fractures: Immobilization in a hinged knee brace, with partial weight bearing.

Displaced fractures:
- 6–12 week period of skeletal traction followed by bracing
- Objective: To restore the normal knee axis with hip and ankle

- Drawbacks:
  - Bed rest
  - Varus
  - Internal rotation deformity
  - Knee stiffness
  - Prolonged hospitalization.

Operative

Open reduction and internal fixation with one of the following:

Screws: interfragmentary screws especially in noncomminuted, unicondylar fractures in young adults with good bone stock.

Plates

- 95° condylar blade plate
- Dynamic condylar screw (DCS)
- Nonlocking periarticular plates (condylar buttress plates)
- Locking plates (with fixed angle screws)

Biological Plating

- Now day's biological techniques of plating are advocating.
- Less invasive stabilization technique (LISS) plate, which uses locked screws and percutaneous fixation
- Basis: Maintain the biological environment without disturbing the fracture hematoma
- Components
  - Minimal incision (percutaneous fixation)
  - Indirect reduction techniques
  - Minimal soft-tissue stripping
  - Gentle retraction
  - Metaphyseal comminution is left *in situ*
  - Regain length and alignment of the fracture
  - Fixation with locking condylar plate.

Intramedullary (IM) Nails

- These implants provide better "biological" fixation than plates because they are load-sharing devices, rather than load-sparing, implants.
- Antegrade inserted or retrograde inserted intramedullary nail (supracondylar nail)
- Other nails such as: Zickel supracondylar device, Ender rods, and Rush rods, have been used with some success
- Major disadvantage: It provides less rigid stabilization of distal femoral fractures than plate fixation

After-treatment:
- The extremity is placed on a continuous passive motion (CPM) device in the immediate postoperative period
- Physiotherapy (active range of motion)
- If fixation is unstable then used cast brace
- Weight bearing: 12 weeks (with radiographic evidence of healing)

External Fixation

- External fixator (knee spanning external fixator) can be used either temporary or definitive fixation device.
- Indication:
  - Open fracture
  - Fracture associated with vascular injury
  - Extensive soft-tissue injury
- Disadvantage
  - Pin track infection
  - knee stiffness

Complication

- Implant failure
- Knee stiffness (post-traumatic osteoarthritis)
- Malunion (unstable fixation or infection; varus is most common deformity)
- Nonunion
- Infection.

Q2. Discuss the management of Unicondylar Fractures of the Femur.

Unicondylar fractures of the lower end of the femur are uncommon injuries that usually occur in the sagittal plane.

Management

- In patients with good bone stock
- Undisplaced
  - Conservatively or
  - Percutaneous fixation with 6.5-mm cancellous lag screws
- Displaced fractures: open reduction and fixation with 6.5 mm cancellous lag screws
- In patients with osteoporotic bone
  - T-buttress plate may be necessary to prevent proximal migration of the condyle

After treatment:

- The injured extremity is placed on removable long leg splint.
- Continuous passive motion (CPM) can be initiated immediately after surgery as tolerated.
- As the swelling subsides start gentle active and active-assisted exercises.
- Start touch down weight bearing with a walker or crutches on postoperative day 2 or 3.
- Start full weight bearing: 12–14 weeks.

Q3. What is a Hoffa's fracture?

Hoffa fracture (coronal fractures of the posterior condyle (AO type B3 or Hoffa fractures)) is an intra-articular fracture of the knee in coronal (tangential) plane analogous to the capitellum fracture of the elbow. The injury is the result of violent force and generally occurs in young adult.

Radiographic Evaluation

- Careful radiographic evaluation, including AP, lateral, tangential patellar, and tunnel views, is necessary.

- CT scan: Helpful especially in cases where antero-posterior and lateral radiographs appear normal.

Management

Open reduction and internal fixation with partially threaded cancellous screws in the lag mode to secure compression across the fractures.

PATELLA AND EXTENSOR MECHANISM INJURIES

Q1. Discuss the clinical features and management of patella fracture.

The patella is the largest sesamoid bone in the body. Its anterior subcutaneous location of the patella makes it vulnerable to direct injuries. Fractures of the patella accounts ~ 1% of all skeletal injuries, resulting from either direct or indirect trauma.

Mechanism of Injuries

Direct trauma such as:
- Knee striking the dashboard of an automobile
- Fall on the anterior knee
- Often results in:
    - Comminuted or displaced fractures
    - It may result in chondral injury to the distal femur or patella

Indirect (most common):
- Violent contraction of the quadriceps (in tetanus or epilepsy) with the knee flexed or semi-flexed position
- Usually results in:
    - Transverse fracture pattern, with variable inferior pole comminution
    - Tears of the medial and lateral retinacular expansions
- Combination of direct and indirect forces:

Effects of fracture of the patella
- Loss of continuity of the extensor mechanism.
- Potential incongruity of the patellofemoral articulation.

Clinical Features

- Pain
- Boggy swelling in the knee joint
- Haemarthrosis
- localized tenderness
- Palpable gap between the fracture fragments
- Inability to extend the knee

Radiographic Evaluation

- Anteroposterior (AP), lateral and axial (sunrise) views of the knee.
- AP view:
    - A bipartite patella (8% of the population) may be mistaken for a fracture
    - It is due to failure of fusion of the superolateral portion of the patella

– It usually occurs in the superolateral position and has smooth margins
– It is bilateral in 50% of individuals.
- Lateral view
  – Displaced fractures usually are obvious.
  – Transverse fractures usually are best seen in this view.
- Axial view (sunrise or merchant): For evaluation of:
  – Osteochondral or vertical marginal fractures
  – Articular incongruity.

Classification

Descriptive

- Open or closed
- Undisplaced or displaced
- Pattern
  – Stellate
  – Comminuted
  – Transverse
  – Vertical (marginal)
  – Polar
- Osteochondral

Patellar classification

- Undisplaced
- Transverse
- Lower or upper pole
- Comminuted undisplaced
- Comminuted displaced
- Vertical
- Osteochondral

Management

Principle of Treatment

- Accurate reduction
- Early mobilization of the knee
- Good quadriceps power for the knee stabilization and movements.

Acute Injury

- Rest
- Ice
- Compression or splinting in extension or slight flexion
- Elevation
- Analgesic

Nonoperative

- Closed fractures with:
  – Minimal displacement (2–3 mm)
  – Minimal articular incongruity (1–2 mm)
  – An intact extensor retinaculum

- Treatment consist of:
  - Immobilizing the knee in extension in a cylinder cast from ankle to groin or knee immobilizer for 4–6 weeks
  - Weight bearing allowed with crutches as tolerated by the patient
  - Progressive active flexion and extension strengthening exercises are encouraged after radiographic evidence of union.

Operative

Goal

- Restoration of articular congruity
- Repair of the extensor mechanism with fixation
- Early motion

Indications

- Fractures associated with retinacular tears
- Open fractures
- Fractures with more than 2–3 mm of displacement
- Incongruity

Open reduction and internal fixation with one of the following techniques:

- Cerclage wiring, alone or in combination
- Tension band wiring, alone or modified with longitudinal Kirschner wires or screws (principle: the distracting or shear forces are converted into compressive forces across the fracture site)
- Magnusson wiring
- Lotke longitudinal anterior band wiring

Open reduction and external fixation

- Used by some authors successfully to treat transverse and comminuted fractures
- Using superior and inferior pins placed transversely, adjacent to the proximal and distal poles and connected externally to compressive

Patellectomy: Partial patellectomy (excision of pole) quadriceps tendon repair:

Indication

- Presence of a large, salvageable fragment in the presence of smaller fragment
- Comminuted polar fragments in which it is impossible to restore the articular surface or to achieve stable fixation

Total Patellectomy with quadriceps tendon repair: Severe Comminution

After-treatment:

- Limb is immobilized in extension in a posterior plaster splint or removable knee brace
- At ~2–3 weeks: when the wound has healed start Active range-of-motion exercises
- 6 to 8 weeks: if there is radiographic evidence of healing, start resistance exercises and discontinued the brace
- 18–24 weeks: when full strength of quadriceps strength has returned encourage unrestricted activity

Complication

- Patellar instability
- Quadriceps wasting

- Knee stiffness
- Early osteoarthritis
- Osteonecrosis (proximal fragment)
- Fixation or implant failure
- Refracture

Q2. Discuss the management of acute and recurrent dislocation of patella.

Patellar dislocation is more common in females, due to physiologic laxity, as well as in patients with hypermobility and connective tissue disorders like Ehlers-Danlos syndrome or Marfan syndrome.

Predisposing Factors

- Incompetence of the medial patellofemoral ligament
- Increase the Q angle (Q-angle: angle formed by the line of pull of the quadriceps mechanism and that of the patellar tendon as they intersect at the center of the patella)
- High-riding patella (patella alta)
- Dysplasia of the femoral condyles
- Hypertrophic lateral retinaculum
- Hypoplasia of the vastus medialis.

Mechanism of Injury

- Lateral dislocation: Internal rotation of the femur on an externally rotated and planted tibia with knee in flexion is the most common cause.
- Medial instability (rare, could be iatrogenic or congenital, traumatic, or may be associated with atrophy of the quadriceps musculature).
- Intra-articular dislocation: Uncommon
- Superior dislocation: Elderly individuals from forced hyperextension injuries to the knee

Clinical Features

- Hemarthrosis
- Inability to flex the knee
- Deformity:
  - Displaced patella (seated on the lateral side of the knee)
  - Prominence of the medial condyle of femur
- Painful restriction of knee joint (both active and passive)
- If it reduced spontaneously:
  - Knee may be swollen
- There may be:
  - Bruising
  - Tenderness over the medial side
- In cases of recurrent dislocation:
  - Symptoms and sign are less marked
  - Apprehension test is positive:
    - Holds the relaxed knee in 20–30° of flexion and manually subluxates the patella laterally.
    - When the test is positive, the patient suddenly complains of pain and tries to resists any further lateral movement of the patella

Radiographic Evaluation

AP lateral views and axial (sunrise) of the knee is obtained.

Other special views:
- Hughston 55° of knee flexion: Patellar index, sulcus angle
- Merchant 45° of knee flexion: Congruence angle, sulcus angle
- Laurin 20° of knee flexion: Patellofemoral index, lateral patellofemoral angle

Lateral radiograph of the knee: Assessment of patella alta or baja by:
- *Blumensaat line*: A line extending through the intercondylar notch should just touch the lower pole of the patella with the knee flexed to 30°. Patella significantly proximal to Blumensaat line is patella alta.
- *Insall-Salvati ratio*: Length of patella tendon (LT) and length of patella (LP) have normal LT-to-LP ratio of 1.0. Variation of more than 20% indicates abnormal position. A ratio of 1.2 indicates patella alta, whereas 0.8 indicates patella baja

Treatment

Acute Dislocation

- Usually managed by closed methods
- Extension of the flexed knee with pressure applied to the lateral margin of the patella results in reduction of patella
- The limb is immobilized in a knee immobilizer or brace for 10–14 days.
- Early range of motion is encouraged:
  - To prevent arthrofibrosis
  - To promote the formation of strong collagen along the lines of stress
- Quadriceps strengthening is continued for 3–4 months

Surgical Intervention for Acute Dislocations

- It is rarely indicated
- Indicated in:
  - Displaced intra-articular fractures
  - In osteochondral fracture
  - Loose body formation
  - Joint incongruity.

Old Unreduced Dislocation of Patella

Old traumatic patellar dislocations may be treated by:
- Observation if function of the knee are satisfactory
- Patellar realignment (open reduction) combine with *VY quadriceplasty* if:
  - Degenerative changes of the patella are minimal or absent
  - Tibiofemoral joint is essentially normal
- Patellectomy: Significant patellar degenerative changes

Recurrent Patellar Dislocation

Operative procedures: These are primarily used with recurrent dislocations.

Procedures generally can be grouped into five categories:
- I: Release of the tightened lateral retinaculum
- II: Proximal realignment of the extensor mechanism

- III: Distal realignment of the extensor mechanism
- IV: Combined proximal and distal realignment of the extensor mechanism
- V: Patellectomy combined with realignment of the extensor mechanism

Operative Procedure	Indications	Techniques
Lateral retinacular release	Recurrent subluxation, relatively normal Q angle	Open
	Tight lateral structures Lateral tilt with minimal lateral sub-luxation on radiograph in combination with realignment procedure	Arthroscopic
Repair of medial patello-femoral ligament and vastus medialis	Acute or subacute dislocation in asso-ciation with osteochondral fracture	Open
Proximal extensor realignment	Subluxation or dislocation, Q angle <20°	Insall, Madigan et al.
Distal extensor realign-ment	Recurrent subluxation or dislocation	Roux-Goldthwait, Galeazzi
	Q angle >20°, skeletally immature (soft-tissue realignment) Q angle > 20°, skeletally mature	Elmslie-Trillat
Proximal and distal realignment	Recurrent dislocations, skeletally mature, Q angle approaching 20°	Hughston, modified Elmslie-Trillat
Patellectomy with extensor realignment	Skeletally mature, salvage procedure	West and Soto-Hall

After treatment:

- Knee is immobilized in a knee immobilizer or brace in full extension.
- Patient should be encouraged to bear weight as tolerated in a knee immobilizer.
- At 2–3 weeks after surgery, the immobilizer is removed and ,gradual passive, active and quadriceps-strengthening exercises are begun.

Complications

- Redislocation
- Patellofemoral pain

Q3. Discuss clinical features and management of rupture of quadriceps tendon.

The most frequent cause of partial or complete rupture of a tendon or muscle is eccentric overload of the muscle-tendon unit. Other causes may include an open lacerations and a direct blow by the sharp edge of an object on an actively contracted muscle

Site of Rupture

It usually ruptures transversely at the osteotendinous junction

Age and Risk Factors

- Rupture typically occurs in patients >40 years old through the degenerative area.
- Rupture occurs at the mid-substance in most patients <40 years old.
- Bilateral quadriceps tendon ruptures in patients with underlying medical conditions, such as gout, diabetes, or steroid use.

- Risk factors for quadriceps rupture
  - Tendinitis
  - Anabolic steroid use
  - Local steroid injection
  - Diabetes mellitus
  - Inflammatory arthropathy
  - Chronic renal failure

Clinical Features

- Acute pain
- Inability or difficulty in weight bearing
- Palpable suprapatellar gap or defect
  - If gap is present but patient able to extend the knee, then intact extensor retinaculum
  - If no active extension, then both retinaculum and tendon are completely torn
- Tenderness at the upper pole of patella
- Inability actively to extend the knee.

Radiographic Evaluation

- AP, lateral, and tangential (Sunrise, Merchant) view
  - Anteroposterior and lateral radiographs may show:
    - Obliteration of the quadriceps tendon shadow
    - Suprapatellar mass (retraction of the ruptured tendon)
    - Suprapatellar calcific densities (avulsed bone fragment or tendon calcifications)
    - Patellar displacement (Patella alta possible with patellar tendon rupture and Patella Baja with quadriceps tendon rupture)
- Ultrasound:
  - Assessment of rupture location
  - Helps in differentiation of partial from complete tears
- MRI:
  - Rupture is partial or complete
  - Help to identify other pathology within the knee

Management

Incomplete Ruptures

- Usually managed conservatively
- Immobilization of the knee in full extension for 6 weeks
- After 6 weeks begun protected physical therapy to regain strength and range of motion

Complete Ruptures

Operative repair should be done as early as possible with one of the following techniques:
- Re-approximate the tendon to bone using non-absorbable sutures after passing through bone tunnels
- Mid-substance tears may undergo end-to-end repair after freshening the edges.
- Scuderi technique:
  - Local flap technique used for reinforcement, from a distally based partial-thickness quadriceps tendon turned down across the repair site and reinforces it with Bunnell

pullout wire in the medial and lateral sides of the proximal tendon, pass them along each side of the patella, and bring them through the skin just distal to the patella.
- Codivilla tendon lengthening and repair:
  - Neglected rupture or chronic tears may require a V-Y plasty of a retracted quadriceps tendon (Codivilla V-Y-plasty technique).

Postoperative Management

- A cylinder cast or knee immobilizer is worn for 4–6 weeks.
- Weight bearing with crutches is allowed at 3 weeks or as tolerated
- At 2–3 weeks, a hinged knee brace is used
- Starting with 45° of active range of motion and gradually progress the range with 10–15° each week

Complication

- Loss of knee motion especially flexion
- Infection (due to subcutaneous placement of non-absorbable sutures or wires)
- Rerupture
- Persistent quadriceps atrophy/weakness and extensor lag

KNEE DISLOCATION AND LIGAMENTOUS INJURY AROUND KNEE

Q1. Discuss the management of knee dislocation.

Knee dislocation is a medical emergency as there is high incidence of neurovascular compromise; immediate reduction is recommended before radiographic evaluation.

Clinical Features

- Pain
- Gross swelling
- Tenderness
- Deformity
- Ligamentous laxity: assess status of ligament
  - Anterior cruciate ligament (ACL): Lachman test at 30°
  - Posterior cruciate ligament (PCL): Posterior drawer test at 90°
  - Lateral collateral ligament (LCL)/Posterolateral corner (PLC): Varus stress at 30° and full extension; Increased tibial external rotation at 30°; Increased posterior tibial translation at 30°
  - Medial collateral ligament (MCL): Valgus stress at 30°
- Neurovascular evaluation pre- and post-reduction is very critical
  - Nerve injuries:
    - In 16% to 43% of cases
    - Most often Peroneal nerve is involved.
    - Prognosis is guarded
  - Vascular injuries:
    - Popliteal artery usually involved (20–60%).
    - Danger signals include:

- Absence of pulses in the pedal vessels
- Tenderness, swelling, and ecchymosis in the popliteal fossa
- Cold, cyanotic foot

Radiographic Evaluation

Immediate reduction should be advised before radiographic evaluation.

X-rays

- AP and lateral
- 45° oblique
- Patellar sunrise
- X-rays shows:
  - dislocation
  - Irregular or asymmetric joint space
  - Lateral capsular sign (Segond fracture)
  - Avulsions
  - Osteochondral defects

Angiography or MRA: If vascular compromise is suspected

MRI

It helps in:
- Preoperative planning
- Identification of ligament avulsions
- Medial Collateral Ligament: injury location
- Lateral structures: popliteus, LCL, biceps
- Identification of any meniscal injury
- Articular cartilage lesions

Classification

Based on the displacement of the tibia in relation to the femur:
- Anterior
- Posterior
- Medial
- Lateral
- Rotary
  - Anteromedial
  - Anterolateral
  - Posteromedial
  - Postero-lateral

Schenck's Anatomic Classification:

- **I:** Single cruciate + collateral (ACL + collateral or PCL + collateral)
- **II:** ACL/PCL (collaterals intact)
- **IIIM:** ACL/PCL/MCL (LCL + PLC intact)
- **IIIL:** ACL/PCL/LCL + PLC (MCL intact)

- **IV:** ACL/PCL/MCL/LCL + PLC
- **V:** Fracture-dislocation
- **C:** Arterial injury
- **N:** Nerve injury

Treatment

Immediate closed reduction is essential

Types of dislocation	Reduction maneuver
Anterior	Axial limb traction + lifting of the distal femur
Medial/lateral	Axial limb traction + lateral/medial translation of the tibia
Posterior	Axial limb traction + extension and lifting of the proximal tibia
Rotatory	Axial limb traction + derotation of the tibia

Post Reduction

Splinted at 20°–30° of flexion in a splint or with external fixator (knee spanner)

Operative

Indications
- Failed closed reduction.
- Soft issue interposition
- Open injuries or fasciotomy
- Vascular injuries or vascular repair
- Head injury
- Open wounds.

Transarticular Pins

- *Transarticular pin* inserted through the intercondylar notch of the femur into the intercondylar eminence of the tibia to provide immediate stability for knees that redislocate after vascular repair or in a splint
- *Disadvantage: Pin track infection and breakage.*

Knee-spanning External Fixator

Indication
- Open injuries
- Knee dislocations with extensive soft-tissue injury
- In unstable knees after vascular repair

Advantage
- Protects vascular repair
- Permits skin care for open injuries and promote soft tissue healing
- Permits easy dressing and wound inspection in an open injury.

Vascular Injury

- Immediate surgical exploration
- It is treated with excision of the damaged segment and re-anastomosis with a reverse saphenous vein graft.

Nerve Injury

- Primary exploration with grafting or repair is not effective
- Secondary exploration (3 months) is associated with poor results.
- Bracing and/or tendon transfer may be necessary for treatment any residual muscular deficiencies

Ligamentous Injuries

- Early ligament repair produced more satisfactory long-term results
- Repair depends upon:
    - Skeletal injuries
    - Vascular deficits
    - Open wounds

Complications

- Posttraumatic arthritis
- Decreased range of motion
- Ligamentous laxity
- Instability
- Neurovascular deficit

Q2. Classify knee joint instability resulting from ligamentous injury.

Classification

One-plane Instability (Simple or Straight)

- One-plane medial
- One-plane lateral
- One-plane posterior
- One-plane anterior

Rotary Instability

- Anteromedial
- Anterolateral
- Flexion
- Approaching extension
- Posterolateral
- Posteromedial

Combined Instability

- Anterolateral-anteromedial rotary
- Anterolateral-posterolateral rotary
- Anteromedial-posteromedial rotary

Q3. Define sprain and classify it.

Sprain is an injury limited to ligaments (connective tissue attaching bone to bone) and a *strain* is a stretching injury of muscle or its tendinous attachment to bone.

Based on tear of fibres and instability sprains are classified into three degrees of severity.

Classification of ligamentous injuries (American Medical Association)

Grade I

- Mild
- Tear of a minimal number of fibres of the ligament
- Localized tenderness
- No instability

Gradd II

- Moderate
- Disruption of more ligamentous fibres
- More loss of function and more joint reaction
- Mild-to-moderate instability

Grade III

- Severe
- Complete disruption of the ligament
- Marked instability
- It can be further classified based on of instability demonstrated during stress testing:
    - + Instability, the joint surfaces separate 5 mm or less
    - ++ Instability, they separate 5–10 mm
    - +++ Instability, they separate 10 mm or more respectively.

Q4. Discuss injuries around the knee (IDK or internal derangement of knee).

This is a group of injuries characterized by pain, swelling, locking, muscle wasting in stability and early osteoarthritis following injury to the knee. The lesion may involve meniscus, collateral/cruciate ligaments.

Mechanism of Injury

Mechanisms capable of disrupting the ligamentous structures around the knee are:
- Abduction, flexion, and internal rotation of the femur on the tibia (most common)
- Adduction, flexion, and external rotation of the femur on the tibia
- Hyperextension
- Anteroposterior displacement

I. CRUCIATE LIGAMENT

a. Anterior Cruciate Ligament (ACL)

Clinical Features

- Pain
- Within a few hours of injury, the knee swells, and aspiration of the joint reveals hemarthrosis.
- Patient often describes the knee as having been hyper-extended or popping out ("giving –way") of joint and then reducing.
- POP is frequently heard or felt (signify ligamentous injury).

Diagnostic Tests

Anterior Drawer Test

Position: patient supine on the couch, the hip is flexed to 45° and the knee to 90°, with the foot placed on the tabletop.
Procedure
- The examiner can sit on the patient's foot to stabilize it and grasp around the patient's calf with both hands.
- Proximal part of the leg then is gently and repeatedly pulled and pushed anteriorly and posteriorly and tibial excursion is compared to the unaffected knee.
- This test done in three positions of rotation, initially with the tibia in neutral rotation and then in 30° of external or internal rotation

Inference: An anterior drawer sign >6–8 mm of the opposite knee indicates a torn anterior cruciate ligament.

Slocum Anterior Rotary Drawer Test

It is valuable in determining rotational instability of the knee.
Procedure
- Anterior displacement of the tibia on the femur is noted and recorded.
- The test is done in 15° of internal rotation, 30° of external rotation, and neutral rotation.
Inference
- Positive test in 15° of internal rotation indicates anteromedial rotary instability.
- Positive test in 30° of external rotation indicates anterolateral rotary instability.

Jerk Test of Hughston and Losee

Procedure
- The knee is flexed to 90°, the tibia is rotated internally and valgus stress is applied over the proximal end of the tibia and fibula.
- The knee is then extended gradually, maintaining the internal rotation and valgus stress.

Inference: If test is positive, the lateral tibia spontaneously subluxates forward in the form of a sudden jerk at ~30° of flexion.

Lateral Pivot Shift Test of Macintosh

Position: Knee extended.
Procedure:
- Foot is lifted and the leg internally rotated, and a valgus stress is applied to the lateral side of the leg (proximal part).
- The knee is then flexed gradually, maintaining the internal rotation and valgus stress.

Inference: the positive test provides the force that reduces the lateral tibial plateau on the lateral femoral condyle.
Note: The pivot shift is tested while the knee is moved from extension to flexion, and the jerk test is performed while the knee is moved from flexion to extension.

Other test includes external rotation–recurvatum test, flexion–rotation drawer test, tibial external rotation test, etc.

Investigations

- Standard AP and lateral radiographs, as well as a tangential view of the patella.
- Arthrography: Replaced by magnetic resonance imaging (MRI).

- KT-1000/2000 (knee ligament arthrometers): A measuring system documents AP tibial displacement by tracking the tibial tubercle in rotation to the patella. The right-left difference is $\leq$3 mm in 90% of knees with an acute anterior cruciate ligament injury. It is more effective in evaluating patients with chronic anterior cruciate ligament disruption.
- Arthroscopy is very useful in precise diagnosis, and subsequent management.
- MRI: Standard imaging study for imaging meniscus pathology and all intra-articular disorders

Treatment

Treatment options include:
- Nonoperative management
- Repair of the anterior cruciate ligament (either isolated or with augmentation)
- Reconstruction with either autograft or allograft tissues or synthetics.

Nonoperative

Reserved for grade I and II tears
- Rest
- NSAIDs
- Functional knee brace for 4–6 weeks
- At 3 weeks:
    - Flexion from 0–90° is allowed in the brace.
    - Isometric quadriceps and hamstring exercises are begun.
- At 6 weeks: Crutches are discontinued.
- 8 weeks: Full active and passive range of motion should be achieved.
- Progressive resistance exercises are continued for at least 3 months.

Operative

- Mostly prefer reconstruction rather than primary repair several weeks after the acute injury.
- Acute repair is appropriate when a bony avulsion occurs with the anterior cruciate ligament attached. The bony fragment is replaced and is fixed with sutures or passed through trans-osseous drill holes or screws.
- In old cases, reinforcement is indicated. It could be intra- or extra-articular or both by using semitendinosus, iliotibial band, etc.
- In chronic ACL insufficiency: reconstruction is indicated. It could be intra- or extra-articular replacement.
- The most common current graft choices are bone–patellar tendon–bone graft (BPTB) and the quadrupled hamstring tendon graft.
- Nowadays, surgeons are using either a triple- or quadruple-stranded semitendinosus graft or a quadruple-stranded semitendinosus-gracilis tendon graft.

b. Posterior Cruciate Ligament

Diagnostic Tests

Posterior drawers test
- *Position:* Patient supine and the knee flexed to 90° with the foot placed on the tabletop.
- *Procedure:*
    - The examiner can sit on the patient's foot to stabilize it and grasp around the patient's calf with both hands and a thumb is placed on each anteromedial joint line.

- A posterior force is applied on the proximal tibia, which is opposite but similar to the force applied in the anterior drawer test.
- *Inference*
  - Posterior movement of the tibia on the femur shows posterior instability compared with the normal tibia (indicates a torn posterior cruciate ligament).
  - Loss of the normal 1-cm anterior step-off of the medial tibial plateau with respect to the medial femoral condyle indicates a torn posterior cruciate ligament or posterior instability.

Tibial Sag Test

- *Position:* patient supine and the hip flexed to 90°. The heels of each extremity are placed in the examiner's hands.
- *Inference*: From the effects of gravity, the tibia sags posteriorly if posterior instability present when sighting across the horizon of the flexed knees.

Quadriceps Active Test

- Normally: In 90° flexion, the patellar ligament is directed slightly posterior, and contraction of the quadriceps does not result in an anterior shift.
- In posterior cruciate deficiency:
  - The tibia sags into posterior subluxation, and the patellar ligament is directed anteriorly.
  - Contraction of the quadriceps muscle in a knee results in an anterior shift of the tibia of ≥2 mm.

Management

Nonoperative

Indications:
- Posterior drawer of <10 mm (grade II) with the tibia in neutral rotation
- <5° of abnormal rotary laxity
- No significant valgus-varus abnormal laxity (no associated significant ligamentous injury).

Operative

Repair:
- Repaired if the ligament is avulsed with a fragment of bone
- Usually delay reconstruction for 1–2 weeks after injury:
  - To allow painful intra-articular reaction to subside
  - To allow the patient to regain full motion and some strength.

Acute PCL avulsion:
- Large fragment: Open reduction and internal fixation
- Small fragment (posterior tibial translation <10 mm): Quadriceps rehabilitation
- Small fragment (posterior tibial translation >10 mm): PCL reconstruction

PCL Reconstruction:
- Extra- or intra-articular
- Use of the lateral meniscus, the medial Gastrocnemius, the semitendinosus and gracilis tendons, and bone–patellar tendon–bone autografts
- Arthroscopic or open techniques

II: MENISCAL INJURIES

Meniscal function is essential to the normal function of the knee joint. They act as joint filler, compensating for gross incongruity between femoral and tibial articulating surfaces.

Important Functions

- Prevent capsular and synovial impingement during flexion-extension movements.
- Joint lubrication function (distribution of synovial fluid and aiding the nutrition of the articular cartilage)
- Stability
- Proprioception (type I and II nerve endings)
- Load transmission

Types

a. Medial Meniscus

- C-shaped structure (semicircular)
- Larger in radius than the lateral meniscus
- Posterior horn being wider than the anterior
- Anterior horn is attached more firmly to the tibia anterior to the intercondylar eminence and to the anterior cruciate ligament
- Most of the weight is borne on the posterior portion of the meniscus
- Its entire peripheral border is attached to the joint (medial) capsule and through the coronary ligament to the upper border of the tibia.
- It is torn more frequently than lateral because it is less mobile (being fixed to the medial collateral ligament)

b. Lateral Meniscus

- More circular and covers around two thirds of the articular surface.
- Smaller in diameter, thicker in periphery, wider in body, and more mobile than the medial meniscus.
- Separated from the lateral collateral ligament by the popliteal tendon.
- Anterior horn is attached to the tibia medially in front of the intercondylar eminence
- Posterior horn inserts into the posterior aspect of the intercondylar eminence and in front of the posterior attachment of the medial meniscus.

Classification of Tears

Based on type of tear found at surgery:
- Longitudinal tears (most common; bucket-handle)
- Transverse and oblique tears
- Combination of longitudinal and transverse tears
- Tears associated with cystic menisci
- Tears associated with discoid menisci (discoid meniscus are abnormal, and because of hypermobility and the bulk they are vulnerable to compression and rotary stresses)

Based on their location in three zones of vascularity
- Red (fully within the vascular area)
- Red-white (at the border of the vascular area)
- White (within the avascular area)

Clinical features and Diagnosis

- History of trauma while playing football with the knee flexed.
- True locking is present in only 30% of cases and its presence clears the diagnosis.
- Locking usually occurs only with longitudinal tears and is much more common with bucket-handle tears, usually of the medial meniscus.
- In absence of locking, the diagnosis is more difficult. The patient may complaint of:
  - Several episodes of trouble (pain, swelling) referable to the knee
  - Effusion (within 6–12 hours of rotational stress)
  - Sensation of "giving way" or snaps, clicks, catches, or jerks
  - Tenderness in the anterior joint space following exertion
  - Localized tenderness (most important physical finding) along the medial or lateral joint line or over the periphery of the menisci.
  - Mechanical block or painful restriction of the range of motion.

Diagnostic Tests

- Noises like clicks, snaps, or catches, either audible or detected by palpation during flexion, extension, and rotary motions of the joint are localized to the joint line, suggest tear in meniscus.
- *McMurray test*
  - *Position*: Patient supine and the knee acutely and forcibly flexed, palpating the posteromedial (medial meniscus) or posterolateral (lateral meniscus) of the joint with one hand
  - *Procedure*: Keeping the knee completely flexed, the leg is externally (medial meniscus) or internally (lateral meniscus) rotated as far as possible and slowly extending the knee while listening and feeling for a click.
  - *Inference*: Click produced by the McMurray test usually is caused by a posterior peripheral tear of the meniscus
- *Apley grinding test*
  - *Position*: prone and knee is flexed to 90° and the anterior thigh is fixed against the examining table.
  - *Procedure*: foot and leg are then pulled upward to distract the joint and rotated to place rotational strain on the ligaments.
  - *Inference*: positive tests results in pain at joint line.
- *Steinmann test:* Tibial rotation is performed with the patient seated and the knee flexed 90° (squatting position). Asymmetric pain is created with external (medial meniscus) or internal (lateral meniscus) rotation.
- *Thessaly test:* It involved the examiner supporting the patient by holding his or her outstretched hands and the patient rotating the knee and body, internally and externally, 3 times, keeping the knee in flexion at 5, and repeating the procedure at 20° medial or lateral joint line discomfort or a sense of catching or locking constitute a positive results.
- *Ege's test:* It is a specific maneuver to detect a meniscal tear. With a patient squatting, an audible and palpable click is heard/felt over the are of the meniscus tear. The patient's feet are turned outwards to detect a medial meniscus tear, and turned inwards to detect a lateral meniscus tear.

Investigations

- Plain radiography: Anteroposterior, lateral, and intercondylar notch views with a tangential view of the inferior surface of the patella view to rule out degenerative joint changes (arthritis) or fractures.

- Arthrography: Replaced by magnetic resonance imaging (MRI).
- Arthroscopy is very useful in precise diagnosis, and subsequent management.
- MRI: Standard imaging study for imaging meniscus pathology and all intra-articular disorders.

Management

Nonoperative

Indication
- Incomplete tears or small peripheral tears (displaced <3 mm)
- Incomplete meniscal tear or a small (5 mm) stable peripheral tear with no other pathological condition
- Stable tears
- Meniscal tears that cause infrequent and minimal symptoms
- Tears associated with ligamentous instabilities (if the patient defers ligament reconstruction or if reconstruction is contraindicated).

Procedure
- In acute cases: Aspiration of effusion and compression bandage.
- Rest and quadriceps exercises.
- Groin-to-ankle cylinder cast or knee immobilizer worn for 4–6 weeks.
- Progressive isometric exercise program
- At 4–6 weeks:
  - Immobilization is discontinued
  - The rehabilitative exercise program for the muscles around the hip and knee is intensified.
- Counsel the patient that if symptoms recur after a period of nonoperative treatment, surgical repair or removal of the damaged meniscus may be necessary.

Operative

Procedures: Repair
- Tears of the menisci can be sutured by open or arthroscopic techniques.
- Rehabilitation program
  - Tear is small and stable
    - knee is placed in a hinged brace
    - Immediate range of motion 0–90° is permitted.
    - Touch-down weight bearing is permitted immediately
    - Full weight bearing is permitted at 6 weeks when the brace and crutches are discarded.
    - No sports are allowed for 3 months.
  - The tear large
    - Knee is placed in a hinged brace that is locked in full extension for 3–4 weeks.
    - Only touch-down weight bearing with crutches is permitted.
    - At 4 weeks, the hinge mechanism of the brace is adjusted, and motion 0–90° is begun.
    - Brace is worn for 6 weeks and then removed.
    - Crutches can be discontinued at 8 weeks.
    - No sports are allowed for 6 months.

- Menisectomy: Subtotal or total
- Meniscal transplant: Ideal candidate is a symptomatic patient with prior menisectomy, persistent pain in the involved compartment.

III: COLLATERAL LIGAMENTS

a. Medial Collateral Ligament

This is due to valgus opening of the knee joint and often associated with tear of medial meniscus.

Clinical Features

- Pain
- Swelling
- Limitation of movements
- Tenderness at the medial joint line, exaggerated on valgus stress
- Instability.

Management

- Conservative: Aspiration and compression bandage with A/K well-moulded POP cast (for I and II degree).
- Surgical: Repair of the torn ligament (for III degree).

b. Lateral collateral ligament:

This is similar to medial collateral, and is due to varus strain.

Q5. What is "the unhappy triad" of O'Donoghue?

Rupture of medial collateral ligament, medial meniscus and avulsion of anterior cruciate ligament constitute triad of O'Donoghue.

When abduction, flexion, and internal rotation of the femur on the tibia occur, supporting structures on the medial side, i.e. the medial collateral ligament and the medial capsular ligament are the injured first and with increasing magnitude of force, the anterior cruciate ligament can be torn. The medial meniscus may be trapped between the condyles of the femur and the tibia, and it may be torn as the medial structures tear, thus producing *"the unhappy triad" of O'Donoghue.*

Q6. What is Pellegrini–Stieda Disease?

Pellegrini–Stieda disease is calcification of tibial or medial collateral ligament secondary to trauma, such as a sprain or tear of the tibial collateral ligament or distal tibiofibular ligaments and interosseous membrane.

Management

Conservative

- Spontaneous recovery may occur without treatment.
- Infiltration with a local anesthetic agent, supplemented by injection of 40 mg of methylprednisolone produces quick relief.
- Ultrasound and extracorporeal shock wave therapy.

Operative

- The calcific deposit should be excised if response to conservative measures is unsatisfactory.

TIBIAL PLATEAU

Q1. Discuss the classification, clinical features and management of tibial plateau fractures.

It constitute 1% of all fractures and 8% of fractures in the elderly.

Mode/Mechanism of Injury

- It is caused by high-energy mechanisms (road traffic accident)
- Motor vehicle accidents or bumper strike injuries
- Varus or valgus forces coupled with axial loading
- It may be associated with:
    - Neurological and vascular injury
    - Compartment syndrome
    - Deep vein thrombosis
    - Contusion or crush injury to the soft tissues, or open wounds.

Clinical Features

- Pain
- Extensive swelling in upper third of the leg
- Haemarthrosis
- Tenderness
- Inability to stand and walk or move the knee
- Neurovascular examination is essential: Always examine for distal pulsations and sensations as incidence of compartmental syndrome is very high.
- Assessment of ligamentous injury is also essential.

Associated Injuries

- Meniscal tears in up to 50% of tibial plateau fractures.
- Ligamentous injury to the cruciate or collateral ligaments in up to 30% of tibial plateau fractures. It occur more frequently in minimally displaced, local compression, and split compression fractures.
- Higher incidences of peroneal nerve or popliteal neurovascular lesions associated with fractures involving the medial tibial plateau.
- Peroneal nerve injuries are caused by traction or stretching (neurapraxia).
- Arterial injuries frequently represent traction induced intimal injuries and may present as thrombosis.

Radiographic Evaluation

- **X-rays**
    - Standard AP and lateral view
    - 40° internal (lateral plate) and external rotation (medial plateau) oblique views

- Signs of associated ligamentous injury:
  - Avulsion of the fibular head
  - Segond sign (lateral capsular avulsion)
  - Pellegrini-Steata lesion (calcification along the insertion of the medial collateral ligament)
- Stress views under sedation to assess the collateral ligamentous injury
- **CT three-dimensional reconstruction**
  - Preoperative planning
  - to assess the degree of comminution or depression
- **MRI:** It is useful for evaluating injuries to:
  - The menisci
  - The cruciate and collateral ligaments
  - The soft tissue coverage
- **Arteriography** or colour Doppler if there is doubtful vascular deficit.

Classification

Hohl and Moore classification
- Type 1: Minimally displaced
- Type 2: Local compression
- Type 3: Split compression
- Type 4: Total condyle
- Type 5: Bicondylar

Schatzker Fracture Classification
- Type I: Pure cleavage; Lateral plateau, split fracture (associated with medial collateral ligament injuries)
- Type II: Cleavage combined with depression; Lateral plateau, split depression fracture
- Type III: Pure central depression; Lateral plateau, depression fracture (usually in older individuals)
- Type IV: Fractures of medial condyle (Medial plateau fracture)
- Type V: Bicondylar plateau fractures
- Type VI: Plateau fracture with dissociation of metaphysis and diaphysis

Hohl and Moore Classification of Proximal Tibial Fracture-Dislocations
- Type I: Coronal split fracture
- Type II: Entire condyle fracture
- Type III: Rim avulsion fracture
- Type IV: Rim compression fracture
- Type V: Four-part fracture

Treatment

Goals of Treatment

Restoration of:
- Articular congruity
- Axial alignment
- Joint stability
- Functional motion

Nonoperative

Indications:
- Undisplaced or minimally displaced fractures
- Patients with advanced osteoporosis
- Medically unfit
- Elderly, sedentary or nonambulatory patient

Nonoperative treatment consisting of:
- Early motion in a hinged knee brace
- Delayed and protected weight bearing (generally at 8–10 weeks)
- Physiotherapy:
    - Isometric quadriceps exercises
    - Progressive passive, active or active-assisted active range-of-knee motion exercises

Operative

Indication
- Presence of varus or valgus instability of 10° or more with the knee flexed less than 20°
- Articular depression >2 mm. Accepted varies range of articular depression from <2 mm to 1 cm.
- Open fractures
- Compartment syndrome
- Associated vascular injury

Operative treatment: Schatzker type I–IV fractures
- Percutaneous screws (cancellous screw fixation) or lateral placed periarticular plate (AO/ASIF T-plates, T-plate for intercondylar and subcondylar fractures).
- Elevation through a cortical window, bone grafting, and fixation with either large cancellous screws or a buttress plate.
- If satisfactory closed reduction (<1 mm articular step-off) cannot be achieved with closed techniques, open reduction and internal fixation are indicated.

Schatzker type V and VI fractures: These can be managed using:
- Plate and screws
- Ring fixator (Ilizarov)
- Hybrid fixator

An avulsed anterior cruciate ligament
- If it is with a large bony fragment should be repaired.
- If the fragment is minimal or the ligament has an intrasubstance tear, reconstruction should be delayed.

Postoperative
- Non-weight bearing with continuous passive motion and active range of motion
- Weight bearing is encouraged at 8–12 weeks.

Complications

- Stiffness of knee and pain due to intra- and peri-articular adhesions
- Instability due to damaged ligaments
- Post-traumatic osteoarthritis
- Malunion or nonunion, especially in *Schatzker VI* fractures at the *metaphyseal-diaphyseal junction*, related to *comminution, unstable fixation, implant failure, or infection.*

- Compartment syndrome
- Peroneal nerve injury
- Popliteal artery laceration.

TIBIA–FIBULA SHAFT

Q1. Discuss the classification, clinical features and management of fracture shaft tibia and fibula.

Tibia is the most commonly fractured long bone as it is exposed to frequent injury. Open fractures are more common in the tibia than in any other major long bone because 1/3rd of the tibial surface is subcutaneous throughout most of its length.

Mode/Mechanism of Injury

Direct

- High-energy: Motor vehicle accident
- Penetrating: Gunshot
- Bending

Indirect

- Torsional mechanisms: Twisting with the foot fixed and falls from low heights
- Stress fractures (military recruits).

Clinical Features

- Pain
- Swelling
- Tenderness
- Deformity
- Blister formation (soft tissue injury)
- Bony crepitus
- Abnormal movements
- Always examine the distal pulsations and sensations
- Monitor for compartment syndrome.

Radiographic Evaluation

- Tibia (AP and lateral views) with visualization of the ankle and knee joints
- Following thing will be appreciated on AP and lateral views:
  - Location and morphology of the fracture
  - Presence of secondary fracture lines
  - Presence of comminution
  - Degree of displacement; widely displaced fragments suggest that the soft tissue compromised and the fragments may be avascular
  - Bone loss
  - Evidence of pathological fracture: Osteopenia, metastases, infection or a previous fracture

– Gas in the tissues: Usually secondary to open fracture but may also signify the presence of necrotizing fasciitis, gas gangrene, or other anaerobic infections.
- Colour Doppler or angiography: If there is vascular deficit.

Classification

OTA Classification

- Type A: Simple
- Type B: Wedge (butterfly fragment)
- Type C: Complex (comminuted)

Descriptive

- Open/closed
- Anatomic location
  - Proximal
  - Middle
  - Distal third
- Fragment number and position
  - Comminution
  - Butterfly fragments
- Configuration
  - Transverse
  - Spiral
  - Oblique
- Angulation
  - Varus/valgus
  - Anterior/posterior
- Shortening
- Displacement
- Rotation.

Treatment

Nonoperative

- Undisplaced and satisfactory alignment: *A/K POP* cast for 12 weeks.
- CR under GA followed by application of a long leg cast for isolated, closed, low energy fractures with minimal displacement and comminution.
- Cast with the knee in 0–5° of flexion to allow for weight bearing with crutches as soon as tolerated by patient
- After 4–6 weeks, the long leg cast may be exchanged for a PTB or patella-bearing cast or fracture brace.

Acceptable criteria for reduction:
- <5° of varus/valgus angulation
- <10° of anterior/posterior angulation is recommended (<5° preferred).
- <10° of rotational deformity is recommended, with external rotation better tolerated than internal rotation.
- <1 cm of shortening.
- >50% cortical contact is recommended

Tibia stress fracture
- Cessation of the offending activity
- Short leg cast may be necessary, with partial-weight-bearing ambulation.

Fibula shaft fracture
- Although not required for healing, a short period of immobilization to minimize pain
- Weight bearing as tolerated
- Nonunion is rare because of the extensive muscular attachments.

Operative

Indication
- Unstable and displaced fractures
- Open fractures
- Polytrauma patient
- Complicated fracture (associated with compartment syndrome or vascular injury)

Intramedullary (IM) Nailing

Interlocking or simple nailing.

Advantages
- Preservation of periosteal blood supply
- Limited soft tissue damage
- Biomechanical advantages of being able to control translation, alignment, and rotation.

Flexible Nails (Enders, Rush Rods)

Indicated only in children or adolescents with open physes.

Plates and Screws

- Dynamic compression plate is reserved for fractures extending into the metaphysis or epiphysis.
- MIPPO preserves the local blood supply and improves healing

External Fixation

Indications
- Primarily used to treat severe open fractures
- Closed fractures complicated by:
  - Compartment syndrome
  - Concomitant head injury
  - Burns

Management of Open Fractures

- If mild infection is present, allow the wound to heal, leg kept in Bohler Braun's splint with lower tibial traction.
- External fixation for compound potentially contaminated injuries, Ilizarov fixator for comminuted fractures and bone loss.

Management of Complicated Fractures

- Management of vascular injuries followed by stabilization of bone
- Fasciotomy of all four muscle compartments of the leg (anterior, lateral, superficial, and

deep posterior) through one or multiple incision techniques is done, if signs of *compartmental syndrome* are obvious.
- External fixator is applied
- Following operative fracture fixation, the fascial openings should not be reapproximated.
- Final management is subsequently done for soft tissue (Local rotational flaps or free flaps may be needed for adequate coverage) and bony injuries.

Complications

- Malunion: Due to poor reduction of fracture fragments and it includes any deformity outside the acceptable range.
- Nonunion: Usually with high-velocity injuries, open fractures (especially Gustilo grade III), inadequate fixation, infection, intact fibula, and initial fracture displacement. It usually occurs in the lower one third due to poor blood supply.
- Infection may occur.
- Soft tissue loss: Secondary suturing for greater than 7–10 days in open fractures has been associated with higher rates of infection in that case local or rotations flap may be indicated.
- Compartmental syndrome *(Involvement of the anterior compartment is most common)* in closed crush injuries of tibia.
- Neurovascular injuries leading to foot drop or gangrene.
- Stiffness at the knee and/or ankle may occur.
- Knee pain: Most common complication associated with IM tibial nailing.
- Reflex sympathetic dystrophy:
  - It is usually occur in those patients who are unable to bear weight early and in those with prolonged cast immobilization.
  - It is characterized by initial pain and swelling followed by atrophy of limb.
  - Radiographic signs are spotty demineralization of foot and distal tibia and equinovarus ankle.
  - It is treated by:
    - Elastic compression stockings
    - Weight bearing
    - Sympathetic blocks
    - Foot orthoses
    - Aggressive physical therapy
- Hardware breakage or implant failures.

ANKLE INJURIES

Q1. Discuss the classification and management of ankle fracture.

Most ankle fractures are isolated malleolar fractures, accounting for 2/3rd of fractures, with Bimalleolar fractures occurring in 1/4th of patients and trimalleolar fractures occurring in the remaining 5–10%.

Mechanism of Injury

The pattern of ankle injury depends on many factors, including:
- Mechanism (axial versus rotational loading)
- Chronicity (recurrent ankle instability)

- Patient age
- Bone quality
- Position of the foot at time of injury
- Magnitude, direction, and rate of loading.

Clinical Features

- History of tortional injury to the foot, fall from height
- Pain
- Swelling
- Blister formation
- Tenderness
- Deformity
- Painful restriction of range of motion
- Careful assessment of neurovascular status.

Radiographic Evaluation

AP, lateral, and mortise views of the ankle.

AP View

- Tibiofibula overlap of less than 10 mm is abnormal and implies syndesmotic injury.
- Tibiofibula clear space of more than 5 mm is abnormal and implies syndesmotic injury.
- Talar tilt: A difference in width of the medial and lateral aspects of the superior joint space of more than 2 mm is abnormal and indicates medial or lateral disruption.

Lateral view

- The dome of the talus should be centered under the tibia and congruous with the tibial plafond.
- Posterior tibial tuberosity fractures and avulsion fractures of the talus by the anterior capsule may be identified.

Mortise View

Positioning: The foot is in 15–20° of internal rotation to offset the intermalleolar axis.

Assessment
- A medial clear space of more than 4–5 mm is abnormal and indicates lateral talar shift.
- Talo-crural angle: The angle subtended between the inter-malleolar line and a line parallel to the distal tibial articular surface should be ranged 8–15°. The angle should be within 2–3° of the uninjured ankle.
- Tibiofibular overlap less than 1 cm indicates syndesmotic disruption.
- Talar shift more than 1 mm is abnormal.

Stress View

A stress view with the ankle dorsiflexed and the foot stressed in external rotation can be used to identify medial injury with an isolated fibula fracture.

CT Scan

It helps delineate bony anatomy, especially in patients with plafond injuries.

MRI

It may be used for assessing occult ligamentous, cartilaginous, or tendinous injuries.

Bone Scan

It is useful in chronic ankle injuries, such as stress fractures, osteochondral injuries, infection, or reflex dystrophies.

Classification

I. Lauge-Hansen Classification

- According to this classification, most fractures are *supination-eversion, supination-adduction, pronation-abduction, and pronation-eversion injuries.*
- First word in the designation refers to the foot's position at the time of injury
- The second word refers to the direction of the deforming force.

Supination-Adduction (SA)

- This accounts for 10–20% of malleolar fractures.
- This is the only type associated with medial displacement of the talus.
- Stage I: Transverse avulsion-type fracture of the fibula distal to the level of the joint or a rupture of the lateral collateral ligaments.
- Stage II: Results in a vertical medial malleolus fracture.

Supination-External Rotation (SER)

- This accounts for 40–75% of malleolar fractures.
- Stage I: Disruption of the anterior tibiofibular ligament with or without an associated avulsion fracture at its tibial or fibular attachment
- Stage II: Spiral fracture of the distal fibula, which runs from anteroinferior to postero-superior
- Stage III: Disruption of the posterior tibiofibular ligament or a fracture of the posterior malleolus
- Stage IV: Transverse avulsion-type fracture of the medial malleolus or a rupture of the deltoid ligament

Pronation-Abduction (PA)

- This accounts for 5–20% of malleolar fractures.
- Stage I: transverse fracture of the medial malleolus or a rupture of the deltoid ligament
- Stage II: rupture of the syndesmotic ligaments or an avulsion fracture at their insertion sites
- Stage III: transverse or short oblique fracture of the distal fibula at or above the level of the syndesmosis; this result from a bending force that causes medial tension and lateral compression of the fibula, producing lateral comminution or a butterfly fragment

Pronation–external rotation (PER)

- This accounts for 5–20% of malleolus fractures.
- Stage I: Transverse fracture of the medial malleolus or a rupture of the deltoid ligament
- Stage II: Disruption of the anterior tibiofibular ligament with or without avulsion fracture at its insertion sites
- Stage III: Spiral fracture of the distal fibula at or above the level of the syndesmosis running from anterosuperior to posteroinferior
- Stage IV: Rupture of the posterior tibiofibular ligament or an avulsion fracture of the posterolateral tibia.

Pronation-dorsiflexion (PD)
- Stage I: Fracture of the medial malleolus
- Stage II: Fracture of the anterior margin of the tibia
- Stage III: Supramalleolar fracture of the fibula
- Stage IV: Transverse fracture of the posterior tibial surface.

II. Danis-Weber Classification

Based on the location and appearance of the fibular fracture the more proximal, the greater the risk of syndesmotic disruption and associated instability.
Three types of fractures are described:

Type A
- caused by internal rotation and adduction
- This involves a transverse fracture of the fibula below the level of the tibial plafond, an avulsion injury that results from supination of the foot and that may be associated with an oblique or vertical fracture of the medial malleolus.
- This is equivalent to the Lauge-Hansen supination-adduction injury.

Type B
- Caused by external rotation
- Oblique or spiral fracture of the fibula occurring at or near the level of the syndesmosis;
- This injury may include rupture or avulsion of the anterior inferior tibiofibular ligament, fracture of the medial malleolus, or rupture of the deltoid ligament.
- This is equivalent to the Lauge-Hansen supination-eversion injury.

Type C
- This involves a fracture of the fibula above the level of the syndesmosis causing disruption of the syndesmosis usually associated with medial injury.
- Type C injuries may involve a medial malleolar fracture or a deltoid ligament rupture. Fracture of the posterior malleolus may accompany any of the three types.
- These injuries are divided into:
- C-1: Abduction injuries with oblique fracture of the fibula proximal to the disrupted tibiofibular ligaments
- C-2: Abduction–external rotation injuries with a more proximal fracture of the fibula and more extensive disruption of the interosseous membrane.

Management

Principles:
- Accurate reduction
- Secure stabilization
- Early mobilization

Nonoperative

Indication
- Undisplaced, stable fracture patterns with an intact syndesmosis.
- Displaced fractures for which stable anatomic reduction is achieved.
- An unstable or multiple trauma patients in whom operative treatment is contraindicated because poor general condition or medical unfitness.

Stable fracture pattern: Below knee cast and allowed to bear weight as tolerated.

Displaced fractures:

- Closed reduction achieved and immobilized in a long leg cast to maintain rotational control for 4–6 weeks with serial radiographic evaluation to ensure maintenance of reduction and healing.
- The patient can be placed in a short leg cast or fracture brace once there is radiographic evidence of an adequate healing
- Patient is allowed to bear weight as tolerated.

Operative

Indications

- Failure to achieve or maintain closed reduction due to interposition of soft tissues.
- Open fractures
- Unstable fractures.
- Fractures that require abnormal foot positioning to maintain reduction (e.g. extreme plantar flexion).

Medial Malleolus:

- Open or closed reduction and fixed it with:
  - Single lag screw through large fragment
  - Two 4 mm cancellous lag screws oriented perpendicular to the fracture
  - Combination of 4 mm lag screw and Kirschner wire for small fragment
  - Tension band wiring for low transverse fracture
  - Vertical countersunk 4-mm lag screw for low transverse fracture.

Lateral Malleolus

- Indications for open reduction are still controversial.
- Fractures distal to the syndesmosis may be fixed using a lag screw or Kirschner wires with tension banding Buttress plating.
- With fractures at or above the syndesmosis, restoration of fibular length and rotation is essential to obtain an accurate reduction.
- Fixation of lateral malleolar done by:
  - 1/3 semitubular 3.5-mm plate and screws
  - Multiple 3.5-mm lag screws
  - Two lag screws for long oblique fracture
  - Single 4.5 mm malleolar screw for low transverse fracture
  - Tension band wiring 4 mm lag screw fixation of associated medial malleolar fracture.
- Acceptable displacement of the fibula:
  - Ranged from 0–5 mm.
  - In most patients, 2–3 mm of displacement is accepted depending upon the demand of the patient

Bimalleolar fracture: Open reduction and internal fixation of both malleoli

Syndesmotic injury: A syndesmotic screw is placed 1.5–2.0 cm above the plafond from the fibula to the tibia (the lateral malleolus and into the distal tibia)

Posterior malleolus fractures: Indications for fixation of include:

- Involvement of more than 25% of the articular surface
- More than 2 mm displacement
- Persistent posterior subluxation of the talus

- Fixation is done by indirect reduction and placement of an anterior to posterior lag screw, or a posterior to anterior lag screw through a separate incision.

After treatment: Stable fixation:

- Ankle is immobilized in a posterior plaster splint with the ankle in neutral position and elevated
- Remove the splint in 2–4 days and range-of-motion exercises are started
- Weight bearing is restricted for 6 weeks
- Full weight bearing is allowed after 12 weeks once there is radiographic evidence of healing.

If skin conditions, bone quality, or other factors have prevented secure fixation:

- The fracture must be immobilized longer.
- The patient is immobilized in either a short leg or a long leg non-weight bearing cast, depending on the stability of the fixation.
- After 4–6 weeks, the long leg cast can be converted to a short leg cast.
- The patient is restricted to bear weight on the ankle until fracture healing is progressing well (8–12 weeks).
- A short leg-walking cast is applied, and weight bearing is progressed.
- The cast is removed when the fracture has united.

Complication

- Malunion
- Nonunion
- Infection
- Wound dehiscence
- Posttraumatic arthritis
- Loss of reduction
- Compartment syndrome (foot)
- Reflex sympathetic dystrophy
- Tibiofibular synostosis
- Loss of ankle range of motion may occur

CALCANEUS FRACTURE

Q1. Discuss the Classification and management of fracture calcaneum.

It accounts for approximately 2% of all fractures. These fractures are associated with numerous complications and poor outcomes due to high rates of complications.

Mechanism of Injury

- Axial loading: Falls from a height are responsible for most intra-articular fractures
- Twisting forces: Usually associated with the extra-articular fractures.
- Tuberosity fractures from avulsion by the Achilles tendon are common in diabetic patient.

Clinical Features

- History of fall from the height
- Inability to stand following a fall
- Pain

- Ecchymosis around the heel
- Swelling
- Tenderness
- Blistering may be present
- Always examine dorsal lumbar spine for wedge compression fracture in a patient with a history of fall from height.

Radiographic Evaluation

It should include five views:

Lateral view:

- To assess height loss (loss of Bohler angle; increase in Gissane (crucial))
  - Bohler angle
    - It composed of a line drawn from the highest point of the anterior process of the calcaneus to the highest point of the posterior facet and a line drawn tangential from the posterior facet to the superior edge of the tuberosity.
    - The angle is normally between 20° and 40°
    - A decrease in this angle indicates collapse of posterior facet of the calcaneum
  - The Gissane (crucial) angle:
    - It is formed by two struts extending laterally, one along the lateral margin of the posterior facet and the other anterior to the beak of the calcaneus.
    - These struts form an obtuse angle usually between 95° and 105°.
    - An increase in this angle indicates collapse of the posterior facet of the calcaneum.
- To assess rotation of the posterior facet.

Axial (or Harris) view: To assess varus position of the tuberosity and width of the heel.

Anteroposterior and oblique views of the foot: To assess the anterior process and calcaneo-cuboid involvement

Borden view:

- Obtained by internally rotating the leg 40° with the ankle in neutral, then angling the beam 10–15° cephalad
- to evaluate congruency of the posterior facet

Computed tomography (CT):

- The images are obtained in 30° semi-coronal, axial, and sagittal planes
- Better delineation of the fracture.

Classification

Extra-articular Fractures (Not Involving the Subtalar Joint)

- These do not involve the posterior facet.
- Account for 25–30% of calcaneus fractures

Types

- Anterior process fractures
- Tuberosity fractures
- Medial process fractures
- Sustentacular fractures
- Body fractures not involving the subtalar articulation

Intra-articular Fractures (Involving the Subtalar Joint)

- Account for approximately 75% of calcaneal fractures
- Associated with poor functional outcome

Essex-Lopresti Classification

Primary Fracture Line

- It extends from the proximal, medial aspect of the calcaneal tuberosity, through the anterolateral wall
- Most critical is its location through the posterior facet of the calcaneus; it can be located in the:
  - Medial third near the sustentaculum tali
  - The central third
  - The lateral third near the lateral wall.

Secondary Fracture Line

Continue axial force results in additional comminution, separating free lateral piece of posterior facet from the tuberosity fragment.

- Tongue fracture:
  - A secondary fracture line appears beneath the facet and exits posteriorly through the tuberosity.
  - Posterior facet fragment exist distal to the Achilles tendon insertion
- Joint depression fracture:
  - A secondary fracture line exits just behind the posterior facet.
  - Posterior facet fragment exist anterior to the attachment of the Achilles tendon.

Sanders Classification

Based on CT scans (location and number of fracture lines through the posterior facet)

- **Type I:** All nondisplaced fractures regardless of the number of fracture lines
- **Type II:** Two-part fractures of the posterior facet; subtypes IIA, IIB, IIC, based on the location of the primary fracture line
- **Type III:** Three-part fractures with a centrally depressed fragment; subtypes IIIAB, IIIAC, IIIBC
- **Type IV:** Four-part articular fractures; highly comminuted

Management

Goals

- Restoration of congruency of the posterior facet of the subtalar joint
- Restoration of the height of the calcaneus (Bohler angle)
- Reduction of the width of the calcaneus
- Decompression of the subfibular space available for the peroneal tendons
- Realignment of the tuberosity into a valgus position
- Reduction of the calcaneocuboid joint if fractured.

Nonoperative

Indications
- Undisplaced or minimally displaced extra-articular fractures.
- Undisplaced intra-articular fractures.

- Anterior process fractures with <25% involvement of the calcaneocuboid articulation.
- Fractures in patients with insulin-dependent or diabetes severe peripheral vascular disease.
- Fractures in medical unfit patients.
- Fractures associated with blistering and massive prolonged edema, severely compromised soft tissue status, large open wounds, or life-threatening injuries.

Treatment comprises of:

- Elevation
- Cold compression
- Below knee POP slab/cast in neutral flexion to prevent an equinus contracture for 3 weeks of non-weight bearing followed by gradual mobilization.

Operative

Indications

- Displaced intra-articular fractures involving the posterior facet
- Anterior process of the calcaneus fractures with more than 25% involvement of the calcaneo-cuboid articulation
- Displaced fractures of the calcaneal tuberosity
- Fracture-dislocations of the calcaneus
- open fractures of the calcaneus

Timing of surgery

- Within the initial 3 weeks of injury, before fracture consolidation occurs.
- Surgery should not be performed until swelling in the foot and ankle has subsided, as indicated by the reappearance of skin wrinkles.

Extra-articular Fracture

Anterior Process Fractures

Indication for surgery: Fractures involving more than 25% of the calcanealcuboid articulation
Treatment: Open reduction and fixed with small or mini-fragment screws.

Tuberosity (Avulsion) Fractures

Due to violent pull of the gastrocnemiussoleus complex
Indication for surgery

- Posterior skin crease is at risk from pressure from the displaced tuberosity
- Prominence of Posterior portion of the bone so that it affect shoe wear
- Gastrocnemius soleus complex function is compromised
- Avulsed fragment involves the articular surface of the joint.

Treatment: Open reduction and fixed with a lag screw fixation with or without cerclage wire.

Medial or Lateral Process Fractures

- Usually nondisplaced
- Undisplaced fractures: Short leg weight-bearing cast for 8–10 weeks (until the fracture heals).
- Displaced fractures: Closed manipulation.

Intra-articular Fractures

Operative goals
- Restore congruity of the subtalar or talocalcaneal articulation
- Restore Bohler angle
- Restoration of the normal width and height of the calcaneum
- Maintenance of the normal calcaneo-cuboid articulation

Treatment
- Open reduction and internal fixation with recon or buttress plate and screws.
- *Essex-Lopresti maneuver*: Using percutaneous axial pin reduction technique for lifting the fragment in tongue-type fractures

After treatment:
- Limb Elevation for 72 hours
- At 3 weeks, the sutures are removed, and a new cast is applied; cast is worn for 4 weeks
- Non-weight bearing for 8–12 weeks.
- Full weight bearing is allowed by 3 months.

Complications

- Wound necrosis
- Dehiscence
- Infection
- Loss of reduction of major fragments
- Mal-reduction
- Sural nerve and peroneal tendon injuries
- Increased heel width
- Loss of subtalar motion
- Posttraumatic arthritis
- Chronic pain
- Reflex sympathetic dystrophy.

TALUS

Q1. Discuss the blood supply, classification and management of fracture talus.

This is an important tarsal bone as it is a link between tibia, the fixed long bone of the lower extremity and the mobile part of the foot. It has no muscle attachments, and is part of the ankle and talocalcaneonavicular joint complex.

Fracture of the talus is peculiar because of its precarious blood supply like that of scaphoid and head of femur.

Blood Supply

- The vascular channels enter the talus from its undersurface of the neck through the vessels passing through the sinus tarsi, which ascend and then pass into the head, neck and the body.
- It consists of:
  - Arteries to the sinus tarsi (Peroneal and dorsalis pedis arteries).
  - Head and neck regions are richly supplied by the superior neck vessels, branching off the dorsalis pedis artery and the artery of the sinus tarsi.

- Artery of the tarsal canal (posterior tibial artery). It is the most consistent major supplier of blood to the body of the talus. In the tarsal canal, it sends four to six direct vessels into the body of the talus. The talar body is vulnerable because of its blood supply.
- The deltoid artery (posterior tibial artery), which supplies the medial one fourth to one-half of the talar body.
- Capsular and ligamentous vessels and intraosseous anastomoses.
- Posterior tubercle of the talus is supplied by direct branches most commonly from the posterior tibial artery or the peroneal artery.
- Any fracture or dislocation causes damage to this vascular channel and is responsible for avascular necrosis and nonunion of the fracture site.

Talar Head Fractures

It constitutes 5–10% of talar injuries.

Mechanism of injury
- Axially directed loading and compression of the talar head
- a dorsal compression fracture of the anterior tibial plafond
- Comminution is common; one must also suspect navicular injury and talonavicular disruption.
- As the recognition of this fracture is difficult, a high index of suspicion should be maintained for *post-traumatic tenderness* in the anterior ankle region.

Radiographic evaluation
- Plain radiographs may define the fracture clearly.
- CT often is necessary for definitive diagnosis and evaluation of displacement.

Treatment
- *Undisplaced fracture*
  - Patient should be immobilized in a well-moulded short leg cast and should be partially weight bearing for 6 weeks.
  - Arch support is worn in the shoe to splint the talonavicular articulation for 3–6 months.
- *Displaced fracture:*
  - ORIF using an anteromedial approach, medial to the anterior tibial tendon
  - Stable fixation with partially threaded cancellous lag screws or with headless, fully threaded compression screws
  - Early motion can be encouraged at ~ 2 weeks after surgery, with delayed weight bearing at a minimum of 6 weeks
- *In osteonecrosis (10%) degenerative arthrosis or for severe fracture:* Arthrodesis of the talonavicular joint.

Talar Neck Fractures

It constitutes 25–30% of talar injuries.

Mechanism of Injury

- Hyperdorsiflexion of the ankle
- Aviator Astraguls: refers to a rudder bar of a crashing airplane impacting the plantar aspect of the foot, resulting in a talar neck fracture

Clinical Features

- An obvious history of injury to the ankle
- Diffuse Swelling involving the ankle and subtalar area
- Foot pain
- Tenderness over the talus and subtalar joint
- Inability to stand and bear weight
- The blood leaks into the soft tissue and all ankle movements are painful and restricted.

Radiographic Evaluation

- Anteroposterior (AP), mortise, and lateral radiographs of the ankle and foot
- Canale view: Optimum view of the talar neck
  - Ankle is in maximum equinus
  - The foot is placed on a cassette, pronated 15°
  - The radiographic source is directed cephalad 15° from the vertical
- Computed tomography (CT): It helps:
  - To characterize fracture pattern and displacement further
  - To assess articular involvement
- Technetium bone scans or magnetic resonance imaging (MRI): to assess occult talar neck fractures

Classification

Hawkins classification of talar neck fractures
- Group I fracture: Nondisplaced vertical fractures of the neck
- Group II fracture: Displaced fractures with subluxation or dislocation of the subtalar joint
- Group III fracture: Fracture with dislocation of the subtalar and the ankle joints (group III fractures)
- Group IV fracture: *(Canale and Kelley)*: Type III with associated talo-navicular subluxation or dislocation

Treatment

Type I Fractures

If the subtalar joint is free of displacement and fragments
- Initially kept in a well-padded slab and subsequently converted into a non-weight bearing cast for 4–6 weeks.
- Non-weight bearing cast is applied with the foot fully plantar flexed (equinus) an unfamiliar and unpleasant position which is essential.

Types II, III, and IV Fractures

- Open reduction and internal fixation
- Early reduction and fixation done in cases of fracture-dislocation.
- *Old unreduced fracture*, dislocations and comminuted burst fractures are best treated by pantalar arthrodesis.

Internal fixation by:
- K-wires

- Two interfragmentary lag screws or headless screws:
  - These are placed perpendicular to the fracture line.
  - These can be inserted in antegrade or retrograde fashion.
  - Posterior-to-anterior directed screws are biomechanically stronger.
- Use of titanium screws allows better visualization and evaluation of subsequent osteonecrosis with MRI.
- Sometimes plate can be used to buttress areas of comminution.

Post-treatment

- The foot is held in neutral position
- Well moulded BK cast is applied
- After 6–8 weeks, depending on radiographic signs of early union, a walking boot is applied, and weight bearing is permitted.
- 3 months after surgery, if union has progressed satisfactorily, the cast is removed.
- *Hawkins sign*: Subchondral osteopenia (seen on the AP ankle radiograph) in the talus at 6–8 weeks tends to indicate talar viability.

Complications

- Infection: Early open reduction and internal fixation with soft tissue coverage for open injuries or waiting until swelling has decreased.
- Osteonecrosis: It increased in frequency with the grade. Maximum with grade IV
- Skin slough or necrosis, especially in displaced fracture dislocations
- Posttraumatic arthritis
- Delayed union and nonunion
- Malunion
- Foot compartment syndrome (Rare)

FOOT

Q1. Write short note on Lisfranc's (Tarsometatarsal) fracture-dislocation.

Tarsometatarsal (Lisfranc) joint injuries are generally considered rare.

Mechanism of Injury

Three most common mechanisms include:
- Twisting (motor vehicle accidents)
- Axial loading of a fixed foot
- Crushing.

Clinical Features

- Swelling
- Ecchymosis over the plantar aspect
- Mid-foot tenderness (palpate each articulation for tenderness and swelling)
- Rotation test: Stressing the second tarso-metatarsal joint by elevating and depressing the second metatarsal head relative to the first metatarsal head elicits pain at the Lisfranc joint.

- Inability to bear weight on the foot (sign of instability).
- Careful neurovascular examination is essential, because dislocation of Lisfranc joint (associated with impingement on or partial or complete laceration of the dorsalis pedis artery (DPA)).

Radiographs

- AP/lateral views in bearing weight
- Following things should be evaluated:
  - AP view: The medial shaft of the second metatarsal should be aligned with the medial aspect of the middle cuneiform.
  - Oblique view: The medial shaft of the fourth metatarsal should be aligned with the medial aspect of the cuboid.
  - First metatarsal–cuneiform articulation should have no incongruency.
  - "Fleck sign": in the medial cuneiform–second metatarsal space. This represents an avulsion of the Lisfranc's ligament.
  - Subluxation of the naviculo-cuneiform articulation
  - Compression fracture of the cuboid.

MRI

- Lisfranc's ligament in acute cases
- If the level of injury cannot be determined by plain radiographs

Classification

Myerson

Based on commonly observed patterns of injury with regard to treatment:
- Total incongruity: Lateral and dorso-plantar
- Partial incongruity: Medial and lateral
- Divergent: Partial and total

Type A

- Displacement of all five metatarsals with or without fracture of the base of the 2nd metatarsal.
- The usual displacement is lateral or dorsolateral, and the metatarsals move as a unit.
- Homolateral

Type B

- One or more articulations remain intact.
- *Type B1* injuries: Medially displaced, sometimes involving the intercuneiform or naviculo-cuneiform joint.
- *Type B2* injuries: Laterally displaced and may involve the 1st metatarsal–cuneiform joint.

Type C

- Divergent injuries and can be:
  - Partial (C1)
  - Complete (C2)
- These generally are high-energy injuries, associated with significant swelling, and prone to complications, especially compartment syndrome.

Ouenu and Kuss

Based on commonly observed patterns of injury.
- **Homolateral:** All five metatarsals displaced in the same direction.
- **Isolated:** One or two metatarsals displaced from the others.
- **Divergent:** Displacement of the metatarsals in both the sagittal and coronal plane.

Associated Injuries

- Fractures of the cuneiforms, cuboid, and/or metatarsals are common.
- Fracture 2nd metatarsal (most frequent).

Treatment

Conservative

Indication: Closed, nondisplaced (<2 mm) injuries
Procedure
- Non-weight bearing cast for 6 weeks
- It is followed by a weight bearing cast for an additional 4–6 weeks.
- Serial radiographs at regular intervals should be obtained to ensure that no displacement is occurring in the cast.

Operative

Indications: Displaced fractures
Procedures
- Closed reduction and internal fixation with Steinmann pins (3/32-inch) or K-wires or 4 mm cannulated or 4 mm standard, partially threaded cancellous screws.
- Open reduction and internal fixation is preferred if reduction is inadequate, or significant comminution is present (especially in partial (type B) or divergent (type C) patterns)

After-treatment
- Bulky dressing
- Posterior splint
- At 7–10 days: Below knee, non–weight bearing cast.
- At 6–8 weeks: Partial weight bearing may be allowed.
- At 8 weeks: Laterally placed implants are removed.
- At 4 months: Medial screws/wires are removed.

Complications

- Posttraumatic arthrosis (managed successfully with tarso-metatarsal and inter-metatarsal arthrodesis)
- Compartment syndrome (although rare and usually seen only with higher energy fracture-dislocations)
- Infection
- Complex mediated regional pain syndrome (RSD)
- Neurovascular injury
- Hardware failure

Q2. Write short note on Jones fracture

Jones Fracture

- Fracture base of fifth metatarsal.
- This is due to inversion injury of foot due to imbalance.
- Usually presents with:
  - Pain
  - Swelling
  - Tenderness over the base of fifth metatarsal

Treatment

- Undisplaced fracture treated by BK POP cast for 6 weeks.
- If avulsion and separation is seen, then open reduction and internal fixation with screw or tension band wiring should be done.

PELVIS

Q1. Discuss the classification and management of pelvic fractures.

Fractures of pelvis accounts for <5% all skeletal injuries, but they are important because of increased incidence of associated soft tissue injury and high risk of *massive blood loss (~3L), shock, sepsis, ARDS (or fat embolism).*

Mechanism of Injury

- Low-energy trauma, such as:
  - Falls in elderly patients
  - Sudden muscular contractions in young athletes that cause an avulsion injury
  - Straddle-type injury
- High-energy pelvic fractures result most commonly from:
  - Motor vehicle accidents
  - Falls
  - Motorcycle accidents
  - Automobile-pedestrian encounters
  - Industrial crush injuries
- Impact injuries
- Injury patterns vary by the direction of force application:
  - *Anteroposterior (AP) force*: Results in external rotation of the hemipelvis
  - *Lateral compression (LC) force*: Most common and results in impaction of cancellous bone through the SI-joint and sacrum.

Clinical Features

- History of major trauma due to vehicular accident, collapse of building or crush injury.
- The patient is usually in shock due to haemorrhage from pelvic venous plexus of veins in unstable pelvic fractures.
- Massive flank or buttock contusions and swelling with hemorrhage indicates bleeding
- Localized tenderness at fracture site and swelling

- Pelvic compression and distraction is painful.
- SLR is zero or decreased on the affected site
- Anuria due to rupture of bladder (20%) or urethra (10%)
- Haematuria due to urethral injury (10%)
- Distension of abdomen due to bladder
- Signs of visceral injury.

Radiographic Evaluation

X-rays

AP of the pelvis for:
- Pubic rami fractures and symphysis displacement
- SI joint and sacral fractures
- Iliac fractures
- Fractures of L5 transverse process

Special Views

Obturator and iliac oblique views: In cases of suspected acetabular fractures.
Inlet radiograph:
- Positioning: the patient supine with the tube directed 60° caudally, perpendicular to the pelvic brim.
- Useful for:
  - Assessment of:
    - Anterior or posterior displacement of the sacroiliac joint
    - Sacrum
    - Iliac wing
  - Determine internal rotation deformities of the ilium and sacral impaction injuries.

Outlet radiograph:
- Positioning: patient supine with the tube directed 45° cephalad.
- Useful for:
  - Determination of vertical displacement of the hemipelvis.
  - Visualization of subtle signs of pelvic disruption

CT scan: Assessing the posterior pelvis, including the sacrum and SI joints

To rule out any visceral injury or other sources of bleeding:
- CT scan of the chest and abdomen
- Supraumbilical peritoneal lavage
- Abdominal ultrasound

Radiographic signs of instability include:
- SI displacement of 5 mm in any plane.
- Posterior fracture gap.
- Avulsion of the L5 transverse process, the lateral border of the sacrum (sacrotuberous ligament), or the ischial spine (sacro-spinous ligament).

Classification

Tiles classification:
- Type A: Stable (posterior arch intact)
  - A1: Avulsion injury

- A2: Iliac wing or anterior arch fracture caused by a direct blow
- A3: Transverse sacro-coccygeal fracture
- Type B: Partially stable (incomplete disruption of posterior arch)
  - B1: Open book injury (external rotation)
  - B2: Lateral compression injury (LC) (internal rotation)
    B2-1: Ipsilateral anterior and posterior injuries
    B2-2: Contralateral (bucket-handle) injuries
    B3: Bilateral
- Type C: Unstable (complete disruption of posterior arch)
  - C1: Unilateral
  - C1-1: Iliac fracture
  - C1-2: Sacroiliac fracture-dislocation
  - C1-3: Sacral fracture
  - C2: Bilateral, with one side type B, one side type C
  - C3: Bilateral

In most easy way: Stable fracture with:
- Intact pelvic ring
- An isolated fracture of ilium (Duverney's), pubic rami ischium

Unstable fracture (bi- and tri- planar): This involves:
- Double lesions like bilateral rami *(saddle fracture)*
- Opening of pubic symphysis and sacroiliac joint
- Ipsilateral fracture of pubic rami with ala of sacrum (Malgaigne's fracture) and contralateral *(Bucket handle fracture)*

Complicated fracture: With visceral damage:
- *Bladder*: Anuria with abdominal distension.
- *Urethra*: Haematuria, anuria or incontinence of urine.
- *Vessels*: Pelvic plexus of veins, causing shock/death.
- *Nerve*: Posterior ring fracture, leading to sciatic nerve damage.

Management

Pelvic Damage Control

Principles of Care
- Resuscitation (ABC)
- Management of shock by replacement of blood, fluids
- Thorough assessment of visceral damage (especially anus, rectum, vagina, and genitourinary system)
- Assessment of any neurologic injury
- Hemorrhage control
- Closed reduction of the pelvis at admission
- External fixation
  - Wrapping pelvis with sheets with inner rotation and slight flexion of knees
  - External fixator
  - Pelvic C-clamp (*Ganz "anti-shock" pelvic fixator* for immediate, provisional stabilization of pelvic fractures)
  - Pneumatic anti-shock garment

- Control of haemorrhage
  - Pelvic packing
  - Angiography
- Control of contamination
  - Repair of genitourinary and rectal injuries
  - Debridement of necrotic tissue in the case of open injury

Factors for increased mortality include:
- Patient's age
- Injury severity score
- Associated head or visceral injury
- Blood loss
- Hypotension
- Coagulopathy
- Unstable or open pelvic fractures

Treatment (in General)

Stable Fracture

Rest for 2–3 weeks followed by mobilization.

Unstable Fracture

- Hammock's sling with traction on both lower limbs for biplanar fractures.
- Hip spica for children with minimal displacement.
- ORIF for fracture of the ilium and acetabulum.
- External fixator or plating for pelvic ring disruption.
- *After treatment*: When the patient's comfort allows, ambulation started with a walker or crutches with touchdown weight bearing on the affected side.

Weight-bearing Status

Weight-bearing status may be encouraged as follows:
- Full weight bearing on the uninvolved limb started within several days.
- Partial weight bearing on the involved extremity is recommended for at least 6 weeks.
- Full weight bearing on the involved extremity without crutches or support started by 12 weeks.

Operative Techniques

External Fixation

- This can be applied as a construct mounted on 2–3.5 mm cancellous shanz pins spaced 1 cm apart along the anterior iliac crest under image intensifier, or with the use of single pins placed in the supra-acetabular area in an AP direction (Hanover frame).
- It is a resuscitative fixation
- Used for definitive fixation of anterior pelvis injuries
- It cannot be used as definitive fixation of posteriorly unstable injuries.

Internal Fixation

Iliac wing fractures: ORIF using lag screws and neutralization plates.

Diastasis of the pubic symphysis: Plate fixation if there is no open injury or cystostomy tube is present.

- Sacral fractures:
  - Plate fixation or sacroiliac screw fixation
  - Transiliac bar fixation may be inadequate or may cause compressive neurologic injury
- *Unilateral sacroiliac dislocation*: Fixation with cancellous screws or anterior sacroiliac plate fixation is used
- *Bilateral posterior unstable disruptions*: Fixation of the displaced portion of the pelvis to the sacral body by posterior screw fixation.

Complication

Early

- Shock due to haemorrhage.
- Visceral damage consisting of urethra, bladder and bowel.
- Damage to important vessels and sciatic nerve.
- Thromboembolism
- Infection (incidence increased with open fractures, presence of contusion or any soft tissue injury)
- Associated fracture of femur, spine and hip dislocation.

Late

- Malunion
- Nonunion (rare)
- Painful gait
- Problems during childbirth.

ANKYLOSIS AND ARTHRODESIS

Q1. Define ankylosis and classify it.

Ankylosis is loss of movement in the joint either by intra-articular (true ankylosis) or by extra-articular involvement (false ankylosis).

Types

I. True Ankylosis

a. *Fibrous variety*
- There occurs fibrosis between the articular surfaces following destruction to the cartilage leading to limitation of movements.
- Pain on using force (or on attempted movements)
- Joint line visible in X-rays
- Two types:
  - *Short fibrous ankylosis*: Jog of movements present and are painful
  - *Long fibrous ankylosis*: Range of movement is slightly better than short fibrous ankylosis and are painful
- Example: It is commonly seen as a sequel of:
  - Tubercular arthritis

- Acute arthritis
- Gonococcal arthritis
- Rarely rheumatoid arthritis

b. *Bony ankylosis*:

- There occurs formation of *bony trabeculae* between the articular surfaces following destruction of the articular cartilage.
- No movements even on using force.
- No pain
- Bony trabeculation across the joint in X-rays.
- Example: It occurs following:
- Suppurative arthritis

II. False Ankylosis:

Extra-articular involvement; causes are:

- Burns
- Myositis traumatica
- Contracture of the soft tissue (ligaments/capsule/muscles)

Q2. Define Arthrodesis. Give the optimum positioning of arthrodesis at different joint.

This is *surgical ablation of movements at a joint* to relieve pain, cure a disease and provide stability. This gives the joint, stability at the cost of mobility.

Indication

- Infection
- Trauma
- Tumors
- Paralytic conditions
- Osteoarthritis
- Rheumatoid arthritis

Technique

The arthrodesis is done by excision of the articular cartilage and the fusion of the joint by:
- Intra-articular technique
- Extra-articular technique
- Combined intra-articular and extra-articular

Modalities Used for Arthrodesis

The stability may be additionally provided by:
- Cortico-cancellous bone grafts
- Plates and screws
- Charnley's compression clamp/Ilizarov apparatus is used for fusion of knee/ankle.

Functional position of arthrodesis

The ideal positions for the common joints are:

Shoulder Arthrodesis

Indications
- Infection
- Paralytic disorders
- Unreconstructable rotator cuff tears
- Combined insufficiency of rotator cuff and deltoid
- Failed shoulder arthroplasty
- Arthritic diseases unsuitable for arthroplasty
- Recurrent dislocations
- Neoplastic lesions

Position: 25–40° of abduction, 20–30° of forward flexion, and 25–30° of internal rotation.

Elbow Arthrodesis

Indications
- Infection
- Failed total joint arthroplasty
- Posttraumatic arthritis
- Arthritic diseases unsuitable for arthroplasty
- Severely comminuted intra-articular fractures

Position
- *Unilateral elbow*: Fusion at 90° was optimal for personal hygiene needs, whereas fusion at 70° was best for extra-personal activities.
- *Bilateral elbow (if indicated)*: One elbow should be placed in 110° of flexion to permit the patient to reach the mouth, and the other should be placed in 65° to aid in personal hygiene.

Wrist Arthrodesis

Indications
- Posttraumatic arthritis
- Neoplastic lesions
- Severely comminuted intra-articular fractures
- Rheumatoid arthritis
- Wrist or hand paralysis
- Spastic hemiplegia
- Failed total joint arthroplasty
- Failed limited arthrodesis

Position:
- 10–20° of extension (dorsiflexion)
- In general, neutral to 5° of ulnar deviation is preferred.
- If bilateral wrist fusions are indicated: the positions should be determined by the needs of the patient

Hip Arthrodesis

- Prerequisites: Normal function of the lumbar spine, contralateral hip, and ipsilateral knee.
- Position: 30° of flexion, 0–5° of adduction, and 0–15° of external rotation.

Knee Arthrodesis

Indications:
- Painful ankylosis (after infection, tuberculosis, or trauma)
- Severe deformity in paralytic conditions
- Neuropathic arthropathy
- Malignant or potentially malignant lesions around the knee
- Failed total knee arthroplasty (most frequent now a days)

Position: 0–15° of flexion, 5–8° of valgus, and 10° of external rotation.

Ankle Arthrodesis

Indications
- Posttraumatic arthritis (most common)
- Rheumatoid arthritis
- Infection
- Neuromuscular conditions
- Salvage of failed total ankle arthroplasty

Position: 0° of flexion, 0–5° of valgus, and 5–10° of external rotation with slight posterior displacement of the talus.

7

Spine Injury

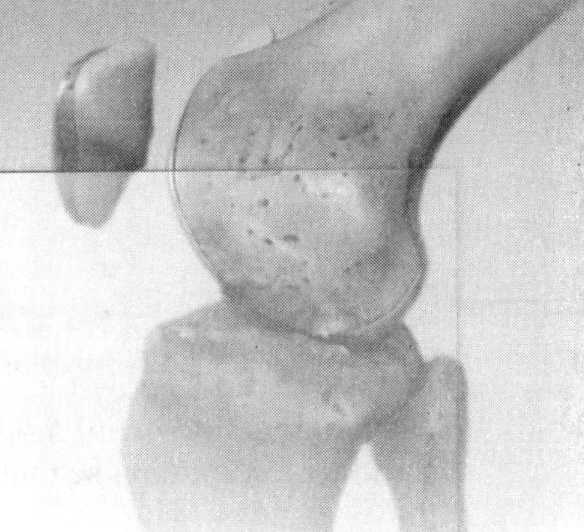

Q1. Discuss the mechanism of injury.

Mechanism of Spinal Injury

Primary

- This refers to physical tissue disruption caused by mechanical forces.
- *Contusion*: Brief compression by a displaced structure
- *Compression*: Occur with translation or angulation of the spinal column
- *Stretch*: Longitudinal traction, as in the case of a flexion distraction
- *Laceration*: By penetrating foreign bodies, missile fragments, displaced bone.

Secondary

- This refers to additional neural tissue damage resulting from the biologic response (inflammation; release of mediators) initiated by the physical tissue disruption.
- Local tissue elements undergo structural and chemical changes.

Pathophysiology

Primary Neurological Damage

- Direct trauma, haematoma and SCIWORA <8 years old
- In 4 hours: Infarction of white matter occurs
- In 8 hours: Infarction of grey matter and irreversible paralysis.

Secondary Damage

- Hypoxia
- Hypoperfusion
- Neurogenic shock
- Spinal shock

Q2. What are different types of spinal cord injury and discuss in brief about various spinal cord syndromes.

Spinal cord injuries can be classified into either complete or incomplete categories.

Complete

- It is characterized by complete loss of both motor and sensory function below the level of traumatic level.

- No evidence of motor/sensory recovery in sacral segments within 48–72 hours post injury.

Incomplete

- It is characterized by variable neurological deficits with partial loss of sensory and/or motor function below the lesion.
- Preservation of partial motor and sensory functions below the level of traumatic level and including sacral segments.

Types of Spinal Cord Paralysis

- Monoplegia—paralysis of one limb
- Diplegia—paralysis of either upper or lower limbs
- Paraplegia—paralysis of both lower limbs
- Hemiplegia—paralysis of upper limb, torso and lower leg on one side of the body
- Quadraplegia—paralysis of all four limbs.

Spinal Cord Syndrome

These syndromes are usually resulting from incomplete traumatic lesions.

Central Cord Syndrome

- Most common.
- Usually results from a hyperextension injury (older individual with preexisting osteoarthritis of the spine) or occur in younger patients with flexion injuries.
- There occurs destruction of the central area of the spinal cord, including gray and white matter.
- Features:
  - Patient presenting with quadriparesis involving the upper extremities more than the lower.
  - Initial flaccid weakness followed by lower motor neuron type of paralysis.
  - Sensory sparing varies, but usually sacral pinprick sensation is preserved.
- Prognosis: Variable.

Anterior Cord Syndrome

- Caused by a hyperflexion injury
- Characterized by: Complete motor loss
  - Loss of pain and temperature discrimination below the level of injury
  - Posterior columns are spared to varying degrees, resulting in preservation of deep touch, position sense, and vibratory sensation
- Prognosis: Poor

Posterior Cord Syndrome

- Syndrome is rare
- Caused by an extension injury
- Involves the dorsal columns of the spinal cord
- Produces loss of proprioception vibrating sense
- Preserving other sensory and motor functions

Brown-Sequard Syndrome

- Injury to either half of the spinal cord
- Result of a penetrating injury, rotational injury or unilateral laminar or pedicle fracture, resulting in a subluxation.
- Characterized by:
  - Motor weakness on the side of the lesion
  - Contralateral loss of pain and temperature sensation
- Prognosis: Good.

Conus Medullaris Syndrome

- Injury of the sacral cord (conus) and lumbar nerve roots within the spinal canal
- Most occur between T11 and L2
- Results in:
  - Flaccid paralysis
  - Areflexic bladder, bowel (loss of all bladder and perianal muscle control)
  - Absence of the bulbocavernosus reflex and the perianal wink (irreversible).

Cauda Equina Syndrome

- Injury between the conus and the lumbosacral nerve roots within the spinal canal
- Results in areflexic bladder, bowel, and lower extremities (flaccid paralysis)
- Bulbocavernosus reflex, anal wink, and all reflex activity in the lower extremities are absent.

Q.3 Discuss classification and instability of spinal injuries.

CERVICAL SPINE INJURY

- *Cervical vertebral* allow movement in the planes of *flexion, extension, lateral bending, and rotation.*
- C_2 and C_5 as the two most common areas of cervical spine injury
- These injuries produce neurological damage in ~ 40% of patients.
- ~10% of traumatic cord injuries have no obvious radiographic evidence of vertebral injury (whiplash injury).

Classification

- There are following six common patterns of injury
- Each of these patterns is further subdivided into stages based on the degree of injury to osseous and ligamentous structures.
  - Compressive flexion (subdivided into five stages)
  - Vertical compression (subdivided into three stages)
  - Distractive flexion (subdivided into four stages)
  - Compressive extension (subdivided into five stages)
  - Distractive extension (subdivided into two stages)
  - Lateral flexion (subdivided into two stages)

Instability

Instability: It is the loss of the ability of the spine under physiological loads to maintain relationships between vertebrae in such a way that the spinal cord or nerve roots are not irritated or damaged, and deformity or pain does not develop.

Instability may be **acute or chronic.**

- *Acute*: it is caused by bone or ligament disruption that places the neural elements in danger of injury with any subsequent deformity or loading.
- *Chronic instability*: it is the result of progressive deformity that may cause neurological deterioration, prevent recovery of injured neural tissue, or cause increasing pain or decreasing function.

White and Panjabi's criteria of instability

Element	Point value
• Anterior elements destroyed or unable to function	2
• Posterior elements destroyed or unable to function	2
• Relative sagittal plane translation >3.5 mm	2
• Relative sagittal plane rotation >11°	2
• Positive stretch test	2
• Medullary (cord) damage	2
• Root damage	1
• Abnormal disc narrowing	1
• Dangerous loading anticipated	1
A score of 5 or more indicates instability	

Radiographically instability is indicated by:

- Horizontal translation >3.5 mm on the lateral flexion-extension view
- >11° of angulation.

Stretch Test

- Determining clinical instability in the lower cervical spine
- Contraindicated in an obviously unstable injury
- It should always be done under supervision of the attending physician
- Use of MRI in combination with reformatted CT has minimized the necessity of this test.

THORACIC AND LUMBOSACRAL FRACTURES

Classification

Nicoll's Classification

- Stable
- Unstable

Holdsworth classified thoracolumbar fractures into five groups according to the mechanism of injury:

- Pure flexion
- Flexion and rotation
- Extension
- Vertebral compression
- Shearing

Denis developed a three-column concept of spinal injury:

- Anterior column: Contains the anterior longitudinal ligament, the anterior half of the vertebral body, and the anterior portion of the anulus fibrosus.
- Middle column consists of the posterior longitudinal ligament, the posterior half of the vertebral body, and the posterior aspect of the anulus fibrosus.

- Posterior column includes the neural arch, the ligamentum flavum, the facet capsules, and the interspinous ligaments.
- Instability exists with disruption of any two of the three columns. Thoracolumbar stability usually follows the middle column: if it is intact, then the injury is usually stable.

McAfee et al.

Wedge Compression Fractures

- Result from forward flexion
- Cause isolated failure of the anterior column
- They rarely are associated with neurological deficit except when multiple adjacent vertebral levels are affected.

Stable Burst Fractures

- Anterior and middle columns fail because of a compressive load
- No loss of integrity of the posterior elements

Unstable Burst Fractures

- Anterior and middle columns fail in compression ·
- Posterior column is disrupted
- Posterior column can fail in compression, lateral flexion, or rotation.
- Tendency for posttraumatic kyphosis and progressive neural symptoms because of instability.

Chance Fractures

- Horizontal avulsion injuries of the vertebral bodies
- Caused by Flexion around an axis anterior to the anterior longitudinal ligament
- Entire vertebra is pulled apart by a strong tensile force.

Flexion Distraction

- Flexion axis is posterior to the anterior longitudinal ligament.
- Anterior column fails in compression, whereas the middle and posterior columns fail in tension.
- Injury is unstable because the ligamentum flavum, interspinous ligaments, and supraspinous ligaments usually are disrupted.

Translational Injuries

- It is characterized by malalignment of the neural canal, which has been totally disrupted.
- Usually all three columns have failed in shear.
- At the affected level, one part of the spinal canal has been displaced in the transverse plane.

Thoracolumbar Injury Classification and Severity Score

- To assess whether the surgery is appropriate or can be managed conservatively.
- Patients with scores of ≤3 should do well with nonoperative treatment, whereas patients with scores of ≥5 require surgery.

	Points
Fracture mechanism	
• Compression fracture	1
• Burst fracture	1
• Translation/rotation	3
• Distraction	4
Neurological involvement	
• Intact	0
• Nerve root	2
• Cord, conus medullaris, incomplete	3
• Cord, conus medullaris, complete	2
• Cauda equina	3
Posterior ligamentous complex integrity	
• Intact	0
• Injury suspected/indeterminate	2
• Injured	3
Interpretation	
• Score of ≤3—nonoperative treatment	
• Score of ≤5—operative treatment	
• Score of 4—either nonoperative or operative treatment, depending on qualifiers such as comorbid medical conditions and other injuries	

Q4. Discuss in brief clinical and radiological evaluation of patient with spinal injuries.

Fractures and dislocations of the spine are serious injuries that usually occur in young people. Any case of spinal injury must be evaluated under following subheadings:

A Case of Spinal Injury

Assess the patient: *Airway, breathing, circulation, disability, and exposure (ABCDE).*

Physical Examination

- Assess mental status
- An assistant should hold the neck steady in a neutral position while inspection and palpation.
- *Attitude*: Elbows may be flexed if a spinal cord injury causes loss of function below the biceps, or they may be extended if the paralysis at higher level.
- *Head*: For lacerations and contusions and palpated for facial fractures
- *Ear canals*: To rule out leakage of spinal fluid or blood behind the tympanic membrane, its presence indicates a skull fracture
- *Spinous processes* (upper cervical to the lumbosacral): Painful spinous process indicates spinal injury
- *Palpable defects* in the interspinous ligaments: If present indicates disruption of ligamentous complex
- *Pain or tenderness* on palpation of the cervical spine: Indicated spinal injury requiring collar immobilization
- *Sensation* to light touch comparing each spinal level
- *Pinprick sensibility* with a sterile needle if necessary

- *Motor strength* should be examined sequentially.
- *Deep tendon reflexes* and pathological reflexes also should be checked.
- *Motor and sensory evaluation* of the rectum and peri-rectal area is mandatory.
- *Penile erection* and incontinence of the bowel or bladder suggest a significant spinal injury.
- *Quadriplegia* is indicated by flaccid paralysis of the extremities.
- *Bradycardia or episodes* of asystole may be the only finding of significant injury to cervical spine.
- *Chest, abdomen,* and extremities should be examined for occult injuries.

Neurological Evaluation

Glasgow coma scale: Determining the level of consciousness

Eyes Open (E)	
Spontaneous	4
To sound	3
To pain	2
Never	1
Best Verbal Response (V)	
Oriented	5
Confused conversation	4
Inappropriate words	3
Incomprehensible words	2
None	1
Best Motor Response (M)	
Obeys commands	6
Localizes pain	5
Flexion withdrawal	4
Abnormal	3
Extension	2
None	1

Sensory Examination

- Start with light touch, then pinpricks (using a sterile needle), beginning at the head and neck and progressing distally, to examine specific dermatome distributions
- Important dermatome landmarks:
    - C_2 and C_3: Posterior head and neck
    - C_4 and T_2: Adjacent to each other in the upper thorax
    - Nipple line T
    - Xiphoid process T_7
    - Umbilicus - T_{10}
    - Inguinal region T_{12}, L_1
    - Perineum and perianal region: S_2, S_3, and S_4
- Upper extremity
    - C_5: Anterior shoulder
    - C_6: Thumb
    - C_7: Index and middle fingers
    - $C_{7/8}$: Ring finger
    - C_8: Little finger

  - T_1: Inner forearm
  - T_2: Upper inner arm
  - $T_{2/3}$: Axilla
- Lower extremity
  - L_1: Anterior upper-inner thigh
  - L_2: Anterior upper thigh
  - L_3: Knee
  - L_4: Medial malleolus
  - L_5: Dorsum of foot
  - L_5: Toes 1–3
  - S_1: Toes 4,5; lateral malleolus
  - S_3/C_1 (coccygeal1): Anus
- Evidence of sacral sensory sparing establishes the diagnosis of an incomplete spinal cord injury

Motor Examination

- Higher motor function (coordination, memory, cranial nerve examination)
- Begin with upper extremity.
- Inspect for muscle wasting
- Evaluate muscle tone
- Test muscle strength:
- MRC grading:
  - Grade 0: No muscle movement
  - Grade 1: Muscle movement without joint motion (flickering)
  - Grade 2: Moves with gravity eliminated
  - Grade 3: Moves against gravity but not resistance
  - Grade 4: Moves against gravity and light resistance
  - Grade 5: Normal strength

Key Muscle Groups used in ASIA Motor Source Evaluation of Cord Injury

Level	Muscle Group
C5	Elbow flexors (biceps, brachialis)
C6	Wrist extensors (extensor carpi radialis longus and brevis)
C7	Elbow extensors (triceps)
C8	Finger flexors (flexor digitorum profundus to the middle finger)
T1	Small finger abductors (abductor digiti minimi)
L2	Hip flexors (Ilio-psoas)
L3	Knee extensors (quadriceps)
L4	Ankle dorsiflexors (tibialis anterior)
L5	Long toe extensors (extensor hallucis longus)
S1	Ankle plantar-flexors (gastrocnemius, soleus)

Reflexes

Superficial Reflexes

- Superficial reflexes are motor responses to scraping of the skin.
- Graded simply as present or absent

Reflex	Sensory (s)/Motor component (m)
Corneal	V (s) and VII (m)
Nose tickle	V (s) and VII + (m)
Gag	IX, X (s, m)
Abdominal	T_7–T_{12} (s, m)
Cremasteric	T_{12}, L_1 (s, m)
Plantar	$S_{1,2}$ (s, m)
Anal wink	$S_{4,5}$ (s, m)

Deep Tendon Reflexes

- These are performed to assess the integrity of the spinal reflex/arc, which is having a sensory component (afferent) and motor component (efferent).

Stretch (deep tendon) reflex	Sensory (s)/Motor component (m)
Biceps	C_{5-6} (s, m)
Triceps	C_{6-7} (s, m)
Brachioradialis	C_{6-8} (s, m)
Finger flexor	C_{6-8} (s, m)
Knee	L_{2-4} (s, m)
Ankle	$S_{1,2}$ (s, m)

- Graded as:
  - 0: Absent
  - 1: Diminished/sluggish as ankle reflex
  - 2: Normal
  - 3: Brisk/exaggerated as knee reflex
  - 4: Clonus

Pathological Reflex

- *Babinski response* (dorsiflexion of the great toe with spreading of the lateral four toes (fanning) upon stroking the plantar surface of the foot) is suggestive of upper motor neuron lesions.
- *Bulbo-cavernosus reflex*: contraction of the anal sphincter in response to stimulation of the trigone of the bladder with either a squeeze on the glans penis, a tap on the mons pubis, or a pull a urethral catheter.
- Although spinal shock generally resolves within 24 hours, it may last longer.
- A positive bulbo-cavernosus reflex or return of the anal wink reflex indicates the end of spinal shock

Involuntary movement: Look for any involuntary movements

Neurogenic shock

- It refers to flaccid paralysis, areflexia, and lack of sensation physiologic spinal cord in response to injury.
- It is usually seen in cervical and upper thoracic injuries.
- It usually resolves within 24–48 hours.
- The bulbo-cavernosus reflex (S_{3-4}) is the first to return

Differentiate between neurogenic shock/hypovolemic shock

Neurogenic shock	Hypovolemic shock
As the result of loss of sympathetic outflow	As the result of haemorrhage
Hypotension	Hypotension
Bradycardia	Tachycardia
Warm extremities	Cold extremities
Normal urine output	Low urine output

To assess cord level:
- C_2–C_7 = add +1 for cord level
- T_1–T_6 = add +2
- T_7–T_9 = add +3
- T_{10}: L_1, L_2 level
- T_{11}: L_3, L_4 level
- L_1: Sacrococcygeal segments

Grading Systems for Spinal Cord Injury

Frankel Classification

- Grade A: Absent motor and sensory function
- Grade B: Absent motor function, sensation present
- Grade C: Motor function present, but not useful (2 or 3/5), sensation present
- Grade D: Motor function present and useful (4/5), sensation present
- Grade E: Normal motor (5/5) and sensory function

American Spinal Injury Association (ASIA) Impairment Scale
- Grade A: Complete: No motor or sensory function is preserved in sacral segments S4-5.
- Grade B: Incomplete: Sensory but not motor function is preserved below the neurologic level and extends through the sacral segment S4-5.
- Grade C: Incomplete: Motor function is preserved below the neurologic level; most key muscles below the neurologic level have a muscle grade <3.
- Grade D: Incomplete: Motor function is preserved below the neurologic level; most key muscles below the neurologic level have a muscle grade >3.
- Grade E: Normal: Motor and sensory function is normal.

Radiological Evaluation

- *X-rays*
  - Lateral view of the cervical spine (ideally down to T1)
  - AP views of the chest and pelvis
  - Lateral radiographic examination of the entire spine
- *CT scan*
  - In cases of questionable or inadequate plain radiographs
  - Excellent bony detail of the fracture pattern usually can be obtained.
  - Helpful in evaluating the degree of compromise of the spinal canal
- *MRI*
  - It is very useful in the evaluation of patients with neurological deficits without obvious fracture.
  - MRI essential to define spinal cord anatomy and also for assessing ligamentous injury.

- Myelography and EMG
- SCIWORA: Spinal cord injuries without radiographic abnormalities:
  - Most common in children younger than 8 years old
  - Inherent elasticity of the juvenile spine make the spinal cord is vulnerable to injury without disrupting the vertebral column.

Q.5. Discuss in brief the management of traumatic paraplegia.

The *primary goals of treatment* are to:
- Realign the spine, obtain and maintain spinal stability
- Prevent loss of function of uninjured neurological tissue
- Improve neurological recovery
- Obtain early functional recovery

Aim

In paraplegia aim must be:
- No bedsores
- No contractures
- An uninfected bladder, with the early onset of reflex micturition in upper motor neurone lesions
- Bowel care
- The patient's ability to support himself with a craft
- Make a paraplegic's life comfortable.

Three Phases

Phase 1: Emergency phase

- Signs of an unconsciousness patient:
  - Diaphragmatic breathing
  - Neurological shock (Low BP and HR)
  - Flexed upper limbs (loss of extensor innervations below C5)
  - Responds to pain above the clavicle only
- Care must start at scene of injury to reduce injury, preserve function
- Rapid assessment of ABC (airway, breathing, circulation)
  - Primary and second survey (discussed previously)
- Avoid any movement of injured spine during transportation; support the neck with cervical collar.
- Log rolling of the patient should be done for change of lateral position
- Strict immobilization (treat all suspected injuries as injured until proven otherwise)
  - Immobilize and stabilize head and neck, use cervical collar before moving patient.
  - Secure head and maintain patient in supine position.
- Avoidance of hypoxia
- Avoidance of hypotension/hypovolaemia
- Catheterization of patient if urinary retention is suspected and also to monitor urine output.
- Screening for concomitant injury to other organ systems and prompt management of any serious injury.

Role of steroid

- When a spinal cord injury is suspected, steroids should be started in the field.
- The steroid dosage and administration schedule was established by three publications of results from three phases of the National Acute Spinal Cord Injury Study (NASCIS I, II, and III).
- *Summary of NASCIS I, II, and III Protocols*:
    - Methylprednisolone bolus 30 mg/kg, then infusion 5.4 mg/kg/hour
    - Infusion for 24 hours if bolus given within 3 hours of injury
    - Infusion for 48 hours if bolus given within 3–8 hours after injury
    - No benefit if methylprednisolone started more than 8 hours after injury
    - No benefit with naloxone
    - No benefit with tirilazad
- Patients who received methylprednisolone infusion within 8 hours of injury showed significantly more improvement in motor function and pinprick and touch sensation at 6 weeks and at 6 months after injury.

Phase 2: Management of Fracture

Cervical Spine Injury

Aim

- To achieve proper alignment of vertebra
- To maintain it in that position till the vertebral column stabilizes
- To realign the spine
- To prevent loss of function of undamaged neurological tissue
- To improve neurological recovery
- To obtain and maintain spinal stability
- To obtain early functional recovery

Nonoperative treatment: Immobilization in a rigid cervical orthosis for 8–12 weeks may be sufficient.

Indication

- Stable cervical spine injury with no compression of the neural elements
- Stable compression fractures of the vertebral bodies
- Undisplaced fractures of the laminae, lateral masses, or spinous processes
- Unilateral facet dislocations: reduced in traction may be immobilized in a halo vest for 8–12 weeks.
- Stable Jefferson fractures, hangman's fractures, and type II and type III odontoid fractures immobilized in a halo vest.

Braces

- Cervical collar: During the phase of acute pain
- Philadelphia collar
- Sternal-occipital-mandibular immobilizer (SOMI)
- 4-poster brace
- Halo device.

Tractions

- Reduced by skull traction: Crutch field tong (CFT); Head-Halter traction.
- Ten lb of traction weight is applied, and then weight is added in 5-lb increments, with lateral radiographs after each addition, until the spine is realigned.

- A general guideline is 10 lb for the head and 5 lb for each additional level of injury.
- Continuous monitoring during reduction is essential to prevent iatrogenic injury
- Traction recommended for different levels of injury

Level	Minimum weight in pounds (kg)	Maximum weight in pounds (kg)
C1	5(2.3)	10 (4.5)
C2	6(2.7)	10-12 (4.5–5.4)
C3	8 (3.6)	10-15 (4.5–6.8)
C4	10 (4.5)	15-20 (6.8–9.0)
C5	12 (5.4)	20-25 (9.0–11.3)
C6	15 (6.8)	20-30 (9.0–13.5)
C7	18 (8.1)	25-35 (11.3–15.8)

Follow up: Serial radiographs should be obtained weekly for the first 3 weeks and then at 6 weeks, 3 months, 6 months, and 1 year.

Operative:

- Open reduction and internal fixation
- Anterior, posterior, or combined approach depends on the pattern of injury

Indications: Unstable injuries of the cervical spine, with or without neurological deficit.

Thoracolumbar Fractures

Nonoperative

- Relive of pain (analgesic)
- Preventive care including thromboembolism prophylaxis, pulmonary toilet, etc.
- Bracing or casting
    - CASH brace (cruciform anterior spinal hyperextension brace)
    - Jewett hyperextension brace
    - Korsain brace
    - Knight-Taylor brace
    - Rigid LSO
- For stable fracture: Continue brace for 3 months (24 × 7); serial lateral skiagram (at 3, 6, 9, 12 weeks) to assess stability:
    - CSTLO: Fracture above T_{1-6}
    - TLSO: Fracture b/w T_6–L_3
    - TLSO with pelvic band: L_{4-5}

Operative

Indications

- Progressive neurological deficit
- Fracture dislocation
- Translational instability
- Progressive kyphosis >30°
- >50% of canal compromise
- Injury to posterior column
- >50% loss of vertebral height
- Worsening of neurological deficit
- Partial neurological deficit with CT proven loose body in canal

Procedures (anterior, posterior, posterolateral (transpedicular))

Principle: Decompression of cord and internal fixation by either posterior or anterior approach with fusion.

Different techniques to restore integrity of the vertebral column:

- *Kyphoplasty and vertebroplasty* are safe and effective and has useful role in painful osteoporotic vertebral compression fractures that do not respond to conventional treatments.
- *Vertebroplasty* is a minimally invasive image-guided procedure involving the injection of bone cement (Polymethyl methacrylate (PMMA)) into a vertebral body fracture in an effort to improve pain and stability of the fracture.
- *Balloon kyphoplasty* is a similar procedure that utilizes an inflatable balloon tamp, in an effort to reduce the fracture and create a space to theoretically allow safer injection of cement into the fractured vertebral body.
- Specific instrumentation
  - Harrington rod
  - Hartshill rectangle fixation sublaminar wire
  - Pedicle screw instrumentation
  - Anterior spinal instrumentation:
    - Kaneda instrumentation
    - Anterior plate fixation
- Anterior vertebral body excision with titanium cage and bone grafts.

Phase 3: Rehabilitation

- The *primary goal* of the rehabilitation is to enable or motivate the patient to *achieve physical, social, emotional, recreational, vocational and functional recovery.*
- It is a team approach and it should begin as early as possible after the injury.

I. Respiratory management

Paraplegics patient have three issues to manage

- *Secretions:* Due to paralysis of abdominal muscles (D6-L1) required for forceful expiration; coughing is ineffective so there occur accumulation of secretions.
- *Atelectasis:* Due to intercostal muscles paralysis the inspiration is dependent on diaphragm which is already weak hence tendency to develop atelectasis.
- *Hypoventilation:* Due to paralysis of respiratory muscles

Nerve supply of diaphragm is C_{3-5} (C_4). Patient with injury C_2 and above may not survive because even diaphragm is paralyzed. Patient with L_1 or lower level are usually no significant respiratory dysfunction.

Respiratory management involves

- Chest physiotherapy: Chest clapping percussion to loosen the secretion and drain clogged lung lobes.
- Suction: Useful for quadriplegics with lot of secretion.
- Assisted coughing
  - Here manual pressure is applied to abdomen timed with patients cough reflex.
  - Palms are placed below the cage between xiphoid process and umbilicus.
  - After a deep breath is taken by the patient, physiotherapist pushes upward and inwards with palm as patient cough.
  - This maneuver helps to mobilize the secretion from the lower portion of the lungs.
- Incentive spirometry
  - Encourage the patient to inhale as deeply as possible.
  - Purpose is to prevent or treat atelectasis.

- Abdominal binder
  - Useful when patient become seated from supine position.
  - Abdominal content are pulled down by gravity and have a tendency to fall forward due to lack of abdominal muscle tone.
  - This also pulls the diaphragm downwards.
  - Therefore, at the start of inspiration diaphragm is at lower level that is the position of mechanical disadvantage.
  - Abdominal binder pushes abdominal content and diaphragm up which improve ventilation.

II. Bowel Management

- *Defecation centre* is located in sacral cord segment (S_{2-4}).
- *Internal anal sphincter*:
  - It is composed of involuntary smooth muscles
  - It provides continence in the resting state by remaining tonically contracted.
- *External anal sphincter*:
  - It is voluntary
  - It is innervated by pudendal nerve (S_{2-4}).
- *Defecation reflex*:
  - It consists of stretching of rectum and puborectalis muscle by the passage of stool in leading to *reflex relaxation of internal anal sphincter*.
  - This causes an urge to defecate but external anal sphincter and puborectalis muscle prevent defecation.
  - Under voluntary control, external anal sphincter and puborectalis muscle relax allowing defecation

UMN Lesion/Spastic Bowel

- When injury occurs above S_{2-4} segment, i.e. conus medullaris, the anal sphincter becomes spastic.
- Voluntary control is lost but reflex evacuation is intact.
- Bowel management in this type consists of:
  - Planned reflex evacuation by digital stimulation or suppositories.
  - Use of stool softeners
  - Bulk forming agents may help maintain adequate stool consistency.

LMN/Flaccid Bowel

- It occurs when injury involves:
  - Reflex center and or
  - Sacral nerve roots
- This is characterized by flaccid rectum with absence of spine mediated reflex activity.
- Management consists of:
  - Manual evacuation
  - Diet management
  - Use of stool softeners
  - Bulk forming agents removal to facilitate easy removal

III. Bladder Management

Automatic/Reflex/UMN or Cord Bladder

- It occurs due to complete transection of the cord above the sacral segments.
- Micturition reflex is intact.
- The bladder is of small capacity.
- It empties reflexely at regular small intervals in response to certain filling pressure.
- Loss of bladder sensation and there is no voluntary control.

Management:

- Intermittent catheterization
- Reflex voiding (condom catheter)

Autonomous/Denervated/LMN/Autonomous Bladder

- It occur injury to conus medullaris or in cauda equina (disruption of either sacral segment S_{2-4} or sacral nerve roots)
- There is no reflex activity.
- Patient has dribbling urine irregularly.
- Bladder is atonic with large amount of residual urine.

Management

- Intermittent catheterization
- Manual compression (Crede's maneuver)

Urine Complication in Paraplegic

- UTI
- Hydronephrosis
- Renal calculi
- Carcinoma of bladder

Management

- Plenty of fluid intakes
- 2–3 hourly clamping of catheter
- Bladder irrigation with normal saline and betadiene
- Change of Ph from acidic to alkaline and *vice versa*.

IV: Sexual Rehabilitation and Fertility

Males

- Psychogenic errection is mediated via sympathetic system (D_{11}–L_2) while reflex errection results from sacral stimulation via a parasympathetic nervous system (S_{2-4}).
- Ejaculation is controlled by both sympathetic and parasympathetic system.
- Patient with spinal cord injury have erectile and ejaculatory dysfunction.
- In UMN, lesion psychogenic errection is lost but reflex errection may be possible although it may be ill sustained.
- In LMN, lesion reflex errection is possible only in small number.

Management

- Intra cavernous papaverine injection can be used for erectile dysfunction. These patient are unable to ejaculate and there may be retrograde ejaculation.
- Electrostimulation may be done for ejaculatory dysfunction.
- Fertility is decreased due to poor semen quality and ejaculatory dysfunction.
- Assisted reproduction techniques like IU insemination and IVF should be tried if patient wants to father the child.

Female fertility
- There is insignificant impact in fertility but pregnancy is going to be a complicated in pre natal, perinatal and postnatal phases.
- CS is indicated, as patient may not have labour pains.

V. Skin Care and Pressure Sores (Bed Sores)

Factors leading to pressure sores (bed sores) include:
- Sensory loss
- Loss of vasomotor control hence low tissue resistance
- Skin maceration due to moisture or urine
- Nutrition deficiency
- Poor general condition

Grading
- Grade 1: Skin intact but hyperemic for >1 hour after relief of pressure
- Grade 2: Blister or break in dermis
- Grade 3: Subcutaneous destruction extending into the muscles
- Grade 4: Involvement of bone and joints

Prevention
Theses can only be prevented by reliving pressure.
Preventive techniques include:
- Patient education regarding frequent changes of posture
- Water/air bed/sponge mattress to distribute evenly pressure over bony points
- Good nutrition
- Use of long handled mirror for self-inspection.

Treatment consists of:
- Thorough debridement and cleaning
- Operative procedures to repair pressure ulcer includes *direct closure, Musculocutaneous and fasciocutaneous flaps,* which are better able to withstand pressure.

Complication of pressure sores includes:
- Endocarditis
- Heterotropic bone formation
- Septicemia
- Abscess
- Osteomyelitis
- Squamous cell carcinoma

VI. Spasticity
- It correspond with the level of injury to the cord. Higher is the level of injury to the spinal cord more is the incidence of spasticity.
- In some cases spasticity may contribute to improve patient function but it needs treatment when it possess risk of developing contractures interfering with functions and causes pain due to spasm.

Causes include:
- UTI
- Bladder calculi

- Impacted bowel
- Irritation from urinary catheter, etc.

Treatment option includes
- Stretching exercise
- Medication (Baclofen BZD and muscle relaxant)
- Nerve block by absolute alcohol or phenol
- Intrathecal baclofen and absolute alcohol in intractable spasticity

VII. Heterotropic Ossification

- Aetiology is unknown but it could be due to spasticity, tissue hypoxia, necrosis or humoral factors
- It is an extra-articular ossification of muscle of paralyzed extremities.
- Hip is most commonly involved though knee, elbow, shoulder may be involved.
- Anteromedial aspect of hip is most commonly involved.

Clinical features in acute phase:
- Fever
- Swelling of soft tissue
- Movements are painfully restricted

Diagnosis in acute stage is by:
- Bone scan
- USG
- CT scan
- ESR, alkaline phosphatase and CRP are elevated.

Management
- There is no definite prophylaxis
- Treatment in acute phase is:
    - Rest
    - Etidronate therapy which inhibits mineralization and ROM exercises.
    - Mature bone may need resection if it is interfering with sitting, positioning or dressing. One should weight 1.5–2 years before resection to allow time for maturation of bone.

Q6. Enumerate the complications following spinal cord injury.

Complications

- Skin breakdown: Skin breakdown (also termed "decubitus ulcers" or "pressure sores") are a major complication associated with spinal cord injury.
    - They occur as a result of excessive pressure, primarily over the bones of buttock.
    - Following a spinal cord injury, there are not only changes in muscle tone and sensation, but shift in the supply of blood to the skin and subcutaneous tissue.
    - Additionally there is a loss of the normal elastic nature of the tissues underlying the skin.
    - Increased stiffness, vascular alteration and alteration in muscle tone combine to significantly reduce the skin's ability to withstand pressure.
- Osteoporosis and fractures
- Pneumonia, atelectasis, aspiration

- Heterotopic ossification
- Spasticity
- Autonomic dysreflexia
- Deep vein thrombosis
- Cardiovascular disease
- Syringomyelia
- Neuropathic pain
- Respiratory dysfunction

Q7. Enumerate few important spine fractures.

These fractures include:

Burst Fracture

- Axial violence
- Fall on heel or buttock
- Body fractures vertically
- Cervical vertebra: Minerva jacket used
- Plaster jacket in extension for 3 months.

Whiplash injury

- Spinal cord injury without any radiological evidence of vertebral fracture
- Extension injury
- Cervical spine (most common)
- Cervical strain: Philadelphia collar.

Jefferson's Fracture

- Burst fracture of atlas
- Vertical compression force

Kummels Disease

- Neglected compression fracture of spine
- Wedging of vertebra
- Intervertebral space normal

Chance Fracture

- Hyper-flexion injury (flexion-distraction spinal injury)
- Most common site: Thoracolumbar region (T10–L2) in most adults
- Horizontal fracture through the posterior elements also known as "seat belt fracture
- Significant physical exam finding to assess for is the *"seatbelt sign,"* which refers to *bruising or abrasion on the abdomen in the distribution of a seat belt.*

Tear Drop Fracture

In cases of lordotic cervical spine, further extension may crush the vertebral body, forcing bone backwards into the cord.

Hangman Fracture

- Neck hyperextension
- Fracture of C_2 vertebra (axis)
- Dislocation between C_2 and C_3

Q8. Enumerate ascending and descending tracts.

Descending Tract

- Lateral corticospinal tract
- Anterior corticospinal tract
- Rubrospinal tract—control muscle tone of flexor muscle groups
- Olivo-spinal tract
- Vestibule-spinal tract-modulate cervical motor neurons
- Tecto-spinal tract-mediates reflex postural movements in response to visual and possibly auditory stimuli.
- Lateral and medial reticulo-spinal tract-produces monosynaptic and polysynaptic excitation of axial (more strongly) and limb muscles.

Ascending Tract

- Post funiculus
- Fasciculus gracilis: Fine touch (upper part of body)
- Fasciculus cuneatus: Fine touch (lower part of body)
- Lateral funiculus
- Lateral spinothalamic tract: Pain and temperature
- Anterior and posterior spino-cerebellar tract: Unconscious proprioceptive of lower limb and trunk
- Spino-olivary tract
- Spino-tectal tract
- Ant funiculus
- Ant spinothalamic tract: Crude touch.

8

Infection

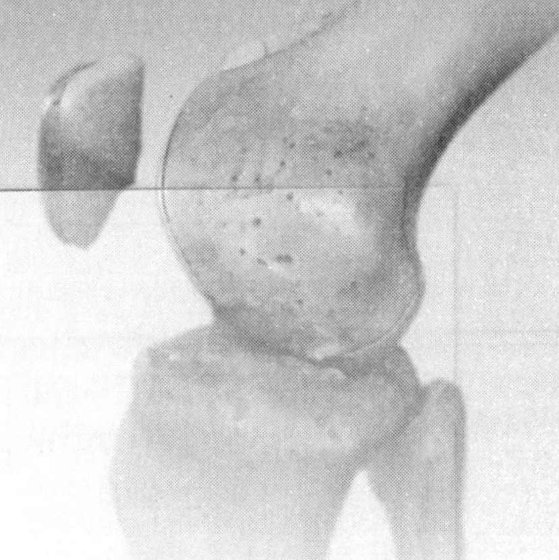

Q1. What is the most common site of involvement of osteomyelitis in long bones in children and why?

Metaphysis is the most common site of involvement of osteomyelitis. It is due to following reasons:

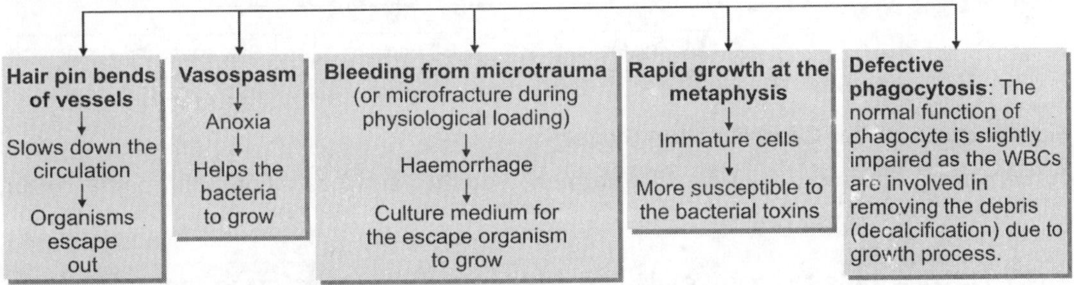

Q2. Write in brief about the classification system used for osteomyelitis.

Classification of osteomyelitis is based on numerous criteria, such as:
- Duration of infection or symptoms (*acute, subacute and chronic*)
- Mechanism of infection (*exogenous or hematogenous*)
- Type of host response to the infection (*pyogenic or nonpyogenic*)

Following systems are generally used for classifying the osteomyelitis:

I. *Waldvogel classification system for osteomyelitis*: Waldvogel classification system divides osteomyelitis into the categories of *hematogenous, contiguous and chronic.*
- Hematogenous osteomyelitis
- Osteomyelitis secondary to contiguous focus of infection
  - No generalized vascular disease
  - Generalized vascular disease
- Chronic osteomyelitis (necrotic bone)

II. *Cierny-Mader staging system for osteomyelitis*: The more recent Cierny-Mader staging system is for *chronic osteomyelitis*, based on physiological and anatomical criteria, to determine the stage of infection.
- In the Cierny-Mader system there are no terms like 'acute' and 'chronic'.
- Stages in this system are dynamic.
- Stages may be altered by changes in the medical condition of the patient (host), successful antibiotic therapy and other treatments.

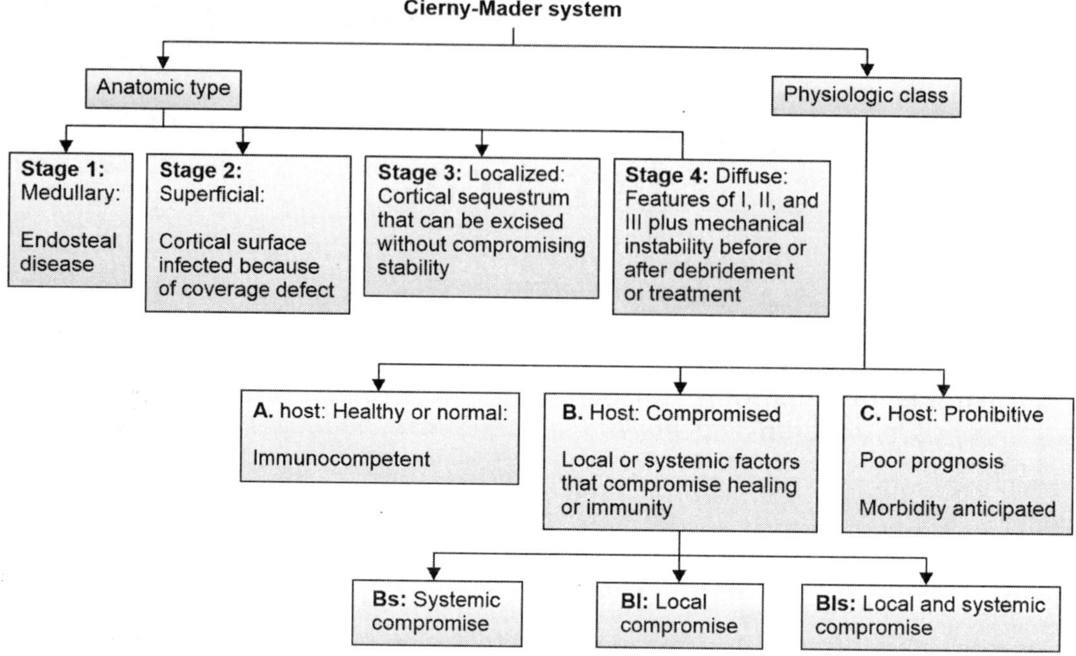

Significance of this Classification System

It help in determining the type of treatment whether simple or complex, palliative or curative or limb ablative or sparing.

Q3. Define acute osteomyelitis. Discuss its clinical features and management.

Acute hematogenous osteomyelitis is the most common type of bone infection and usually is seen in children.

Acute Osteomyelitis

It is a disease of *infancy* and *childhood*, due to pyogenic infection of the metaphysis, may go for septic course and is occasionally fatal.

Aetiology

Host Factors

Age: Bimodal (generally affecting children younger than 2 years and children 8–12 years old).

Sex: Male: female 4:1

Site:

- Infection usually involves a single bone, most commonly the tibia, femur, or humerus in children and vertebral bodies in older adults and injection drug users.
- Trauma causes haematoma formation, which is a good culture medium for organism to grow. Antecedent focus of primary infection (boils) may be present.

Agent factors

Microorganisms

- More than 95% of cases of hematogenous osteomyelitis are caused by a single organism. *Staphylococcus aureus* accounts for 50% of isolates.

- Other common pathogens include group B streptococci and *E. coli* during the newborn period and group A streptococci in early childhood.
- Vertebral osteomyelitis is due to *E. coli* and other *enteric bacilli* in ~25% of cases.
- *S. aureus, Pseudomonas aeuroginasa,* and *Serratia* infections are associated with intravenous drug users, and may involve the sacroiliac, Sternoclavicular, or pubic joints as well as spine.
- *Salmonella* spp. are the major causes of long bone osteomyelitis complicating sickle cell anaemia and other haemoglobinopathies. This infection tends to be diaphyseal rather than metaphyseal.
- *Tuberculosis* and *brucellosis* affect the spine more often than other bones.
- *Proteus, Pseudomonas* and *Bacteroides* seen in soft tissue damage and anaerobic areas,
- Fungal osteomyelitis is seen increasingly in chronically ill patients receiving long-term intravenous therapy or parenteral nutrition
- Development of fungal infection after thorn pricks injury to the foot, etc.

Pathology
- **Infective organisms,** in neonates, are close to the joint, hence epiphyseal damage and growth disturbance is rapid and frequent.
- In a child, organisms reach the traumatized metaphyseal zone and they multiply in this zone of slow blood flow *(due to hairpin capillary flow)* and form a small medullary abscess, which soon expands, but the growth plate acts as a barrier and prevents the spread of abscess towards the joint.
- The bone is:
  - Destroyed by proteolytic enzymes.
  - Necrosed by arterial thrombosis.
  - Decalcified by hyperemia.
  - Absorbed by activity of osteoclast.
- The medullary abscess can spread to:
  - Subperiosteal space
  - Epiphysis
  - Joint cavity or medullary cavity
  - Through skin

Clinical Features

The child has all the features of a febrile illness.

General

- Fever
- Irritability
- Restlessness
- Headache
- Convulsions
- Vomiting
- Tachycardia
- Tachypnoea

Local

- Pseudoparalysis (due to severe pain, the limb is kept motionless)
- Swelling

- Tenderness
- Redness
- Raised temperature around the metaphyseal area
- Diffuse oedema over the extremity
- Sympathetic effusion of the neighbouring joints
- Tender regional lymphadenopathy

Investigations

- *For early diagnosis*
    - MRI (early inflammatory changes in bone marrow and soft tissue)
    - Radioactive isotope uptake (Technetium-99 m bone scans can confirm the diagnosis 24–48 hours after onset in 90–95% of patients)
    - CT scan to see for early signs of bone destruction
- *X-ray*
    - Plain radiographs obtained early in the course of infection may show soft tissue swelling, but the first change in bone—*a periosteal reaction*—is not evident until at 10 (10–12 days) days after the onset of infection.
    - Later on, metaphyseal abscess.
    - Periosteal lifting giving an onion peel appearance, moth eaten erosion of medulla and cortex with sequestrum formation.
    - Lytic changes can be detected after 2–6 weeks, when 50–75% of bone density has been lost.
    - Rarely, a well-circumscribed lytic lesion, or Brodie's abscess, is seen in a child who has been in pain for several months but has had no fever.
- *Blood*
    - Culture is invariably positive
    - Polymorphonuclear leukocytosis
    - Raised erythrocyte sedimentation rate (ESR)
    - C-reactive protein is positive
- *Pus:* Aspiration of abscess and culture of organism (sample is sent to the laboratory for Gram stain, culture, and sensitivities).

Treatment

Conservative

- Intravenous fluids
- Antibiotics (The choice is based on the highest *bactericidal activity, the least toxicity, and the lowest cost*).
- Anti-inflammatory
- Mag-Sulf dressings
- Rest to the part (comfortable positioning of the affected limb) with the help of a splint or traction

Nade's principles for the treatment of acute hematogenous osteomyelitis

- An appropriate antibiotic is effective before pus formation.
- Antibiotics do not sterilize avascular tissues or abscesses, and such areas require surgical removal.
- If such removal is effective, antibiotics should prevent their reformation, and primary wound closure should be safe.

- Surgery should not damage further already ischemic bone and soft tissue.
- Antibiotics should be continued after surgery.

Surgical

Objective: To drain any abscess cavity and remove all non-viable or necrotic tissue.

Indications
- The patient is presenting late (>48 hours) or failure of the patient to improve despite appropriate intravenous antibiotic treatment
- The presence of an abscess requiring drainage

Once pus has formed, it should be removed by:
- Aspiration
- Incision drainage
- If necessary drill holes (4 mm in diameter through the cortex into the medullary canal) in the cortex to decompress medullary abscess and irrigation (at least 3 L of saline with a pulsatile lavage system) of the cavity is done.
- If pus escapes through these holes, use a drill to outline a cortical window 1.3 × 2.5 cm, remove the cortex with an osteotome and evacuate the pus.

In nutshell:

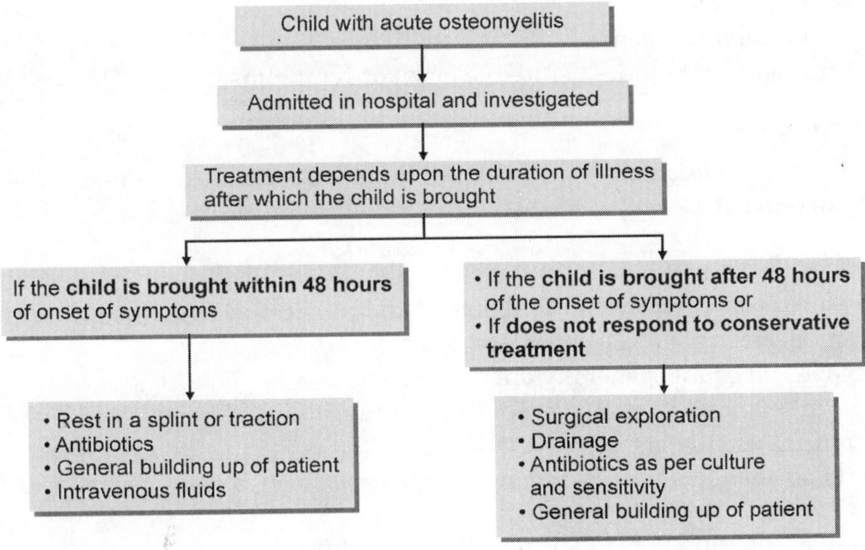

Postoperative Care
- Long leg posterior plaster splint is applied with:
    - The foot in a neutral position
    - The ankle at 90°
    - The knee at 20° of flexion
- Once the wound has healed, the splint is removed, and protected weight bearing with crutches is begun
- 6-week course of intravenous antibiotics should be given
- Follow-up is continued for at least 1 year

Complications

General

- *Anaemia*
- *Amyloidosis*
- Septic embolization leading to *septicaemia or pyaemia* (blood poisoning)

Local

- Acute osteomyelitis, if inadequately treated progresses to *chronic osteomyelitis*.
- *Pathological fracture* due to corticomedullary erosion
- Spreads to joints and causes *septic arthritis* especially in hip and shoulder since the metaphysis is intra-articular.

Q4. Define subacute osteomyelitis and discuss its classification.

In comparison to acute osteomyelitis, subacute hematogenous osteomyelitis has a more indolent course and lacks the severity of symptoms. Therefore, diagnosis typically is delayed for > 2 weeks.

Pathology

Indolent course of subacute osteomyelitis is due to:

- Increased host resistance
- Decreased bacterial virulence
- Administration of antibiotics before the onset of symptoms

Microorganisms

S. aureus and *Staphylococcus epidermidis* are the predominant organisms identified in subacute osteomyelitis.

Important Features

- Temperature is only mildly elevated if at all.
- Mild-to-moderate pain (only consistent signs)
- White blood cell counts generally are normal.
- Erythrocyte sedimentation rate is elevated in only 50% of patients
- Blood cultures usually are negative.
- Even with an adequate bone aspirate or biopsy specimen, a pathogen is identified only 60% of the time.
- Plain radiographs and bone scans usually are positive.

Classification (radiographic classification of subacute hematogenous osteomyelitis by Gledhill and modified by Roberts et al.)

Type	Gledhill classification	Robert et al. classification	Differential diagnosis
I	Solitary localized zone of radiolucency surrounded by reactive new bone formation	Ia—Punched-out radio-lucency	Langerhans' cell histiocytosis
		Ib—Punched-out radiolucent lesion with sclerotic margin	Brodie abscess
II	Metaphyseal radiolucencies with cortical erosion	–	Eosinophilic granuloma; osteogenic sarcoma

(Contd.)

Type	Gledhill classification	Robert et al. classification	Differential diagnosis
III	Cortical hyperostosis in diaphysis; no onion skinning	Localized cortical and periosteal reaction	Osteoid osteoma
IV	Subperiosteal new bone and onion skin layering	Onion skin periosteal reaction	Ewing sarcoma
V	–	Central radiolucency in epiphysis	Chondroblastoma
VI	–	Destructive process involving vertebral body	Tuberculosis; osteogenic sarcoma

Management

Simple Lesion

- In the epiphysis or metaphysis, biopsy is not recommended.
- IV antibiotics for 48 hours followed by a 6-week course of oral antibiotics.

Aggressive lesion or lesions that do not respond to antibiotic treatment alone: Biopsy and curettage followed by treatment with appropriate antibiotics.

Q5. Write short note on Brodie's abscess.

Brodie's abscess is a localized form of subacute osteomyelitis that usually occurs in the long bones of the lower extremities of young adults.

Microorganism

- Organisms of low virulence are believed to cause the lesion.
- *S. aureus* is cultured in 50% of patients; in 20%, the culture is negative.

Age: 11–20 years

Site: Upper end of tibia and lower end of femur

Location: Metaphysis (most common); in adults (metaphyseal-epiphyseal)

Complaints

- Intermittent pain of long duration
- Local tenderness over the affected area

X-rays

It appear as oval lytic lesion surrounded by dense fibrous tissue and sclerotic bone (*lytic lesion with a rim of sclerotic bone*).

Treatment

It is best treated by curettage and bone grafting

Q6. Define chronic osteomyelitis.

Osteomyelitis (*osteo- derived from the Greek word osteon, meaning bone, myelo, meaning marrow, and -itis meaning inflammation*) is the chronic infection of the bone involving the osteoid as well as myeloid tissue.

Q7. What is a sequestrum and what are its different types?

Sequestrum is microscopic or macroscopic *avascular, dead fragment of parent bone surrounded by pus and granulation tissue.* It is *hallmark* of chronic osteomyelitis.

- The surface in contact with the *granulation tissue is rough* and the other *surface is smooth and shiny.*
- *In children,* the periosteum can get lifted easily resulting in a *large diaphyseal sequestrum,* whereas in *cases of adults* the periosteum is firmly adhere and cannot get lifted easily resulting in multiple discharging sinuses.
- *Blood supply* to a part of bone cut off by septic thrombosis of vessels.
- Ischemic bone dies and separate as sequestrum within 3–12 weaks.
- Separation of sequestrum is by osteoclastic activity and granulation tissue.
- If the sequestrum is not separated, it is replaced by creeping substitution when infection is eradicated usually in children.
- Lighter than normal bone
- Denser than normal bone
- Sprouting granulation indicates presence of sequestrum inside.
- Antibiotics cannot sterilise a sequestrum because it is a dead bone devoid of vascular supply.

Types of Sequestra

Disease	Type of sequestra
Tuberculosis	Feathery, flake, coarse sand like, coke and rice grain, coraliform, tubular kissing sequestrum (TB knee and spine)
Mycotic	Bombay nigra, coloured
Syphilis	Ivory
Pin tract infection	Ring sequestrum
Amputation stump	
Children	Tubular, diaphyseal
Actinomycosis	Black granular
Amputation stump	Crown, shell sequestrum
Pyogenic osteomyelitis	Coraliform sequestrum; tubular
Open fracture	Coloured sequestrum (due to deposition of ferrous sulphide)

Q8. Define involucrum and cloacae

Involucrum is a layer of *new bone growth* outside existing bone resulting from the stripping off of the periosteum by the accumulation of pus within the bone, and new bone growing from the periosteum.

Cloacae are small openings in involucrum or cortex through which sequestra, granulation tissue, pus or necrotic bone debris is extruded.

Q9. Describe the pathophysiology, clinical features and diagnosis of chronic osteomyelitis.

Pathophysiology

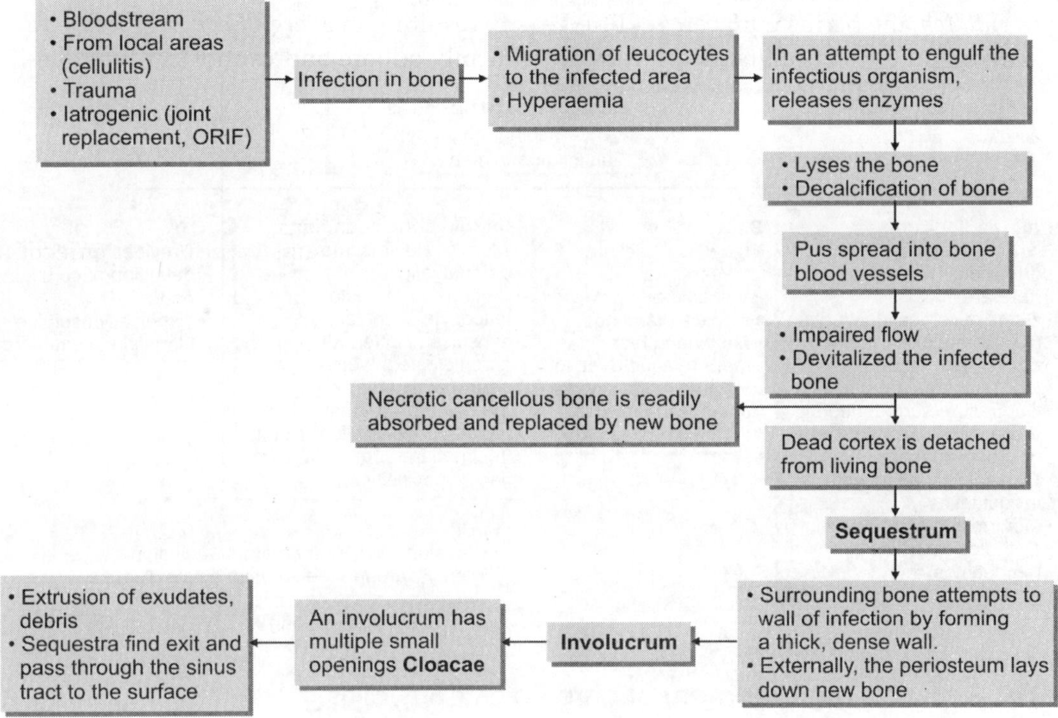

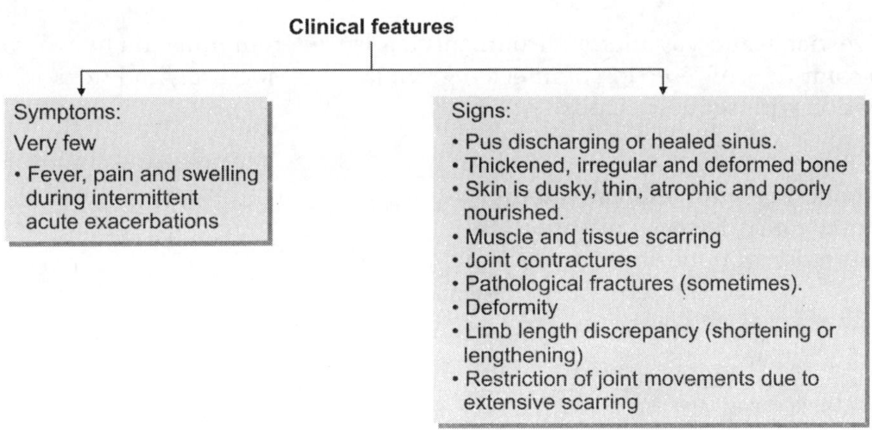

Investigations

Laboratory

Blood:
- Haemoglobin (%) is decreased.
- ESR is increased.
- C-reactive protein is elevated.
- Lymphocytes count is increased.

Pus:
- Culture and sensitivity test to decide appropriate antibiotic

Biopsy with cultural and sensitivity:
- Histological and microbiological evaluation
- Gold standard
- It is helpful in:
  - Establishing a diagnosis
  - Determining the proper antibiotic regimen

Imaging

Imaging aid:
- In confirmation of the diagnosis
- To prepare for surgical treatment

Plain radiographs:
It should be the initial study performed
There are:
- Signs of cortical destruction (corticomedullary moth-eaten destruction)
- Periosteal reaction
- Sequestra (surrounded by a zone of translucency (pus or granulation tissue))
- Cortical thickening and irregularities
- Deformity
- Pathological fracture (sometimes)

Sinography:
- If a sinus track is present
- Valuable adjunct to surgical planning
- Methylene blue or radio-opaque dyes to stain and differentiate dead tissue from live during sinus excision

Isotopic bone scanning:
- More useful in acute osteomyelitis
- Indium-111-labelled leucocyte scans are sensitive in differentiating chronic osteomyelitis from neuropathic arthropathy in the diabetic foot than technetium or gallium scans
- Technetium-99m bone scans lack specificity.

CT:
- Provides excellent definition of cortical bone
- Especially useful in identifying sequestra

MRI:
- Rim sign: Well-defined rim of high signal intensity around the focus of active disease
- Sinus tracks and cellulitis: Increased intensity on T_2-weighted imaging.

Q10. Describe management of chronic osteomyelitis.

Chronic osteomyelitis usually cannot be eradicated without surgical treatment.

Goal

To achieve viable and vascular environment that is free from infection by way of radical debrima comprises of resection of infected granulation tissue, scar, and thick involucrum in association with sequestrectomy.

Principles

- Radical debrima with sequestrectomy
- Appropriate broad spectrum antibiotics
- Reconstruction of bone and soft tissue defects if needed.

Methods

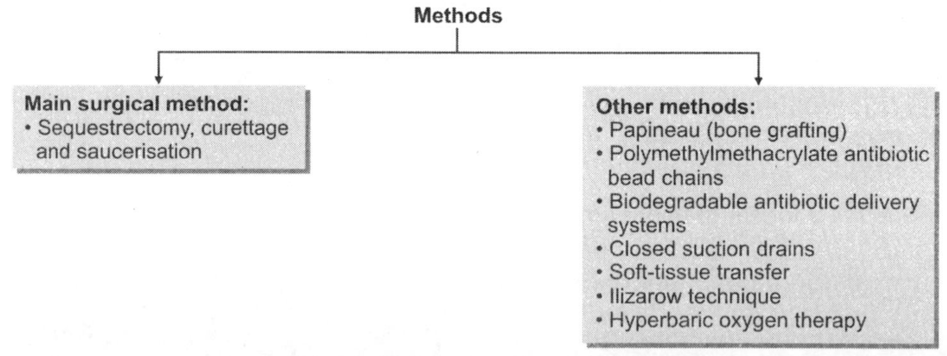

Let us consider each one by one.

Sequestrectomy, Curettage and Saucerisation

- Exposure
- Excision of all sinus tracts
- With the help of multiple drill holes a sufficient section of cortex is removed; so as to permit the free flow.
- The edges are saucerised so as to convert a deep cavity into a shallow one which again facilitates drainage.
- Sequestrectomy done.
- Radical debrima done comprises of excision of all purulent material, scarred and necrotic tissue. Proper curettage done until a bed of raw, bleeding bone remains.
- Opening of medullary canals in both directions which allow the neovascularisation.

Now assess the two things: *Depth of cavity or dead space resulting from sequestrectomy and stability of bone.*

If there is a *cavity or dead space*; there are few methods of immediate biological obliteration of it. These are:
- Local closure (if space is small)
- Packing with cancellous bone grafts
- Muscle pedicle graft (vastus lateralis for femur and brachialis for humerus)
- Free vascularised tissue or bone transfer

If bone is *unstable* then must be stabilized, preferably with an *Ilizarov-type external frame (ring fixator) or Orthofix (Railroad)*.

In the end assess the closure:
- If possible do it in layers over drain.
- If not possible pack the wound open loosely or apply an antibiotic bead pouch and plan for secondary closure.

After procedure:
- The limb is splinted to hasten the soft tissue healing and also to prevent pathological fracture.
- Appropriate antibiotics should be used during preoperative, intraoperative and post-operative phase.

Other Methods

Papineau (Open Bone Grafting)

Papineau et al. described an open bone grafting procedure for the treatment of chronic osteomyelitis.

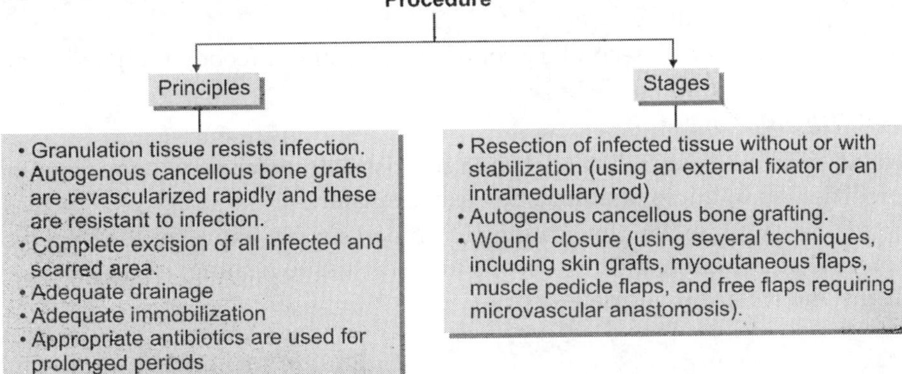

Polymethylmethacrylate (PMMA) Antibiotic Bead Chains

Aim: To deliver levels of antibiotics locally so that its concentration exceed the minimal inhibitory concentrations.

Prerequisites

- All infected, scarred and necrotic tissue should be excised adequately.
- All foreign material should be removed.

Antibiotic used: Thermostable and well eluted antibiotic like aminoglycosides, penicillins, cephalosporins, and clindamycin. Vancomycin elutes much less effectively but it used most commonly in methacillin-resistant *S. aureus*.

Implantation

- Short term: Beads are removed within 10 days
- Long-term implantation: These beads may be left for 80 days

After treatment

- Appropriate immobilization of limb.
- Chain of beads should be changed every 72 hours with repeat wound debrima and irrigation until the wound is ready for secondary coverage.

Biodegradable Antibiotic Delivery Systems

- Bioabsorbable substrates (calcium sulfate or calcium phosphate) allow the surgeon to mix powdered antibiotics (generally vancomycin or tobramycin) to produce resorbable beads.
- By about 8 weeks after surgery these beads are completely resorbed.

Advantage over PMMA beads

- Being biodegradable second procedure is not required to remove the implant.
- These system can also be mixed with some osteoinductive and osteoconductive material to promote new bone formation and thus can be used as bone graft substitute.

Disadvantage: Patients develop an asymptomatic purulent discharge that appears nearly identical to the drainage of a bacterial infection.

Closed Suction Drains

Aim: Closed suction irrigation (Lautenbach continuous irrigation) to avoid collection of blood and pus.

In cases of extensive osteomyelitis continuous ingress and egress irrigation with appropriate antibiotic, detergent and saline is done with intermittent suction till the outflow is sterile for three consecutive days.

Disadvantage: There is risk of secondary contamination and infection with new organisms.

Soft-tissue Transfer

To fill a dead space left after radical debrima soft tissue transfer may range from localized muscle pedicle flap to microvascular free tissue transfer.

Aim: Vascularized muscle flaps by bringing in a blood supply improves the local biological environment that is significant for osseous and soft-tissue healing, in the host's defense mechanisms and for antibiotic delivery

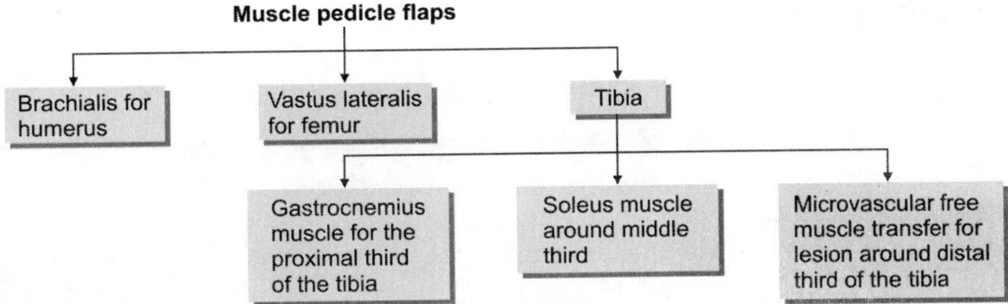

Ilizarov Technique

Ilizarov technique allows radical resection of the infected bone and reconstruction to achieve stability simultaneously.

Advantages
- Promotes Soft tissue healing
- Provides Stability (secure and rigid fixation)
- Bone transport to fill the defect (allows radical resection of the infected bone)
- Correction of complex deformities
- Early ambulation and joint mobilization

Disadvantages
- Pin tract infections
- Patient noncompliance
- Cumbersome and heavy (new light weight carbon rings are available in the market but are very expensive)
- Soft tissue management (secondary procedure) is very difficult

Q11. Write short note on sclerosing osteomyelitis of Garré.

It is chronic form of disease in which the bone is thickened and distended, but sequestra and abscesses are absent. It is also known as idiopathic cortical sclerosis.

Aetiology

- Unknown
- Thought to be an infection caused by a low-grade, possibly anaerobic bacterium

Age: Affects children and young adults

Presentation

- Intermittent pain of moderate intensity and usually of long duration
- Swelling
- Tenderness over the affected bone

Investigations

- X-rays: shows expanded bone with generalized sclerosis
- Erythrocyte sedimentation rate usually is slightly elevated.
- Biopsy specimens show only chronic, low-grade, nonspecific osteomyelitis
- Cultures usually are negative.

Differential Diagnosis

- Osteoid osteoma
- Paget's disease

Treatment

- No specific treatment.
- Fenestration of the sclerotic bone and antibiotics are advisable.

Q12. Discuss in brief iatrogenic or postoperative osteomyelitis.

Osteomyelitis can occur after any operation on bone but more after operating an open fracture and after procedures involving the use of foreign implants.

Incidence

- Reported incidence of postoperative osteomyelitis varies from 0.2 to 10%.
- The incidence depends on the criteria for diagnosing postoperative infection.
- The true incidence is probably around 5%.

Risk Factors

Risk considerably greater in:
- The elderly
- Obese
- Those with diabetes or other chronic diseases
- Patients on steroids or immunosuppressive therapy

Classification

Early Infection

- Superficial infection
- Deep infection
- Superficial and deep infection

Late Infection

- Following early infection
- Covert infection appearing later
- Following a long period of normality

Microorganism

Invasion

The organism may be introduced:
- Directly into the wound from:
    - Atmosphere
    - The instruments
    - The patient or the surgeon
- Indirectly by hematogenous spread from the distant focus.

Local factors that favor bacterial invasion are:
- Soft tissue damage
- Haematomas formation
- Bone death

Types

The organism in postoperative osteomyelitis are usually a mixture of pathogenic bacteria (*S. aureus, Proteus, E.coli, Pseudomonas*) and other that are not normally pathogenic (*Staph. epidermidis*) but may become so in the presence of foreign implant.

Clinical Feature

Early postoperative infection (within 1 month)
- The patient complaints of persistent pain and may have fever.
- The skin over the implants is inflamed, and there may be a purulent discharge from the bone.
- The ESR and white cell count are elevated, the blood culture may be positive.
- Bacteriological examination of the wound discharge will help to identify the organism and establish the antibiotic sensitivity.

Intermediate postoperative infection (1 month – 1 year after operation): There is a history of wound problems in the early postoperative period followed by a long quiescent period and spread when local condition favour.

Late postoperative infection
- It is much more difficult to diagnose.
- Several years may have elapsed since the operation, during which the patient was completely asymptomatic.
- Pain usually starts insidiously and may never become acute.
- Local examination, X-ray signs of bone resorption and increased activity on radionuclide scanning may equally fail to distinguish between aseptic loosening of the implant and infection.
- Confirmation of the diagnosis is obtained by aspirating purulent material from the area, or by culturing the organism in washings taken after attempted aspiration.

Prevention

The risk of implant-mediated infection can be reduced by:
- Avoiding operations on immunosuppressed patients
- Eliminating any focus of infection before operation
- Insisting on optimal operative sterility
- Giving prophylactic antibiotics
- Handling soft tissue gently
- Using high quality implant material
- Ensuring close fit and secure fixation of the implant
- Preventing or counter acting later intercurrent infection.

Treatment

- Appropriate antibiotic given intravenously and in large doses are the first line of defense.
- If there is an abscess, it should be drained and the wound left open until it is clean.

- If these measures fail excision of infected and necrotic material followed by intermittent antibiotic irrigation and suction drainage, may yet control the infection and prevent it from becoming an intractable chronic osteomyelitis.
- If possible, the fixation device should be retained until the fracture has united or if the implant has to be removed in order to achieve adequate debridement, the fracture should be held securely with an *external fixator*.

Q13. Write short note on maduromycosis.

Mycetoma is a chronic, deep, progressively destructive, and deforming infection of skin, subcutaneous tissues, fascia, bone, and muscle following localized trauma.

Mycetoma, also termed *Maduromycosis or Madura foot*, is named after the Indian region where it was first described.

Microorganism

- Mycetoma caused by filamentous bacteria is termed actinomycetoma.
- Actinomycetoma can be caused by *N brasiliensis, N asteroides, Nocardia madurae, Streptomyces somaliensis, Streptomyces pelletieri, and Actinomyces israelii.*

Presentation

- The disorder occurs most commonly on the extremities, especially the foot.
- Mycetoma manifests as a tumor-like area of localized oedema or massive enlargement, with erythema and multiple draining sinus tracts.
- Often, mycetoma is described as a triad of:
  - Tumefaction
  - Sinus tract formation (often multiple)
  - Grains (sulfur granules: Black or yellow granules in the discharge, which is very typical)
  - Sulfur granules (grains) examination:
    - The size, shape, and colour of the grains can help determine the causative agent in mycetoma.
    - Grains can vary from 0.2–5 mm.
    - *White-to-yellow grains*: in association with *Nocardia, Actinomyces, Streptomyces somaliensis, Pseudallescheria boydii,* and *Cephalosporium.*
    - *Brown-to-black grains*: only in association with true dematiaceous fungi, such as *Madurella* and *Phialophora jeanselmei.*
    - *Red grains*: in association with *Streptomyces pelletieri.*

Differential Diagnosis

- Cutaneous tuberculosis
- Dermatologic manifestations of pulmonary disease
- Ecthyma
- Leishmaniasis
- *Mycobacterium marinum* infection of the skin
- Sporotrichosis

Treatment

- Antifungal
- Antibiotics

- Local debridement
- Often amputation has to be done to get rid of the fulminating and extensive tarsal destruction.

Q14. Discuss the aetiology, clinical features and management of acute septic arthritis.

Septic arthritis is a pyogenic infection of the joint as a result of hematogenous transmission or occasionally due to external source as in penetrating wounds.

Mode of Invasion

- Hematogenous spread
- Direct inoculation from trauma or surgery
- Contiguous spread from an adjacent site of osteomyelitis or cellulitis

Aetiopathology

- Age is an important factor in determining the causative agent in bacterial infection.
- Usually, predisposing conditions are associated with particular types of causative organisms.

Organisms Found in Common Clinical Settings of Infectious Arthritis

Clinical factor	Organism
Patient age	
Neonate	*Staphylococcus aureus*
<2 years	*Haemophilus influenzae, S. aureus*
>2 years	*S. aureus*
Young adults (healthy, sexually active)	*Neisseria gonorrhoeae*
Elderly adults	*S. aureus* (50%), streptococci, gram-negative bacilli
Structural abnormalities	
Aspiration or injection	*S. aureus*
Trauma	Gram-negative bacilli, anaerobes, *S. aureus*
Prosthesis	
Early infection	*S. epidermidis*
Late infection	Gram-positive cocci, anaerobes
Medical conditions	
Injecting drug use	Atypical gram-negative bacilli (e.g., *Pseudomonas* species)
Rheumatoid arthritis	*S. aureus*
Systemic lupus erythematosus, sickle cell anaemia	*Salmonella* species
Hemophilia	*S. aureus* (50%), streptococci, gram-negative bacilli
Immunosuppression	*S. aureus, Mycobacterium* species, fungi

Pathology

There is initially synovial effusion followed by synovial proliferation, subsequent purulent collection and necrosis of articular cartilage and other joint structures.

The joint may be in the phase of:
- Synovial effusion
- Arthritis and joint erosion
- Destruction and dislocation.

Clinical Features

General

- Fever
- Pain
- Features of toxaemia.

Local

- Joint effusion
- Tender
- Red-hot swelling with diffuse oedema
- Muscle spasm
- Gross restriction of joint movements occurs.

Investigations

MRI, CT scan and Tc-99 uptake for early diagnosis.

X-ray

Early

- Increased joint space due to effusion
- Soft-tissue swelling
- Displacement of the fat pad.

Late

- Erosion of articular margins
- Diminished joint space
- Subluxation
- Subchondral cysts
- In case of involvement of hip joint, there may be destruction of the femoral head and pathological dislocation.

Ultrasonography

Ultrasonography, in contrast to radiographs, can be used to detect even small collections of fluid deep in the joints.

Radionuclide Scans

- Technetium-99 m methyldiphosphonate scan shows increases in isotope accumulation in areas of osteoblasts and increased vascularity but may be normal in early stage.
- Radiopharmaceuticals, including *gallium citrate* and *indium-111 chloride*, and *gallium and indium scans* are more specific and sensitive in the detection of active infection than technetium-99 m methyldiphosphonate scans.

Blood

Culture is positive and increased polymorphonuclear cells.

Pus

Pus aspiration from the joint is positive for smear and culture.

Management

Nade's Principle

Nade suggested three essential principles:
- The joint must be adequately drained.
- Antibiotics must be given to diminish the systemic effects of sepsis.
- The joint must be rested in a stable position.

Early

- Broad-spectrum antibiotics, analgesics are recommended.
- Traction to relieve the pain, spasm and deformity.
- Aspiration/incision and drainage of abscess, followed by continuous suction irrigation with suitable antibiotic.
- In acute septic arthritis, usually arthrotomy or arthroscopic drainage and antibiotic treatment are adequate.

Late

Minimal and early joint damage: Wilkinson's joint clearance (synovectomy, debridement of joint), lavage, irrigation and early mobilization.

Extensive joint damage
- *For stable fixed joint*: Arthrodesis, the surgical immobilization of a joint is done.
- *For mobile joint*: As in cases of hip and elbow involvement, excision arthroplasty and joint replacement later.
- *For deformity*: Corrective osteotomy and functional restoration of joint.
- *For shortening*: Shoe raise/limb lengthening is done.

Complications

- Pathological dislocation
- Pelvic abscess
- Persistent infection
- Osteomyelitis
- Deformity
- Shortening
- Instability
- Secondary osteoarthritis
- Ankylosis

Q15. Write short note on Tom Smith arthritis.

Tom Smith arthritis is a septic arthritis of hip during infancy and childhood, and usually follows infected umbilical cord.

The child is usually brought late or remains undiagnosed due to the cartilaginous head of femur, which is not visualized in X-ray and needs ultrasound with a 7.5 Hz probe to see the outline of the head of femur in a neonate.

Source of Infection

- It is usually blood borne.
- Primary focus of infection being in the:
  - Skin
  - Upper respiratory tract
  - Paranasal sinuses
  - Umbilicus in the newborn

Microorganism

- *Staphylococcus aureus* (most common)
- *Streptococcus haemolyticus*
- Occasionally *pneumococcus, Bacillus coli* or *Haemophillus*

Involvement of Joints

- In infants, *acute suppurative arthritis* most commonly affects hip, the knee and the shoulder joint.
- Rarely multiple joints are involved.
- Amongst all joints, hip joint is most commonly affected.

Presentation

- The head and neck undergoes rapid destruction (due to proteolytic enzymes present in the pus) with resulting pathological dislocation of hip joint, this damage is irreparable, and a lifetime of *suffering, limp and shortening occurs.*
- On examination:
  - Child walks with unstable gait.
  - Shortening
  - Hypermobility-hip movements are increased in all directions
  - Telescoping is present.

Diagnosis

- For early diagnosis, help of MRI, CT scan, T-99 uptake study should be done.
- The delay in treatment is responsible for the destruction.

X-ray

Initially increased joint space and later destruction of head and neck of femur, with dislocation and high riding greater trochanter; the roof of acetabulum remains normal.

Management

Early: Broad-spectrum antibiotics, traction and aggressive joint drainage at the earliest should take place.

Late: Osteotomy for stabilizing the hip.

Complications

General

- Septicaemia
- Embolism

Local

- Destruction of head and pathological
- Dislocation
- Limp
- Shortening

Q16. Write in short clinical features of syphilitic, tubercular, sickle cell and *Brucella* osteomyelitis

Important feature can be summarized as below.

Type of osteomyelitis	Important features

***Brucella* osteomyelitis**	• Most common site: Spine
	• X-rays:
	  – Destruction of opposing surfaces of adjacent vertebral bodies
	  – Narrowed disk space
	  – Intervertebral bridging
	• *Treatment*: Chlortetracycline or streptomycin plus tetracycline for 3 weeks

Typhoid osteomyelitis	• Most common bone: Rib and tibia • Infection is limited to cortex
Tubercular osteomyelitis	• Most common bones: Ends of long bone and short bones of hand and foot • X-ray: Osteoporosis is the first sign

Sickle cell osteomyelitis	• Most common organism: *Salmonella*
	• Most common in children
	• Multifocal
	• Most common site: Diaphysis
	• Cause: Due to infection of bony infarct
	• Sickle cell dactylitis (common in infants)
	• Aseptic necrosis of femoral head
	• Acute synovitis and joint effusion
	• X-ray:
	  – Fish mouth or biconcave vertebrae
	  – Crew hair cut-skull

Syphilitic osteomyelitis	*Congenital*: • Most common bone: Nose and lower leg bones • *Osteochondritis*: At the junction of epiphysis and metaphysis • Sequestrum does not occur • Periosteitis of tibia: *Saber shin* • Destruction of nose: *Saddle nose* • Early congenital syphilis: *Parrot's pseudoparalysis* • *Onion peel appearance*: periosteal reaction and new bone

(Contd.)

Type of osteomyelitis	*Important features*

	• *Wimberger's sign*: rarefaction of upper medial parts of both knees
	• *Clutton's joint*: symmetrical bilateral hydra-arthrosis of knees
	• *Hutchinson's triad*: Late congenital syphilis
	  – *Interstitial keratitis*
	  – *Hutchinson's teeth* (peg shaped, upper, Permanent central incisors)
	  – *8th nerve deafness*
	Acquired syphilis:
	• Manifestation of tertiary syphilis
	• Most common bones: tibia, clavicle and sternum
	• Characterized by *gumma* formation
	• Gumma is a hypersensitivity reaction
	• Gummatous ulcer—punched out with wash leather base
	• X-rays
	  – Punched out lesions in medulla
	  – Periosteal new bone
	  – Crew haircut—skull

Fungal osteomyelitis (Actinomycosis)	• Most common bone: mandible • Hard mass with multiple discharging sinus • X-ray: Honeycomb appearance with reactive sclerosis • Treatment: Penicillin (DOC)

Skeletal Tuberculosis

Q1. Discuss pathology, clinical features and stages of tuberculosis of hip joint in brief.

Hip joint is the commonest extraspinal site of osteoarticular tuberculosis.

Incidence

- The involvement of hip joint is next to spinal involvement.
- It accounts for 15% of all cases of osteoarticular TB.

Initial Focus of Infection

Initial focus of lesion may start in *(in decrease frequency):*

- Acetabular roof
- Epiphyses
- Metaphyseal region (Babcock's triangle)
- Greater trochanter
- Synovium (rarely)
- Synovial membrane hypertrophy
- Tubercle formation

Pathogenesis

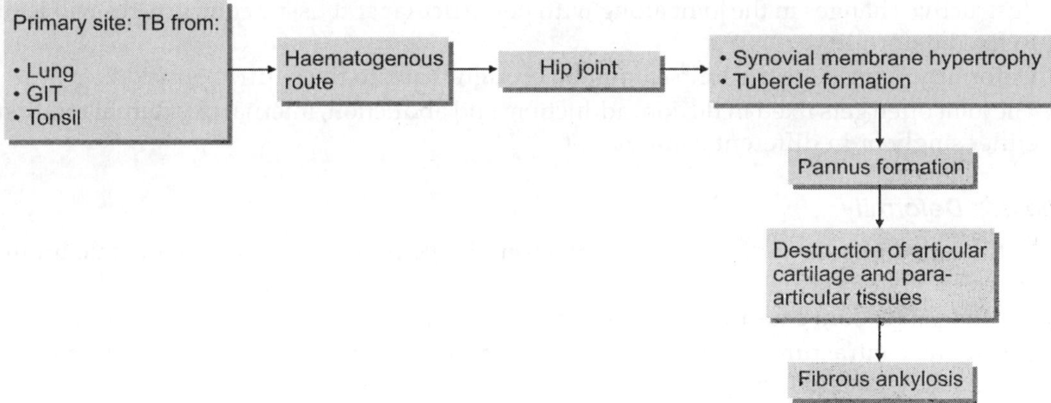

Clinical Features

- *Age*: During first three decades.
- *Onset*: Usually insidious in onset.

- Pale and apathetic appearance.
- Constitutional symptoms like malaise, loss of weight, evening rise of temperature and night sweating.
- *Pain, limping, deformity* and fullness around the hip joint during active phase.
- Disproportionate/gross wasting of thigh and gluteal muscles.
- There may be discrepancy of limb length.
- ~ 8% of patients have clinically palpable cold abscess.
- *Abscess*: It could be mid-inguinal, trochanteric, gluteal with active/healed multiple discharging sinuses.
- ~ 10% of patient may present with pathological dislocation/ subluxation.
- Bitrochanteric compression test is positive with local tenderness below the mid-inguinal point.
- *Gauvian's sign* positive (rotation of lower limb causes abdominal spasm).
- Proximal shift of the trochanter as measured by the Brayant's triangle.

Limp

- Earliest and commonest symptom.
- Antalgic gait with positive Trendelenburg's test in old cases (stance phase on the affected side is decreased).

Pain

- Referred/radiate to the medial aspect of the knee joint.
- Worse in intensity toward the end of the day.
- Disturb the sleep; child may wake from sleep due to night cries (in night *voluntary spam* does not exist and the opposing surfaces moves against each other, this give rise to intense pain at night, the patient suddenly wake up and cries. This is *Night cries*).

Deformity

- Deformity developed as the disease/pathology progresses through different stages.
- Persistent muscular spasm, posture assumed to avoid pain or conceal any deformity, destructive changes in the joint along with periarticular soft tissue contractures will lead to fixed deformity.
- Deformity is fixed, as the limb cannot be brought back to the neutral position.
- The joint often gets fixed in flexion, adduction, and abduction, internal or external rotation either singly or in different combination.

Flexion Deformity

- In the initial phases of disease, the joint assumes *"position of ease"* to provide maximum space.
- Attitude is flexion, external rotation and abduction.
- Soft tissue contracture (spasm of flexors of hip) in due course will turn flexion attitude into fixed flexion deformity.
- In order to gain assess to ground due to loss of extension and soft tissue contractures, the pelvis tilts forward in sagittal plane. This exaggerates the lumber lordosis and concealing the fixed flexion deformity.
- Measured by *Thomas test* (angle subtended by the long axis of bone with the bed).

Abduction Deformity

- During early phases due to joint effusion the limb, assume an attitude of flexion, external rotation and abduction.
- Fibrotic periarticular soft tissue contracture will lead to fixed abduction deformity.

Deformity is compensated by:
- Tilting pelvis downward on the affected side. It is evidenced by ASIS lying at lower level on the affected side.
- Scoliosis of spine with convexity towards the affected side.

Measurement
- The deformity is revealed by squaring of pelvis.
- It is measured by drawing a vertical line from the ASIS after squaring of pelvis. The angle between this line and the long axis of the thigh will give you the *angle of fixed abduction deformity.*
- It can also be measured without squaring the pelvis by *Kothari's angle.*

Adduction Deformity

- As the disease progresses, there occur actual destruction of articular cartilage.
- Severe spasm of flexors and adductors following destruction of cartilage will lead to flexion, adduction and internal rotation deformity.

Deformity is compensated by:
- Tilting pelvis upward on the affected side. It is evidenced by ASIS being at higher level on the affected side.
- Scoliosis of spine with convexity towards the unaffected side or away from the affected side.

Measurement
- The deformity is revealed by squaring of pelvis.
- It is measured by drawing a vertical line from the ASIS after squaring of pelvis. The angle between this line and the long axis of the thigh will give you the angle of fixed adduction deformity.
- It can also be measured without squaring the pelvis by Kothari's angle.

Stages of TB Hip

Stage I or Stage of Synovitis

- The disease is synovial with the joint in "position of ease".
- Attitude is flexion, abduction and external rotation (intra-articular volume has the maximum capacity).
- There is apparent lengthening.
- No true/real shortening.
- Only extreme of movements (both active and passive) are painful.

Stage II or Stage of Early Arthritis

- As the disease progresses, there occur actual destruction of articular cartilage, as a result the friction between the opposing surfaces will give rise to severe pain.
- To prevent this, muscle around the hip joint especially the flexors and adductors go into spasm.

- Muscle spam in turn forces hip to assume a deformity of flexion, adduction and internal rotation.
- There is true/real shortening.
- Significant muscle wasting.
- Limitation of hip movements in all direction.

Stage III or Stage of Advanced Arthritis

- With progression of disease, symptoms and signs are exaggerated.
- Gross destruction of articular cartilage further increases the flexion, adduction and internal rotation deformity.
- The adduction deformity is further exaggerated by the tendency of the patient ot lie on the side of the unaffected hip.
- Gross restriction of movements in all direction.
- True shortening.

Stage IV or Stage of Advanced Arthritis with Sequel (Subluxation or Dislocation)

- With further destruction of articular cartilage and para-articular structures, the proximal femur may displace upwards and dorsally in the migrating or wandering acetabulum.
- Shenton's line is broken.
- There may *pathological dislocation* of femoral head.
- Occasionally the hip may show *protrusio acetabuli.*

Q2. Discuss the diagnosis and management of tuberculosis hip joint.

Investigations

Blood: Low Hb, high ESR, high TLC, increased lymphocytes, L/M (lymphocytes/monocytes) ratio should be 5, if less, it shows poor immune status (avoid surgery).

Urine

- RBC in urine shows silent haematuria and nephritic TB.
- RBC+ albuminuria shows UTI.
- Sugar indicates diabetes mellitus.

Biopsy

Lymph node, synovial biopsy from the hip joint.

Mantoux Test

- Mantoux test: 1TU of PPD in 0.1 ml injected subcutaneously. Horizontal transverse diameter of induration is measured. It is positive if this diameter is >10 mm is positive, it is <6 mm then it is –ve.
- Positive result shows prior sensitization to tuberculous bacilli.

Pus: AFB staining.

Culture: LJ media.

Inoculation

- Disease material (pus, joint aspirate, granulation tissue from the depth of sinus) may be injected into Guinea pig intraperitoneally.
- Positive cases show tubercles on the peritoneum after 5–8 weeks.

X-ray of the Hip Joint

Early: Increased joint space with para-articular osteoporosis.
Late
- Decreased joint space, erosion of articular margins
- Osteoporosis
- Break in Shenton's line
- Wandering acetabulum.

Radiological Classification

Shanmugasundaram TK (1983) for lesion in advance cases of arthritis in *children (C)* and *adult (A)* proposed a new classification for tuberculosis of hip joint.
Radiological types includes:
- Normal type (C)
- Travelling or Wandering acetabulum type (C, A)
- Perthes type (head is dense and collapse) (C)
- Dislocated type (pathological dislocation) (C)
- Protrusio acetabuli type (head threatens to protrude into the pelvic cavity through acetabulum) (C, A)
- Atrophic type (small and atrophic)(A)
- Mortar and pestle type (C,A)

X-ray of chest: For pulmonary Koch's.
MRI/CT scans: For early diagnosis especially in children.
Ultrasonography: For neonates to see the cartilaginous head.

Management
General

- Improve general condition of patient.
- Improve hemoglobin, protein status
- Drugs: ATT for 15 months/DOTS (Cat I or II)

Local

Conservative: Skin traction to the patient:
- To prevent or correct deformity
- Decreases muscle spasm
- Distracts inflamed joint surface
- Avoids subluxation
- Minimizes development of migrating acetabulum
- Permits close observation of the hip

Cold Abscess

Aspirated and instillation of streptomycin with or without isoniazid.
If response is favorable with traction and multidrug chemotherapy then:
- *After 4–6 months*: Ambulation with suitable calipers and crutches
- *First 12 weeks*: Ambulation should be non-weight bearing
- *Next 12 weeks*: Partial weight bearing
- *After 12 months*: Crutches or calipers may be discarded
- *After 18–24 months*: Unprotected weight bearing.

Surgery

I. Active lesions

Stage of Synovitis

Arthrotomy and synovectomy

Stage of Early Arthritis

Wilkinson's joint clearance: Removal of rice bodies/loose bodies, pannus covering the articular cartilage, sequestra, granulation tissue, debris, loose articular cartilage and curettage of juxta-articular osseous foci.

Advanced Arthritis

For a mobile joint: For satisfying the customary needs of sitting cross-legged, squatting, and kneeling.

Girdlestone excision arthroplasty: Excision of the femoral head, femoral neck, proximal trochanter and the Acetabular rim for chronic deep-seated infections.

Postoperatively

- Skeletal traction in 30–50° of abduction for 3 months (aim of giving traction: To develop a layer of fibrous tissue between the acetabulum and cut proximal end of femur and thereby providing ideal surface for pseudoarthrosis).
- During period of traction advised active and assisted physiotherapy.
- After 3 months, the patient should be encouraged to walk using either crutches or weight relieving calipers.
- After 6–9 months, the crutches or calipers were discarded and encouraged the patient to walk with a stick usually in opposite hand.

Complications

- Shortening
- Instability (managed with pelvic support osteotomy).

Interposition Arthroplasty

Vishwakarma et al. reported interposition arthroplasty employing multilayered amniotic membrane.

Replacement Arthroplasty

- Total hip arthroplasty should be considered only after a safe period of absolute disease quiescence.
- Reactivation of infection after joint replacement has been reported in 10–30% of cases.

For a stable fixed joint: **Arthrodesis** (best position): 30° of flexion (depending upon age), no abduction or adduction in adult and 5–10° of external rotation)

Healed Lesions

- *Shortening*: Lengthening of bone
- *Deformity*: Corrective osteotomy
- *Ankylosis*: Total hip replacement

Q3. Discuss pathology, clinical features and stages of tuberculosis of knee joint in brief.

Tuberculosis of knee joint rank third for osteoarticular tuberculosis after spine and hip joint.

Incidence

- It accounts for ~10% of all cases of skeletal tuberculous lesions.
- It is always secondary and the primary is usually in the lymphactics.

Sites

- The joint is involved by haematogenous dissemination/blood-borne infection.
- Initial focus start in:
  - Synovium
  - Subchondral bone (lower femur, upper tibia or patella)
  - Juxta-articular osseous focus

Pathology

Lesion may start as tubercular synovitis.

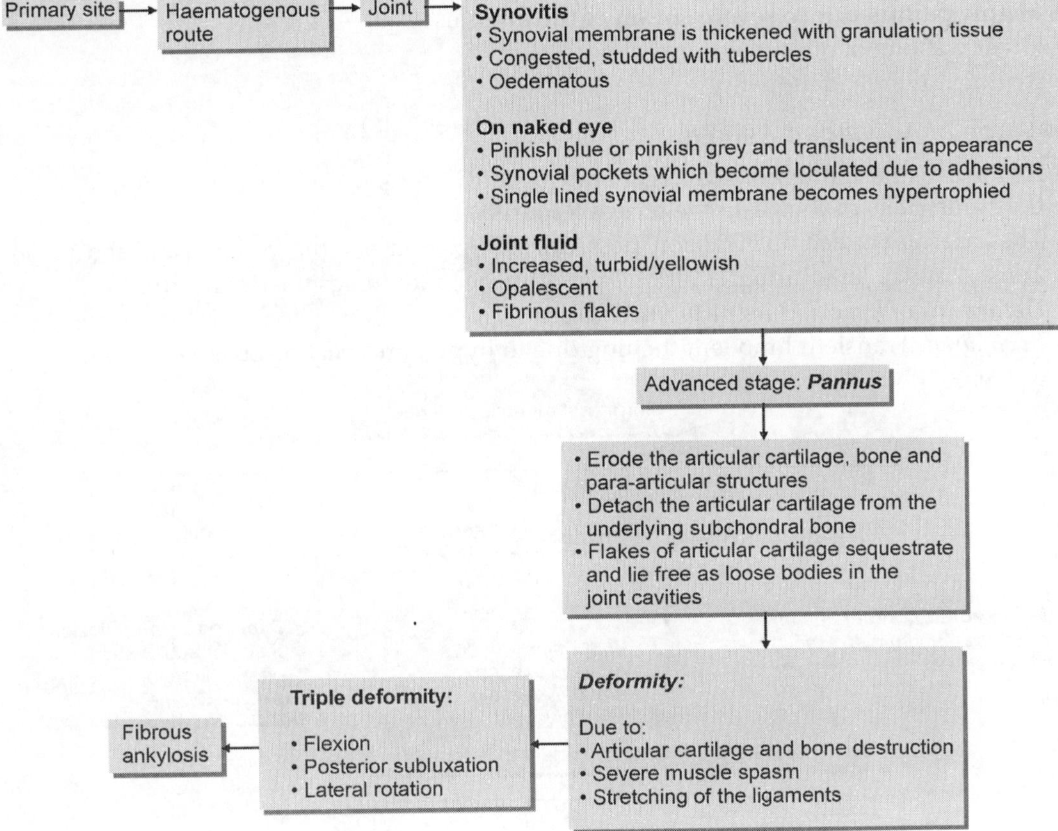

Clinical Features

- Onset: Insidious
- Constitutional features like:
  - *Pain*
    - Mild
    - Night cries common
    - Limping
  - *Swelling*
    - Diffuse, filling up all parapatellar fossae

- Warm
- Tender
- Synovial thickening (boggy or doughy) can be appreciated as semi-elastic tissue between the fingers
- Patellar tap
- Swelling looks exceptionally white "tumor alba or white swollen knee"
• Tender joint line
• Gross muscle wasting

In Stage of Synovitis

Only terminal restriction of movements.

In Stage of Early Arthritis

• Gross restriction of movements
• Highly painful due to severe spasm of the muscles
• Gross wasting of quadriceps muscles
• Regional lymphadenopathy

In Stage of Advanced Arthritis

• As the capsule and ligaments degenerates, there occur severe spasm and contracture of the hamstrings particularly the biceps femoris
• The knee joint pulled up in flexion, posterior subluxation, external rotation and abduction.
• Tensor fasciae lata through iliotibial band further extenuates the deformity.
• *Deformity of knee and its pathomechanics*
• *In children*: Transient limb lengthening due to hyperemia may be observed.

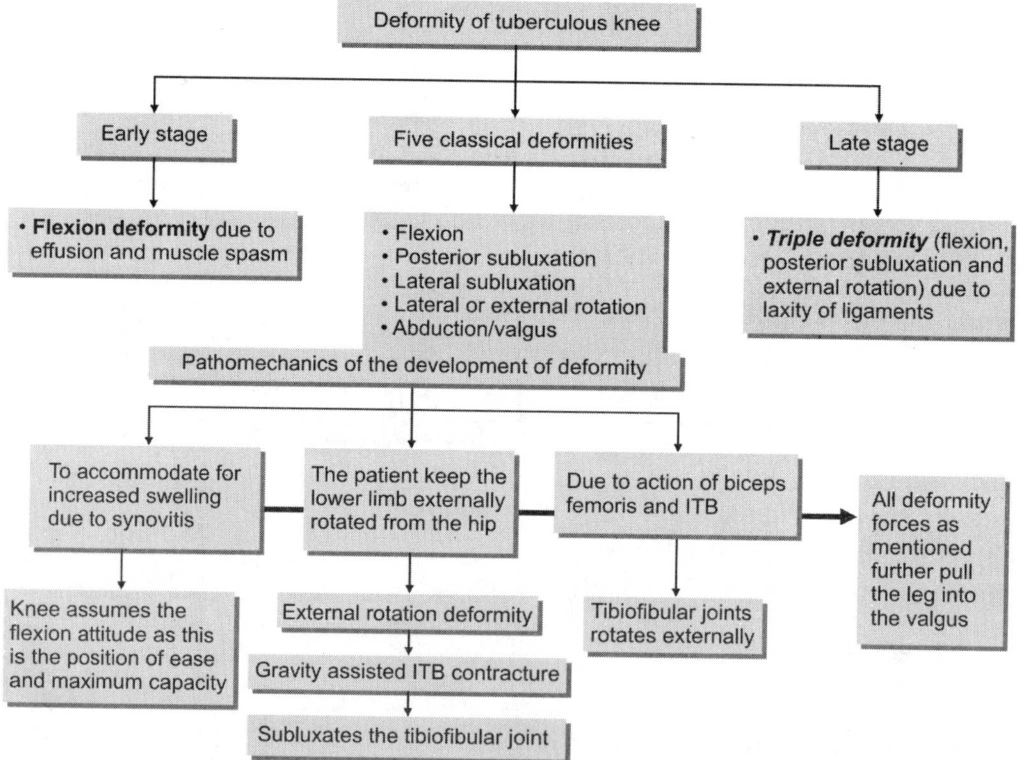

Investigations

Blood: Low Hb, high ESR, high TLC, increased lymphocytes, L/M (lymphocytes/monocytes) ratio should be 5, if less, it shows poor immune status (avoid surgery).

Urine

- RBC in urine shows silent haematuria and nephritic TB.
- RBC+ albuminuria shows UTI.
- Sugar indicates diabetes mellitus.

Biopsy: Lymph node, synovial biopsy from the knee joint.

Mantoux Test

- Mantoux test: 1TU of PPD in 0.1 ml injected subcutaneously. Horizontal transverse diameter of induration is measured. It is positive if this diameter is >10 mm is positive, it is <6 mm then it is –ve.
- Positive result shows prior sensitization to tuberculous bacilli.

Pus: AFB staining.

Culture: LJ media.

Inoculation

- Disease material (pus, joint aspirate, granulation tissue from the depth of sinus) may be injected into Guinea pig intraperitoneally.
- Positive cases show tubercles on the peritoneum after 5–8 weeks.

X-rays

Early stage

- Generalized osteopenic changes
- Increased soft tissue swelling
- Enlarged ossification center (due to para-articular hyperaemia)

Late stage

- Loss of articular cartilage
- Marginal erosion
- Diminution of joint space
- Destruction of the bone
- Osteolytic cavities
- Tubercular sequestra
- Triple deformity
- Sometimes extra-articular focus of infection may be seen in the tibial condyles ends as ankylosis.

Differential Diagnosis

- Rheumatic arthritis (in children)
- Chronic traumatic synovitis (meniscal tear)

- Loose bodies
- Osteochondritis dissecans
- Rheumatoid arthritis in adults
- Subacute pyogenic arthritis/synovitis
- Hemarthrosis
- Villonodular synovitis
- Synovial chrondromatosis
- Synovioma
- Foreign body granuloma

Treatment

General

- Improve general condition of patient.
- Improve haemoglobin, protein status
- Drugs: ATT for 15 months/DOTS (Cat I or II)

Local

Conservative: Skin traction to the patient
- To prevent or correct deformity
- Decreases muscle spasm
- Distracts inflamed joint surface
- Avoids subluxation
- Minimizes development of migrating acetabulum
- Permits close observation of the knee

Aspiration: Aspiration of joint (in cases of effusion) followed by instillation of streptomycin/ INH I/A once weekly.

For deformity: 90°–90° traction to correct triple deformity.

If response is favourable with traction and multidrug chemotherapy then:
- Gentle active and assisted knee bending exercises intermittently (5–10 min).
- After 4–6 months: Ambulation with suitable calipers and crutches.
- First 12 weeks: Ambulation should be non-weight bearing.
- Next 12 weeks: Partial weight bearing.
- After 12 months: Crutches or calipers may be discarded.
- After 18–24 months: Unprotected weight bearing.

Operative

Early
- Synovial excision.
- Wilkinson's joint clearance.

Late: Arthrodesis:
- *Indication*
  - Advanced tubercular arthritis
  - Tubercular arthritis with triple arthritis
  - Gross instability
  - Painful ankylosis

- *Technique*
  - Charnelys compression clamps
  - Other includes: Bone grafts, arthrodesis nail, Steinman pins
- *Position*: In position of 15° of flexion
- *Advantage*: Pain free stable joint.

Joint replacement

Total knee replacement for ankylosing joint.

Q4. Discuss pathology, clinical features and management of Pott's spine.

Pott's spine or osteitis or caries of the vertebrae, usually occurring as a complication of tuberculosis of the lungs. *Sir Percival Pott* first described it as the most crippling lesion characterized by *pain, spinal deformity, cold abscess* and *paralysis.*

This is a disease, which if diagnosed early, can avoid a lot of complications and morbidity.

Incidence

- *Age*: 5–35 years
- *Sex*: Males are more prone to this disease than females due to activities.
- *Location*
  - The commonest site is thoracolumbar junction, followed by cervical.
  - Reasons for frequent involvement of thoracolumbar junction include:
    - Mobility
    - High degree of weight bearing
    - Large amount of spongy tissue
    - Presence of cysterna chylii (abdominal Koch's: Infection can spread easily through cysterna chylii)
  - 7–10% have skipped lesion, 40% have extra-articular lesion.

Types

- *Central*: less common and this know to result in concertina collapse of involved vertebrae.
- *Intervertebral, paradiscal, or metaphyseal*
  - Most common: 95% (tubercular spondylitis)
  - Embryological reason for this, lower half of one vertebra and upper half of adjacent vertebra and the intervertebral disc developed from single sclerotome, has common source of blood supply. Therefore, prone for infection.
- *Anterior or periosteal*: Anterior surface of the vertebrae is involved and results in anterior wedge compression.
- *True tubercular arthritis*: It is usually seen in atlanto-axial and atlanto-occipital joints.
- *Appendiceal*: Involving pedicle, laminae, spinous process or transverse process.
- *Posterior facet joint involvement* (this has presentation like spinal cord tumour syndrome).

Pathology

Essential pathology: Tubercular endarteritis (*see* Flowchart on next page).

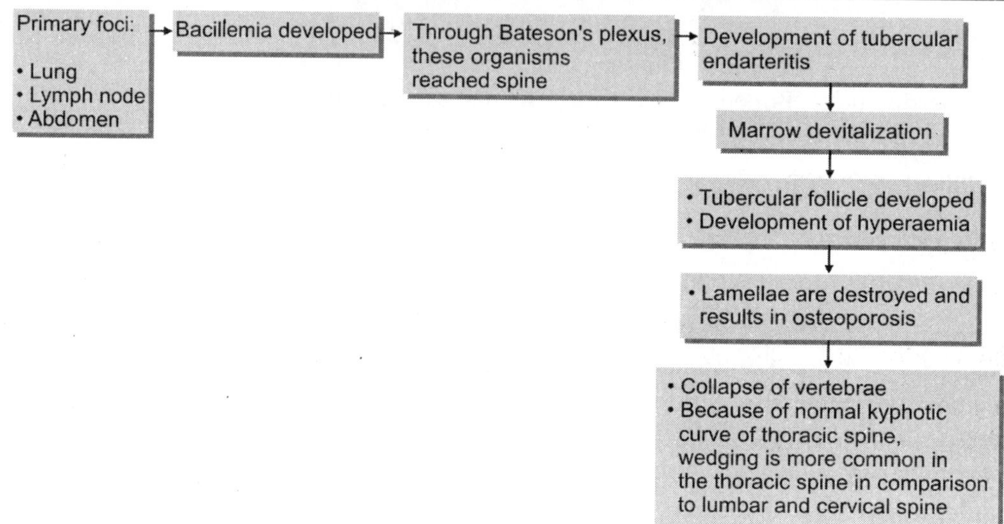

Clinical Features

- Constitutional symptoms like malaise, loss of weight, evening rise of temperature and night sweating.
- *Pain*: Usually in the evening after day's activity, night cries.
- *Muscle spasm* (*back stiffness*): Earliest complaint
  - Cervical zone: Rust sign (chin supporting).
  - Thoracic: Military man attitude.
  - Lumbar: Alderman's gait (pregnant type).
- *Radicular pains*: This is due to posterior facet tubercular lesion.
- *Deformity*:
  - Kyphosis, scoliosis, lumbar lordosis.
  - *Knuckle deformity* (due to collapse of one intervertebral disc space).
  - *Gibbus deformity* (due to collapse of more than two vertebrae).
  - *Scoliosis* (due to collapse of several vertebrae).
- *Abscess* (*cold abscess*):
  - Travels along sheath of vessels, nerves, muscles and facial tracts.
  - *Cervical*: Retropharyngeal and paravertebral, post border of sternomastoid, back of the neck and may travel along the brachial plexus into axilla and paravertebral fascia into mediastinum.
  - *Thoracic*: Intercostal nerves, paraspinal (postspinal nerves), along the rectus sheath, along paravertebral zones.
  - *Lumbar*: Psoas muscle—iliac fossa, mid-inguinal point and femoral triangle.
  - *Obturator nerve*: Popliteal fossa.
  - *Aorta, pudendal artery*: Ischiorectal fossa.
- *Paraplegia*: This is the most dreaded complication of Pott's spine, occurs in 15% of the patients. This is classified into following four grades:
  - Grade I: Patient is unaware of his problem and is diagnosed by the physician. Examination reveals extensor plantar and ankle clonus.
  - Grade II: Patient walks with support and has spastic gait.
  - Grade III: Patient is bedridden with paralysis in extension and sensory deficit less than 50%.

– *Grade IV*: Flaccid paralysis with extensive sensory deficit and bladder/bowel involvement.
- Paraplegia of *early onset* is usually due to inflammatory oedema, granulation tissue or cold abscess and prognosis is good.
- Paraplegia of late onset is usually due to mechanical factors and cord damage, the recovery is poor.

Investigations

Blood: Low Hb, high ESR, high TLC, increased lymphocytes, L/M (lymphocytes/monocytes) ratio should be 5, if less, it shows poor immune status (avoid surgery).

Urine
- RBC in urine shows silent haematuria and nephritic TB.
- RBC+ albuminuria shows UTI.
- Sugar indicates diabetes mellitus.

Biopsy
Lymph node or infected granulation tissue under CT control.

Mantoux test
- Mantoux test: 1TU of PPD in 0.1 ml injected subcutaneously. Horizontal transverse diameter of induration is measured. It is positive if this diameter is >10 mm is positive, it is <6 mm then it is –ve.
- Positive result shows prior sensitization to tuberculous bacilli.

Pus: AFB staining.

Culture: LJ media.

Inoculation
- Disease material (pus, joint aspirate, granulation tissue from the depth of sinus) may be injected into Guinea pig intraperitoneally.
- Positive cases show tubercles on the peritoneum after 5–8 weeks.

X-ray

Spine: AP view
- To see para-vertebral abscess.
- *V-shaped shadow* in upper thoracic abscess.
- *Fusiform-shape shadow (bird nest shadow)* below the level of fourth dorsal vertebrae.
- *Globular shape* when the abscess is in tension.
- *Psoas abscess: Unilateral or bilateral widening of the psoas shadow.*

Lateral
- Reduced intervertebral joint space (earliest sign).
- Erosion of adjoining surface.
- Collapse of vertebra (kyphosis).
- Parafocal osteoporosis.
- To see skip lesions in the vertebra above/below.

Chest: To rule out pulmonary tuberculosis.

CT scan

Destruction of intervertebral disc and adjoining vertebra.

MRI

- For early diagnosis, to see the extent of osseous destruction as well as cold abscess.
- For diagnosis of tubercular infection of difficult and rare site like craniovertebral region, cervicodorsal region, disease of posterior elements and vertebral appendages.
- It is an excellent modality to study the status of the cord.

Treatment

Conservative

- Patient should rest on hard bed.
- Antitubercular drugs
- Spinal braces

Middle Path Regime (Tuli and Kumar)

I: Bed rest

II: Chemotherapy: It comprises of:
  - *Intensive phase* (for 5–6 month) targeting sensitive bacteria
  - It comprising of daily dosage of:
    - INH 300–400 mg
    - Rifampicin 450–600 mg
    - Ofloxacin 400–600 mg
  - *Continuation phase* (for 7–8 months) targeting persisters, slow growing or intermittently growing or dormant or intracellularly bacteria.
  - It comprising of:
    - INH and pyrazinamide (1500 mg daily) for 3–4 month followed by INH and Rifampicin for another 4–5 months
  - *Prophylactic phase* (4–5 months): It is the time when the treated patient is return to his normal environment.
  - It comprises of
    - INH and ethambutol (1200 mg)
    - Dose of the drug can be titrated according to the weight of the patient, co-morbidities and adverse reaction of the drugs
    - For hospitalized patient streptomycin replaces any one of the drug except the INH
  - *Supportive treatment*: comprises of
    - Multivitamins
    - Haematinics
    - High protein diet

III: Radiographs and ESR:
  - 3–6 month interval
  - Kyphosis was measured radiologically

IV: *Gradual mobilization* of the patient in absence of any neurological deficit with the use of spinal braces as early as possible.

V: *Back extension exercise*: After 3–9 weeks of treatment for 5–10 min/day.

VI: *Spinal braces*: continued for 18–24 months and then gradually discarded.

VII: *Abscess are aspirated* followed by instillation of INH streptomycin with or without INH

VIII: *Sinuses heals* within 6–12 weeks.

IX: *Decompression*: It is indicated if there occurs neurologic deficit despite conservative treatment or in those who did not show progressive recovery after trial of conservative therapy.

X: *Excisional surgery*: It is recommended for posterior spinal disease.

XI: *Operative debridement*: It is advised in those who do not show arrest of activity of spinal lesion or pathology even after 3–6 months of chemotherapy or when there is recurrence of the disease. Indication for surgery have been discussed below.

XII: *Postoperative*
- Bed rest for atleast 2–3 weeks and in case of any neural deficit 3–5 months.
- If there is good recovery gradually mobilize the patients with spinal braces
- In absence of any neurological deficit mobilizes the patient with spinal braces 3–5 months after the operative procedure
- After 12–24 months after the operative procedure spinal braces are gradually discarded.

Surgery

Indication for various operations:
- Decompression ± fusion for neurological complication failed to respond to conservative therapy
- Decompression ± fusion in failure of response after 3–6 months of conservative treatment
- Doubtful diagnosis
- Fusion for mechanical instability
- Debridement ± decompression ± fusion in cases of recurrence of disease or of neurological complication
- Prevention of kyphosis by Decompression ± fusion
- Anterior transposition of the cord for neural complications due to severe kyphosis

Types of procedures:
- Drainage of cold abscess
- Spinal decompression
- Spinal fusion
- Laminectomy has no role in Potts spine. It is indicated only in:
  - Spinal tumor syndrome
  - Vertebral canal stenosis
  - Posterior spinal disease

Management of paraplegia (*already discussed under traumatic paraplegia*)
- Care of back
- Bowel and bladder
- Rehabilitation

> **Q5. Discuss the classification, sign, symptom, and management of Pott's paraplegia.**

Most dreaded and crippling complication of Potts spine.

Incidence: Overall incidence is 10–30%

Age: It is more common during first three decade of life.

Type: Paraplegia can be of two types (*Griffths, Seddon and Roaf*).

Early Onset Type

- Comes on during the active phase of the disease
- It occurs within 2 years of the onset.

Underlying Pathology

- Inflammatory edema
- Tubercular granulation tissue
- Tuberculous abscess
- Tubercular caseous tissue
- Rarely ischemic lesion of the cord
- Thrombus

Late Onset Type

- Appearance many years after the disease (>2 years).
- Associated with:
  - Recrudescence of the disease
  - Mechanical pressure

Underlying Pathology

- Recrudescence of the disease
- Holdworth ridge (Gliosis due to constant friction against Holdworth ridge)
- Tubercular caseous tissue
- Tubercular debris
- Sequestra from vertebral body and disc
- Internal gibbus
- Stenosis
- Severe deformity.

Classification (Goel, Tuli and Kumar)

Staging	Grading	Features
I	Negligible	• Patient is not aware of his weakness • Extensor plantar response • Ankle clonus
II	Mild	• Patient is aware of his weakness, complaining of clumsiness, or spasticity or jumpiness of the limb while walking • He is able to walk with support • Clinical features: all sign of spastic paresis
III	Moderate	• Bed ridden • Cannot walk because of severe weakness • Spastic paraplegia in extension • Sensory deficit if present<50%
IV	Severe	• III+ flexor spasm/paralysis in flexion/flaccid • Sensory deficit >50% (usually with bed sores) • Sphincter involved

Pathology

Essential Pathology

- Pressure on the tissue of cord.
- The primary error is tubercular endarteritis.

Inflammatory Edema

- Due to:
  - Vascular stasis
  - Toxins from tuberculous inflammation
- Quick recovery after a simple procedure like draining a paravertebral abscess or rest in bed

Extradural Mass

- Tuberculous osteitis of the vertebral bodies with an abscess in the extradural space.
- Causing compression of the cord from the anterior aspect.
- The abscess may be composed of fluid pus, granulation tissue or caseous material
- The Nature and extent can be best delineated by MRI.

Bony Disorders

- Sequestra may be responsible for:
  - Narrowing of the spinal canal
  - Pressure on the cord
- Angulation of the spine may lead to the formation of a bony ridge or spur called internal gibbus *(Holdworth ridge)*
- Pathological dislocation

Meningeal Changes

Peridural fibrosis may be responsible.

Infarction of the Spinal Cord

- Unusual but an important cause.
- Infarction is caused by an *endarteritis, periarteritis or thrombosis* of an important tributary to the anterior spinal artery or other spinal artery caused by inflammatory reaction.
- Irreparable.
- Because of its extreme rarity spinal angiography does not seems to be justified.
- Obstruction of the spinal artery indicates poor prognosis but it does not obviate the necessity of providing decompression.
- On MRI ischemic necrosis is seen as an area of high intensity in T_2.

Changes in spinal cord (Hughes 1966)

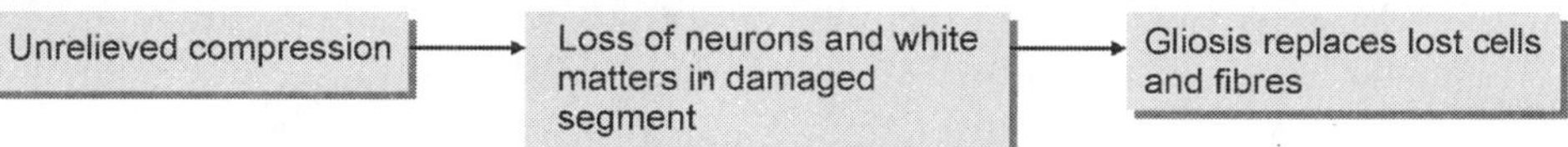

- In patients who did not recover after adequate surgical decompression MRI has revealed:
  - Myelomalacic changes
  - Syringomyelic changes
- Up to 50% reduction in the diameter of the cord substance is often compatible with good cord function.

Extradural Granuloma and Tuberculoma

Very rarely, it is responsible for neurological complications without any radiological evidence of tuberculous involvement of the vertebrae. Such cases may present as *"spinal tumour syndrome"*.

Sign and symptoms: Commonly it is associated with the known lesion of the vertebral column.

- In paralysis of slow onset the first sign of interference with the conduction of the cord may be:
  - Spontaneous twitching of the muscles
  - Clumsiness while walking
  - Extensor plantar response
  - Exaggerated reflexes
  - Sustained clonus of ankle and of patella may be present.
- Motor functions are usually affected before and to a greater extent than the sensory functions because the diseased area in spine lies anterior to the cord thus being nearer to the motor tracts.
- *Stages of paralysis*

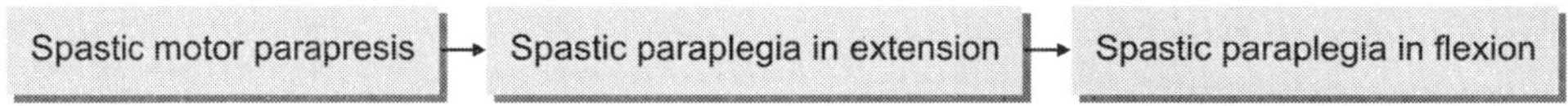

- *In very advanced stage*
  - Bladder and bowel/anal sphincter may be involved and there may a varying degree of sensory deficit.
  - Sense of position and vibration are last to disappear.
- *In extremely severe cases*: All spasticity disappears and the paralysis becomes flaccid (areflexic paraplegia) with anesthesia and loss of sphincter control.
- *Exceptionally*
  - The patient presents with sudden, complete flaccid paralysis like the clinical picture of "spinal shock".
  - Sudden complete paralysis may be caused by:
    - Ischaemia of the cord due to thromboembolic phenomenon
    - Transection of the cord due to pathological dislocation
    - Extremely rarely due to rapid accumulation of the infected material.
- *On rare occasion*: Patient may present like spinal tumor syndrome due to a localized tuberculoma or diffuse granuloma or due to Peridural fibrosis

Investigation

General investigation: As discussed above.

X-ray

Spine

AP view

- To see para-vertebral abscess.
- *V-shaped shadow* in upper thoracic abscess
- *Fusiform-shape shadow (bird nest shadow)* below the level of fourth dorsal vertebrae
- *Globular shape* when the abscess is in tension
- *Psoas abscess: unilateral or bilateral widening of the Psoas shadow*

Lateral

- Reduced intervertebral joint space (earliest sign)
- Erosion of adjoining surface
- Collapse of vertebra (kyphosis)
- Parafocal osteoporosis
- To see skip lesions in the vertebra above/below

Chest: To rule out pulmonary tuberculosis.

CT Scan

Destruction of intervertebral disc and adjoining vertebra.

MRI

- For early diagnosis, to see the extent of osseous destruction as well as cold abscess.
- For diagnosis of tubercular infection of difficult and rare site like craniovertebral region, cervicodorsal region, disease of posterior elements and vertebral appendages.
- It is an excellent modality to study the status of the cord.

Myelography

- Light lipiodol is introduced through lumbar puncture needle or heavy lipiodol injected by cisterna puncture into subarachnoid space. X-rays pictures are taken to find out if there is any filling defect.
- It is helpful in determining the level:
  - Paraplegia without the radiological evidence of the disease as in *"spinal tumor syndrome"*.
  - In cases with multiple vertebral lesions.
  - When a patient has not recovered after decompression procedure.

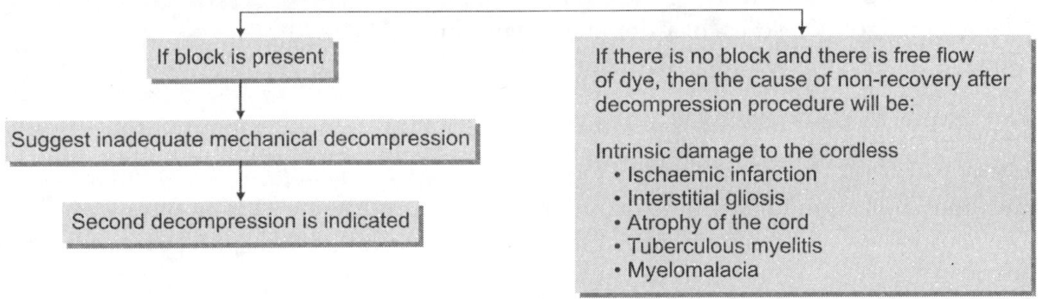

  - It helpful in differential diagnosis; revealed the picture of arachnoiditis.

Prognosis

Factors influencing prognosis in cord involvement:

Involvement of cord	Better prognosis	Relatively poor prognosis
• Degree	Partial	Complete (grade IV)
• Duration	Shorter	Longer (>1 year)
• Type	Early onset (<2 years)	Late onset (>2 years)
• Speed of onset	Slow	Rapid
• Age	Younger	Elder
• General condition	Good	Poor
• Vertebral disease	Active	Healed
• Kyphotic deformity	<60°	>60°
• Cord on MRI	Normal	Myelomalacia/syringomyelia
• Pre-operative	Wet lesion	Dry lesion

Treatment

The key word in the management when the patient is admitted to the hospital is "prevention". It includes:
• Prevention of deformity
• Prevention of pressure areas
• Prevention of further loss of muscle power
• Prevention of debilitation
• Prevention of urinary infection
• Prevention of respiratory and thrombotic episodes

Treatment of paraplegia: It is the treatment of tuberculosis of spine with the added approach of mechanical decompression of cord by removing the diseased granulation tissue.

Prevention is very important. This can be done by:
• Early diagnosis
• Prompt and suitable treatment

Best is Middle Path régime (as discussed above)

General
• Improve general condition of patient.
• Improve hemoglobin, protein status

Conservative
• Chemotherapy (ATT/DOTS)
• Immobilization and bed rest
• Management of bed sores, bladder and bowel care
• Once recovered mobilization with braces
• Physiotherapy
• Rehabilitation

Surgery
Indication: Indication for various operations:
• Decompression ± fusion for neurological complication failed to respond to conservative therapy
• Decompression ± fusion in failure of response after 3–6 month of conservative treatment
• Doubtful diagnosis

- Fusion for mechanical instability
- Debridement ± Decompression ± fusion in cases of recurrence of disease or of neurological complication
- Prevention of kyphosis by decompression ± fusion
- Anterior transposition of the cord for neural complications due to severe kyphosis
- Recurrence of disease

Surgical procedures
- Costotransversectomy
- Anterolateral decompression
- Anterior decompression
- Laminectomy

Flow chart showing the approach of treatment of vertebral tuberculosis with neurological complication:

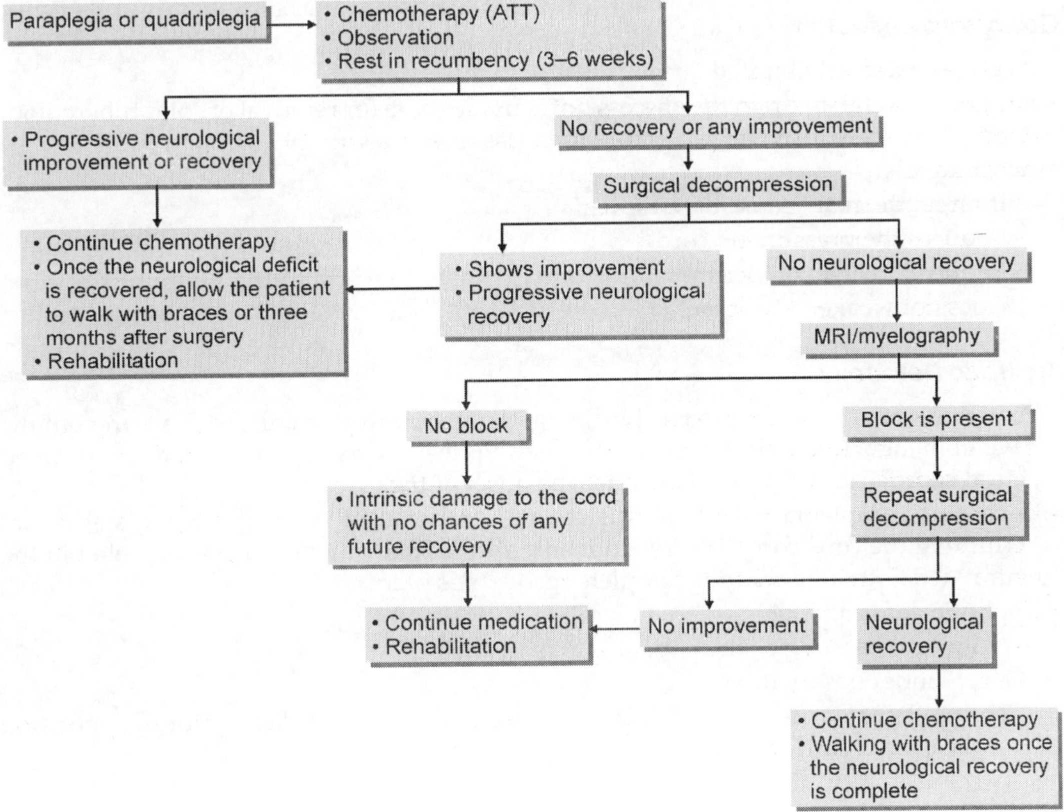

Few Important Points Regarding the Treatment

In the usual Paradiscal lesion
- The compression of the cord is mainly and maximally anteriorly.
- Therefore, it is essential to adequately decompress the cord anteriorly either by anterior approach or anterolateral approach.

Role of Laminectomy

- It is contraindicated as far as decompression is concerned, as it is inadequate for decompression of the anterior part of the cord.
- It removes the healthy part of the vertebrae and thus rendering the spine unstable and liable to pathological dislocation.
- Ill-advised laminectomy may lead to :
  - An increase in kyphotic deformity
  - Deterioration of neural status.
- Absolute indication of laminectomy are:
  - Posterior spinal disease
  - Cervical Potts
  - Spinal tumor syndrome
  - Cauda equine lesion
  - Vertebral canal stenosis

Costotransversectomy

- Its role is extremely limited.
- It is good enough to drain the abscess but is inadequate for removal of solid tuberculous debris, thick caseous material, granulation tissue, sequestra, etc.
- Advantages
  - It target the main cause of paraplegia
  - Reduces the pressure on cord
  - Reduced toxicity of focus
  - Does not weaken the spine.

Kyphotic Deformity

- Posterior spinal fusion for extensive spinal disease during childhood may prevent the development of kyphotic deformity because kyphosis of $\leq 60°$ as a rule produces delayed neural complications 10–15 years after the onset of the disease.
- In case of paraplegia with kyphosis of $\leq 60°$, removal of internal gibbus is essential permitting the cord complete freedom anteriorly. This may produce some relief in the neural deficit though seldom-complete recovery is seen.
- Kyphotic deformity $\leq 45°$
  - No surgery as long as the patient is able to walk
  - Keep under observation
  - The moment a patient shows deterioration and unable to walk, anterior transposition of the cord is carried out.

Sequence of Recovery of Neural Reflexes (Irrespective the Modality of Treatment)

- Vibration and joint sensation
- Temperature
- Touch
- Pain
- Voluntary power activity
- Sphincter functions
- Wasting of muscles

Q6. Discuss the rehabilitation of spinal injury patients.

The *primary goal* of the rehabilitation is to enable or motivate the patient to *achieve physical, social, emotional, recreational, vocational and functional recovery*. It is a team approach and it should begin as early as possible after the injury.

I. Respiratory Management

Paraplegics patient have three issues to manage:
- *Secretions:* Due to paralysis of abdominal muscles (D_6–L_1) required for forceful expiration; coughing is ineffective so there occur accumulation of secretions.
- *Atelectasis:* due to intercostal muscles paralysis the inspiration is dependent on diaphragm which is already weak hence tendency to develop atelectasis.
- *Hypoventilation:* Due to paralysis of respiratory muscles

Nerve supply of diaphragm is C_{3-5} (C_4). Patient with injury C_2 and above may not survive because even diaphragm is paralyzed. Patient with L_1 or lower level are usually no significant respiratory dysfunction.

Respiratory Management Involves

- *Chest physiotherapy:* Chest clapping percussion to loosen the secretion and drain clogged lung lobes.
- *Suction:* Useful for quadriplegics with lot of secretion.
- *Assisted coughing*
  - Here manual pressure is applied to abdomen timed with patients cough reflex.
  - Palms are placed below the cage between xiphoid process and umbilicus.
  - After a deep breath is taken by the patient, physiotherapist pushes upward and inwards with palm as patient cough.
  - This maneuver helps to mobilize the secretion from the lower portion of the lungs.
- *Incentive spirometry*
  - Encourage the patient to inhale as deeply as possible.
  - Purpose is to prevent or treat Atelectasis.
- *Abdominal binder*
  - Useful when patient become seated from supine position.
  - Abdominal content are pulled down by gravity and have a tendency to fall forward due to lack of abdominal muscle tone.
  - This also pulls the diaphragm downwards.
  - Therefore, at the start of inspiration diaphragm is at lower level that is the position of mechanical disadvantage.
  - Abdominal binder pushes abdominal content and diaphragm up which improve ventilation.

II. Bowel Management

- *Defecation centre* is located in sacral cord segment (S_{2-4}).
- *Internal anal sphincter*
  - *It* is composed of involuntary smooth muscles
  - *It* provides continence in the resting state by remaining tonically contracted.
- *External anal sphincter*
  - It is voluntary
  - It is innervated by pudendal nerve (S_{2-4}).

- *Defecation reflex*
  - It consists of stretching of rectum and puborectalis muscle by the passage of stool in leading to *reflex relaxation of internal anal sphincter.*
  - This causes an urge to defecate but external anal sphincter and puborectalis muscle prevent defecation.
  - Under voluntary control, external anal sphincter and puborectalis muscle relax allowing defecation.

UMN Lesion/Spastic Bowel

- When injury occurs above S_2 to S_4 segment i.e. conus medullaris, the anal sphincter becomes spastic.
- Voluntary control is lost but reflex evacuation is intact.
- Bowel management in this type consists of:
- Planned reflex evacuation by digital stimulation or suppositories.
- Use of stool softeners
- Bulk forming agents may help maintain adequate stool consistency.

LMN/Flaccid Bowel

- It occurs when injury involves:
  - Reflex center and or
  - Sacral nerve roots
- This is characterized by flaccid rectum with absence of spine mediated reflex activity.
- Management consists of:
  - Manual evacuation
  - Diet management
  - Use of stool softeners
  - Bulk forming agents removal to facilitate easy removal.

III. Bladder Management

Automatic/reflex/UMN or cord bladder

- It occurs due to complete transection of the cord above the sacral segments.
- Micturition reflex is intact.
- The bladder is of small capacity.
- It empties reflexely at regular small intervals in response to certain filling pressure.
- Loss of bladder sensation and there is no voluntary control.

Management
- Intermittent catheterization
- Reflex voiding (condom catheter)

Autonomous/denervated/LMN/autonomous bladder

- It occur injury to conus medullaris or in Cauda equina (disruption of either sacral segment S_{2-4} or sacral nerve roots).
- There is no reflex activity.
- Patient has dribbling urine irregularly.
- Bladder is atonic with large amount of residual urine.

Management
- Intermittent catheterization
- Manual compression (Crede's maneuver)

Urine complication in paraplegic

- UTI
- Hydronephrosis
- Renal calculi
- Carcinoma of bladder

Management
- Plenty of fluid intakes
- 2–3 hourly clamping of catheter
- Bladder irrigation with normal saline and betadiene
- Change of pH from acidic to alkaline and vice versa.

IV. Sexual rehabilitation and fertility

Males

- Psychogenic errection is mediated via sympathetic system (D_{11}–L_2) while reflex errection results from sacral stimulation via a parasympathetic nervous system (S_{2-4}).
- Ejaculation is controlled by both sympathetic and parasympathetic system.
- Patient with spinal cord injury have erectile and ejaculatory dysfunction.
- In UMN, lesion psychogenic errection is lost but reflex errection may be possible although it may be ill sustained.
- In LMN, lesion reflex errection is possible only in small number.

Management
- Intracavernous papaverine injection can be used for erectile dysfunction. These patient are unable to ejaculate and there may be retrograde ejaculation.
- Electrostimulation may be done for ejaculatory dysfunction.
- Fertility is decreased due to poor semen quality and ejaculatory dysfunction.
- Assisted reproduction techniques like IU insemination and IVF should be tried if patient wants to father the child.

Female Fertility

- There is insignificant impact in fertility but pregnancy is going to be a complicated in prenatal, perinatal and post natal phases.
- CS is indicated, as patient may not have labour pains.

V. Skin care and pressure sores

Factors leading to pressure sores includes:
- Sensory loss
- Loss of vasomotor control hence low tissue resistance.
- Skin maceration due to moisture or urine
- Nutrition deficiency
- Poor general condition

These can only be prevented by reliving pressure.

Preventive techniques includes:
- Patient education regarding frequent changes of posture
- Water/air bed to distribute evenly pressure over bony points
- Good nutrition
- Use of long handled mirror for self-inspection.

Treatment consists of:
- Thorough debridement and cleaning
- Operative procedures to repair pressure ulcer includes *direct closure, musculocutaneous and fasciocutaneous flaps*, which are better able to withstand pressure.

Complication of pressure sores includes:
- Endocarditis
- Heterotropic bone formation
- Septicemia
- Abscess
- Osteomyelitis
- Squamous cell carcinoma

VI. Spasticity

- It correspond with the level of injury to the cord. Higher is the level of injury to the spinal cord more is the incidence of spasticity.
- In some cases spasticity may contribute to improve patient function but it needs treatment when it possess risk of developing contractures interfering with functions and causes pain due to spasm.

Causes
- UTI
- Bladder calculi
- Impacted bowel
- Irritation from urinary catheter, etc.

Treatment option
- Stretching exercise
- Medication (Baclofen BZD and muscle relaxant)
- Nerve block by absolute alcohol or phenol
- Intrathecal baclofen and absolute alcohol in intractable spasticity

VII. Heterotropic Ossification

- Aetiology is unknown but it could be due to spasticity, tissue hypoxia, necrosis or Humoral factors
- It is an extra-articular ossification of muscle of paralyzed extremities.
- Hip is most commonly involved though knee, elbow, shoulder may be involved.
- Anteromedial aspect of hip is most commonly involved.

Clinical features in acute phase:
- Fever
- Swelling of soft tissue
- Movements are painfully restricted

Diagnosis in acute stage is by:

- Bone scan
- USG
- CT scan
- ESR, alkaline phosphatase and CRP are elevated.

Management

- There is no definite prophylaxis
- Treatment in acute phase is:
  - Rest
  - Etidronate therapy which inhibits mineralization and ROM exercises.
  - Mature bone may need resection if it is interfering with sitting, positioning or dressing. One should weight 1.5–2 years before resection to allow time for maturation of bone.

Q7. Discuss the aim and principles of antitubercular drugs chemotherapy.

Aims of Chemotherapy

- To cure patients
- To avoid relapse
- To prevent chronic disease
- To reduce the period of infectivity thereby halting transmission of infection to others.

Principles of Chemotherapy

- Patients with higher bacillary burdens (i.e. patient with active disease) should receive an intensive phase of treatment with at least three drugs, to rapidly decrease the bacillary burden and to prevent the emergence of drug resistance.
- Drugs must be given in adequate dosages, adequate duration without interrupting the treatment.
- Combinations must be given; single drugs administration will result in the development of drug resistance.
- It is preferable to give drugs in single doses, as peak concentration at one particular point is more bactericidal rather than having uniform concentration.
- Simultaneously two aminoglycosides should not be given.
- In short course chemotherapy, in the intensive phase bactericidal and sterilizing drugs should be given.
- Monitoring of therapy to watch for tolerance and adverse reactions and their treatment is necessary.
- In reserve chemotherapy, care must be taken to use two or three drugs that were not used in the past preferably bactericidal drugs.
- Interactions between antitubercular drugs and other drugs given simultaneously, must be kept in mind and dosages adjusted accordingly.
- Treatment must not be started without confirmation of diagnosis as it is a social stigma and there is a risk of drug toxicity.
- In doubtful diagnosis, pure tuberculostatic drugs such as *INH, Ethambutol* must be given and not antitubercular antibiotics, as they act on other organisms and confuse the picture.
- Interactions between antitubercular drugs and other drugs given simultaneously must be kept in mind and dosages adjusted accordingly.

- According to latest recommendations, SCC is the treatment of choice both in pulmonary and extrapulmonary tuberculosis not only in adults but also in children.
- Only regimens that were tested in controlled clinical trials or other studies must be given.
- Simultaneous administration of corticosteroids if necessary, should be given under the coverage of antituberculosis treatment only.

Q8. Discuss in brief the classification and important characteristic features and side effects of first line antitubercular drugs.

Classification of Antitubercular Drugs

First-line Drugs

- Rifampin
- Isoniazid
- Ethambutol
- Pyrazinamide
- Streptomycin

Second-line Drugs

- Thiacetazone
- Para-aminosalicylic acid
- Cycloserine
- Ethionamide
- Amikacin
- Kanamycin
- Capreomycin

Newer Drugs

- Fluoroquinolones:
  - Ciprofloxacin
  - Ofloxacin
- Macrolides:
  - Clarithromycin
  - Azithromycin
- Rifamycins: Rifabutin
- Oxazolidinones: Linezolid
- Nitroimidazopyrans and diarylquinolines

Antibiotics

- Streptomycin
- Aminoglycosides
- Rifampicin
- Cycloserine

Chemotherapeutic Agents

- INH
- Ethambutol

- TZA
- PZA
- Ethionamide
- PAS

Bactericidal

- Killing of rapidly multiplying bacteria
- INH, rifampicin, PZA, streptomycin, ethambutol

Bacteriostatic

- Inhibition of multiplication of organisms
- PAS, TZA, ethionamide, cycloserine

Sterilizing

- Killing of persistors or slow multiplying organisms.
- Rifampicin, PZA, INH

Essential antitubercular drugs as classified by WHO

- INH
- SM
- Ethambutol
- Rifampicin
- Pyrazinamide
- Thiacetazone

Drugs that prevent emergence of drug resistance to another drug:
- INH
- Rifampicin

Antitubercular Drugs

I. Rifampin

- Most potent.
- Active against some gram-positive and gram-negative bacteria, *Legionella* spp., atypical mycobacteria.
- Mechanism of action: Inhibits RNA synthesis. It inhibits DNA dependent RNA synthesis. Rifampin resistance is nearly always due to mutation in the repo-B gene (for the β subunit of RNA polymerase the target of rifampin action).
- Both intracellular and extracellular, bactericidal activity.
- Distributes throughout most body tissues, including meninges.
- Turns body fluids (urine, saliva, sputum, tears) a red-orange colour.
- Metabolise in liver.
- Excreted through the bile and the kidneys.
- Rifampin is also available for IV administration.

Side Effects

- Hepatitis (dose related)
- Respiratory syndrome
- Purpura

- Haemolysis
- Shock and renal failure
- Cutaneous syndrome
- Flu syndrome
- Abdominal syndrome
- Urine and secretions may become orange red but this is harmless.
- Potent inducer of microsomal enzymes and thereby decreases the half-life of a number of drugs, e.g. clarithromycin, the HIV protease inhibitors, the HIV nonnucleoside reverse transcriptase inhibitors.

II. Isoniazid

- Should include in all regimens unless the organism is resistant.
- Bacteriostatic against resting bacilli and bactericidal against rapidly multiplying organisms.
- Mechanism of action: Inhibits cell wall synthesis
- Act extracellularly and intracellularly.
- Equally acting in acidic and alkaline medium.
- Diffuses well throughout the body and reaches therapeutic concentrations in serum, cerebrospinal fluid (CSF), and infected tissue, including caseous granulomas.
- Metabolized in the liver.
- Excreted into the urine.

Side Effects

Hepatotoxicity: Hepatitis increases in incidence with:
- Age
- Alcohol consumption
- Concomitant rifampin administration
- Active hepatitis B infection
- In women who are pregnant or in the immediate postpartum period (up to 3 months after delivery).
- The Centers for Disease Control and Prevention (CDC) and the American Thoracic Society (ATS) recommend that it should be discontinued whenever:
  - An asymptomatic elevation of the ALT level exceeds five times the upper limit of normal or
  - The ALT is three times the upper limit of normal in conjunction with hepatitis symptoms or jaundice.

Peripheral neuropathy
- Relates to interference with pyridoxine (vitamin B_6) metabolism.
- The prophylactic administration of 25–50 mg of pyridoxine daily should be considered.

III. Ethambutol

- Least potent
- Bacteriostatic
- Mechanism of action: Inhibits cell wall synthesis
- Distribution throughout the body is adequate except in the CSF.
- Excrete via kidney.

Side Effects

- Retrobulbar optic neuritis is the most serious adverse effect.
- The risk of optic neuritis depends on the dose and duration of therapy; usually reversible, but recovery may take >6 months.
- Other adverse effects are
- Hyperuricemia but asymptomatic.
- Peripheral sensory neuropathy rare .

IV. Pyrazinamide

- Bactericidal drug
- More active to intracellular bacilli
- Mechanism of action: Unclear; disrupt plasma membrane, disrupt energy metabolism
- It is active only at a pH of <6.0 (acidic medium)
- It highly active at the site of inflammation, because at inflammation medium is acidic. So it is highly active during first 2 months of therapy, when inflammation is high.
- Well distributed throughout the body. Levels in CSF are excellent. So drug of choice in tubercular meningitis.
- Metabolized in the liver.
- It is excreted in urine.
- Can use in pregnancy.

Side Effects

- Hepatotoxicity at the high dosages.
- Hyperuricaemia can leads to clinical gout rarely.
- Polyarthralgias .

V. Streptomycin

- An aminoglycoside isolated from *Streptomyces griseus*.
- Streptomycin is available for IM and IV administration only.
- *Mechanism of action:* Inhibits protein synthesis by disruption of ribosomal function.
- Bactericidal for rapidly dividing extracellular mycobacteria but is ineffective in the acidic environment within the macrophage.
- It diffuses poorly into the meninges.
- Eliminated exclusively by the kidneys, the dosage must be lowered and the frequency of administration reduced (to only two or three times per week) in most patients >50 years of age and in any patient with renal impairment.

Side Effects

- Ototoxicity
  - Hearing loss and vestibular dysfunction
  - Vestibular dysfunction is more common and includes loss of balance, vertigo, and tinnitus.
- Renal toxicity
- Other includes perioral paresthesia, eosinophilia, rash, and drug fever.

Doses

- Adult dose is 0.5–1.0 g (10–15 mg/kg)
- The pediatric dose is 20–40 mg/kg daily, with a maximum of 1 g/day.

Dosage for Adults

Drug	Dosage	
	Daily dose	*Thrice-weekly dose*
• Isoniazid	5 mg/kg, max 300 mg	15 mg/kg, max 900 mg
• Rifampin	10 mg/kg, max 600 mg	10 mg/kg, max 600 mg
• Pyrazinamide	20–25 mg/kg, max 2 g	30–40 mg/kg, max 3 g
• Ethambutol	15–20 mg/kg	25–30 mg/kg

Q9. What are current WHO guidelines regarding treatment of TB.

The WHO has ranked TB patients from category I (highest priority) to category IV (lowest priority).

• Disease categorization is based on the severity of the disease judged by:
  – The patient's sputum smear status
  – Clinical condition and radiological extent of the disease
  – The site of the disease (pulmonary or extrapulmonary)
• Whether or not the patient had received prior treatment for TB.

Significant modifications in the WHO guidelines of 2003 from the previous guidelines of 1997 are:

• TB patients with concomitant HIV infection are included in category I
• The treatment for category III patients is the same as that for category I patients.

WHO Recommended Regimens for Different Categories

Disease category	Tuberculosis patient definition	Regimen initial (daily or three phase times weekly)	Continuation phase (daily or three phase times weekly)
I	• New smear-positive • New smear-negative with extensive parenchymal involvement • New severe extrapulmonary tuberculosis or severe concomitant HIV infection	2 HRZE	4 HR or 6 HE daily
II	Previously treated sputumsmear-positive pulmonarytuberculosis – relapse – treatment after interruption – treatment failure	2 HRZES/ 1 HRZE	5 HRE
III Osteoarticular TB	New smear-negative pulmonary tuberculosis Extra-pulmonary tuberculosis	2 HRZE	4 HR or 6 HE daily
IV	Chronic and MDR tuberculosis	Specially designed standardized or individualized regimens	

Q10. Write short note on DOTS.

Purpose of directly observed therapy for TB patients
• To provide extra support to patients to assist with the administration of TB treatment
• To provide the correct dosage of TB drugs at the same time each day, without missing any doses.
• Successful treatment and cure of TB disease

The entire approach comprises of:
- Treatment of tuberculosis in RNTCP is done in two phase.
  - Intensive phase (IP)
  - Continuation phase (CP).
- Every dose of medicine in *intensive phase* and at least the first dose every week in continuation phase are directly observed.
- After patients swallow their drugs in presence of a DOT provider, those receiving streptomycin should be given an injection.
- Any patient who has stopped taking drugs is traced and brought back under treatment.
- Drugs are supplied in *patient wise boxes* containing the full course of treatment and packaged in blister packs.
- Box have a colour code indicating category:
  - Red: Cat-I
  - Blue: Cat-II
  - Green: Cat-III
- Each PWB have two pouch, one for IP(A) and one for CP(B)
- For IP each blister pack contains one day's medication.
- For CP each blister pack contains one week's supply of medication.
- Drugs for prolongation phase/pouches are supplied separately.

Dosage Strength

- (H) Isoniazid 600 mg—2 pills
- (R) Rifampicin 450 mg—1 pill
- (Z) Pyrazinamid 1500 mg—2 pills
- (E) Ethambutol 1200 mg—2 pills
- (S) Streptomycin 750 mg
- If patients >60 kg additional rifampicin 150 mg
- If patients >50 years streptomycin 500 mg
- If patients <30 kg Received drugs as per body weight.

DOTS Regime

Category	Type of patient	Regimen	Pre-treatment	Test at month	IF result is	Then →
I	New sputum smear positive	2(HRZE)₃	+	2	−	Start continuation phase, test sputum again at 4/6 months
	Seriously ill sputum smear −ve seriously ill extrapulmonary	4(HR)₃			+	Continue intensive phase for 1 more month
			−	2	−	Start continuation phase, test sputum again at 6 monthn
					+	continue intensive phase for 1 more month, test sputum again at 3, 4 and 7 months

Category	Type of patient	Regimen	Pre-treatment	Test at month	IF result is	Then →
II	Sputum smear positive relapse	2(HRZES)₃	+	3	−	Start continuation phase, test sputum again at 5/6 months
	Sputum smear positive failure	1(HRZE)₃			+	Continue intensive phase for 1 more month, test sputum again at 4,6 and 9 months
	Sputum smear positive treatment after default	5(HRE)₃				
III	New sputum smear −ve, not seriously ill	2(HRZ)₃	−	2	−	Start continuation phase, test sputum again at 6 month
	New extrapulmonary, not seriously ill	4(HR)₃			+	Reregister the patient and begin Cat II

Benefits of DOTS

- Produces cure rates of up to 95%
- Prevents new infections
- Prevents the development of MDR-TB
- Cost effective

Q11. Write short note on: a. Spina ventosa; b. Caries sicca.

a. Spina ventosa

- This is tubercular involvement of proximal phalanx (short tubular bones).
- Presenting as:
    - 'Spindle' shaped deformity of the finger
    - Tenderness
    - Swelling
    - Cold abscess or multiple discharging sinuses (may present)
    - Shortening
- *Radiologically*: Honeycombing; soft coke-like sequestra; lytic lesion or diffuse uniform infiltration.
- Biopsy revealed typical tubercular features.
- *Effective treatment requires*:
    - Rest in functional position
    - Chemotherapy
    - Early active exercise
    - If not responding to above: chemotherapy plus evacuation of abscesses and sequestrectomies.
    - If ankylosed in awkward position: Excisional arthroplasty or corrective osteotomy.

b. Caries sicca

- It is common *dry atrophic form* of *tubercular disease of the shoulder.*
- More frequent in adults.

- Incidence of concomitant pulmonary tuberculosis is high.
- *Presentation*:
  - Synovitis (very rarely)
  - Usually present with painful restriction of abduction and external rotation
  - Marked wasting of the muscles around the shoulder joint.
  - Swelling or cold abscess or sinus formation (very rarely)
  - With the advance diseases, there occur marked destruction and atrophy of the proximal humerus and glenoid cavity and finally the shoulder undergoes fibrous ankylosis.
  - In neglected cases, the shoulder is fixed in adduction.
- *Biopsy*: Sent for bacteriological and histological examination.
- Radiologically:
  - Generalized rarefaction of bones
  - Varying degree of erosion of the articular margins
  - Destruction of the proximal humerus and of glenoid cavity
  - Some periosteal reaction (in absence of sinus formation)
  - Inferior subluxation of joint (in some cases)
- *Biopsy*: bacteriology and histological examination
- *Effective treatment requires*:
  - Chemotherapy.
  - Immobilized in shoulder spica (70-90° of adduction, 30° forward flexion and about 30° of internal rotation).
  - After 3 months, remove the spica and abduction frame is applied.
  - Not responding to the conservative therapy (few cases)/painful, unstable joint: arthrodesis of joint.

10

Diseases of Joints

The normal synovial fluid has the following characteristics:

Characteristics	Normal synovial fluid
Gross appearance	• Clear, viscous (due to presence of hyaluronate)
Colour	• Clear or pale straw colour
Amount	• 0.13–3.5 ml
Intra-articular pressure	• –8 cm to –12 cm
Culture	• Sterile
Clotting	• Does not clot
Immune antibodies	• Identical with those of blood serum
Specific gravity	• 1.008–1.015
Cytology	• WBCs are less than 200/mm^3
	• Mostly lymphocytes and monocytes
	• Less than 25% are neutrophils (acute inflammation will evoke a response of polymorphs)
Protein	• 2g/dl, consisting of albumin, mucin and globulin
Mucin	• Firm mucin clot
	• (*Rope test:* an examination of the integrity of hyaluronic acid–protein (mucin) complex. There is a formation of tight ropy clot (does not break up on agitation) on addition of acetic acid in normal synovial fluid.)
	• A poor mucin clot, that breaks up easily indicates destruction or dilution of hyaluronate
Glucose	• Same as that in the blood
Enzymes	• Lipase, amylase, protease
	• Extremely low alkaline phosphatase

Ans: In cases of an acute monoarthritis, infectious or crystal induced arthropathies, arthrocentesis and analysis of synovial fluid are always indicated.

Joint Fluid Characteristics

Characteristics	Inflammatory	Non-inflammatory	Septic or infectious
Colour	Yellow or opalescent	Amber	Variable-may be purulent
Clarity	Translucent	Transparent	Opaque

(Contd.)

Characteristics	Inflammatory	Non-inflammatory	Septic or infectious
Viscosity	Low	High	Typically low
Mucin clot (Rope test)	Friable	Firm	Friable
WBCs/mm^3	2,000–100,000	200–2000	>50,000 usually >100,000
Polymorphonucleo-cytes (%)	>50	<25	>75
Culture (Gram stained)	Negative	Negative	Usually positive (pathologic organism)
Conditions	RA, Gout and other	Osteoarthritis, trauma and other	Acute (*Streptococcal, Staphylococcus, gonococcus*) Chronic (*Tubercle bacillus*)

Crystal's arthropathy: Synovial fluid should be analyzed immediately for the presence of crystals (polarized light) as for appearance, viscosity, and cell count.

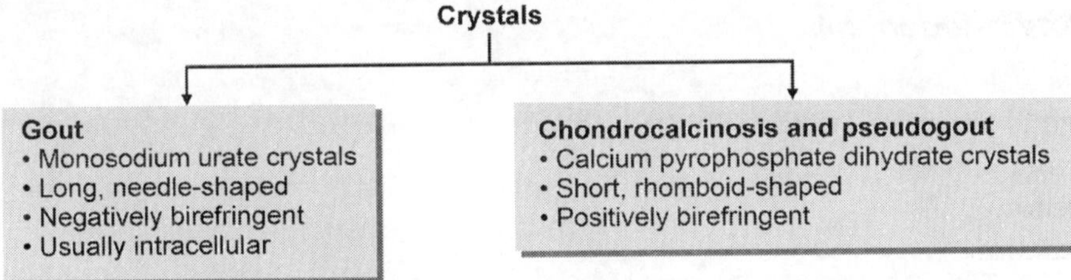

Always remember when you are sending samples of synovial fluid for:

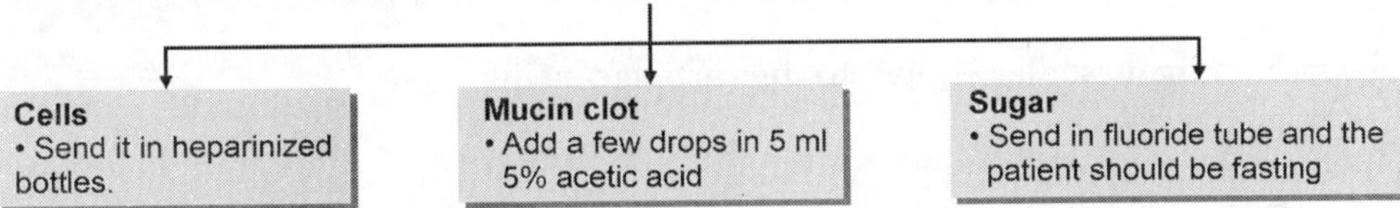

Q3. Write a short note on Haemarthrosis.

Haemarthrosis is a bleeding into joint spaces or simply it is collection of blood in the joint.

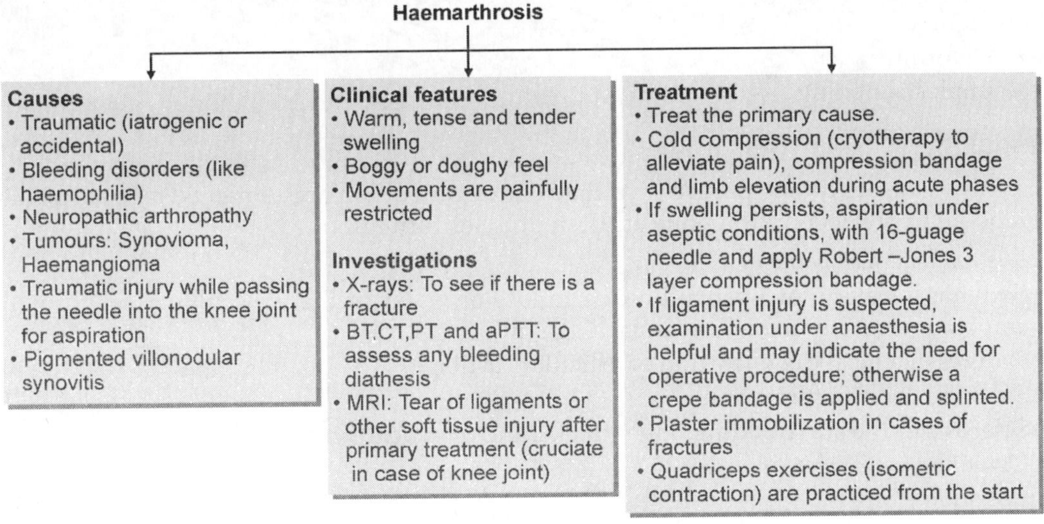

Q4. Discuss in brief osteoarthritis or degenerative joint disease.

Osteoarthritis (OA) is a *degenerative, non-inflammatory joint disease* affecting the articular cartilage and subchondral bone. It is a slowly progressive degenerative disease of diarthrodial (synovial) joints.

This is the commonest cause of morbidity after the age of 45, involving 60% of the population, characterized by *joint pains, reduced mobility, instability and crippling deformity.*

Aetiology

It may be primary (idiopathic) or secondary due to overweight, diabetes or post-traumatic.

Primary osteoarthritis

This is age-related and gradually progressive.

Secondary osteoarthritis

This is due to:
- Damage to the articular cartilage due to:
  - Trauma
  - Infection
  - Irradiation
  - Gout
  - Steroids
  - Alcohol
- Alteration in the vascular supply to the cartilage as in:
  - Storage diseases
  - Haemoglobinopathies
  - Paget's disease
  - Caisson sickness (disease caused by nitrogen bubbles in deep sea divers)
  - Osteoporosis
  - Osteomalacia
- Alteration in joint alignment/bio-mechanics following:
  - Injury
  - Deformity
  - Limb shortening

Pathology

The basic cause is due to progressive articular degeneration accompanied by poor repair, remodelling of subchondral bone and osteophytes formation.

OA is characterized pathologically by:
- Softening, fraying or fibrillation due to loss of water of the weight bearing normally smooth and glistening articular cartilage (initial event)
- Progressive focal degeneration of articular cartilage.
- Subarticular cyst formation.
- Sclerosis of the surrounding bone (thickening of subchondral bone).
- Osteophytes formation.
- Capsular fibrosis.
- Joint deformity.

Diagnosis

This is based on:
- History
- Clinical examination
- Corroborative findings on X-ray

History

- Pain in relation to the joint activity and relief by rest
- Grinding and joint crepitus
- Gradually progressive loss of joint movements
- Recurrent swellings and crippling deformities

Examination

- The patient shows obvious signs of ageing, wrinkles on the face and arcus senilis.
- Examination of joints in general reveals:
    - Joint line tenderness
    - Palpable crepitus (osteophytes)
    - Reduced mobility
    - Joint instability
    - Deformity and muscle atrophy.
    - There may be associated neurological signs depending on root involvement especially the cervical and lumbar zone.
- *Hand*: Osteoarthritis here occurs more common in females with classical signs of **Heberden's nodes** on the distal interphalangeal joints or **Bouchard's nodes** over proximal interphalangeal joints.
- *Knee*: This causes pain during routine activities of life, stiffness, instability and progressive varus deformity leading to bowlegs.
- *Hip*: This presents as groin pain and progressive antalgic gait.
- *Spine*: The degeneration may involve intervertebral disc, facet joints or exiting nerves and presents as radicular pains as well as local stiffness.

Investigations

- **X-ray** of shows:
    - Reduction of joint space
    - Increased density of subchondral bone
    - Osteophytes/loose bodies
    - Joint subluxation
    - Deformity
    - Malalignment of joint
- Synovial fluid, blood and urine examination is necessary to rule out secondary causes.

Treatment

This is based on the severity of the disease and demands of the patients

Conservative

- Exercises to improve the joint movements and muscle power.
- Reduce weight so as to cut down the load on the major weight-bearing joints.

- Local therapy by hot fomentation, massage and anti-inflammatory liniments.
- Supportive aids like splints, braces, canes, and crutches.
- Change in lifestyle and joint demands.
- Drugs: Analgesic/anti-inflammatory drugs, cartilage rejuvenators like glucosamine.

Surgery

- Joint realignment by osteotomies around hip and knee
- Stability of joint by arthrodesis in the hand and knee
- Joint replacement especially hip, knee, elbow, shoulder, and small joints of the fingers.

Q5. Discuss the clinical features and management of osteoarthritis of knee joint.

Osteoarthritis (OA) is a degenerative, non-inflammatory joint disease affecting the articular cartilage and subchondral bone. It is a slowly progressive degenerative disease of diarthrodial (synovial) joints. The knee is the commonest of the large joints to be affected.

It may be primary (idiopathic) or secondary due to overweight, diabetes or post-traumatic.

Pathology

OA is characterized pathologically by
- Softening, fraying or fibrillation due to loss of water of the weight bearing normally smooth and glistening articular cartilage (initial event)
- Progressive focal degeneration of articular cartilage
- Subarticular cyst formation
- Sclerosis of the surrounding bone (thickening of subchondral bone)
- Osteophytes formation
- Capsular fibrosis
- Joint deformity

Clinical Features

- Onset is insidious.
- Progressive, continuous, usually mild, aching pain. Pain is mild in the morning but increases with activity and is relieved by rest.
- Swelling
- Limitation of knee movements while squatting, going up and down a stairs
- Minimal tenderness can be elicited.
- Minimal effusion
- Movements are often accompanied by patellofemoral crepitus.
- Instability gradually limits the mobility of the patient in due course of time.
- If there are loose bodies in the joint then patient give history of locking or giving way of the joint.
- Deformity (genu varum or bow legs).

Investigations

X-rays: Radiological assessment of the knee joint in the most important diagnostic tool. The anteroposterior X-ray must be taken with the patient standing and weight bearing. The following radiological features can be appreciated:
- Reduction of joint space *(usually of medial tibiofemoral compartment)*
- Increased density of subchondral bone *(subchondral sclerosis)*
- Subchondral cyst *(resulting from synovial fluid intrusion into the bone)*
- Osteophytes *(resulting from revascularization of remaining cartilage)*
- Loose bodies *(resulting from fragmentation of osteochondral surface)*
- Joint subluxation *(resulting from destruction of capsule and ligaments)*
- Deformity *(resulting from destruction of capsule and ligaments)*
- Malalignment of joint *(resulting from destruction of capsule and ligaments).*

Radiological Classification to Assess the Severity of Knee OA

Kellgren and Lawrence (1957) and **Ahlback (1968)** are most commonly employed grading system for knee OA. The two grading systems are compared in table below.

Ahlback grade	Ahlback definition	Kellgren and Lawrence grade	Kellgren and Lawrence definition
		Grade 1 "Doubtful"	*Minute osteophytes, doubtful significance*
		Grade 2 "Minimal"	*Definite osteophytes, unimpaired joint space*
Grade 1	*Joint space narrowing (joint space <3 mm)*	**Grade 3 "Moderate"**	*Moderate diminution of joint space*
Grade 2	*Joint space obliteration*	**Grade 4 "Severe"**	*Joint space greatly impaired, with sclerosis of subchondral bone*
Grade 3	*Minor bone attrition (0–5 mm)*	**Grade 4**	*As above*
Grade 4	*Moderate bone attrition (5–10 mm)*	**Grade 4**	*As above*
Grade 5	*Severe bone attrition (>10 mm)*	**Grade 4**	*As above*

- *Routine blood investigations:* Sedimentation rate is normal, blood profile is normal, febrile agglutination tests are negative.
- *Synovial fluid analysis:* Shows non-inflammatory picture.
- *Radionuclide scanning with Tc^{99m}-HDP:* Shows increased uptake due to increased vascularity and new bone formation during the bone phase in the subchondral regions of affected joints.
- *MRI and CT scan:* Sometimes used to diagnose subchondral cysts, osteophytes, status of ligaments or meniscus, etc.
- *Arthroscopy:* May show articular cartilage damage, osteophytes and loose bodies.
  For OA X-rays are so characteristic that other forms of imaging are seldom necessary.

Management

Principles of Treatment

- Relieve pain
- Maintain movements and muscle strength.
- Increase mobility.
- Protect the joint from 'overload'
- Modify daily routine activities.

Treatment

- Conservative
- Surgery

Conservative

Relieve pain

- *Rest* to reduce compression and shear stress. It also allows the synovial inflammation to subside.
- *Analgesics*: Salicylates are the preferred drugs (used for their analgesic and anti-inflammatory property).
- Chondroprotective drugs
- *Intra-articular* injection of corticosteroids
- *Physical therapy*: Like moist heat, SWD (short wave diathermy), etc.
- *Vertical load reduction*: By weight reduction and use of a walking stick in hand opposite to the affected joint.
- *Precautions*: Like avoiding climbing stairs, squatting position and sitting cross-legged. Prefer use of commode for toilet.

Increase mobility

- *Graduated isometric exercises and physiotherapy*: To improve and balance muscle power acting about the joint.
- *To prevent capsular contracture*: The joint is moved through a full range of motion several times daily.
  Reduces instability: Braces.

Surgery

Aim

- Relieving pain
- Improving and maintaining joint movements.
- Correcting deformity and malalignment.
- Reducing vertical loads and shear stresses.
- Removing the intra-articular cause of erosion of articular surface.

Indications

- Persistent pain failure to respond to conservative treatment.
- Progressive deformity.
- Gross instability of joint.
- Progressive painful restriction of movements.

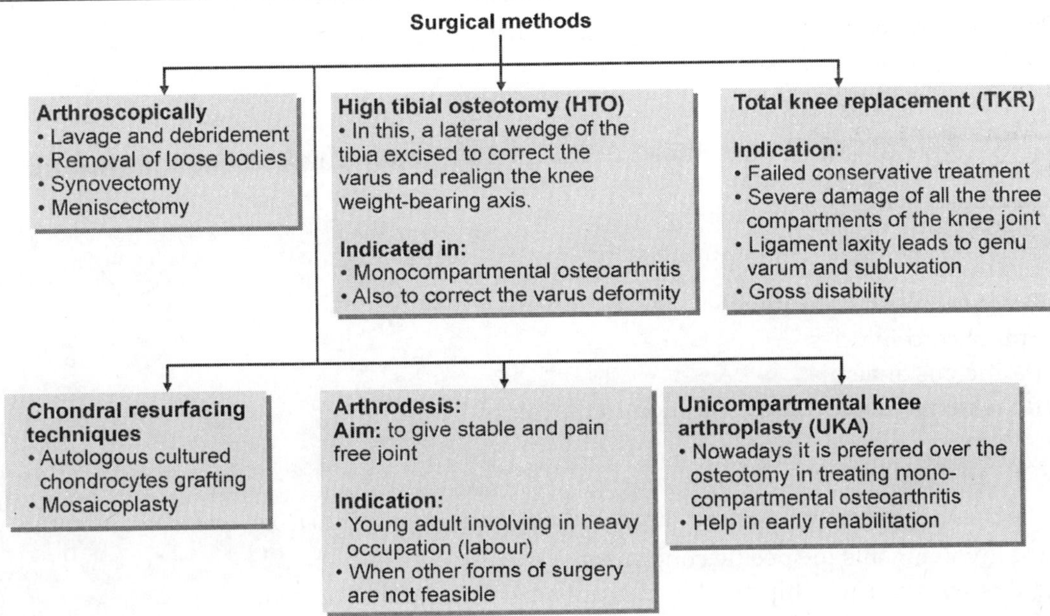

Recent in OA Knee

Viscosupplementation

It involves the injection of *gel-like substances (hyaluronates)* into a joint to supplement the viscous properties of synovial fluid.

- *Aim*: Replacing the osteoarthritic synovial fluid with a product made of *HA (hyaluronan (natural) and hylan G-F 20 (synthetic))*, that is closer to normal synovial fluid.
- *Indication*: In all patients who have significant residual symptoms despite *traditional non-pharmacologic and pharmacologic treatments*.
- *Mechanism of action*: Restoration of the elastoviscous properties of synovial fluid
- *Benefit*: the patient experiences pain relief due to the presence of a new "lubricant" in the knee that is also acting as a shock absorber.

Other includes
· Ozone therapy
· Bone marrow infusion
· Stem cell infusion
· Cultured autologous chondrocytes

Q6. Write a short note on Charcot's joint or Neuropathic arthropathy or neuro-pathic joint.

This is a *degenerated painless joint* due to loss of pain, temperature and proprioceptive sensation to the joint. *Jean Mortin Charcot* first described it in 1868 in patients with *Tabes arthropathy*.

Neuropathic joint is associated with:

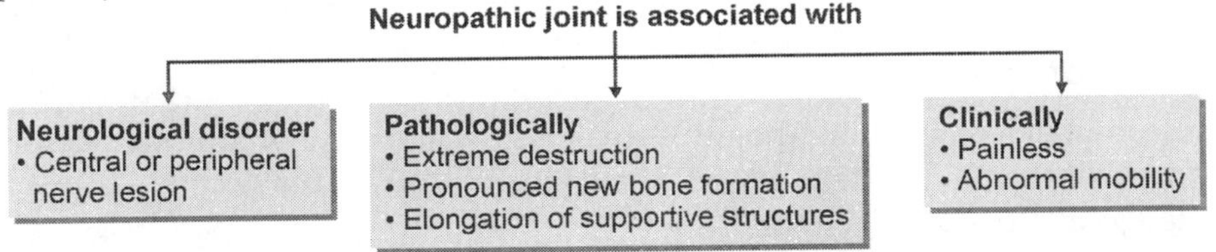

Disorders associated with neuropathic joint disease:
- Tabes dorsalis
- Diabetes mellitus
- Meningomyelocele
- Syringomyelia
- Multiple sclerosis
- Amyloidosis
- Leprosy
- Peroneal muscle atrophy
- Spinal cord injuries
- Pernicious anaemia
- Repeated hydrocortisone injection in the joints.

Areas of Predilection

In decreasing order of frequency are *knee, foot, ankle, hip, spine, elbow, shoulder,* and *wrist.*

Joint involvements in specific conditions:
- *Tabes dorsalis*: Knee, hips and ankles are most commonly affected.
- *Syringomyelia*: Glenohumeral joint, elbow and wrist.
- *Diabetes mellitus*: Tarsal and metatarsal joints.

Types

- Charcot originally described the *benign* and the *malignant* types.
- At present, the commonly described types are the **hypertrophic or proliferative** (*excess bone formation in the form of osteophytes, sclerosis and parosteal ossification*) and **atrophic or degenerative forms** (*destruction and osteoporosis predominate*).

Pathological Stages

Brailsford has recently claimed that neuropathic joints pass through four distinct stages:
- Stage of hydroarthrosis
- Stage of disintegration
- Stage of hypertrophy
- Stage of atrophy

Pathogenesis

In these joints, the subchondral bone disintegrates with an alarming speed as these *lacks the normal reflex safeguard* against the abnormal stress or injury.

Clinical Features

General examination

Reveals features of underlying neurological disorders.

Local Examination

- Patient complains of swelling (boggy), weakness, instability, progressive deformity of joint and laxity.
- Repeated joint effusion

- Pain is characteristically absent
- Painless abnormal mobility
- Palpation of the soft, thickened capsule reveals numerous intra-articular bodies (loose bodies) just like *"bag of bones"*.
- In worst cases, the joint is flail.

Investigations

- *X-rays*: Shows gross joint swelling, erosion of articular surface with osteophytes, multiple loose bodies and displacement of the joint.
- *Synovial fluid analysis*: Abundant, yellow, and viscous and clots rapidly. The cell count is 500–2000/mm^3 with predominance of lymphocytes.

Treatment

Mainly conservative and consist of:
- Splintage of unstable joint (braces)
- Joint should be shielded from trauma of ordinary motion and weight bearing.
- Analgesics and other medications.

Treat the primary cause.

Surgical Method

Arthrodesis may be attempted in conditions where the joints are so unstable that the splintage is useless.

> ## Q7. Discuss the aetiology, pathology, clinical features, diagnosis and management of haemophilic arthritis or bleeders joint.

It is a hereditary bleeding diathesis characterized by recurrent bleeding into large joints, usually spontaneous or following trivial trauma. It is an X-linked recessive trait, and thus manifests in males and in homozygous females.

Aetiology

- It is X-linked recessive genetic disorder of coagulation due to mutations in the F8 gene (hemophilia A or classic hemophilia) or F9 gene (hemophilia B).
- It results from a reduction in the amount or activity of factor VIII, which serves as a cofactor for factor IX in the activation of factor X in the coagulation cascade
- Haemophillia A is by far the most common type, constituting 85% of cases.

Classification

Based on the residual activity of factor VIII in blood, haemophillia A can be classified as:

Severity	Activity of factor VIII
• Severe	Less than 1% of normal activity
• Moderate	1–5% of normal activity
• Mild	More than 5% of normal activity (6–30%)

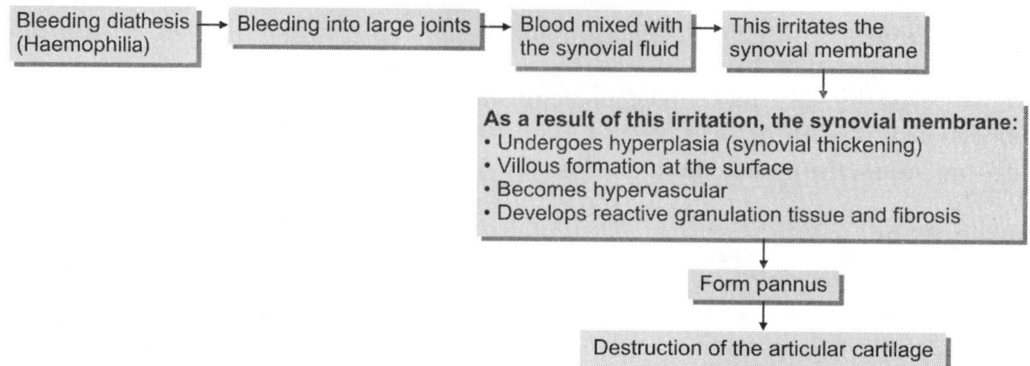

Areas of Predilection

In order of frequency, the joint most commonly involved/affected are the *knees, ankles, elbows, shoulders, and hips*. Small joints of the hands and feet are occasionally.

Clinical Features

- History is typical (*bleeding occurring spontaneously or following trivial trauma; repeated episodes of bleeding from gums and cuts*)
- Patient is exclusively man (*only homozygous female are affected*).

Acute Phase

- Rapid effusion (*within minutes to several hours*)
- Marked swelling (*within minutes to several hours*)
- Severe pain
- Joint is warm and tender
- Joint acquire a position of maximal relaxation of capsule (*e.g. Partial flexion and slight abduction and external rotation at the hip; Partial flexion at the knee and elbow.*)
- This phase subsides over a period of few days to several weeks.

Chronic Phase

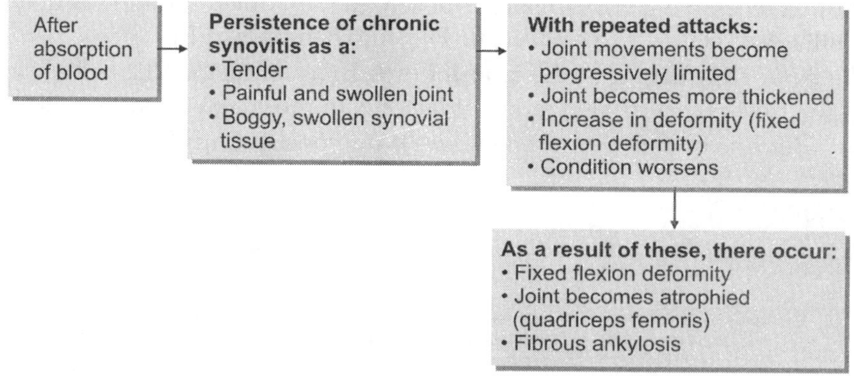

Consequence of spontaneous bleeding

- Bleeding into joint (haemoarthrosis) causing damage to articular cartilage, deformity and later ankylosis of the joint
- Secondary osteoarthritis

Haemophilic pseudotumour or haemophilic cysts:
- Intramuscular bleeding that covers the bone produces the characteristic haemophilic pseudotumour or haemophilic cysts.

Most often occurs in:
- Iliopsoas
- Quadriceps femoris
- Triceps surae
- Gluteus maximus
- Forearm muscles

Most common location:
- Anterior thigh
- Calf
- Inner aspect of the ilium
- Volar aspect of the forearm

Consequences:
- Involvement of associated nerve and causes paralysis (bleeding into the iliacus sheath may cause femoral nerve paralysis or into forearm compartment leading to median and ulnar nerves damage)
- Myostatic contracture (bleeding into firm fascial compartment like volar compartment of forearm and posterior compartment of leg→ ischaemic necrosis → severe pain → as it recedes, it leaves weak, fibrotic and contracted muscle)

Others:
- Easy bruising
- Intra-abdominal, retroperitoneal and mesenteric bleeding
- Intracranial haemorrhage (intracerebral haemorrhage and subdural haematoma)
- Bleeding from socket following dental extraction.
- Haematuria
- Ureteric colic

Investigations

Coagulation Profile

- Prolongation of the *aPTT (activated partial thromboplastin time)* assay.
- *Bleeding time, prothrombin time and platelets count* are normal.
- Specific factor VIII assay can confirm the diagnosis.

X-rays: features/changes may be categorized roentgenographically as:

Early stage:
- Rounded bulged out synovium
- No para-articular bony abnormality

Chronic intermediate stage:
- Osteoporosis (epiphysis esp.)
- Subchondral cavities (cysts)
- Squaring of the patella
- Widening of intercondylar notch of femur
- Widening of the trochlear notch of ulna
  (Up to this stage, the arthropathy is reversible)

Late stage:
- Narrowing of the joint space
- Increases irregularities of subchondral cortex
- Subchondral cyst becomes conspicuous.
- Sclerosis
- Osteophytes formation
- Fibrous ankylosis

Treatment

Medical Management

Replacement Therapy
- *Aim*: to correct deficiency of factor VIII or IX
- *Agent used*: Lyophilized cryoprecipitate containing either factor VIII or factor IX.

Indications
- Control of bleeding during trauma and surgery
- Prolonged or severe tissue and wound bleeding
- Early treatment of episodes of spontaneous bleeding.

Dose

- As per general rule, one unit of factor VIII/kg will raise the plasma level by 2%. Ones aim is to raise the factor levels to at least 50%.
- Dose of factor VIII = Desired factor level (%) × Weight in kg × 0.5.

Non-transfusion Therapy in Hemophilia

- Desmopressin (DDAVP (1-deamino-8-D-arginine vasopressin)): It is given at doses of 0.3 μg/kg body weight infused over a 20-min period.
- *Antifibrinolytic drugs*: ε-aminocaproic acid (EACA) or tranexamic acid to control local hemostasis. Tranexamic acid is given at doses of 25 mg/kg three to four times a day.

Orthopaedics Treatment

Non-surgical: For Acute Haemoarthrosis

- Single infusion of deficient/appropriate factor to achieve a plasma level of 40–50%
- Ice bags
- Limb elevation
- Immobilization

Aspiration of the joint *should be avoided* for fear of:
- Reducing the intra-articular counter pressure
- Introducing infection to the joint

Aspiration if attempted then plasma level of factor should be at least 30% and should be done under aseptic condition.

Precaution while Splinting the Limb

- Constant monitoring of the skin
- Monitoring of neurovascular status
- Muscle atrophy should be prevented (first isometric exercises and then graduated range of motion exercise)
- Joint motion should be encouraged in order to prevent contractures
- Repeated hemarthrosis controlled

Contractures
- Gentle traction and by turnbuckle cast with semicircular fixed hinge (for knee flexion contracture)
- Physiotherapy

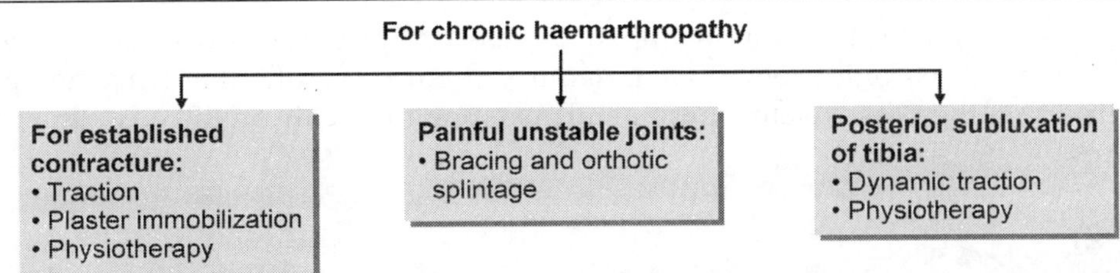

Surgical

Indications	*Surgical procedure*
• Chronic synovitis • Repeated uncontrollable hemarthrosis	• Synovectomy
Fractures • Stable fractures	• Immediate replacement of deficient factor • Maintenance of haemostasis • Absolute immobilization
• Unstable fractures	• Especially in adult; treated by internal fixation only once the adequate level of deficient factor has been achieved.
• Severe flexion contracture of the knee joint (not responding to the conservative modality)	• Supracondylar osteotomy
• Severely painful destroyed joints • Sever pain (not due to bleeding but is the result of mechanical changes in the joint) and advanced arthropathy	• Arthrodesis • Total joint replacement
• Contracture of the triceps surae • Equines deformity	• Achilles tendon lengthening
• Neuropraxia (nerve involved in decreasing order of frequency are femoral, peroneal, sciatic, median and ulnar nerve)	Usually non surgical comprises of: • Replacement therapy • Splintage • Physical therapy • Electrical stimulation If hyperplasic synovium causes compression then: • Decompression by synovectomy

Q8. What are seronegative spondyloarthropathies and writes in brief about the clinical features, diagnosis and management of ankylosing spondylitis?

The *Spondyloarthritides* are a group of inflammatory arthritides that share certain clinical features and genetic associations.

Ankylosing spondylitis (or Marie-Strumpell disease or Bechterew's disease): *Ankylosing spondylitis* (AS) is a chronic progressive inflammatory disorder of unknown aetiology that primarily affects the axial skeleton; peripheral joints and frequently involved extra-articular structures.

Aetiology

- Unknown aetiology *(exact cause of ankylosing spondylitis (AS) is unknown)*
- Striking correlation with the histocompatibility antigen *HLA-B27 (90% in patients with AS)*
- The disease usually begins in the second or third decade
- Male to female prevalence is between 2:1 and 3:1.

Pathogenesis

- Incompletely understood, but it is almost certainly *immune-mediated.*
- Integrative concept is that the AS disease process begins at sites *where ligaments, articular cartilage, and other structures attach to bone.*
- *Tumor necrosis factor α (TNF-α)* plays a central role in the immunopathogenesis of AS.

Pathology

The pathology of AS include the following process:
- Synovitis
- Enthesopathy
- Capsular inflammation cartilage destruction and bony erosion
- Ossification
- Ankylosis

Clinical Features

- Symptoms usually first noticed in *late adolescence or early adulthood.*
- Initial symptom is usually dull pain, insidious in onset, over gluteal or lower lumbar region.
- Low-back morning stiffness last for few hours' duration *that improves with activity.*
- *Nocturnal exacerbation* of pain (disturbs the sleep and force the patient to rise and move around).
- Loss of spinal mobility, with limitation of anterior and lateral flexion and extension of the lumbar spine.
- Progressive *limitation of chest expansion (due to involvement of costovertebral joint).*
- Neck pain and stiffness from involvement of the cervical spine are usually late manifestations.
- *Enthesitis* and usually manifests as heel pain.
- With progression of disease, the patient patient's posture undergoes characteristic changes, *with loss of lumbar lordosis, buttock atrophy, and exaggerated thoracic kyphosis (Stooped-over position; poker's back).*
- Hips, knee and shoulder joint become swollen and painful.
- Muscle acting over these joint undergo spasm and produces *flexion and internal rotation at the shoulders; flexion at the knees and flexion-adduction at the hip*

Extra-articular Features

- Acute anterior uveitis (most common; 40%)
- Inflammation in the colon or ileum
- Psoriasis
- Aortitis
- Third-degree heart block may occur alone or together with aortic insufficiency.
- Conduction defects
- Pulmonary effusion and pleural thickening
- Apical fibrobullous lesion (aspergillosis)
- Myelopathy secondary to atlanto-axial subluxation
- Retroperitoneal fibrosis
- Prostatitis
- Amyloidosis.

Different Tests to Assess the Restriction of Mobility

Cervical spine involvement spine:
- *Tragus to wall test*: For the flexion deformity, measurement can be made from the wall behind and the tragus of the ear.
- *Fleche test*: This test detects an early involvement of the cervical spine.

   Ask the patient to stand on the heel and back touched on the wall and then ask the patient to touch his back of the head to the wall and at the same time the chin is not moved upward. If the patient is unable to do this, shows the involvement of the cervical spine.

Thoracic Spine Involvement

Chest expansion: It is measured as the difference between maximal inspiration and maximal forced expiration in the fourth intercostals space in males or just below the breasts in females.

Interpretation

- Normal chest expansion is $\geq$5 cm.
- If it is less than 5 cm; it is suggestive of AS (due to involvement of costovertebral joint).

Lumbosacral Spine Involvement

Schober test: It is a useful measure of lumbar spine flexion.

Test

- The patient stands erect, with heels together.
- The examiner makes a mark approximately at the level of L5 (fifth lumbar vertebrae).
- Then the examiner marks over the spine 5 cm below and 10 cm above the lumbosacral junction (identified by a horizontal line between the poster superior iliac spines).
- The patient then bends forward maximally, and the distance between the two marks is measured.

Interpretation

- If the distance between the two *marks increases by $\geq$5 cm; indicates normal spinal mobility.*
- If the distance between the *two marks increases by <4 cm; indicates decreased spinal mobility.*

Sacroiliac Joint Involvement

- *Gaenslen's sign*: Instruct the patient to lie supine on the edge of the examining table with knee and hip flexed over the edge to fix the pelvis. Ask the patient to drop the unsupported leg off the table; this procedure will elicit pain in the contralateral SI joint by stretching it.
- *SLR test (straight leg raising test)*: The patient is in supine lying position and then asked to lift the leg up with his knee extended. By this, pain is felt on the affected side at the SI joint.
- *Pump handle test*: The patient is in supine lying and then, do the flexion of the hip and knee and then give some extrapressure as to touch the knee to the opposite side of the shoulder (across the chest). By this procedure, the pain is felt on affected side.

Diagnosis

The widely used *modified New York criteria* (1984) these consist of the following:
1. A history of inflammatory back pain
2. Limitation of motion of the lumbar spine in both the sagittal and frontal planes
3. Limited chest expansion
4. Definite radiographic sacroiliitis

Criterion 4 plus any one of the other three criteria is sufficient for a diagnosis of definite AS.

Investigations

- *Erythrocyte sedimentation rate* is raised
- *HLA-B27 test:* This is positive in about 90–95% of patients.
- *Haemoglobin: Normochromic or normocytic anaemia* may occur but in contrast to RA, patients with active disease often have a normal hemoglobin and blood film.
- *Synovial fluid analysis:* Contains a moderate number of mononuclear leucocytes in contrast to the increased polymorphonuclear leucocyte count of RA fluid.
- *Rheumatoid factor:* Rheumatoid factors are absent.
- *Pulmonary function tests*: Flow measurements are usually normal. In patients with thoracic involvement usually show:
  - Diminished vital and total lung capacity
  - Increased residual volume and functional residual volume
- *Nuclear scans:* Tc^{99} stannous pyrophosphate bone scans, can often *detect areas of active inflammation in AS, before standard changes are present.*
- *Roentgenographic findings:* The features of different sites are:

Sacroiliac joint:	Spine: Spinal changes include:	In advance disease:
• Sclerosis of the subchondral bone (ilium and sacrum) on either side of the joint (*earliest sign*). • Haziness of the joint margins • Pseudo-widening of the joint space, which may progress to fusion. • When ankylosis is complete, the periarticular sclerosis fades. Sometimes leaving the evidence of the previous joint line, known as *Ghost joint*.	• Squaring of the vertebral bodies (*earliest sign*) • Syndesmophyte formation • Arthritic changes and later apophysial joint fusion occurs • Atlantoaxial subluxation. • Calcification of the paraspinal ligaments • The Romanus sign (*"Shiny corner sign"*) is the erosion surrounded by sclerosis at the vertebral body margin. • Normal lumbar lordosis lost	• Characteristic *bamboo spine* results from syndesmophyte or paraspinal ligament calcification around the normal disc space.

Management

Aim:
- To control pain
- Maintain maximum skeletal mobility
- Prevent deformity

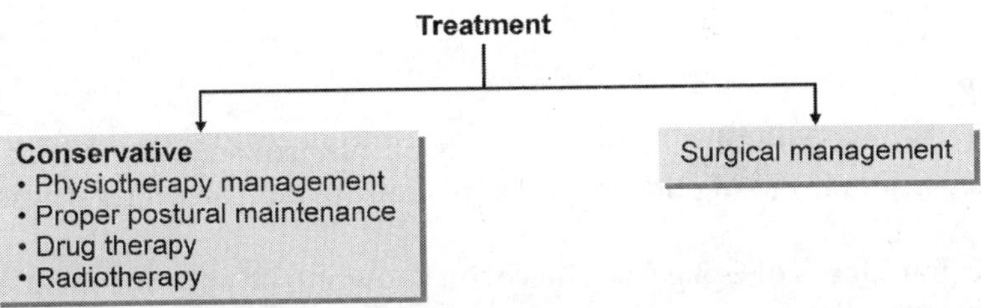

Conservative Management

Physiotherapy Management

Aims:
- Relieve pain.
- Maintain the mobility of joints affected like spine, hip, thorax, shoulder, etc.
- Prevent and correct deformity
- Increase chest expansion and vital capacity
- Attention to posture
- To maintain and improve physical endurance.

Pain relief: Pain and muscle spasm are treated by the following modalities and the relaxation is advised.

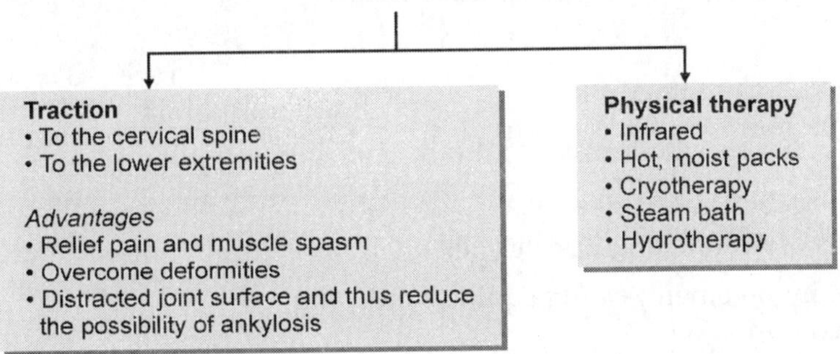

Increase chest expansion and vital capacity
- Deep breathing exercises
- Apical breathing exercises.
- Diaphragmatic breathing exercises.
- Lateral costal breathing exercises.
- Ballooning exercise

Proper postural maintenance
- Patient should maintain the erect posture during sitting, standing and walking. This helps to prevent and correct deformity.
- Recumbency in prone position or supine on a firm mattress with a thin or no pillow by this, the spine remains in extended position and not in flexion.

- Particularly for those who spend most of their working hours sitting at desk the design of chairs is important. An upright chair with some cushioning to support the lower lumber spine is better than low armchair and is better to be avoided,
- Avoidance of prolonged immobilization or bed rest, because of this, the spinal extensors become weak and by this the extended position of the spine is not retained
- Adjust the height of the working table and ensure that the patient does not stoop on that.

Drug Therapy

- *Non-steroidal anti-inflammatory drugs (NSAIDs)*: Naproxen (Naprosyn) 500 mg bid, Indomethacin (Indocin) 25 mg tid. These agents reduce pain and tenderness and increase mobility.
- *Sulfasalazine*: It in doses of 2–3 g/day has been shown to be of modest benefit, primarily for peripheral arthritis.
- *Methotrexate*, although widely used is of questionable benefit.
- *Local glucocorticoid* with mydriatic agents: Managed attacks of uveitis.
- *Recent therapy (anti- TNF-α therapy)*: Infliximab (chimeric human/ mouse anti-TNF-α monoclonal antibody: A dose of 3–5 mg/kg body weight, and then repeated 2 weeks later, again 6 weeks later, and then at 8-week intervals), etanercept (soluble p75 TNF-α receptor IgG fusion protein: Subcutaneous injection in a dose of 25 mg twice weekly or 50 mg once weekly), or adalimumab (human anti-TNF-α monoclonal antibody: Given by subcutaneous injection in a dose of 40 mg biweekly.)

Radiotherapy

It is not curative but relieves pain quickly, presumably by lessening muscle spasm. Relief lasts for 6 month and treatment is given every 2–3 days.

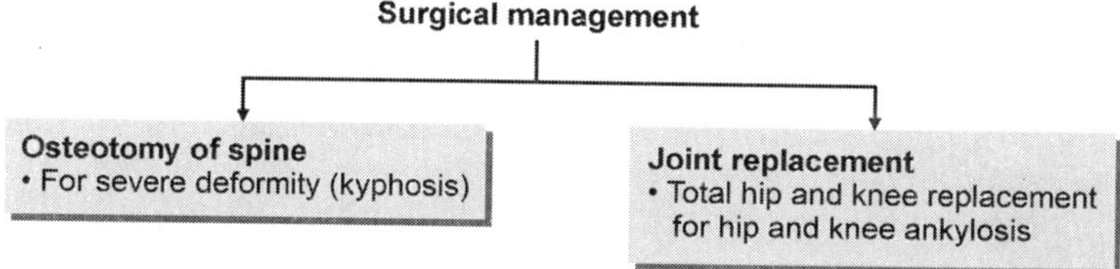

Complications of Ankylosing Spondylitis

- Neurological involvement/cauda equina syndrome
- Spinal cord compression
- Spinal fracture
- Amyloidosis
- *Romanus lesions* (on lateral radiograph; a rim of sclerosis develops on the vertebral side of the enthesis, also referred to as "*Shiny corner sign*")
- Painful heel or Achilles tendinitis
- Reduced chest expansion and vital capacity
- Chest infection
- Osteoporosis

Q9. Write a short note on pigmented villonodular synovitis.

Pigmented villonodular synovitis (*synovial xanthoma; villous synovitis; diffuse type giant cell tumor*): It is an idiopathic, uncommon, intra-articular benign lesion *associates to a villous overgrowth and proliferation of synovial membrane (tendon sheaths, joints, and bursae) most commonly affects the knee or hip joint in young adults. Its diagnosis usually delayed because complaints and symptoms are nonspecific.*

Aetiology

Unknown: Theories regarding the aetiology of PVNS include the following:

- Localized lipid metabolic derangement
- A benign neoplastic process
- Repeated non-traumatic inflammation
- A response to blood or blood products within the joint
- Rearrangements of 1p11-13 and 16q24, as well as translocation of t (1; 2) (p22; q35-37) have been reported.

Pathology (Gross/Microscopic)

- Grossly, multifocal or diffuse synovial lesion, chocolate colored mass
- Synovial hyperplasia, hypervascularity (dilated blood capillaries) and accumulation of histiocytes
- Multinucleated giant cells, lipid-laden macrophages (foam cells) or xanthoma cells, fibroblasts, intra- and extracellular haemosiderin are characteristic features.
- Ubiquitous presence of haemosiderin lends the tissue a characteristic pigmented appearance
- Mitotic figures are common.

Classification

- *Diffuse*: Diffuse or villous PVNS affects the entire synovium and typically occurs in large joints such as the knee or hip; occurs in second and third decades.
- *Localized*: Localized, or nodular, PVNS is less common than the diffuse form and typically occurs in smaller joints such as the hands and feet; occurs in third to fifth decades.

Clinical Features

- Usually seen in young adult from 20 to 40 years
- More in men than women
- Typically intra-articular and are most commonly seen in the knee. Other sites in decreasing order of frequency include the lower extremity, foot and ankle, hand and wrist, hip, shoulder and elbow.
- Gradual onset of pain, which is mild to moderate in intensity, intermittent and associated with limp
- Swelling
- Joint effusion
- Mechanical interference causes stiffness, limitation of movements usually in extension, locking and snapping sensation.

Physical Examination Reveals

- One or more palpable nodules or diffuses joint swelling.
- Swelling may feel warm.

Investigations

Laboratory findings	**X-rays**	**Aspiration**	**CT scan**
• Not diagnostic • Blood cholesterol level is raised (upper normal limit)	• Signs similar to joint effusion or soft-tissue swelling • Foci of dystrophic calcification may be seen • Periarticular lucencies **Arthroscopy** • Visualize the gross pathologic picture of PVNS	• Aspirated synovial fluid is typically xanthochromic or serosanguinous **Biopsy**: To confirm the diagnosis	• High attenuation because of the haemosiderin content **MRI** • MRI findings are diagnostic in more than 95% of patients • The signal intensity is decreased (due to the presence of haemosiderin within tissue) in both T1 and T2 weighted images • Areas of high signal on T1 sequences represent either lipid laden macrophages or haemorrhage

- Patella tap present
- Moderate generalized tenderness

Treatment

- Arthroscopic or open synovectomy.
- Low-dose radiation therapy (RT) in the treatment of diffuse PVNS.
- Combined partial arthroscopic synovectomy and radiation therapy.
- Joint replacement indicated for PVNS with joint destructive changes.
- Recurrences are common.

Q10. What are the types of psoriatic arthritis. Discuss the features and management of psoriatic arthropathy in brief.

Psoriatic arthritis is an inflammatory erosive arthritis usually seronegative, often involved the distal interphalangeal (DIP) joints of the fingers and the spine and sacroiliac joints that characteristically occurs in individuals with psoriasis. It develops in 5–30% of cases of psoriasis of skin.

Aetiology

- Family history
- HLA associations have been found. The HLA-Cw6 gene is directly associated with psoriasis, HLA-B27 is associated with psoriatic spondylitis.
- Typically begins in the fourth or fifth decade, at an average age of 37 years.

Pathology

- Chronic synovitis with edema and round cells infiltrations
- Inflammation is followed by extensive fibrous replacement (synovial fibrosis).
- Erosion of the cortex and articular cartilage
- Inflammatory tissues cause erosion from without, causing the characteristic scalloped appearance.
- Fibrous ankylosis with dislocation and subluxation is more common.

Pathogenesis

- It is almost certainly immune-mediated.
- Synovium shows infiltration with T cells, B cells, macrophages, and NK receptor–expressing cells.
- Cytokine production in the synovium (predominantly a T_H1 pattern)
- Interleukin (IL) 2, TNF-α, interferon γ, and IL-1β, -6, -8, -10, -12, -13, and -15 are found in synovium or synovial fluid.
- Marked increase in osteoclastic precursors in peripheral blood and up-regulation of RANKL (receptor activator of NF-$\kappa\beta$ ligand) in the synovial lining layer.

Classification

Wright and Moll described five patterns:
- Arthritis of the DIP joints (5%)
- Asymmetric oligoarthritis (70%)
- Symmetric polyarthritis similar to RA (15%)
- Axial involvement (spine and sacroiliac joints) (5%)
- Arthritis mutilans (a highly destructive form of disease) (5%)

Clinical Features

- Psoriasis usually precedes arthritic manifestations.
- Progressive asymmetrical oligoarthritis, affecting proximal and distal interphalangeal joint with generalized swelling of the finger producing characteristic "sausage-like digits".
- Sacroiliitis (asymmetric) or spondylitis develops in approximately half the cases of psoriatic arthritis, causing pain, stiffness of the lower back and tenderness over sacroiliac joint.
- Shortening of digits because of underlying osteolysis (telescoping)
- Dactylitis occurs in >30%.
- Enthesitis and tenosynovitis are also common.
- Nail changes (six patterns: horizontal ridging, onycholysis, yellowish discoloration of the nail margins, dystrophic hyperkeratosis, and combinations of these findings) in the fingers or toes occur in 90% of patients.
- Eye involvement, either conjunctivitis or uveitis (often bilateral, chronic, and/or posterior).
- Aortic valve insufficiency (<4% of patients).

Investigations

Laboratory Findings

- ESR and CRP are often elevated.
- Uric acid may be elevated (reflecting increased purine metabolism in skin).
- HLA-B27 is found in 50–70% of patients with axial disease, but $\leq$15–20% in patients with only peripheral joint involvement.
- Anaemia is common.
- Low titers of antinuclear antibodies.
- Test for rheumatoid factor is usually negative.

Radiographic Findings

- Asymmetry and destruction of small isolated joints.
- DIP involvement, including the classic *"pencil-in-cup"* deformity
- Dissolution of terminal phalangeal tufts *(acro-osteolysis)*
- Marginal erosions with adjacent bony proliferation *("whiskering")*
- Small-joint ankylosis
- Osteolysis of phalangeal and metacarpal bone, with *telescoping* of digits
- Periostitis and proliferative new bone at sites of *enthesitis.*
- Asymmetric sacroiliitis.

Diagnostic Features

- History of trauma to an affected joint preceding the onset of arthritis
- Asymmetrical joint involvement
- Involvement of DIP joint
- Presence of sacroiliitis or spondylitis
- Absence of rheumatoid nodules
- Characteristic skin lesions.

Treatment

- Majority of the patient respond to *NSAIDS* and small dose of corticosteroid (2.5 mg or 5 mg prednisolone) at night.
- *Methotrexate* in doses of 15–25 mg/week and sulfasalazine (usually given in doses of 2–3 g/day) found to have clinical efficacy.
- Other agents found to be beneficial includes *cyclosporine, retinoic acid derivatives, and psoralen plus ultraviolet light (PUVA).*

Recent therapy: All of these treatments require careful monitoring.

- Use of the anti-TNF-α agents like *etanercept, infliximab,* and *adalimumab.*
- Anti-T cell biologic agent *alefacept*, in combination with methotrexate.
- Pyrimidine synthetase inhibitor *leflunomide.*

Q11. Discuss the aetiology, clinical manifestation, diagnosis and management of gout.

Gout (also known as podagra when it involves the big toe) is a hereditary disorder of purine metabolism (hyperuricaemia) most often affecting middle-aged to elderly men and postmenopausal women.

It is typically, characterized by *recurrent attack of acute arthritis*, deposition of *monosodium urate monohydrate* (MSU) crystals in articular, peri-articular and connective tissue tophi, and in late stages, by *renal dysfunction, uric acid urolithiasis, cardiovascular lesions* and crippling deforming arthritis.

Aetiology

Exact cause is unknown.

Predisposing causes includes:

- Hereditary
- Age: 2nd to 4th decades.
- Sex: Predominantly male; females, usually at menopause.

- *Cortisol steroid* counteracts the gouty attack (depletion will precipitate the attack).
- *Vascular changes* (increased blood flow and amplitude during attack), *disturbed electrolyte equilibrium* (marked dieresis before an acute attack) and *decreased urinary 17-ketosteroids* (reduction <3 mg/24 hours is a constant finding).

Pathophysiology

There is an *increase in uric acid level leading to deposits of MSU crystals* in the synovial fluid, capsule, ligaments, kidney, pinna, etc. either because of:

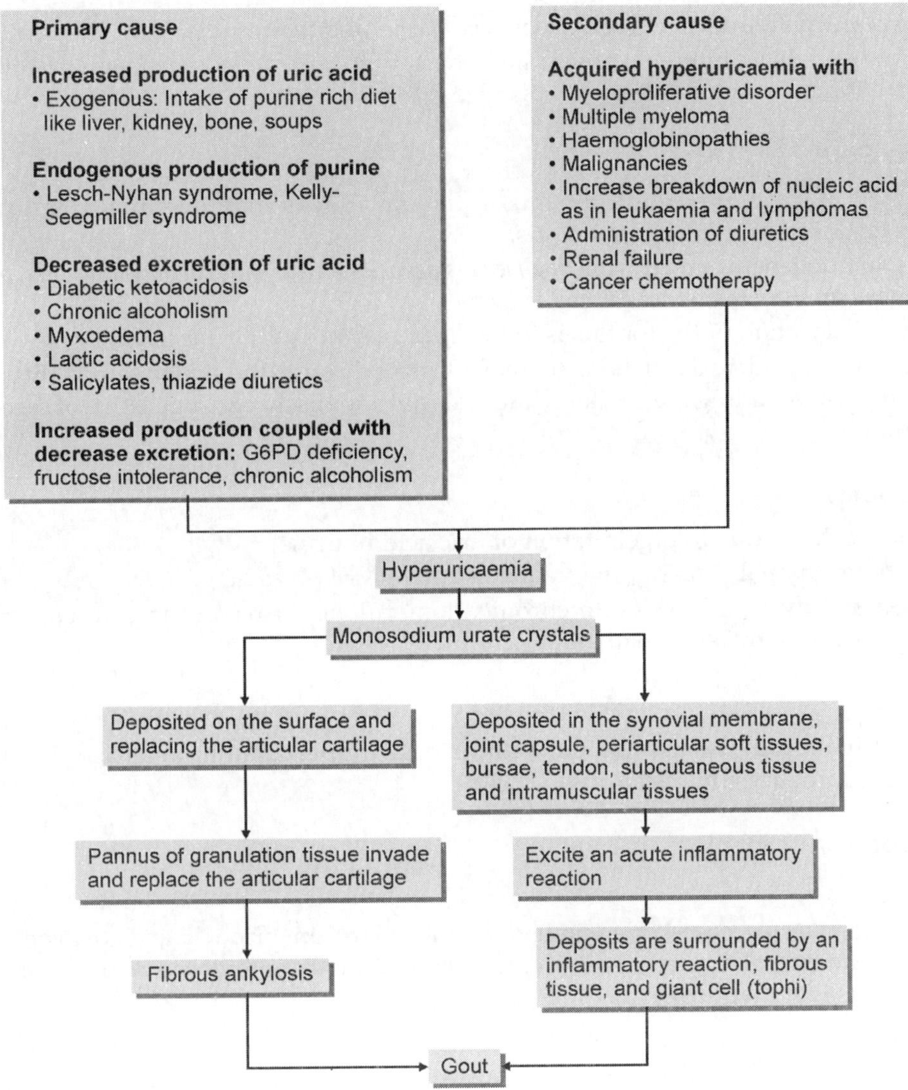

Clinical Features

Acute Gout

- Acute onset usually monoarticular.
- Sudden in onset without any warning and often preceded by *provocative factors (trauma, surgery, dietary excess, hypouricemic therapy, excessive ethanol ingestion, and serious medical illnesses such as myocardial infarction and stroke)*

- The patient has a *nice party with lots of drink and non-veg diet*, gets up at midnight or morning with *acute excruciating pain, redness, swelling involving the metatarsophalangeal joint of great toe.*
- Next in frequency most affected are the *intertarsal joints, Tendo-Achilles, ankle, the fingers and the wrist.*
- The affected joint *is warm, red, swollen and tender.* The swelling is extreme and simulate the cellulitis.
- The inflammation subsides spontaneously within 3–10 days and the overlying skin desquamates subsequently.
- There is always associated *fever, malaise, headache,* and *tachycardia.*
- Most patients have intervals of varying length with *no residual symptoms (asymptomatic or intercritical phase)* until the next episode.

Chronic Gout

- Repeated many acute mono- or oligoarticular attacks may eventually merge into polyarticular nonsymmetric synovitis.
- Secondary degenerative arthritis, *tophaceous deposits* in the *joint cartilage, capsule, over the olecranaon, in the pinna of the ear and tendons.*
- The classic location of the tophus is in the *helix and anti-helix of the ear.*
- These tophi may increase in diameter may ulcerate through the skin to form a chronically draining sinus exuding the chalky white material and discharge suggestive of secondary infection.

Nephropathy

- Uric acid calculi (due to precipitation of uric acid in urine)
- Renal parenchymal disease (due to deposition of MSU crystals)
- Severe renal dysfunction due to chronic glomerulonephritis and interstitial nephritis may leads to uremia and death.

Other

Gouty arthritis may be associated with arterial hypertension, arteriosclerosis and consequent coronary complications.

Investigations

Blood

- Hyperuricemia: Increased uric acid level >7 mg/dl (serum uric acid levels can be normal or low at the time of the acute episode, as inflammatory cytokines can be uricosuric. This limits its use for diagnosis).
- ESR is raised
- WBCs count is increased.
- Increased in urea and serum creatinine in patients with decreased renal function.

Synovial fluid analysis:

- Synovial fluid cell
- Thick pasty or chalky joint fluid
- Counts are elevated from 2000 to 60,000/µl.

- Polarizing light microscopy shows strongly *birefringent needle-shaped monosodium urate crystals with negative elongation both intracellularly and extracellularly (these crystals are digest by uricase).*

Chemical Test or Murexide Test

Suspected substance + nitric acid → evaporated to dryness → then moistened with ammonium hydroxide → purple color (due to murexide) will indicate the presence of uric acid.

X-rays

- Early, joint appear normal shows only soft tissue swellings.
- Later, urate deposition produces characteristic *"punched-out"* cyst.
- Para-articular cystic lesion
- Joint space decreased
- Degenerative arthritis.

Treatment

Prevention

- Increased urine output by increased water intake
- Alkalinize the urine with soda-bicarbonate
- Decrease purine rich diet
- Avoid alcohol, thiazide diuretics, fasting and dehydration

Acute Gouty Arthritis

- Ice pack applications
- rest of the involved joints.

Drugs

- *Colchicine*: 0.6 mg tablets every 6–8 hours till the pain decrease or first sign of loose stool (diarrhea)
- *NSAIDs*: Most effective drugs indomethacin, 25–50 mg tid; ibuprofen, 800 mg tid; or diclofenac, 50 mg tid
- *Oral glucocorticoids* such as prednisone, 30–50 mg/day as the initial dose and gradually tapered.
- For single or few involved joints intra-articular triamcinolone acetonide, 20–40 mg, or methylprednisolone, 25–50 mg
- In acute polyarticular refractory gout or in those where colchicines is contraindicated: **Adrenocorticotropic hormone (ACTH)** as an intramuscular injection of 40–80 IU in a single dose or every 12 hours for 1– 2 days.

Chronic Gouty Arthritis

Hypouricaemic Therapy

Aim

- Attempts to normalize serum uric acid to <300–350 μmol/L (5.0–6.0 mg/dl)
- To prevent recurrent gouty attacks.
- Eliminate tophaceous deposits.

Indications

- Number of acute attacks (urate lowering may be cost effective after two attacks).
- Serum uric acid levels [progression is more rapid in patients with serum uric acid >535 µmol/L (>9.0 mg/dl)].
- Patient's willingness to commit to lifelong therapy.
- Presence of uric acid stones
- Any patient who already has tophi or chronic gouty arthritis.

Uricosuric Drugs

- *Probenecid*: 250 mg twice daily and increased gradually as needed up to 3 g in order to maintain a serum uric acid level <300 µmol/L (5 mg/dl).
- *Sulfinpyrazone* 100–200 mg/day.

Precautions while using uricosuric drugs
- Urine volume must be maintained by ingestion of 1500 ml of water every day and pH >4.
- Avoid using salicylates (antagonistic).

Drugs used to lower serum urate: *allopurinol and benzbromarone*

Indications

- Overproducers
- Urate stone formers
- Patients with renal disease [serum creatinine levels of >177 µmol/L (2.0 mg/dl)]

Drugs

- *Xanthine oxidase inhibitor allopurinol (most common)*: Single morning dose, 100–300 mg initially and increasing up to 800 mg if needed.
- *Most serious side effects* include skin rash with progression to life-threatening toxic epidermal necrolysis (TEN), systemic vasculitis, bone marrow suppression, granulomatous hepatitis, and renal failure.

Prophylaxis

Colchicine prophylaxis in doses of 0.6 mg one to two times daily is usually continued, along with the hypouricemic therapy, until the patient is normouricaemic and without gouty attacks for 6 months or as long as tophi are present.

Recent Therapy

New urate-lowering drugs undergoing investigation include a *PEGylated uricase* and a new specific *xanthine oxidase inhibitor, febuxostat.*

Febuxostat

- It is a *non-purine selective inhibitor of xanthine oxidase.*
- Use in the treatment of *hyperuricemia* and *gout* and people who are *intolerant of allopurinol.*
- It is recommended at *40 mg or 80 mg* once daily.
- Adverse effects includes: *nausea, headache, diarrhea, arthralgia, increased hepatic serum enzyme levels* and *rash*

Q12. Write a short note on pseudogout or calcium pyrophosphate dihydrate (CPPD) deposition disease.

Pseudogout is a rheumatologic disorder resulting due to the accumulation of crystals of calcium pyrophosphate dihydrate in the connective tissues. Calcium pyrophosphate crystals laid down in the cartilage and act as an irritant to the joint.

Acute CPPD arthritis was originally termed pseudogout by McCarty because of its striking similarity to gout.

Aetiology

- In most cases, cause of CPPD deposition is uncertain
- Diseased cartilage or biochemical changes in aging favor crystal nucleation
- Mutations in the ANKH gene described in both familial and sporadic cases
- Most of the patients are female over the age 60 years.

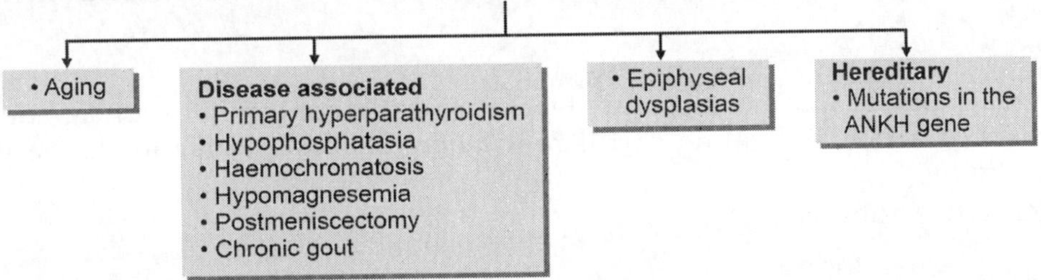

Pathophysiology

There is an increased production of inorganic pyrophosphate due to enhanced activity of ATP pyrophosphohydrolase and 5'-nucleotidase and decreased levels of pyrophosphatases in cartilage extracts.

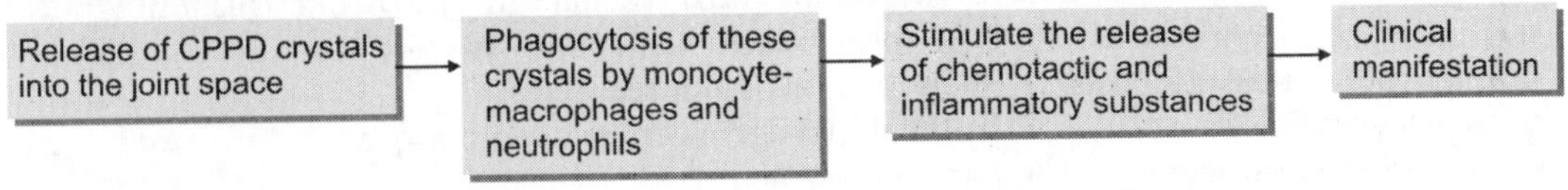

Area of Predilection

- *Knee joint* most commonly
- Other sites include the *symphysis pubis, wrist, shoulder, ankle, elbow, and hands.*
- Rarely, the *temporomandibular joint* and *ligamentum flavum* of the spinal canal are involved.

Clinical Features

- Acute attacks of CPPD arthritis precipitated by trauma, surgery, sprain or sudden fall of serum calcium concentration (severe medical illness or after surgery (especially parathyroidectomy)
- Severe joint pain, redness, swelling and tenderness; recurring at varying interval and lasting for several weeks.

Other clinical manifestations of CPPD deposition include:

- Induction or enhancement of *osteoarthritis*
- Induction of *severe destructive disease* that may mimic neuropathic arthritis radiographically

- Production of *symmetric proliferative synovitis*, simulating to rheumatoid arthritis clinically and frequently seen in familial forms with early onset
- *Ligament and intervertebral disk calcification* with restriction of spine mobility, mimicking ankylosing spondylitis (especially in familial form)
- *Spinal stenosis* in the elderly (rarely).

Investigation

Definitive diagnosis requires demonstration of crystals in synovial fluid or articular tissue.

Synovial fluid analysis

- Inflammatory characteristics, WBCs ranging from 1,000 to 100,000 cells/μl with predominance of neutrophils.
- Examination under polarized light microscopy reveals *rhomboid, square,* or *rod-like crystals with weak positive birefringence inside tissue fragments and fibrin clots* and in *neutrophils*

X-rays

- Punctuate and/or linear radiodense deposits (calcification) in fibrocartilaginous joint menisci or articular hyaline cartilage (*chondrocalcinosis*) (diagnostic feature on radiography)
- Degenerative arthritis.

Treatment

No definitive treatment:

Condition	Treatment
• Untreated acute attacks	• Joint aspiration
	• NSAIDs or by intra-articular glucocorticoid injection
• Frequent recurrent attacks	• Daily prophylactic treatment with low doses of colchicine
• Severe polyarticular attacks	• Short courses of glucocorticoids.
• Persistent synovitis	• Antimalarial agents or even methotrexate
• Progressive destructive	• Joint replacement
• large-joint arthropathy	

Q13. Briefly, comment on the difference between the gout and pseudogout.

Characteristics	Gout	Pseudogout
• *Sex*	Usually men	Usually female
• *Pain*	Intense	Moderate
• *Joint inflammation*	Marked	Only swollen
• *Joint involvement*	Smaller joints	Large joints
• *Pathology*	Hyperuricaemia	Chondrocalcinosis
• *Crystals*	Birefringent needle-shaped mono-sodium urate crystals with negative elongation	Rhomboid, square, or rod-like crystals with weak positive bire-fringence

Q14. Discuss the aetiology, pathology, clinical features and diagnosis of rheumatoid arthritis.

Rheumatoid arthritis (RA) is a chronic inflammatory multisystem disease of unknown cause characterized by progressive, destructive, symmetric inflammation and deformity involving the small joints of the hand, fingers, large joints, soft tissue and always associated with constitutional symptoms.

Cartilage damage and bone erosions by synovial inflammation and subsequent changes in joints integrity is the hallmark of the disease.

Aetiology

- It is unknown.
- Family studies indicate a *genetic predisposition* (class II major histocompatibility complex allele *HLA-DR4 (DRβ1*0401)* known to be major genetic risk factors).
- In a genetically susceptible host, it may be a manifestation of the response to an *infectious agent.* Though no convincing evidences are available, a number of possible causative agents have been suggested, including *Mycoplasma, Epstein-Barr virus (EBV), rubella virus, parvovirus, and cytomegalovirus.*
- Other probable causes would be *allergic* (RA frequently exhibit different allergic manifestations; Eosinophilia is common), *metabolic and endocrinal* (response to adrenocortical steroids).
- *Smoking* has clearly been identified as a risk for RA in genetically susceptible individuals.
- Onset is most common during the fourth and fifth decades of life.
- Female predominate (Women: men (3:1)).

Pathology

- The most widely accepted theory of pathogenesis is that the propagation of RA is an *immunologically mediated event or responses* take place in synovium.
- The disorder is basically, a synovitis.
- Rheumatoid synovitis; characterized by infiltration of *T-lymphocytes, infiltration of variable numbers of B cells and antibody-producing plasma cells.*
- T lymphocyte constitutes the major infiltration. CD4+ T cells predominate over CD8+ T cells
- The *autoantibody rheumatoid factor and polyclonal immunoglobulin,* produced within the synovial tissue leads to the formation of immune complexes.
- Recent studies indicates that the *antibodies to CCP,* which are generated within the synovium, may contribute to RA synovitis
- *Inflammation of synovium, → immunological mediators → Pannus (granulomatous mass) → destroys cartilage, tendons, and ligaments.*
- Systemic manifestations of RA may be due to release of inflammatory effector molecules including IL-1, TNF, and IL-6 from the synovium.

Stages of Rheumatoid Arthritis

- Initiation phase of nonspecific inflammation.
- Amplification phase resulting from T cell activation (promotion of local rheumatoid factor, other autoantibody production and enhanced capacity to mediate tissue damage).
- Stage of chronic inflammation with tissue injury.

Joint Involvement

- Symmetric arthritis with characteristic involvement of *proximal interphalangeal and metacarpo-phalangeal joints.*

- *Distal interphalangeal joints* are rarely involved.
- Synovitis of the *wrist joints* is a uniform feature and may lead to *median nerve entrapment (carpal tunnel syndrome), deformity, and limitation of motion.*
- Involvement of *elbow joint* often leads to *flexion contractures.*
- *Knee joint* is commonly involved with effusion, synovial hypertrophy, and frequently ligamentous laxity.
- Involvement of the lumbar spine is infrequent (usually not seen); axial involvement is confined to upper cervical spine.

Clinical Features (Sign and Symptoms of Articular Disease)

- It is a chronic polyarthritis, which is insidious in onset.
- Begins with, constitutional symptoms like generalized *weakness, fatigue, anorexia, weight loss and vague musculoskeletal symptoms* until the appearance of synovitis becomes apparent.
- *Symmetric pattern* of involvement of joint is more typical.
- Morning stiffness of >1 hour duration is an almost invariable feature, encountered.
- Pain in the affected joint that is aggravated by activity is the most common manifestation.
- Clinically, synovial inflammation in the affected joint causes warmth, swelling, tenderness, and limitation of motion.
- The affected inflamed joint usually held in position of flexion in order to maximize joint volume and minimize distention of the capsule. Later, soft tissue contractures or fibrous or bony ankylosis leads to fixed deformities.

  A variety of characteristic joint changes or deformities develop with persistent inflammation.

Hand

- *Swan-neck deformity:* It is hyperextension of the proximal interphalangeal joints, with compensatory flexion of the distal interphalangeal joints.
- *Boutonniere deformity:* it is flexion of the proximal interphalangeal joints and extension of the distal interphalangeal joints.
- *Loss of thumb mobility and pinch:* due to hyperextension of the first interphalangeal joint and flexion of the first metacarpophalangeal joint

Wrist

- *Bent fork deformity:* It is due to collapse of the carpal bones and subluxation of intercarpal joints.
- *'Z' deformity:* It is radial deviation at the wrist joint with ulnar deviation of the digits, usually associated with palmar subluxation of the proximal phalanges.

Elbow and Shoulder

Effusion and later contracture and degenerative changes.

Knee

- Swelling, flexion contracture and later ankylosis.
- *Baker's cyst:* Extension of inflamed synovium into the popliteal space (Baker's cyst) causes pain and swelling behind the knee.

Feet

- Hallux valgus.
- Widening of the forefoot.
- Eversion at the hind-foot (subtalar joint).
- Plantar subluxation of the metatarsal heads.
- Lateral deviation and dorsal subluxation of the toes.

Others

- Tenosynovitis involving the extensor tendons of the hand, tendo-Achilles and later contractures.
- Later in the disease, disability and deformity is due to structural damage to articular structures.

Extra-articular Manifestations

- Approximately 40% of patients may have these manifestations and in 15%, these are severe with increased morbidity.
- These show the disease activity.
- These are frequent in individuals with high titres of autoantibodies to the Fc component of IgG (rheumatoid factors) or with antibodies to CCP.

Rheumatoid Nodules

- Develops in 20–30% of persons with RA.
- Usually found on *extensor surfaces, periarticular structures, or areas subjected to mechanical pressure*, but also develop elsewhere, including the *pleura and meninges*.
- Common sites include *the proximal ulna, the olecranon bursa, the Achilles tendon, and the occiput*.
- Variable in sizes and consistency.
- Usually asymptomatic, but occasionally they break down due to trauma or become infected.
- Found in almost every patient with circulating rheumatoid factor.
- Histologically, rheumatoid nodules consist of:
  - Granulation tissue in outer zone.
  - Palisading macrophages that express HLA-DR antigens in mid-zone.
  - Central zone of necrotic material (collagen fibrils, noncollagenous filaments, and cellular debris).

Weakness and Atrophy of Muscles

- Frequent in skeletal muscle.
- Atrophy evident within weeks of the onset of RA and is more common in musculature approximating affected joints.
- Biopsy, show type II fibre muscle atrophy and necrosis with or without mononuclear cell infiltrate.

Rheumatoid Vasculitis

- It is seen in patients with severe disease activity and high titers of circulating rheumatoid factor.

- In its severe form, it may cause *polyneuropathy and mononeuritis multiplex, digital gangrene, cutaneous ulceration and dermal necrosis, and visceral infarction (lymph nodes, pancreas, lungs, bowel, liver, spleen,* and *testes.).*
- Renal vasculitis is rare.

Pleuropulmonary Manifestations

- Includes *pleuropulmonary nodules, pleural disease, pneumonitis, interstitial fibrosis,* and *arteritis.*
- Characteristically, the pleural fluid contains very low levels of glucose in the absence of infection.
- Pulmonary fibrosis can impair the diffusing capacity of the lung.
- Pulmonary nodules:
    - Appears singly or in clusters.
    - When associated with pneumoconiosis, may cause *Caplan's syndrome (diffuse nodular fibrotic process).*
    - It may undergo cavitation and produce a bronchopleural fistula or pneumothorax.
- Pulmonary vasculitis on rare occasion causes pulmonary hypertension.

Cardiac Manifestation

- Although rare but evidence of *asymptomatic pericarditis* is found at autopsy in 50% of cases.
- *Chronic constrictive pericarditis* may occur occasionally.
- Recent evidence of *congestive cardiac failure* and death due to cardiovascular disease has been associated with RA.

CNS Manifestations

- Usually it spares the CNS (not affect directly) but *peripheral neuropathy* may occur.
- *Entrapment neuropathies* of median, ulnar, radial (interosseous branch), or anterior tibial nerves may occur secondary to proliferative synovitis or joint deformities.
- *Atlantoaxial or midcervical spine subluxations* may also produces neurological manifestations.

Ophthalmic Manifestations

- Involves the eye in <1% of patients.
- Two principal manifestations are *episcleritis* (mild and transient) and *scleritis* (more serious inflammatory process).
- *Scleromalacia perforans:* Thinning and perforation of the globe as a result of pathological process.
- 15–20% of patient develops *Sjögren's syndrome with attendant keratoconjunctivitis sicca.*

Felty's Syndrome

- It consists of triad of *chronic RA, splenomegaly, neutropenia,* and, on occasion, anaemia and thrombocytopenia.
- These patients usually have systemic manifestation of RA, subcutaneous nodule and high titers of rheumatoid factors.
- Increased frequency of infections usually associated with neutropenia.

Osteoporosis

It is common, secondary to rheumatoid involvement and aggravated by glucocorticoid therapy.

Others

There is increased incidence of *lymphoma, especially large B cell lymphoma* especially in those with persistent inflammatory disease.

Diagnosis

Features, which help in diagnosis, are:

- *Bilateral symmetric* inflammatory polyarthritis involving small and large joints in upper and lower extremities.
- *Sparing of the axial skeleton* except the cervical spine.
- Constitutional features like morning stiffness support the diagnosis.
- Subcutaneous nodules are a helpful diagnostic feature.
- Presence of rheumatoid factor, anti-CCP antibodies, inflammatory synovial fluid with increased numbers of PMNLs.
- Radiographic findings of Juxta-articular osteopenia and erosions of the affected joints.

Guidelines for establishing the diagnosis: The 1987 Revised Criteria for the Classification of RA:

Guidelines for classification
a. Four of seven criteria are required to classify a patient as having rheumatoid arthritis (RA).
b. Patients with two or more clinical diagnoses are not excluded.

Criteria
a. Morning stiffness: Lasting 1 hour before maximal improvement.
b. Arthritis of three or more joint areas: At least three joint areas. The 14 possible joint areas involved are right or left proximal interphalangeal, metacarpophalangeal, wrist, elbow, knee, ankle, and metatarsophalangeal joints.
c. Arthritis of hand joints: Arthritis of wrist, metacarpophalangeal joint, or proximal interphalangeal joint.
d. Symmetric arthritis
e. Rheumatoid nodules: Subcutaneous nodules over extensor surfaces, bony prominences, or juxta-articular regions observed by a physician.
f. Serum rheumatoid factor
g. Radiographic changes: Typical changes of RA on posteroanterior hand and wrist radiographs showing juxta-articular osteopenia.

Note
- Criteria a–d must be present for at least 6 weeks

- *Classic case* should have seven criteria for atleast 6 weeks.
- *Definite case* should have five criteria for 6 weeks.
- *Probable case* should have atleast three criteria for a minimum of 4 weeks.

Investigations

Laboratory Findings

- *Rheumatoid factors* (autoantibodies reactive with the Fc portion of IgG) are found in more than two-thirds of patient with RA.
- It is not specific for RA as:
  - 5% of healthy individuals are positive for rheumatoid factor.
  - There are number of conditions besides RA that are positive for rheumatoid factor. These include *systemic lupus erythematosus (SLE), Sjögren's syndrome, chronic liver disease,*

interstitial pulmonary fibrosis, sarcoidosis, infectious mononucleosis (IM), hepatitis B, tuberculosis, leprosy, syphilis, subacute bacterial endocarditis (SABE), visceral leishmaniasis, schistosomiasis, and *malaria.*

- The *anti-CCP test* has a similar sensitivity and a better specificity for RA than rheumatoid factor. It correlates with the disease activity. It not only confirms the diagnosis of RA but also estimate the prognosis. Patient with *positive anti-CCP are prone for developing bone erosions.*
- Normochromic, normocytic anaemia is frequently present.
- Mild leukocytosis may be present.
- Leukopenia may present without the full-blown picture of Felty's syndrome. Eosinophilia, if present, usually reflects severe systemic disease.
- Erythrocyte sedimentation rate (ESR) is invariably increased.
- Acute phase reactants like *ceruloplasmin and C-reactive protein* are also elevated, reflecting disease activity.
- *Synovial fluid analysis*
    - Confirms the presence of inflammatory arthritis (WBCs >2000/µl with >75% PMNLs is highly characteristic of inflammatory arthritis)
    - Turbid
    - Reduced viscosity
    - Protein content is increased
    - Glucose concentration is slightly decreased or normal
    - WBCs varies between 5 and 50,000/µl PMNLs predominate.
    - Diminished Total hemolytic complement, C3, and C4.

Radiographic Evaluation

- AP view
    - Soft tissue swelling and joint effusion (initial findings)
    - Symmetric involvement
    - Juxta-articular osteopenia
    - Loss of articular cartilage
    - Decreased joint space
    - Bone erosions and subchondral cyst
    - Deformed, ankylosed joint
- ^{99m}Tc bisphosphonate bone scanning and MRI: Detecting early inflammatory changes that is not apparent on standard radiography; not necessary for routine evaluation.

Q15. Discuss the management of the rheumatoid arthritis.

Management of patients with RA involves an interdisciplinary approach, which deals with functional as well as psychosocial problems of these individuals.

Goals of Therapy

- Ameliorate pain, swelling and joint stiffness
- Reduction of inflammation thereby preserving joint motion
- Protection of articular structures thus preventing secondary joint stiffness and deformity
- Maintenance of health of muscles supplying motor power about the joint
- Control of systemic involvement and other constitutional defects.

Conservative

Nonpharmacological treatment

- *Rest*: Physical, emotional and articular ameliorates symptoms.
- *Physical therapy*: Hot moist packs, fomentation, infra-red, short wave diathermy reduces muscle spasm.
- *Exercise*: Graduated isometric exercises to build muscle power while minimizing joint stress; thus maintains muscle strength and joint mobility.
- *Traction*: During the acute inflammatory phase, especially of weight, bearing joints to keep the joint surface distracted and to stretch the contracted capsule until the inflammatory phase subsides.
- *Splinting* of inflamed joint in functional position relieves pain and reduces inflammation quickly.
- *Education and counseling* of the patient and the family members to aware them about the potential complication/impact of the disease and to encourage making necessary accommodation in lifestyle to maximize the level of satisfaction.

Pharmacological Treatment

Involves five general approaches.

1. Nonsteroidal anti-inflammatory drugs (NSAIDs)

- First line drug.
- Rapidly effective at mitigating signs and symptoms.
- Minimal effect on the progression of the disease.

Mechanism of action: Inhibition of PG synthesis.

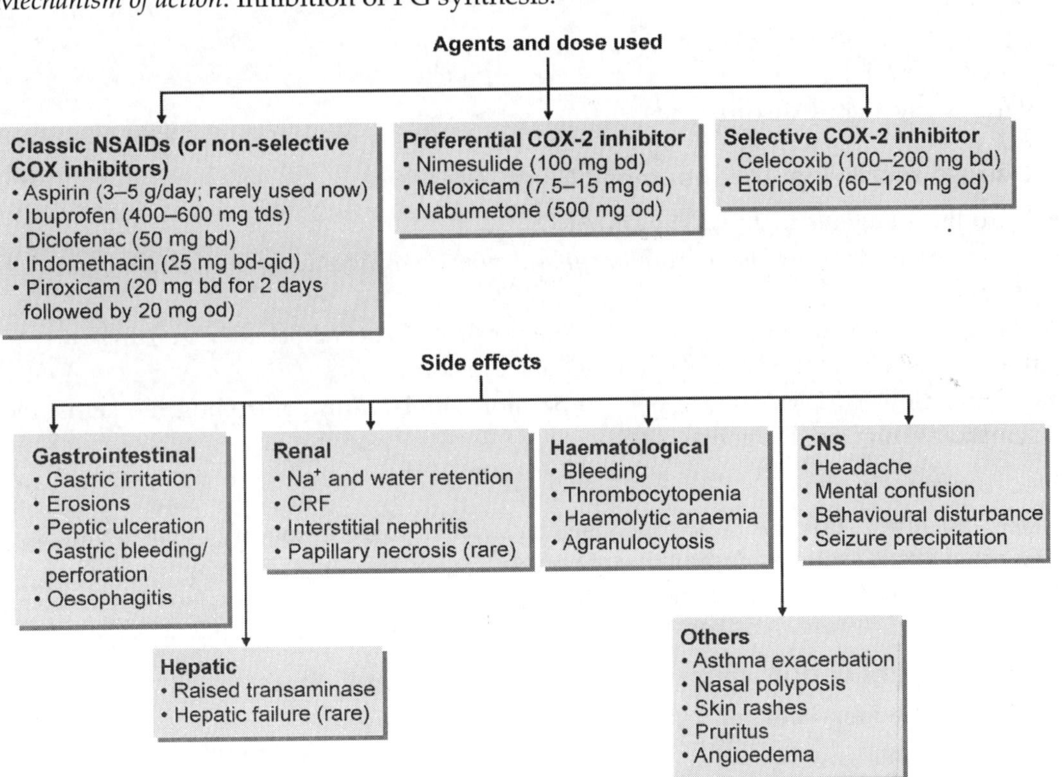

2. Steroids

- Second line of therapy involves use of low-dose oral glucocorticoids.
- These agents have potent immunosuppressant and anti-inflammatory activity.
- Suppress signs and symptoms of inflammation.
- Retard the development and progression of bone erosions.
- Increases the anti-inflammatory effects of agents such as methotrexate and the protective effect of these agents on bone damage as well.
- *Low dose* should be considered in patient either alone or when therapy with disease modifying anti-rheumatic drugs (DMARDs) is considered.
- *High doses of steroids* are employed over short periods in cases with severe systemic manifestations.
- In cases where systemic therapy failed to resolve inflammation *intra-articular glucocorticoids* can often provide transient symptomatic relief.
- Low-dose (<7.5 mg/day) prednisone should be considered.

Disadvantages

Long-term administrations of steroids are associated with serious disadvantages like
- Osteoporosis
- Cushing's habitus
- Suppression of hypothalamic-pituitary adrenal axis (HPA)
- Myopathy
- Glaucoma
- Posterior subcapsular cataract
- Peptic ulceration
- Various psychiatric disturbances.

3. Disease-modifying Anti-rheumatic Drugs (DMARDs)

- Third line of agents includes the DMARDs.
- These agents include *methotrexate, sulfasalazine, hydroxychloroquine, gold salts, or D-penicillamine.*
- Therapy should started as early as the diagnosis of RA established as starting early in the course, retards the development of bone erosions.
- Combinations of DMARDs appear to be more effective in controlling the signs and symptoms than single agents.

Mechanism of action

- Decrease elevated levels of acute-phase reactants; thought to modify the inflammatory component and thus its destructive capacity.
- Exert minimal direct nonspecific anti-inflammatory or analgesic effects (so NSAIDs must be continued during their administration).

Appearance of benefit

Usually delayed for weeks or months.

Agents and doses

Agent	Dose	Side effects
Methotrexate (MTx), DRAMDs of choice	• Weekly schedule of 7.5–25 mg given either orally in divided doses or, if necessary, sc or im	Dose related and reversible: • Gastrointestinal upset • Oral ulceration • Liver function abnormalities • Hepatic fibrosis • Drug-induced pneumonitis • Low doses causes megaloblastic anaemia • High doses causes pancytopenia **Note:** Concurrent administration of folic acid or folinic acid may diminish the frequency of some side effects
Sulfasalazine (compound of sulfapyridine and 5-amino salicylic acid)	• 1–3 g/day in 2–3 divided doses	• Neutropenia/thrombocytopenia occurs in 10% of cases • Hepatitis
Chloroquine and hydrooxychloroquine	• Chloroquine 150 mg (base) per day • Hydrooxychloroquine 400 mg/day for 4–6 weeks, followed by 200 mg/day for maintenance	• Retinal damage • Corneal toxicity • Rashes • Graying of hairs • Irritable bowel syndrome • Myopathy • Neuropathy **Note:** Retinal damage and corneal opacity is less common with hydroxy-chloroquine therefore it is preferred over chloroquine
Leflunomide (immunomodulator)	• Loading dose of 100 mg daily for 3 days followed by 20 mg od	• Diarrhoea • Headache • Nausea • Rashes • Loss of hair • Thrombocytopenia • Leucopenia • Chest infection • Raised hepatic transaminase **Note:** Contraindicated in children and pregnant/lactating women
Gold (Auranofin) rarely used now-a-days	• Auranofin (orally active) 6 mg/day in 1 or 2 doses	Parenteral • Hypotension • Dermatitis • Stomatitis· Kidney and liver damage Oral: • Diarrhoea • Abdominal cramps • Pruritus • Taste disturbances • Mild anaemia • Alopecia
d-Penicillamine	· Start with 125–250 mg od, then 250 mg od	• Loss of taste • Systemic lupus • Myasthenia gravis

4. Biologic Response Modifiers

Fourth group of agents are the biologics, which include IL-1-neutralizing agents (anakinra), TNF-neutralizing agents (infliximab, etanercept, and adalimumab), those that deplete B cells (rituximab), and those that interfere with T cell activation (abatacept).

Agent and dose

Agent	Dose	Side effects
TNF-neutralizing agents:		
• Etanercept (it is a recombinant fusion TNF type II receptor fused to IgG1)	• SC injection 50 mg weekly	At the injection site: • Pain • Redness • Itching • Swelling **Others:** • Chest infection may be increased.
• Infliximab (chimeric mouse/human monoclonal antibody to TNF)	• 3–5 mg/kg infused every 4–8 weeks	Acute reaction comprise of: • Fever • Chills • Urticaria • Bronchospam • Renal anaphylaxis **Others:** • Chest infection is increased • Worsening of CHF
• Adalimumab (fully human antibody to TNF)	• SC 40 mg every 2 weeks	• Injection site reaction • Respiratory infections
IL-1 antagonist • Anakinra (less effective than TNF inhibitors)	• 100 mg sc daily	• Local reaction and chest infection
Agents that deplete B cells: • Rituximab, a chimeric antibody directed to CD20 that depletes mature B cells	• Optimal regimen has not been established • Repeated usually at 6-month intervals when circulating B cells return	• Transfusion reactions
Agents that interfere with T cell activation: • Abatacept is a fusion protein consisting of CTLA4 and the Fc portion of IgG1		• More adverse events, including serious infections, and, therefore, is not recommended.

5. Immunosuppressive Therapy

- Fifth group of agents are the immunosuppressive and cytotoxic drugs.
- Immunosuppressive drugs *azathioprine, leflunomide, cyclosporine, and cyclophosphamide.*
- These agents are less effective than the DMARDs.
- Associated with serious toxicities.

Indications

- Rheumatoid vasculitis.
- Patients who have clearly failed therapy with DMARDs and biologics.

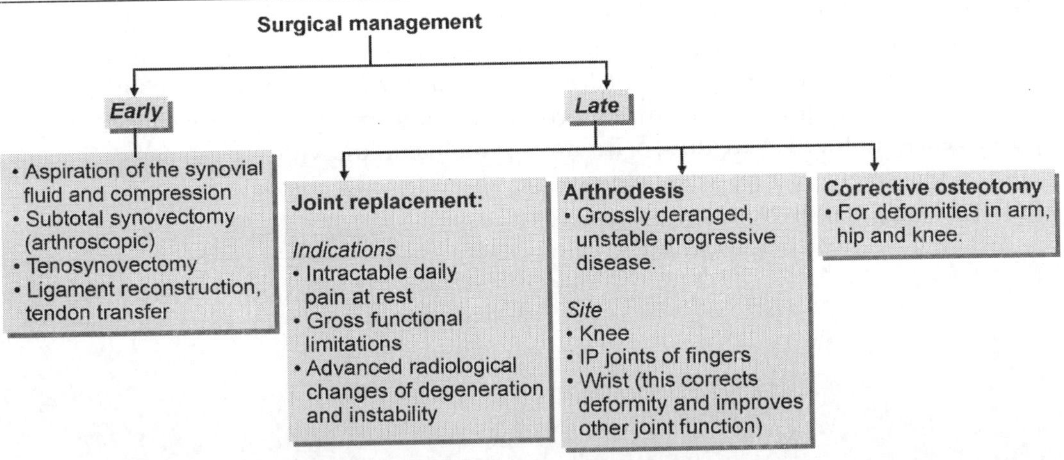

Q16. Write in short about ochronotic arthritis (alkaptonuric arthritis).

Ochronosis is the connective tissue manifestation of alkaptonuria related to an autosomal recessive mutation of the *HGA gene located on 3q chromosome* caused by deficiency of homogentisate 1,2-dioxygenase activity. Alkaptonuria is a rare metabolic disorder characterized by a triad of *degenerative arthritis, ochronotic pigmentation,* and *homogentisic aciduria.* Alkaptonuria affects both men and women with ochronotic arthropathy; the trend is more severe and more frequent for men than for women. Ochronotic arthropathy usually involves the *large weight-bearing joints (knee and hip joints)* rather than the small joints of the hand and foot.

It affects *hyaline cartilages, intervertebral discs, skin and sclera.* The cardiovascular, genitourinary and respiratory systems at times affected.

Clinical Presentation

- Black discoloration of urine when exposed to air
- Brownish-grey color of the sclera
- Dark skin
- Kidney stones
- Aortic calcifications
- *Ochronotic arthropathy* (degenerative and destructive damage of the spine and the peripheral joints): Symptoms typically of osteoarthritis (pain, crepitus, clicking and locking knee joint, backache, stiffness of spine; Spine radiograph shows *intra-discal calcifications* giving a "doubling" of the outline, which confirmed the diagnosis of ochronosis)

Diagnosis

Chromatographic, enzymatic or spectrophotometric determinations of HGA are confirmatory tests.

Treatment

- Patients with alkaptonuria are usually asymptomatic, and the ochronotic arthropathy appears after the fourth decade.

- Currently, there is no definitive cure for alkaptonuric ochronosis. Symptomatic treatment of the complications of alkaptonuria is the only option, including *pain management, physiotherapy, chiropractic care, and instruction regarding a home exercise program*
- High dose of vitamin C and nitisinone have some promising role; however, the effectiveness of these in treating ochronosis remains unknown.
- Total replacement of hip, knee, elbow, and shoulder can alleviate pain and increase patient's daily activities

11

Congenital Anomalies and Development Disorders

The anomalies may be broadly grouped as under.

Absence:

Amelia:
The congenital absence of a limb or limbs

Phocomelia:
A congenital malformation in which limb represented as short stubs — only hand, fingers.

Hemimelia:
Absence of part of limb transverse, axial-medial, lateral or ectromelia

Extra:

Polydactyly:
A developmental anomaly characterized by extra fingers, toes, thumb.

Syndactyly:
A common congenital anomaly characterized by fused fingers and toes.

Upper Limb

Cleidocranial dysostosis:
There is defective ossification of the membranous bones involving vault of skull, maxilla, clavicle, etc.

Lobster claw hand:
Cleft hand

Radioulnar synostosis:
Fusion of radioulnar joint completely/incompletely

Sprengel's deformity:
Undescended scapula or congenital elevation of scapula.

Syndactyly or polydactyly

Radial club hand:
Absence of radius and radial ray, i.e. thumb

Lower Limb

CDH: Dysplastic hip joint
Tibia hemimelia: Congenital absence of tibia
CTEV
Coxa vara: Reduced neck shaft angle.

Pseudoarthrosis of tibia: Kyphoscoliotic tibia with nonunion of fractured tibia.

Flat foot: A condition in which the medial arch of the foot is flat developmentally or due to congenital vertical talus.

Spine:

Torticollis: Damaged sternomastoid muscle leading to bent, rotated neck.
Klippel–Feil syndrome: Fused lamina of cervical spine with short webbed neck.

Spina bifida:
Developmental anomaly in the spinal column, involving the posterior arch of vertebra

Joints:

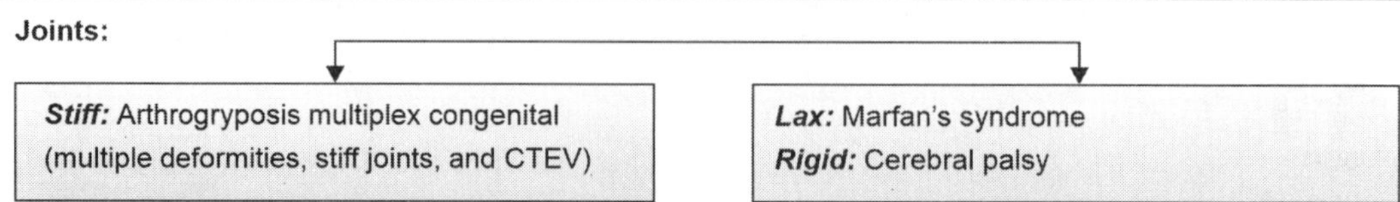

Q2. Define CTEV and discuss the relevant anatomy of various joint, ligaments and tendons involved in the deformity.

Relevant Anatomy

To understand the aetiology and/or management of clubfoot, it is essential to know relevant anatomy, which can be divided into related *joints, ligaments, and tendons.*

Joints

Joints related to clubfoot are:

Ankle joint: It is a synovial joint of hinge variety. The upper articular surface comprises of:
- Lower end of tibia including the medial malleolus.
- Lateral malleolus of the fibula.
- Inferior transverse tibiofibular ligament.

The inferior articular surface comprises of articular areas on the upper, medial and lateral aspects of talus.

Subtalar or talocalcanean joint: It is a plane synovial joint between the concave facet on the inferior surface of the body of the talus and the convex facet on the middle one-third of the superior surface of the calcaneum

Talonavicular joint: It is between the talus and navicular.

Calcaneocuboid joint: This is a saddle joint. The opposed articular surfaces of the calcaneum and cuboid are concavoconvex.

Ligaments

The related ligaments are:

Spring Ligament (or Plantar Calcaneonavicular Ligament)

- It is a powerful ligament.
- It is attached posteriorly to the anterior margin of the sustentaculum tali, and anteriorly to the plantar surface of the navicular bone between its tuberosity and articular margin.
- This is the most important ligament for maintaining the medial longitudinal arch of the foot.

Deltoid Ligament (Medial)

This is a very strong triangular ligament present on the medial side of the ankle. The ligament is divided into superficial and deep part.

Capsular Ligaments

Play important role in pathology of clubfoot.

Plantar Ligament (Long and Short)

- Strong ligament whose importance in maintaining the arches of foot is surpassed only by the spring ligament.

- It is attached posteriorly to the plantar surface of the calcaneum, and anteriorly to the lips of the groove on the cuboid bone, and to the bases of the middle three metatarsals.

Tendons

Mainly on medial side of foot.

Tibialis Posterior

- The most important muscle in causing deformity.
- The tibialis posterior is inserted chiefly into the tuberosity of the navicular bone
- The tendon also gives off slips to all tarsal bones except talus and to 2nd, 3rd, and 4th metatarsal bone, it is an invertor and powerful flexor.

Other being: Flexor hallucis longus, flexor digitorum longus
On the posterior side: Tendon Achilles (is the thickest and strongest tendon of the body).

Q3. Define various deformities of foot.

The various deformities in clubfoot that usually encountered are:
- *Equinus*: The foot is fixed in plantar flexion (walk on toes with the heel raised).
- *Calcaneus*: The foot is fixed in dorsiflexion.
- *Varus*: The foot is inverted and adducted at the mid-tarsal joint. The plantar surface faces medially.
- *Valgus*: The foot is everted and abducted at the midtarsal joint. The plantar surface faces laterally.
- *Planus*: Absence or collapse of the arches leads to flat foot
- *Cavus:* The longitudinal arch of the foot is exaggerated.

Talipes equinovarus and *talipes calcaneovalgus* are the two common combinations and among the mixture of two different deformities stated above, *talipes equinovarus* is the commoner of the two.

Q4. Discuss the aetiology, pathological changes and clinical features in CTEV.

Talipes equinovarus is the most common congenital foot abnormality, accounts for over 50% of foot deformities and described by Hippocrates in the year 400 BC.

Clubfoot is a complex congenital anomaly still incompletely understood and hence a wide-ranging aetiopathology and equally large number of surgical variations are seen.

Incidence

- Approximately 1 per 1000 live births
- Male: Female 2:1
- Bilateral in 30–50% of cases
- Most cases are sporadic
- Positive Family history in few (autosomal dominant trait with incomplete penetrance)
- 10% chance of subsequent child being affected if positive family history; 2.3% if no family history

Aetiology

It could be:
- *Congenital:*
  - Idiopathic (most common)
  - Dysplastic

- Neuropathic/neuromuscular
- Osseous
- *Acquired*
  - Spastic
  - Post-traumatic
  - Postinfective
  - Paralytic

Theories

Numerous theories of the aetiology have been postulated. Some of the most accepted theories relative to the development of CTEV are:

- Hereditary influences
- Medial displacement of the navicular and calcaneus around the talus *(Turco)*
- Intrauterine mechanics or pressure-related theories *(Hippocrates)*
- Three-dimensional aspect of bony deformity of the subtalar complex in clubfoot*(McKay)*
- Arrest of embryologic or fetal development *(Bohm)*
- Nerve abnormalities with muscle contractures or neuromuscular theory *(Ponseti and Uhthoff; Isaacs H,)*
- Circulatory abnormalities of tarsal precursors
- Rotational and torsional abnormalities
- Primary osseous deformation (most widely accepted)
- Defective cartilaginous anlage of the talus *(Irani and Sherman)*
- Retracting fibrosis : Increased fibrous tissue in muscles and ligaments *(Ippolito and Ponseti)*
- Anomalous tendon insertions *(Inclan)*

Other Condition Associated with CTEV

- Arthrogryposis multiplex congenita (multiple joint contractures, muscle weakness and fibrosis)
- Cerebral palsy
- Polio
- Myopathy
- Developmental dysplasia of hip (DDH or CDH)
- Peripheral nerve injury
- Amyotrophic lateral sclerosis
- Infantile spastic Hemiplegia
- Spina bifida
- Meningomyelocele
- Friedreich's ataxia

Pathology

The three basic components of clubfoot are *equinus, varus,* and *adduction* deformities. Clubfoot is accompanied by internal tibial torsion. The ankle, mid-tarsal, and subtalar joints, all are involved in the pathological process.

Bony and Soft Tissue Changes in CTEV

Bony Changes

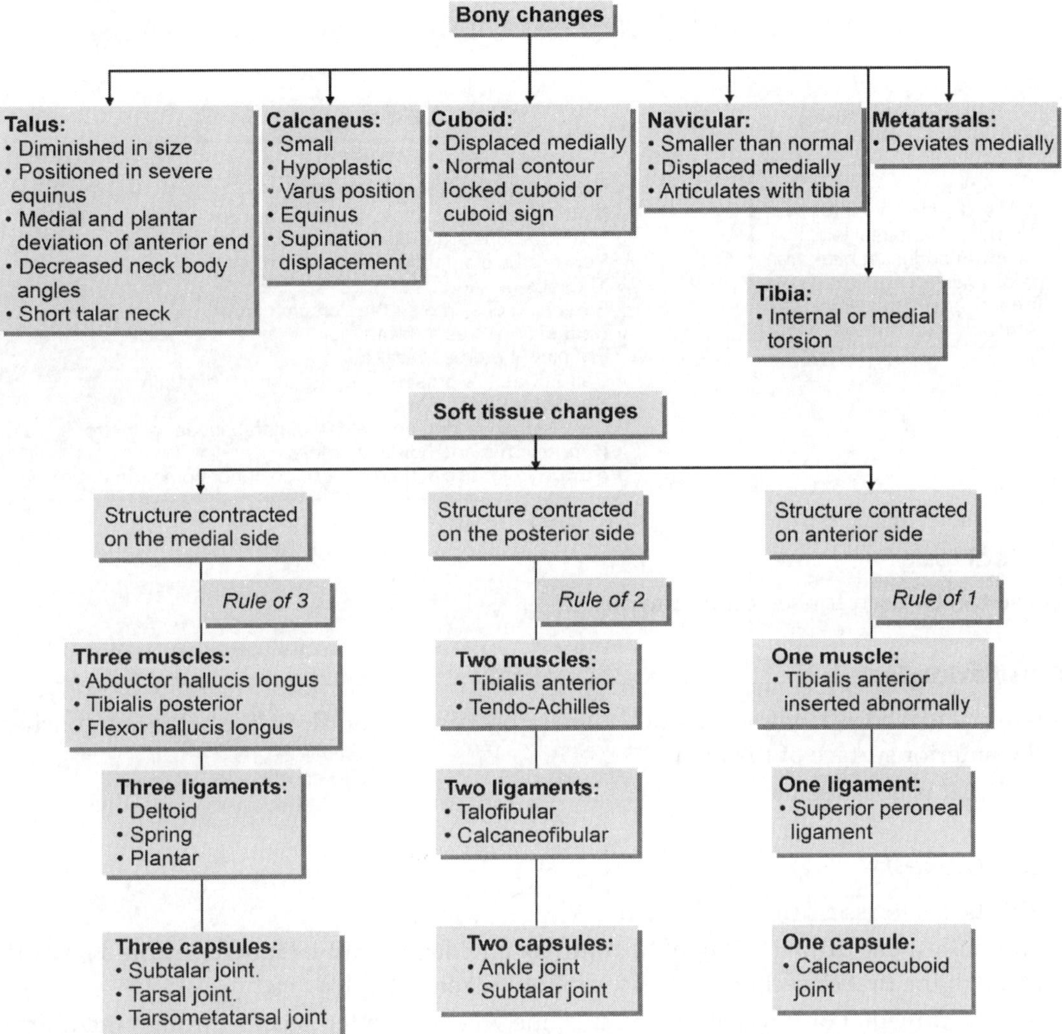

Clinical Features

In a patient of CTEV always do general examination to rule out other deformities / anomalies.

Features

- The foot is small with up drawn heel
- A thin calf and tight tendo-Achilles
- Sole faces inwards with deep furrows along the medial border
- The toes are adducted and as the child starts walking on the dorsolateral aspect of the foot,

- Callosities develop on the skin
- Other features and primary deformities as shown in flowchart:

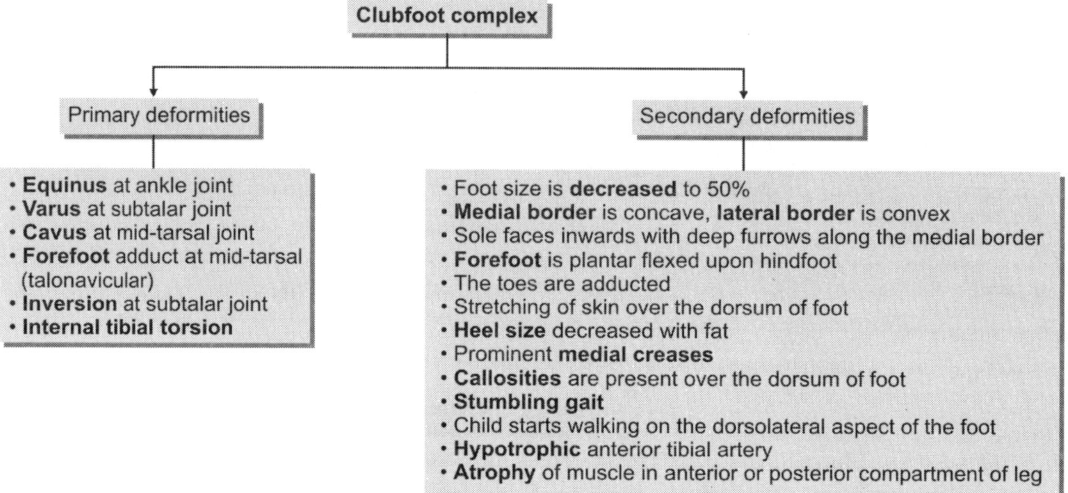

Clinical Tests

These can be used for screening purposes.

Dorsiflexion Test

- Normal newborn: Complete dorsiflexion is possible, i.e. dorsal surface of the foot touches the anterior surface of the tibia.
- CTEV: It is not possible.

Plumbline Test

- This test is to assess the tibial torsion.
- Normally a line drawn through the centre of patella to the tibial tubercle should passing through the first or second web space in foot when extended.
- In case of medial or internal torsion this line when extended passes through the fourth or fifth web space.

Scratch Test

- This test is to assess the muscle imbalance in newborn.
- Eversion of foot on medial scratching of sole tests the peroneal.
- Inversion of foot on lateral scratching of the sole tests the invertors.

Q5. Discuss the various classifications or scoring system of CTEV.

Two of the more recent classifications by Diméglio et al. and Pirani et al. depends solely on physical examination and require no radiographic measurements or other special studies.

Pirani's System

- Comprises of 10 different physical examination findings, each scored 0 for no abnormality, 0.5 for moderate abnormality, or 1 for severe abnormality.
- Each foot is assigned a total score, the maximum being 10 points, with a higher score indicating a more severe deformity

Pirani Classification of Clubfoot Deformity

Physical examination findings	*Score of 0*	*Score of 0.5*	*Score of 1*
Curvature of lateral border of foot	Straight	Mild distal curve	Curve at calcaneocuboid joint
Severity of medial crease (foot held in maximal correction)	Multiple fine creases	One or two deep creases	Deep creases change contour of arch
Severity of posterior crease (foot held in maximal correction)	Multiple fine creases	One or two deep creases	Deep creases change contour of arch
Medial malleolar–navicular interval (foot held in maximal correction)	Definite depression felt	Interval reduced	Interval not palpable
Palpation of lateral part of head of talus (forefoot fully abducted)	Navicular completely 'reduces'; lateral talar head cannot be felt	Navicular partially 'reduces'; lateral head less palpable	Navicular does not 'reduce'; lateral talar head easily felt
Emptiness of heel (foot and ankle in maximal correction)	Tuberosity of calcaneus easily palpable	Tuberosity of calcaneus more difficult to palpate	Tuberosity of calcaneus not palpable
Fibula-Achilles interval (hip flexed, knee extended, foot and ankle maximally corrected)	Definite depression felt	Interval reduced	Interval not palpable
Rigidity of equinus (knee extended, ankle maximally corrected)	Normal ankle dorsiflexion	Ankle dorsiflexes beyond neutral, but not fully	Cannot dorsiflex ankle to neutral
Rigidity of adductus (forefoot is fully abducted)	Forefoot can be overcorrected into abduction	Forefoot can be corrected beyond neutral, but not fully	Forefoot cannot be corrected to neutral
Long flexor contracture (foot and ankle held in maximal correction)	MTP joints can be dorsiflexed to 90°	MTP joints can be dorsiflexed beyond neutral but not fully	MTP joints cannot be dorsiflexed to neutral

Diméglio et al.

In this system, four parameters are assessed on the basis of their reducibility with gentle manipulation as measured with a handheld goniometer:

- Equinus deviation in the sagittal plane
- Varus deviation in the frontal plane
- Derotation of the calcaneopedal block in the horizontal plane
- Adduction of the forefoot relative to the hindfoot in the horizontal plane

Classification of Clubfoot Severity by Diméglio et al.

Parameters Measured	Reducibility (degrees)	Score
• Equinus deviation in sagittal plane	90–45	4
• Varus deviation in frontal plane	45–20	3
• Derotation of calcaneopedal block in horizontal plane	29–0	2
• Adduction of forefoot relative to hindfoot in horizontal plane	0–20	1
	<20	0
		16
Other elements considered		
• Posterior crease marked		1
• Mediotarsal crease marked		1
• Plantar retraction or cavus		1
• Poor muscle condition		1
• Possible total score		20

Grade	Type	Frequency (%)	Score	Reducibility
I	Benign	20	1–4	>90% soft-soft, resolving
II	Moderate	33	5–9	>50% soft-stiff, reducible, partially resistant
III	Severe	35	10–14	>50% stiff-soft, resistant, partially reducible
IV	Very severe	12	15–20	<10% stiff-stiff, resistant

Q6. Discuss the radiographic assessment and management of clubfoot.

Radiographic evaluation not only helps in assessing the severity of the deformity but also to measure the correction and prediction of the recurrence.

Investigations

Cardiac: To rule out anomalies and fitness for surgery.
CNS: For secondary causes of CTEV, e.g. meningocele, Friedreich's ataxia.
Spine: For Spina bifida, etc.

X-ray

These are essential to:
• Assess the severity of the deformity
• Amount of correction achieved
• Prediction of the recurrence.

Foot: This is done before and after the correction.

• In a non-ambulatory child, standard radiographs include *anteroposterior and stress dorsiflexion lateral* radiographs of both feet
• Anteroposterior and lateral standing radiographs may be obtained for an older child.
• Both, AP and stress dorsiflexion lateral view for talocalcaneal axis, known as KITE'S angle (25°–55°)

Important Angles to Consider in the Evaluation

• Talocalcaneal angle on the anteroposterior radiograph
• Talocalcaneal angle on the lateral radiograph and the talus—first metatarsal angle
• Tibiocalcaneal angle on the stress lateral radiograph

Values of these Angles

Talocalcaneal Angle

- It is the angle between the long axis of the talus and calcaneum.
- These angles are to assess the extent of varus deformity.
- Anteroposterior view: 30–55° (normally)
- Dorsiflexion lateral view: 25–50° (normally)
- In CETV, theses angles are reduced

Tibiocalcaneal Angle

- It is the Angle between the long axis of the tibia and calcaneum.
- This angle indicates the degree of equinus.
- Stress lateral view: 10–40° (normally)
- In CTEV it is negative

Talus–first Metatarsal Angle

- It is the angle between the long axis of the talus and first metatarsal.
- This angle indicates the extent of forefoot adduction.
- Anteroposterior view: 5–15° (normally)
- In CTEV it is 0° to negative

Management

The principles of management are correction of the deformity and subsequent maintenance of the correction achieved by appropriate footwear, until the child starts walking and regains the muscle balance.

- *Conservative*: Manipulations and serial corrective POP casts
- *Surgery*:
  - Soft tissue release.
  - Tendon transfer.
  - Bony operations.
- *JESS distractor*, correction by *differential distraction*

Conservative

Manipulative correction

By mother.

Serial manipulation and Corrective cast:

- Order of correction by serial manipulation and casting should be as follows:
  - First, correction of forefoot adduction
  - Next, correction of heel varus
  - Finally, correction of hindfoot equinus
- The cast is well padded with cotton and applied above knee, knee flexed at 90° to avoid slipping out, extending up to the toe tips.
- The cast is changed every three weeks until maximum correction is achieved.

Caution: Do not forcefully dorsiflex the foot initially otherwise complication of ROCKER BOTTOM may occur due to break in the mid foot.

Ponseti technique: A New Technique of Corrective Cast

This method is particularly suited for developing countries where there are few economical and easy on the babies. If well implemented, it will greatly decrease the number of clubfoot cripples.

First Four or Five Casts (More if Necessary)

- Start as soon after birth as possible.
- Make the infant and family comfortable.
- *First cast*: The first element of management is correction of the cavus deformity by positioning the forefoot in proper alignment with the hind foot.
- Second, third, and fourth casts: During this phase of treatment, the adductus and varus are fully corrected.

Manipulation

The manipulation consists of abduction of the foot beneath the stabilized talar head. Locate the head of the talus (which is the fulcrum for correction). All components of clubfoot deformity, except for the ankle equinus, are corrected simultaneously

Equinus Correction and Fifth Cast

Perform the tenotomy approximately 1.5 cm above the calcaneus with the foot held in maximal dorsiflexion by the assistant and maintain the corrected position in fifth cast.

Maintenance Phase

- When the final or last cast is removed, the infant is placed in a brace that maintains the foot in its corrected position *(abducted and dorsiflexed)*.
- The brace (foot abduction orthosis) consists of shoes mounted to a bar in a position of 70° of external rotation and 15° of dorsiflexion.
- The distance between the shoes is set at about 1" wider than the width of the infant's shoulders.
- This brace is worn 23 hours each day for the first 3 months after casting and then while sleeping for 2–3 years.

Surgery

A fair trial of corrective POP cast must always be done before embarking on any surgical intervention, nevertheless, I agree with suggestion of Lovell [1970] who suggested that if correction is not achieved within 3 months of conservative management, then surgery should be done.

Ideal time for soft tissue release is 3 months to 1 year.

Aims of surgical management are To provide a painless plantigrade and flexible foot with near normal gait and lasting correction of the deformity.

The surgical options available are depending on the deformity and age of the child.
- Posteromedial soft tissue release (3 months to 1 year).
- Tendon transfer (5–8 years).
- Soft tissue differential distraction by JESS/Ilizarov apparatus (3 months to adulthood).

Bony Procedures

- Immature foot: Evans/Dwyer's osteotomy (5–10 years).
- Mature foot: *Triple arthrodesis* (Surgical fusion of the subtalar, talo-navicular, and calcaneo-cuboid joints)/ talectomy (>15 years).

Posteromedial Soft Tissue Release

The structures released are as follows.

Posterior

Z-Plasty lengthening of tendo-Achilles, capsule/ligaments of ankle and subtalar joint.

Medial

Tibialis posterior tendon insertions, abductor hallucis deltoid ligament (superficial layer).

Plantar

Plantar fascia, spring ligament.

Shortcomings of Posteromedial release are:
- Mild forefoot adduction (because of unattended T/M and calcaneocuboid joints).
- Heel varus (due to subtotal release of subtalar joint).

Tendon Transfer

- The principle is to transfer the deforming force of tibialis posterior as an inverter to the dorsum of the foot so that it works as a dorsiflexor.
- Tibialis posterior is transferred anteriorly and attached to the dorsum of 3rd cuneiform, this transfer is done after the child is 5 years old and mature enough to understand tendon retraining.

Bony Operations

Required to correct residual deformity.
Forefoot adduction:
- Cuboid decancellation <3 years.
- Evan's procedure (dorsolateral wedge resection of calcaneocuboid joint) >5 years.
- Tarsometatarsal capsulotomy <5 years.
- Metatarsal osteotomy >5 years.

Heel Varus

Dwyer's osteotomy of the calcaneum—3–10 years.

Treatment of Resistant Clubfoot

Deformity	Treatment
· Metatarsus adductus	>5 years: metatarsal osteotomy
· Hindfoot varus	<2–3 years: modified McKay procedure 3–10 years: Dwyer's osteotomy (isolated heel varus) Dillwyn-Evans procedure (short medial column) Lichtblau procedure (long lateral column) 10–12 years: triple arthrodesis
· Equinus	Achilles tendon lengthening plus posterior capsulotomy of subtalar joint, ankle joint (mild-to-moderate deformity) Lambrinudi procedure (severe deformity, skeletal immaturity)
· All three deformities	>10 years: triple arthrodesis

Neglected CTEV

Early: JESS/Ilizarov distracters to stretch out the contracted soft tissues.
Late: Triple arthrodesis/talectomy with resection.

Criteria for Correction

Clinical Features

- The child walks with a full plantigrade foot
- No limp/in-toeing
- Painless cosmetic scar
- The child can wear normal footwear.

Radiological Features

- Restoration of normal talocalcaneal angle in both AP and lateral view
- Talocalcaneal index >40

Maintenance of Correction Achieved

Non-ambulatory Child

- NOVA shoes
- Dennis Browne night splint

Ambulatory Child

Surgical shoes with broad toe box:
- Straight medial border of sole.
- Thomas heel (lateral wedge extension)
- Inside iron and outside T-strap.

Q7. Discuss the aetiology, clinical features, investigation and management of Congenital Dislocation of Hip or Developmental Dysplasia of Hip.

It is a *disabling disorder* present at birth, which is invariably missed, if diagnosed early and treated adequately can provide good long-term result.

Definition

- The term *"developmental dysplasia of the hip"* has replaced the term "congenital dislocation of the hip" because it more accurately reflects the full spectrum of developmental abnormalities of the hip joint.
- *Developmental dysplasia of the hip* can result in both *subluxation* and *dislocation of the hip* and can predispose to the development of early degenerative changes.
- A *subluxated hip* is one in which the femoral head is displaced from its normal position but still makes contact with a portion of the acetabulum.
- With a *dislocated hip,* there is no articular contact between the femoral head and the acetabulum

Component of congenital dysplasia of hip:
- Subluxation (partial dislocation) of the femoral head
- Acetabular dysplasia
- Complete dislocation of the femoral head from the true acetabulum

Incidence

- 1 in 1000 live births
- It is uncommon in Asian and African countries where it is habit of the mother to carry the child cross-legged, which is in itself a good corrective mode of treatment.
- It is common in girls (5:1) and often unilateral.
- Family history increases the likelihood of this condition to approximately 10%
- More common in white children than in black children
- More common in firstborn children than in subsequent siblings
- Breech presentation to result in congenital dysplasia of the hip in 1:35
- Left hip is more commonly involved than the right

Association with other conditions:
- Congenital torticollis
- Metatarsus adductus
- Talipes calcaneovalgus

Several theories regarding the aetiology:
- Mechanical factors (Breech delivery)
- Hormone-induced joint laxity (maternal hormones released during delivery)
- Primary acetabular dysplasia
- Genetic inheritance (70% incidence of a positive family history)

Pathologic Changes

Pathologic changes in the *newborn* are predominantly related to:
- A shallow acetabulum
- Laxity of the capsule
- Soft-tissue interposition

Older children show pathologic changes in both the soft tissues and the osseous architecture.
- Delay in the ossification of the acetabulum
- Acetabulum is often abnormally   shallow, anteverted, and deficient anterolaterally.
- Delay in ossification of the femoral head
- Exaggerated femoral anteversion

Obstacles to a concentric reduction may classified as:
- Extra-articular or intra-articular
- Extra-articular obstacles includes:
    - Tight psoas tendon, which can constrict the anterior capsule to create an "hourglass" narrowing of the capsule, which prevents reduction.
    - Tight adductor muscles
- Intra-articular obstacles that may impede reduction include:
    - Constricted joint capsule
    - Fibrofatty pulvinar
    - Hypertrophied ligament teres
    - An infolded labrum
    - Hypertrophied transverse Acetabular ligament
    - Located in the inferomedial portion of the acetabulum

Clinical Features

In newborns (≤6 months old):

An observant mother notices the limb

- Length discrepancy
- An extra groin crease
- A click during hip massage

Clinical screening includes:

- Ortolani test
- The provocative manoeuvre of Barlow

Age 6–18 months and adolescent:

- Limitation of abduction
- Asymmetrical skin folds
- Galeazzi sign is positive
- In a child of walking age:
    - Trendelenburg gait pattern
    - "Waddling" type of gait (if bilateral)
    - Positive telescoping test
- Vascular sign of Narath is positive
- Supratrochanteric shortening present
- Limb length discrepancy

Adults:

- All sign seen during adolescent age
- Pain
- Features of secondary degenerative changes:
    - Pain
    - Limp
    - Crepitations
    - Stiffness
    - Restriction of movements

Diagnosis

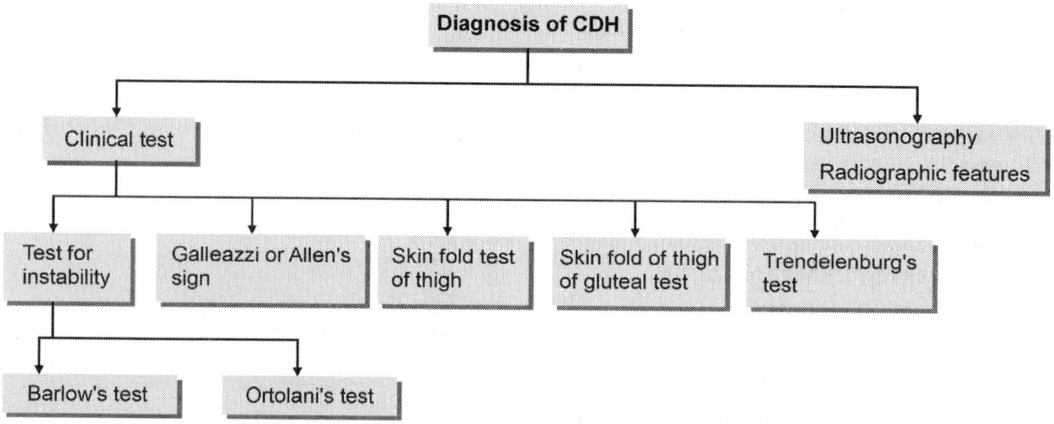

Ortolani's test: *Test of entry: Relocates a dislocated hip*

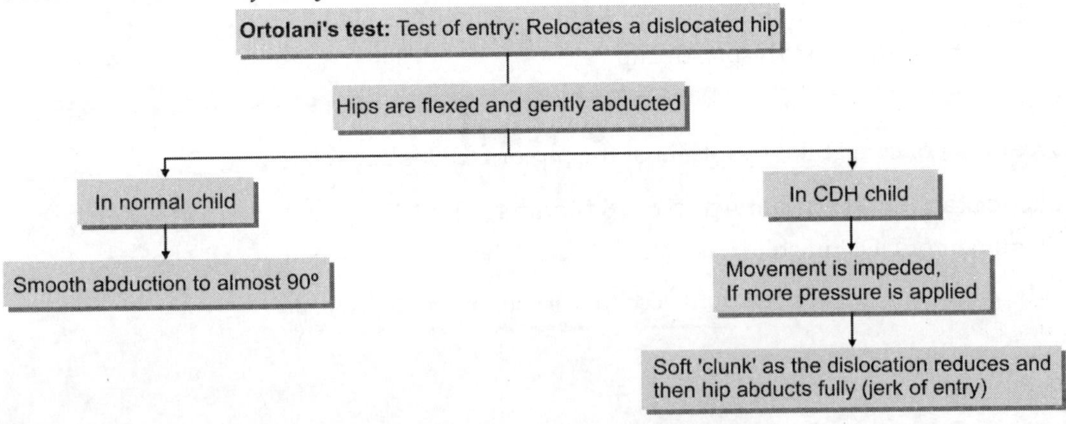

Barlow's Test

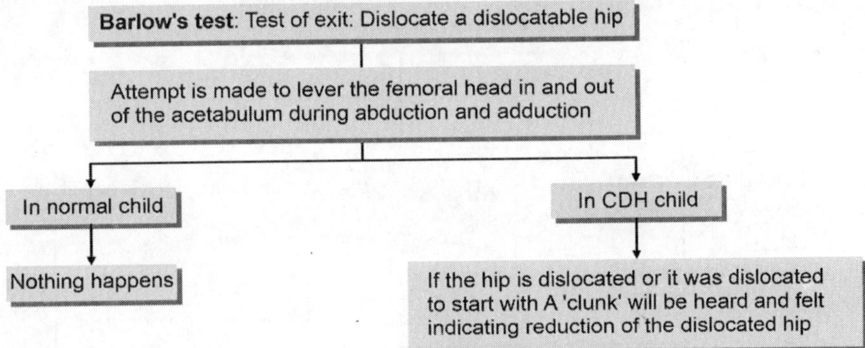

Other Tests

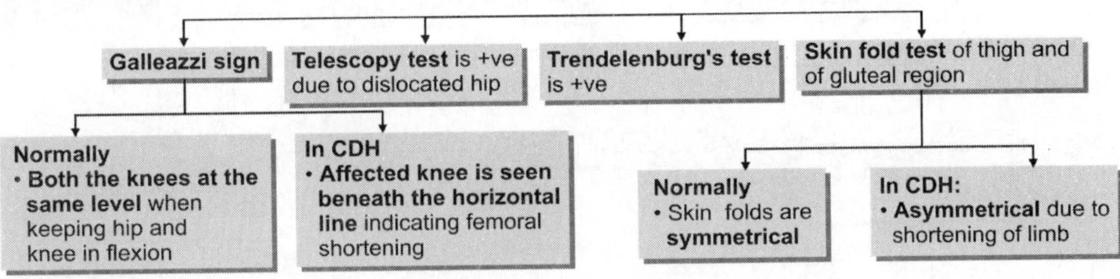

Sonography

Since the head of the femur is visible only after a year, it is better to do an ultrasonography to see the position of the head in neonates.

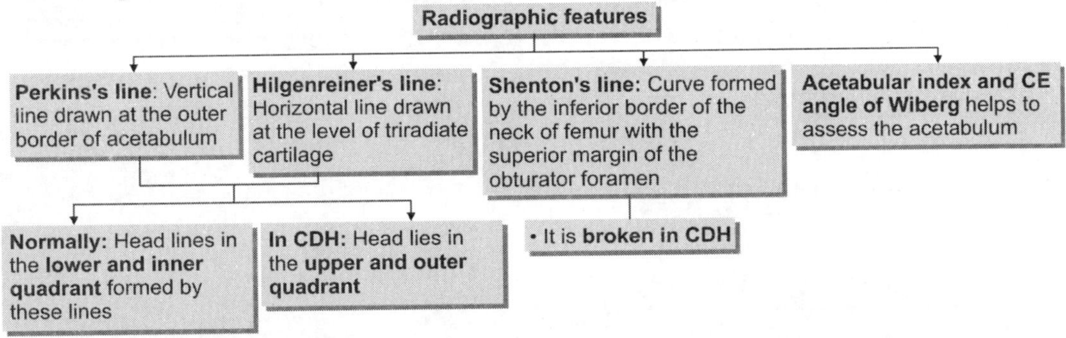

Other Features

Ossific nucleus usually Present in normal hip by 4–6 months while it is small and show delayed appearance in dysplastic hip

Treatment

Treatment of congenital dysplasia of the hip or DDH is age related

Dislocated Hip in Patient Aged 6–18 Months

Treatment of DDH in children aged 6–18 months is shown schematically below.

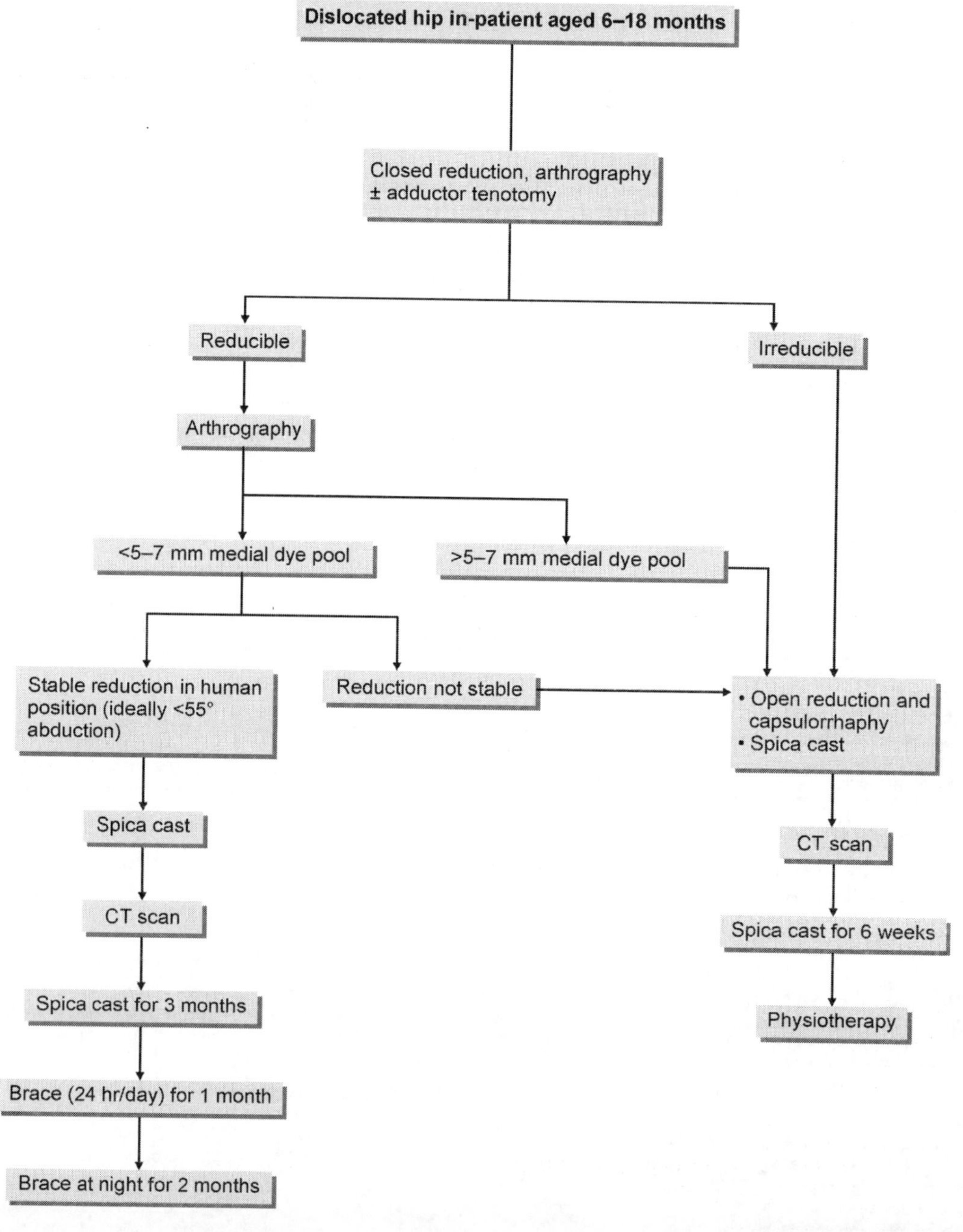

Dislocated Hip in Patient Aged 18–48 Months

Treatment of DDH in children aged 18–48 months show schematically below.

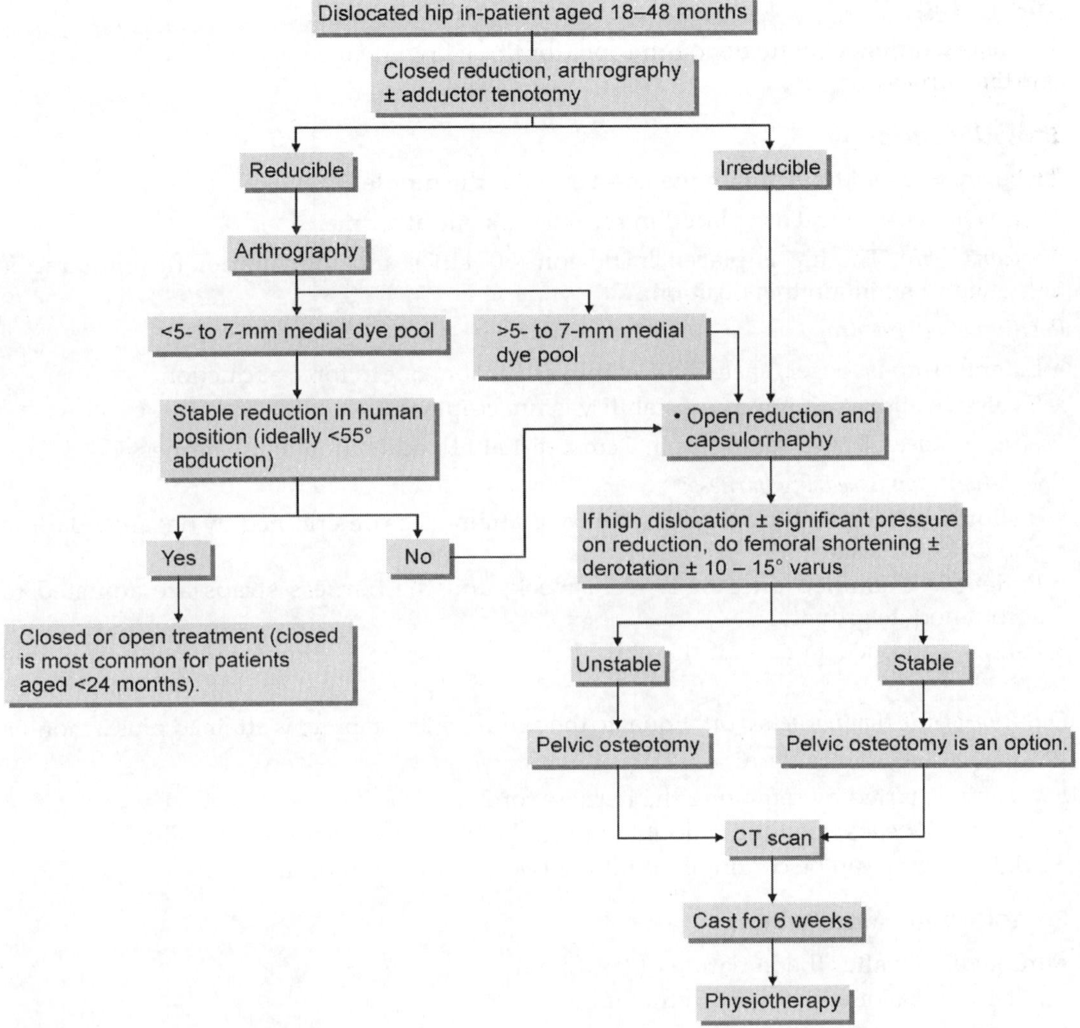

In short

Neonates

- In children > 6 months of age, closed reduction of a dislocated hip can usually be achieved by use of the Pavlik harness. *Pavlik harnesses* keep the hip in abduction.
- Double diapers/von Rosen's splint

Pavlik Harness

It is a *dynamic flexion-abduction* orthosis

Component of Pavlik harness are:
- Chest strap
- Two shoulder straps
- *Two stirrups*: Each stirrup has an anteromedial flexion strap and a posterolateral abduction strap.

Position

Harness is applied with the child supine and in a comfortable undershirt.

Chest Strap

It is fastened first, allowing enough room for three fingers to be placed between the chest and the harness.

Shoulder Straps

These are buckled to maintain the chest strap at the nipple line.

Position of feet: The feet are placed in the stirrups one at a time.

Position of hip: The hip is placed in flexion (90–110°), and the anterior flexion strap is tightened to maintain this position.

Position of lateral strap:

- Lateral strap is loosely fastened to limit adduction, not to force abduction.
- Excessive abduction to ensure stability is unacceptable.

Position of knees: Knees should be 3–5 cm apart at full adduction in the harness

Precautions while wearing harness:

- It should be worn full-time until stability is attained, as determined by negative Barlow and Ortolani tests.
- Patient is examined once or twice a week, and the harness straps are adjusted to accommodate growth.
- Family is trained in care of the child in the harness, including *bathing, diapering, and dressing*

Duration of full-time harness wear: Equal to the age at which stability is attained plus 2 months

Weaning of harness:

- Weaning started by removing the harness for 2 hours each day.
- Every 2–4 weeks this time is doubled until the device is worn only at night.
- Night bracing can be continued until the hip is normal radiographically

Radiographic Monitoring

- Immediately after the initiation of treatment
- After any major adjustment in the harness
- 1 month after weaning begins
- At 6 months old
- At 1-year-old

6 Months

- Abduction hip spica (*human position*: spica cast is applied with the hip joint in 95° of flexion and 40–45° of abduction; this position is best for maintaining hip stability and minimizing the risk of osteonecrosis)
- Splint
- Frejka pillow

12 Months

- Traction, closed reduction, arthrography ± adductor tenotomy followed by hip spica.

3 years

With neck in valgus and anteversion requires a *femoral varus derotation osteotomy*

5 years

- Femoral osteotomy or Salter's innominate
- To provide an acetabular roof:
  - By Pemberton pericapsular (Shelf) osteotomy
  - By Chiari's pelvic osteotomy

In General

Indication for open reduction: It is indicated for any hip in which a *concentric, stable reduction* cannot be achieved by closed means

Criteria for open reduction:

- Hip stable in neutral position—*no osteotomy*
- Hip stable in flexion and abduction—*innominate osteotomy*
- Hip stable in internal rotation and abduction—*proximal femoral derotational varus osteotomy*
- "Double-diameter" acetabulum with anterolateral deficiency—*Pemberton-type osteotomy*

Recommended Osteotomies for Congenital or Developmental Dislocation of the Hip:

Osteotomy	Age	Indications
• Salter innominate osteotomy	18 months–6 years	Congruous hip reduction <10–15° correction of acetabular index required
• Pemberton acetabuloplasty	18 months–10 years	>10–15° correction of acetabular index required small femoral head, large acetabulum
• Steel or Ganz osteotomy	Late adolescence to skeletal maturity	Residual acetabular dysplasia symptoms; congruous joint
• Shelf procedure or Chiari osteotomy	Adolescence to skeletal maturity	Incongruous joint symptom other osteotomy not possible

Complications

- Chronic dislocations
- Osteonecrosis of the femoral head (most devastating)
- Osteoarthritis

Q8. Write short note on Sprengel's shoulder.

This is a failure of the descent of the scapula from the neck downward during the development, it may be associated with Klippel-Feil syndrome *(the fusion of cervical vertebrae with a short neck and low hair line)*.

Incidence

- *Sprengel's deformity* is the most common congenital malformation of the shoulder girdle.
- The condition is sporadic. Rarely, it may run in families (autosomal dominant pattern of inheritance)
- The male-to-female ratio is 3:1.

Gross Pathology

Scapula

- The scapula is dysplastic
- It is located higher than normal in the neck or upper thoracic region
- Inferior angle is rotated medially, causing the glenoid to face inferiorly

Omovertebral Connection

- An omovertebral connection, which may be fibrous, cartilaginous, or bony, may exist in about one third of cases
- Usually unilateral
- It attaches the superomedial angle of the scapula to the spinous process, lamina, or transverse process of the cervical vertebrae and it may be the prime cause of limited shoulder motion in patients with a Sprengel's deformity

Periscapular Muscles

- The spino-scapular muscles may be fibrotic and contracted
- the trapezius muscle is most commonly affected

Condition Associated with Sprengel's Shoulder

- Klippel-Feil syndrome (most common)
- Greig syndrome
- Poland syndrome
- VATER association (i.e. vertebral defects, imperforate anus, tracheoesophageal fistula, and radial and renal dysplasia)
- Velocardiofacial syndrome
- Floating-harbor syndrome
- Goldenhar syndrome
- X-linked dominant hydrocephalus, skeletal anomalies, and mental disturbance syndrome

Cavendish Grades

Based on the severity of the condition, a Sprengel's deformity can be classified as follows.
- **Grade 1:**
  - The deformity is very mild.
  - The shoulders are almost level, and the deformity cannot be appreciated with the clothes on.
- **Grade 2:**
  - The deformity is mild.
  - The shoulders are almost level, but the superomedial portion of the high scapula is visible as a lump.
- **Grade 3:**
  - The deformity is moderate.
  - It is visible, and the affected shoulder is elevated 2–5 cm higher than the opposite shoulder.
- **Grade 4:**
- The deformity is severe.
- The scapula is very high, with the superomedial angle at the occiput, with neck webbing and brevicollis

Presentation

- Shoulder asymmetry
- Restriction of shoulder abduction
- On examination:
  - The affected scapula usually is adducted and elevated 2–10 cm, and its inferior pole is rotated medially
  - A prominence in the suprascapular region due to upwardly rotated superomedial angle of the scapula
  - Scapula is hypoplastic.
  - The length of the vertebral border is decreased.
  - Scapulothoracic movements may be severely limited.

Radiographs

- Anteroposterior (AP) view of the chest and both shoulders
- A lateral view of the cervical and thoracic spine to rule out associated spinal anomalies

Treatment

If deformity and impairment are mild, no treatment is indicated.

Non-operative Treatment

- Physical therapy
- Exercises are used:
  - To maintain an individual's range of motion
  - To strengthen the weak periscapular muscles

Surgery

Indications:
- Significant cosmetic concerns
- Significant restriction of shoulder abduction in children age <6 years

Surgical options include:
- Subperiosteal resection of part of the scapula
- Extraperiosteal release
- Transplantation of the muscular origins of the scapula
- Excision of the superomedial portion of the scapula
- Vertical scapular osteotomy
- Morcellization of the Clavicle

Green (Modified Green scapuloplasty) and the Woodward procedures remain the criterion standards for correction of the Sprengel's deformity

Brachial plexus palsy is the most severe complication of surgery for Sprengel's deformity.

Q9. Write short note on: a. Congenital radioulnar synostosis; b. Radial club hand; c. Mirror Hand; d. Congenital vertical talus; e. Spina bifida

a: Congenital Radioulnar Synostosis

Congenital radioulnar synostosis is a bilateral congenital fusion of the superior radioulnar joint.

Synostosis, or osseous union, of any two adjacent bones can involve any part of the upper extremity. Synostosis between the radius and ulna can be congenital and post-traumatic

Congenital Types

Wilkie described two types of *congenital synostosis,* based on the proximal radioulnar junction:
- Type I:
  - Complete synostosis
  - The medullary canals of the radius and ulna are joined.
  - The proximal end of the radius is malformed
  - Proximal end is fused to the ulna for several centimeters
  - Radius is longer and larger than the ulna, and its shaft arches anteriorly more than normally
- Type II:
  - Often is unilateral
  - The radius is fairly normal
  - The fusion is neither as extensive nor as intimate as in the first type
  - Its proximal end is dislocated either anteriorly or posteriorly.
  - Proximal end is fused to the proximal ulnar shaft.
  - Sometimes another deformity, such as a supernumerary thumb, absence of the thumb, or syndactylism, also is present.

Cleary and Omer

Divide into four different types:
- Fibrous synostosis
- Bony synostosis
- Associated posterior dislocation of the radius
- Associated anterior dislocation of the radius

Associated Conditions

About 1/3 of cases are associated with general skeletal abnormalities, such as:
- Hip dislocation
- Knee anomalies
- Clubfoot
- Polydactyly
- Syndactyly
- Madelung deformity
- Ligamentous laxity
- Thumb hypoplasia
- Carpal coalition
- Problems of the cardiac, renal, neurologic, and GI systems

Post-traumatic Radioulnar Synostosis

Most common cause of post-traumatic radioulnar synostosis is an operatively treated forearm fracture.

It could be based on location:
- Type 1: Least common; occurs in the distal forearm
- Type 2: Occurs in the mid-forearm
- Type 3: Occurs in the proximal forearm

Salient Features

- It is more often bilateral than unilateral.
- Familial predisposition is frequent.
- It usually involves the proximal ends of the radius and ulna.
- It is most often fixing the forearm in pronation.
- The child is being unable to supinate the forearm.
- An abnormal carrying angle of the elbow or a shortening of the forearm may be observed.

Radiograph

Standard AP and lateral view of elbow, forearm and wrist joint are essential.

Treatment

Problems in treatment:
- Fascial tissues are short and their fibres are abnormally directed.
- The interosseous membrane is narrow.
- The supinator muscles may be abnormal or absent.
- Widespread anomalies.

Osteotomy

- Treatment is restricted to osteotomy so as to place the forearm in functional position.
- Derotation osteotomy of the radius can be tried.
- Percutaneous drill-assisted osteotomies (Lin et al.) followed by manipulation of the forearm into the desired functional position.

b: Radial Club Hand

Radial aplasia or radial club hand is congenital absence of part or whole of the radius and thumb leading to deviation of the wrist outwards with curved overgrown ulna and subluxated wrist. The muscles on the radial side may be absent.

Incidence

- It occurs in 1/100,000 live births
- It is bilateral in 50% of children affected

Classification

- Type 1: Short radius
- Type 2: Hypoplastic radius (radius growth substantially retarded)
- Type 3: Partial absence of the radius (miniature radius)
- Type 4: Completely absent radius (most common)

Associated Anomalies

- The condition is frequently associated with thumb hypoplasia or complete thumb absence.

- In types 2–4: Hypoplastic or absent radial-sided structures including:
  - Radial artery
  - Flexor carpi radialis tendon or the radial wrist extensors

Other Conditions

- Holt-Oram syndrome
- TAR syndrome (thrombocytopenia absent radius)
- VATER (vertebral defects, anal atresia, tracheoesophageal atresia, esophageal atresia, and renal defects)
- Fanconi's anaemia

Treatment

Two staged treatment:
- First is correction of the soft tissue contractures by JESS distracters, or by ring external fixator application.
- Second stage consists of centralization of the carpus on the ulna with pin stabilization and few cases require ulnar osteotomy.

Contraindications to Surgical Correction

- Poor general health
- Severely compromised overall functional ability
- Ipsilateral elbow extension contracture. In cases of the elbow extension contracture, the radial club hand allows the patient to reach the mouth.

c. Mirror Hand

Mirror hand or ulnar dimelia is the rarest congenital anomaly characterized by symmetric duplication of the upper limb in the midline. There is absence of the radius, duplication of the ulna, and polydactyly with 7–8 digits in mirrored symmetry about the middle finger.

Aetiology

Replication of zone of polarizing activity (ZPA) signaling center.

Types

There are two types of ulnar dimelia:
- Type I: Characterized by duplication of ulna, presence of 5 proximal carpal bones (*2 triquetral, 2 pisiform and 1 lunate*) and 5 distal carpal bones (*2 hamate, 2 capitate and 1 trapezoid*) one index finger in the middle and three other fingers (M, R and L) on both side of index
- Type II: Differs from the type I in presence of 2 lunate and 2 trapezoid bones in wrist as well as 2 index fingers in the hand.

Features

- Skeletal malformation
- Arterial anomalies as an absence of the radial artery, duplication of the ulnar artery, presence of abnormal arterial arches in the hand
- Nervous anomalies shortening of radial nerve, duplication of ulnar nerve

Management

- *Aim*: To achieve a functional and aesthetic upper limb
- Involve a number of complex and multiple surgeries.
- The treatment is designed to reduce the number of digits to four
- Reconstruct a thumb from one of the most functional radial digit

d. Congenital Vertical Talus

Congenital vertical talus, congenital rigid flatfoot or rocker-bottom flatfoot, commonly seen in infants and children. It must be distinguished from flexible pes planus.

Associations

It is associated with numerous neuromuscular disorders, such as:
- Arthrogryposis
- Myelomeningocele

Clinical Finding

- It can be detected at birth by the presence of a rounded prominence of the medial and plantar surfaces of the foot produced by the abnormal position of the head of the talus.
- The talus is almost vertical.
- Calcaneus is in an equinus position although to a lesser degree.
- Forefoot is dorsiflexed at the midtarsal joints
- Navicular lies on the dorsal aspect of the head of the talus
- Sole is convex
- There are deep creases on the dorsolateral aspect of the foot anterior and inferior to the lateral malleolus
- As the weight bearing begun adaptive changes occurs; talus becomes shaped like an hourglass, calcaneus remains in an equinus
- Callosities develop along the medial border of the foot superficial to the head of the talus and beneath the anterior end of the calcaneus
- There occur contraction of Capsules, ligaments, and tendons on the dorsum of the foot.
- The posterior tibial and peroneus longus and brevis tendons act as dorsiflexors rather than plantar flexors as they come to lie anterior to the malleoli.

Radiographs

Routine radiographs should include AP and plantar flexion lateral views (for confirming the diagnosis of congenital vertical talus)

Treatment

- It is difficult to correct Congenital vertical talus
- It has tendency to recur
- For a young child (1–4 years) with a *mild or moderate deformity*: Open reduction and Realignment of Talonavicular and subtalar Joints.
- *Children 4–8 years old* can be treated by open reduction and soft-tissue procedures combined with extra-articular subtalar arthrodesis
- For an older child with a *more severe or a recurrent deformity*, open reduction and a Grice extra-articular subtalar fusion.
- For a *child 12 years old or older* with functional symptoms, a triple arthrodesis is preferred.

e. Spina Bifida

Spectrum of conditions develops due to *failure of fusion of the posterior part of the spine* resulting in a defect through which *membranes and even the spinal cord herniate.*
Most common site: lumbosacral region

Varieties

Spina bifida occulta:
- Defect in the posterior vertebral elements that includes the spinous process and often part of the lamina
- Most commonly affects the fifth lumbar and first sacral vertebrae
- Usually asymptomatic and is often an incidental finding on X-rays
- Seen in ~10% of adult spines
- Rarely associated with any neurological involvement
- Detected by presence of dimple, tuft of hairs, dilated vessels or a naevolipoma

Meningocele:
- Cystic distention of the meninges through unfused vertebral arches
- Spinal cord remains in the vertebral canal
- Most lesions are posterior
- It contains only CSF.

Meningomyelocele

- Most common
- Protrusion of dura and arachnoid through the deficit in the vertebral arches.
- Cord and nerve roots are carried out through this defect in the vertebral arches
- Most commonly in the lower thoracic and lumbosacral regions
- Skin over a myelomeningocele is almost always absent
- Neurological deficits
- Dark shadow of cord or nerves on transillumination
- Rachischisis: nerve roots exposed outside
- Diastematomyelia: cord is bifurcated by bone projecting backwards from vertebral body.

Syringomyelocele

- Rarest type
- Central canal of the spinal cord is dilated
- Cord lies within the sac
- Asomia: agenesis of vertebral body

Myelocele

- Central canal of the cord opens on the surface and discharges CSF continuously
- Neurological deficits like paralytic deformities of foot and incontinence of urine and feces are always associated with it.

Management

Multidisciplinary approach/team effort by:
- Counselor
- Neurosurgeon

- Neurophysician
- Orthopaedician
- Urologist
- Paediatrician
- Physiotherapist
- Orthotist.

Important Facts

- Splints: Prevent soft tissue contractures and maintain correction.
- Orthotic treatment is aimed at obtaining effective mobility with minimal restriction.
- Paralysis may require permanent splintage in a caliper, and crutch walking for life.
- Scoliosis is common and is treated in a brace until the child is old enough for fusion.
- Kyphosis: if severe; require localized vertebral resection and arthrodesis.
- Muscles imbalance: Maintain by tendon transfer
- Joint deformities:
- Corrected by: Gentle physiotherapy
- Splintage with lightweight orthosis
- Corrective osteotomies (if required).

Q10. Write short note on: a. Achondroplasia, b. Enumerate types of Mucopoly-saccharidosis, c. Chondro-osteodystrophy, d. Hurler's Disease

a. Achondroplasia

Achondroplasia (Dwarfism): Achondroplasia is the most common type of short-limbed (disproportionate short stature) dwarfism. The word achondroplasia literally means *"without cartilage formation.* It occurs in 1:26,000–1:28,000 live births. It is inherited as autosomal dominant trait, although most cases are sporadic and due to new *fibroblast growth factor receptor 3 (FGFR 3)*, inhibit chondrocytes proliferation in the growth plate. The abnormal proliferation at the growth plate leaving other areas relatively unaffected in the tubular bones, causes production of short bones that are proportionately thick (*these children are often seen as jokers in the circus*).

Clinical Features

Features that may be seen at any age:
- Disproportionate short stature
- Macrocephaly with frontal bossing
- Midface retrusion and depressed nasal bridge
- Rhizomelic (proximal) shortening of the arms with redundant skin folds on limbs
- Limitation of elbow extension
- Brachydactyly
- Trident configuration of the hands (*trident hand*)
- Genu varum (bowlegs)
- Thoracolumbar kyphosis (principally in infancy)
- Exaggerated lumbar lordosis, which develops when walking begins.
- The length of spine is almost always normal.

- Those who survive infancy usually have normal sexual and mental development and life span may be normal.
- Spinal deformity (Spinal stenosis) nevertheless may lead to a cord compression and nerve root encroachment.
- Obstructive sleep apnoea is common.
- Middle ear dysfunction is frequently a problem (conductive hearing loss).

Radiographic Findings

- Short, robust tubular bones
- Narrowing of the interpedicular distance of the caudal spine
- Square ilia and horizontal acetabula
- Narrow sacrosciatic notch
- Proximal femoral radiolucency
- Mild, generalized metaphyseal changes.

Diagnosis

Usually on basis of clinical and radiographic features. Molecular confirmations do not require, but it may aid in receiving new treatment.

Treatment

Currently there is no treatment for achondroplasia, it is usually symptomatic. Certain aspects of the condition can be corrected with orthotics, bracing, physical therapy or surgery.

b. Types of Mucopolysaccharidosis (MPS)

Abnormal metabolism of glycosaminoglycans (GAGs) due to inherent deficiency of lysosomal degradation enzymes leads to their intracellular and extracellular accumulation in various tissues of the body. These are multi-systemic disease and inherited as an autosomal recessive trait except type II, the Hunter's syndrome, which has an X-linked inheritance.

Various Types of MPS

- MPS 1 H/S (Hurler/Scheie syndrome): deficiency of an enzyme, *alpha-L-iduronidase*
- MPS I H (Hurler disease): deficiency of an enzyme, *alpha-L-iduronidase*
- MPS I S (Scheie syndrome): deficiency of an enzyme, *alpha-L-iduronidase*
- MPS II (Hunter syndrome): due to the deficiency of enzyme *iduronate-2-sulfatase*
- MPS III A, B, C, and D (Sanfillipo syndrome): Involves multiple enzyme deficiencies involving *heparan-N-sulfatase (IIIA), α-N-acetylglucosaminidase (IIIB), α-glucosaminide acetyltransferase (IIIC), and N-acetylglucosamine-6-sulfatase (IIID)*
- MPS IV A and B (Morquio syndrome): *Type IVA* occurs due to deficiency of *N-acetylgalactosamine-6-sulfatase* (accumulation of keratan sulfate and chondroitin-6-sulfate) and *Type IVB* which occurs due to the *deficiency of β-galactosidase enzyme* (accumulation of keratan sulfate)
- MPS VI (Maroteaux-Lamy syndrome): deficiency of the enzyme *N-acetylgalactosamine-4-sulfatase*
- MPS VII (Sly syndrome): Due to β-galactosidase deficiency
- MPS IX: due to hyaluronidase deficiency

c. Chondro-osteodystrophy

It is a type of *Mucopolysaccharidosis type IV (MPS IV)* also known as **Morquio-Brailsford disease** and is a hereditary dysplasia of growing bones due to excessive storage of *mucopolysaccharides* in which there is a defect in degradation of glycosaminoglycans, is inherited as an autosomal recession trait. There is deficiency of major enzyme *galactose-6-sulfatase*, which leads to imperfect processing of and leads to *abnormal deposition of keratin sulfate in tissues, distorting upper airways.* There is defective maturation of chondroblast of the epiphyseal plate leading to broadening and fragmentation of the epiphyseal zone of the spine and limbs leading to **dwarfism.**

Clinical Features

The child is mentally normal and physically healthy but suffers from severe skeletal defects:
- Short stature
- Short neck
- Large head
- Sunken eyes (with corneal opacities)
- Angulated chest (*a marked manubriosternal angle almost 90° is pathognomonic*)
- Prominent mandible and lower face
- Spine with ligament laxity
- Atlanto-axial instability with risk of quadriparesis
- Knock-knee
- Flat feet
- Spinal kypho-scoliosis
- Kyphosis

Radiographic Findings

- Odontoid hypoplasia
- The vertebral bodies are flattened, tongue shaped, best seen in the mid-thoracic area (*platyspondyly*).
- The femoral epiphyseal shows flattening and fragmentation with deformed acetabulum (acetabular dysplasia).
- Goblet shaped flared iliac wings, increased acetabular angles
- Bilateral hip coxa vara
- Genu valgum
- Hand shows short metacarpals and wide metacarpals with proximal pointing of index to little finger.

Urine

Urine examination shows excessive excretion of keratan sulfate.

Treatment

- Symptomatic
- Regular neurologic assessment and radiologic imaging
- Surgical stabilization of upper cervical spine before the development of myelopathy is lifesaving.

d. Hurler's Disease:

Hurler syndrome, was formerly known as *gargoylism* is a type of MPS (Type I). It is an inherited lysosomal disorder caused by the ***deficiency of alpha-L-iduronidase***, an enzyme responsible for the degradation of glycosaminoglycans (GAGs or mucopolysaccharides).

It is characterized by *dwarfism, multiple skeletal deformities with mental retardation, corneal opacity and hepatosplenomegaly*. The child has a frog like look due to enlarged head with prominent frontal bones, wide set eyes, broad nose bridge and low set ears. The average age of mortality is 5 years, and nearly all patients die before 10 years of age. The treatment modalities are directed towards treatment of complications.

Q11. Write short note on: a. Osteogenesis imperfecta (Fragilitas ossium), b. Osteopetrosis, c. Fibrous Dysplasia, d. von Recklinghausen's Disease

a. Osteogenesis Imperfecta (Fragilitas Ossium)

This is also known as **'Fragilitas ossium'**.

This is a familial disease characterized by fragile bones due to defective osteoid and failure of maturation of collagen leading to poor, thin cortex, which easily bends and breaks (*bone fragility*).

Major Clinical Features

- Increased bone fragility
- Decreased bone mass
- Blue sclera
- Dentinogenesis imperfecta (normal enamel with dentin abnormality)
- Short stature
- Hearing loss
- Ligament laxity and increased joint mobility
- Easy bruising

Sillence (1981) classify four clinical types of osteogenesis imperfecta:

- Type I (Mildest)
  - The most common variety; over 50% of all cases
  - Autosomal dominant inheritance
  - Fractures usually appear at 1–2 years of age.
  - Healing is reasonably good.
  - Deformities are not marked.
  - Sclerae deep blue
  - Teeth usually normal but some have dentinogenesis imperfecta.
  - Impaired hearing in adults (conductive deafness).
  - Quality of life good; relatively normal life expectancy
- Type II (most severe type)
  - 5–10% of cases
  - Most due to new dominant mutations; some autosomal recessive
  - Extreme bone fragility (accordion femur)
  - Intrauterine and neonatal fractures
  - Large skull and wormian bones.
  - Sclerae grey

- Rib fractures and respiratory difficulty.
- Stillborn or survive for only a few weeks.
- Type III (severe deforming)
  - The 'classic', but not the most common
  - Sporadic, or autosomal recessive inheritance
  - Fractures often present at birth.
  - Large skull and wormian bones; pinched-looking face (triangular facies)
  - Coxa vara, marked deformities and extremely short stature
  - Early onset scoliosis; kypho-scoliosis by 6 years
  - Frontal bossing, basilar invagination
  - Sclerae grey, becoming white
  - Dentinogenesis imperfecta
  - Marked joint laxity
  - Respiratory problems
  - Poor quality of life; few survive to adulthood.
- Type IV (moderately severe)
  - Uncommon(< 5 %)
  - Autosomal dominant inheritance
  - Frequent fractures during early childhood
  - Deformities common.
  - Sclerae pale blue or normal.
  - Dentinogenesis imperfecta.
  - Survive to adulthood with fairly good function.

Cole further added types V to XI to the original Sillence classification (type V with autosomal dominant and types VI to XI with autosomal recessive transmissions)

Looser et al.: Classified osteogenesis imperfecta (OI) into two types: *OI congenita* (presence of numerous fractures at birth); and *OI tarda* (fractures occur after perinatal period)

Diagnosis: Based on:
- Clinical (*most common bone fragility*) and family history
- Bone mineral density (lumbar vertebra)
- Bone biochemistry and radiographic features

Treatment:
- General measures to prevent recurrent trauma, maintain movement and promote social adaptation are very significant.
- Children with severe osteogenesis imperfecta may be treated medically with cyclical bisphosphonates to improve bone mineral density and lessen the tendency to fracture.

Treatment of orthopaedics problems: This is aimed at prevention of fractures and correction of deformities. Correction of gross deformities of long bones is done:

Infants and children:
- Closed osteo-clasis without intramedullary fixation
- Closed osteo-clasis with percutaneous intramedullary fixation
- Open osteotomy with internal fixation (*Sofield and Millar procedure*): Rush nail, Williams rod

Young adult patient: External fixation with ring or uni-planar constructs with osteotomy.

Prophylactic intramedullary rod:
- For children who repeatedly fracture their long bones.

- Different types of rods according to bone size and skeletal maturity:
- Osteotomy and fixation with telescoping rod: (Sheffield rod, Fassier-Duval rod, Bailey-Dubow rod,)
- Osteotomy and fixation with a non-telescoping rod (K-wire, Steinmann pin, Williams rod, fixed-length rods)

Orthotic devices: Walking aids, orthosis, wheelchairs

Physical therapy (PT): Aims to increase strength, flexibility and range of motion

b. Osteopetrosis

Osteopetrosis, derived from the Greek words for *'bone' (osteo) and 'stone' (Petros)*. It is also known as *'**Marble bone disease**'* or *'**Albers-Schoenberg's disease**'*. This is characterized by sclerosis and thickening of bones. This occurs due to imbalance between the bone formation and resorption.

Reduced osteoclastic bone resorption results in a high bone mass that appears with increased radiographic density. The bone appears *hard, chalky and brittle*. The medulla is also obliterated leading to *aplastic anaemia (myelophisthic anaemia) with hepatosplenomegaly*.

The disturbance of normal bone modeling and remodeling can leads to skeletal deformity and dental abnormalities and can interfere with mineral homeostasis. The child is brought with *pathological fracture* of brittle bones or *neuropathy* due to osteosclerosis of optic and cranial nerve foramina leading to *blindness* and *deafness*.

Osteopetrosis Tarda

- Common, benign form
- Autosomal dominant disorder
- Usually *pathological fracture* is the presenting feature or detected when an X-ray is taken for other reasons—hence the term *tarda*
- *Blindness* and *deafness (due to bone encroachment on foramina)*
- Prone to bone infection (*Mandible*)
- *X-rays:* Increased density of all bones (*bone-within-bone* or *endobones*); Vertebrae: Uniformly dense or take on a *"sandwich vertebrae"* or *"rugger-jersey"* appearance (when a normal-appearing vertebral mid-body is sandwiched between dense bands along the superior and inferior endplates). *Erlenmeyer flask bone deformity. If periosteal reaction appears as flowing down of molten wax from a candle then it is known as **melorheostosis**.*
- Treatment: only if complications occur.

Osteopetrosis Congenita

- Rare, autosomal recessive form
- Causes severe disability
- Bone encroachment on marrow results in *pancytopenia, haemolysis, anaemia and hepato-splenomegaly*.
- Foraminal occlusion due to bone encroachment may lead to optic or facial nerve palsy *(compressive neuropathies)*.
- *Osteomyelitis* following, for example, tooths extraction or internal fixation of a fracture is quite common.
- Repeated haemorrhage or infection usually leads to death in early childhood
- Treatment: bone-marrow transplantation form normal donor, long-term treatment by *interferon gamma*

c. Fibrous Dysplasia

First described by von Recklinghausen in 1891, *fibrous dysplasia* is a developmental skeletal disorder defect characterized by thinning of the cortex and replacement of the marrow with fibro-osseous tissue that demonstrates characteristic ground-glass appearance on X-rays. The underlying defect in fibrous dysplasia is a mutation of the *GNAS1 gene. Pain, fracture and deformity* are common clinical features.

Sites most commonly involved: The skull base and proximal metaphysic of femora.

Types

Fibrous dysplasia presents in monostotic and polyostotic forms:

Monostotic:
- Common (70–85% of cases) and affects one bone
- Manifests later in life usually between 20 and 30 years of age
- Most commonly affects: Femur or the ribs
- Mostly the lesions are asymptomatic and found incidentally on imaging

Polyostotic:
- Less common and affects several bones
- Manifests earlier, usually in children <10 years; has a more serious prognosis
- Frequently affects: Maxilla or other craniofacial bones, ribs, femur, or tibia
- 3% of polyostotic cases are associated with **cafe-au-lait spots** (*cutaneous pigmentation; jagged, irregular borders (Coast of Maine)*) and a *hyper-functional endocrine state* characteristic of **McCune-Albright syndrome**. This is more common in females than males (10:1) and more likely to cause *precocious puberty* in girls. Malignant transformation occur 5% of patients with *Albright's syndrome.*

Craniofacial FD

- Involvement of multiple bones in the craniofacial skeleton
- 90% of these presenting before the age of 5 years

Mazabraud syndrome is the combination of fibrous dysplasia with intramuscular myxoma.

Malignant Transformation

- Rarely, about 0.4–4%.
- Usually in polyostotic disease and Mazabraud's syndrome
- Most common histological types: *Osteosarcoma, fibrosarcoma* and *chondrosarcoma.*

X-ray

It shows a corticomedullary destruction, which is *ground glass in appearance* and causes thinning and expansion of the cortex with a *multilocular appearance*. It may produce bending of the bone (the weight bearing bone may be bent; and one of the classic feature is the 'shepherd's crook' deformity of proximal femur) and *pathological fracture*. Radio-scintigraphy shows marked activity in the lesion

Laboratory test: It shows normal serum calcium which differentiates it from hyperparathyroidism.

Treatment

- Treatment is usually required when patients present with pain and pathological fractures.
- Bisphosphonates were postulated to inhibit osteoclastic resorption.

- Deformities: requires corrective osteotomy
- Surgical treatment is directed towards curettage of the cavity and cancellous bone grafting.
- For very large lesions, the grafts can be supplemented by methylmethacrylate cement (PMMA).

d. von Recklinghausen's Disease (Multiple Neurofibromatosis)

Neurofibromatosis type 1, also known as von Recklinghausen's disease, is a neurodermal dysplasia. This is a rare genetic disorder characterized by *multiple fibromatosis* along the cutaneous nerves with *scoliosis, café-au-lait spots with skin nodules* and occasional *hypertrophy of one limb* with strange skeletal disturbances of growth, and *Pseudoarthrosis of tibia* (Rule out other causes like congenital defect, fibrous dysplasia and acquired tibia defects following fracture).

Types

Type 1 (NF-1): Also known as *von Recklinghausen's disease*:
- More common
- Incidence ~1 in 3500 live births
- The abnormality is located in the gene which codes for neurofibromin on chromosome 17.
- Transmitted as autosomal dominant, with almost 100% penetrance, but more than 50% of cases are due to new mutation.
- The most characteristic lesions are *neurofibromata (Schwann cell tumours)* and patches of *skin pigmentation (café au lait spots)*
- *Musculoskeletal manifestation* are present in nearly 50% of cases

Type 1 (NF-2):
- Less common
- Incidence of 1 in 50,000 births
- The abnormality is located in the gene which codes for which codes for schwannomin, located on chromosome 22. Transmitted as autosomal dominant
- Intracranial lesions (e.g. acoustic neuromas and meningiomas) are usual.
- Musculoskeletal manifestations are rare.

Clinical Features

- Café-au-lait spots
- Axillary and inguinal freckling
- Optic gliomas
- Lisch nodules (pigmented hamartomas of the iris)
- Spinal and peripheral nerve neurofibromas
- Neurological or cognitive impairment
- Scoliosis (most common skeletal abnormality)
- Abnormalities in the oral and maxillofacial region
- Malignant tumors of the nerve sheath, pheochromocytoma
- Vasculopathy
- Congenital tibial dysplasia and pseudarthrosis

X-ray shows *kyphoscoliotic deformity of tibia* and *nonunion* following fracture (pseudoarthrosis of tibia). Pressure erosion of bone, and sometimes one of the tumours may undergo malignant change.

Treatment

- Excision of painful nodules in the limbs and vertebrae with spinal decompression and fusion for scoliosis
- Pseudoarthrosis of tibia requires excision of fibrous defect and bone grafting as given below:
  - Boyds Dual onlay bone graft.
  - Mac Farland's by-pass bone grafting
- Sofield's osteotomy and rotation of the fibrous defect
- Excision of the nonunion, acute docking of the refreshed site and proximal osteotomy lengthening by Ilizarov apparatus
- Elephantiasis requires soft tissue dissection. These patients are prone to fatal haemorrhage during surgery.

Q12. Write short note on: a. Marfan's syndrome, b. Down syndrome.

a. Marfan's syndrome (Arachnodactyly)

Marfan's syndrome (MFS) is a pleiotropic connective tissue disorder with a reported incidence of 1 in 3000 to 5000 individuals affecting the *skeletal, joint ligaments, eyes* and *cardiovascular structures.* There is a defect of cross-linkage in collagen and elastin. The genetic abnormality has been mapped to the defect is in the *FBN1 gene (encoding fibrillin 1)* on chromosome 15 (15q21.1). It is transmitted as *autosomal dominant* but sporadic cases also occur. Males and females are equally affected.

It is characterized by three clinical criteria (*thoracic aortic aneurysm* and/or *dissection* (TAAD]), *ectopia lentis* (EL), and systemic features [SFs, multisystemic manifestations] with score ≤7) and two genetic criteria (the presence of a first-grade relative with Marfan's syndrome diagnosed according to revised Ghent-2 criteria and presence of a pathogenic mutation in *FBN1 gene* in presence of *TAAD or EL*)

Clinical Features

- Patients are tall, with disproportionately long legs and arms
- Flattening or hollowing of the chest (*pectus excavatum*)
- Upper body segment is shorter than the lower (ratio <0.8 is suggestive) & arm span exceeds height by 5 cm or more.
- Digits are unusually long (*spider finger; arachnodactyly*)
- Scoliosis, spondylolisthesis
- Slipped upper femoral epiphysis
- Generalized joint laxity
- Protrusio acetabuli
- Flat feet
- Dislocation of patella or shoulder
- High arched palate
- Hernias
- Lens dislocation, retinal detachment, cataract, myopia
- Aortic aneurism and mitral or aortic incompetence.

X-rays

Bone structure appears normal but may reveal *scoliosis, spondylolisthesis or slipped epiphysis*.

Diagnosis

- There is no specific laboratory test except for molecular genetic testing for the diagnosis of MFS
- *Marfanoid features* along with *ophthalmic and cardiovascular defects* are diagnostic.

Management

- There is no specific treatment that cures MFS
- Medical therapy with *beta-blockers* and other after load-reducing agents: reducing stress on the aortic valve, mitral valve, and aortic root
- Beta-blockers, noninvasive aortic imaging, and elective aortic root repair: improves the survival rates.
- Patients occasionally need treatment for progressive scoliosis or flat feet. The heart should be carefully checked before operation.

b. Down Syndrome (Trisomy 21)

This is a genetic disorder results from having an *extra copy of chromosome 21*. It is the *most common chromosomal abnormality* occurring in humans. Characteristic features at birth includes head is fore shortened eyes slant upward, prominent epicanthal fold; nose is flattened, lips are parted, tongue protrudes, abnormal palmar creases, clinodactyly, spreading of first and second toes, reduced muscle mass, hypotonicity, increased joint laxity and delayed skeletal development. Children are short with varying degrees of mental retardation and joint laxity. Adults have atlantoaxial instability, cardiac defects, and decreased resistance to infection. *Hypothyroidism* is more common than hyperthyroidism. *Neutrophilic, thrombocytopenia, and polycythemia* are the most common haematological abnormalities. Patients with Down syndrome are 10-time more at risk of developing *leukemia. Atrioventricular septal defect (AVSD)* is the most common cardiac defect and the others are *secundum atrial defect (10%), tetralogy of Fallot (6%)*, and *isolated PDA (4%)*.

Diagnostic Method

Amniocentesis is the most conventional invasive prenatal diagnostic method.

Treatment

- There is no specific treatment but surgery can offer considerable cosmetic improvement.
- *Atlanto axial* fusion is occasionally needed for patients with neurological symptoms.
- Speech therapy, physical therapy and occupational therapy.

12

Metabolic Diseases

Q1. Discuss in brief the aetiology, pathology, clinical and radiological features of scurvy.

Scurvy (scorbutus) is a nutritional disorder resulting from a deficiency of *vitamin C*, which is required for the synthesis of collagen in humans and characterized clinically by *generalized bleeding tendency.*

Importance of Vitamin C

- Three enzymes participate in collagen hydroxylation.
- These reactions add hydroxyl groups to the *amino acids lysine or proline* in the collagen molecule *via lysyl hydroxylase and prolyl hydroxylase,* both requiring *vitamin C* as a cofactor.
- *Hydroxylation* allows the collagen molecule to assume its triple helix structure and making vitamin C essential to the *development and maintenance of scar tissue, blood vessels, and cartilage.*

Aetiology

- Insufficient intake (*ignorance, famine, anorexia, restrictive diets*) of vitamin C (ascorbic acid).
- Artificially fed infants (5–10 years of age).
- Those with poor access to fresh fruit and vegetables, such as remote, *isolated sailors and soldiers.*
- Combination of *scurvy and rickets* is known as *Barton's disease.*
- *Infantile scurvy* is sometimes referred to as *Barlow's disease.*

Clinical Features

Mild forms of scurvy are more common. Adults usually present with pain and tenderness over the bony structures while infant presents with restlessness, irritability, night cries, pseudoparalysis and tenderness over the epiphyseal-metaphyseal region.

Important Features

- Infant is *pale, febrile, irritable and restless.*
- Severe muscle spasm, child is reluctant to move his limb. This involuntary immobilization of limb is termed as *pseudoparalysis.*
- Palpable swellings due to *subperiosteal hemorrhage.*
- Swelling are tender, associated with excruciating pain and are fixed to the bone.
- *Scorbutic rosary*: sharp anterior ends of the bony ribs that protrudes anteriorly due to costochondral separation.

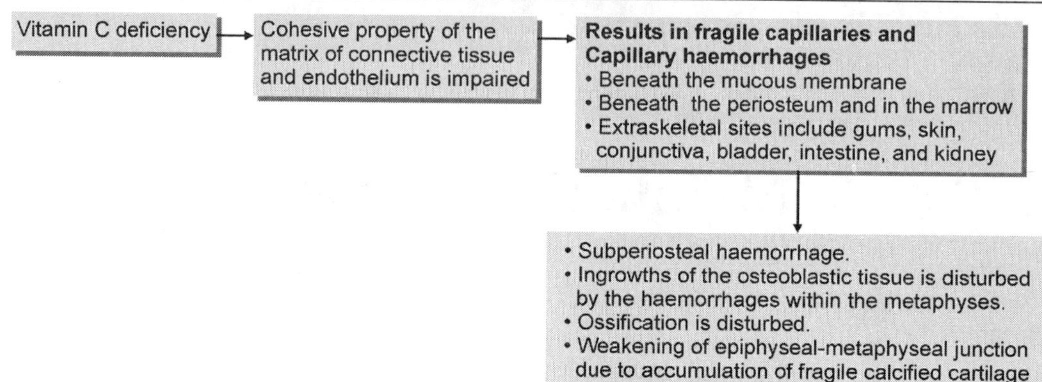

- Epiphyseal fracture/separation often occurs at lower end femur, upper tibia and upper humerus.
- Teeth loosen and gums display a *bluish spongy swelling* commonly around the upper central incisor.
- *Ecchymoses or petechiae* are found in the mucous membrane or skin.
- Sometime there may be *Hematuria* and *haematemesis*.
- There occur *weight loss, anorexia, progressive anaemia, pneumonia, pyrexia* with the worsening of the disease.
- In severe cases, sometime even death may ensue.

Investigations

Laboratory Findings

- Anaemia
- A plasma ascorbate concentration <0.2 mg/dl indicate vitamin C efficiency.
- Leukocyte concentration $<10 \ \mu g/10^8$ WBCs (most sensitive indicator) indicates latent deficiency even in the absence of clinical features.

Roentgenographic Findings

Following features are characteristic:

- *White line of Fraenkel*: Radio-opaque (calcified cartilage) line between the epiphyses and metaphyses.
- *Pelkan spur*: it is a bony spur protruding from the lateral border (occasionally medial) of the metaphyses near its junction with the epiphyses.
- *Scurvy line*: it is zone of radiolucency due to deficient ossification in the metaphyseal region just adjacent to the *white line of Fraenkel.*
- *Wimberger's line*: calcified cartilage accumulates around the bony centrum within the epiphyses itself. This dense ring is termed as *Wimberger's line.*

- Osteoporosis.
- Ground glass appearance.
- Thin cortices.
- Epiphyseal fracture/separations.
- Periosteum is elevated due to subperiosteal haemorrhages (soft tissue shadow), which subsequently ossify.
- Subperiosteal fractures.
- Vertebral and costochondral angulation of the rib.

Treatment

- Essentially conservative.
- Supplementing diet with vitamin C. Good dietary sources of vitamin C include citrus fruits, green vegetables (especially broccoli), tomatoes, and potatoes.
- Vitamin C supplements of 100–200 mg orally or parenterally.
- Processed Milk is prohibited.
- Fractures and painful joints need to be immobilized with splints.

Q2. Write short note on Fluorosis.

In many parts of the country like *Andhra Pradesh (Nellore, Nalgonda), Punjab, Haryana, Karnataka, Kerala and Tamil Nadu* where *fluorine concentration exceeds 3–5 mg/L **fluorosis** is endemic.* It is an important public health problem.

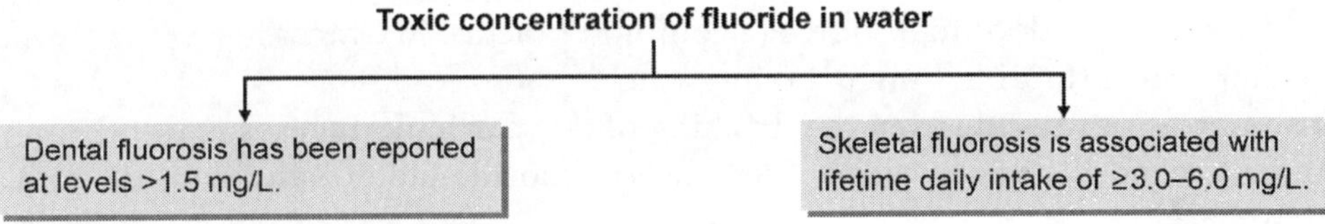

Pathology

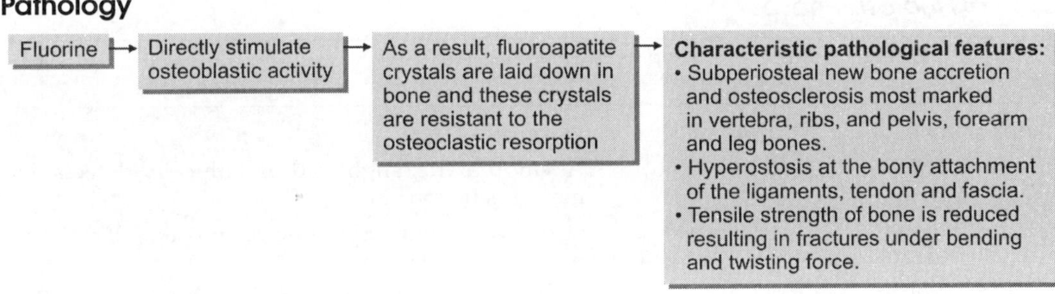

Clinical Features

Dental Fluorosis

- Occurs when excess of fluoride is ingested during the period of tooth calcification (the first seven year of life).
- Observed at a level >1.5 mg/l.
- It is characterized by "mottling" of the dental enamel, which is best seen on the upper incisors. It is usually confined to the permanent teeth and develops only during the years of formation.
- In severe cases, it results in destruction of tooth.

Deans Index

- In 1942, HT Dean's fluorosis index was developed; It is currently the most universally accepted classification system.
- Presence of most severe form of fluorosis on two or more teeth forms the basis of individual's fluorosis score.

Classification	Criteria – description of enamel
Normal	Smooth, glossy, pale creamy-white translucent surface
Questionable	Few white flecks or white spots
Very mild	Small opaque, paper white areas covering less than 25% of the tooth surface
Mild	Opaque white areas covering less than 50% of the tooth surface
Moderate	All tooth surfaces affected; marked wear on biting surfaces; brown stain may be present
Severe	All tooth surfaces affected; discrete or confluent pitting; brown stain present

Skeletal Fluorosis

It is associated with lifetime daily intake of $\geq$3–6 mg/L.

Causes

- Inhalation of fluoride dusts/fumes by workers in industry.
- Use of coal as an indoor fuel source (a common practice in China).
- Consumption of fluoride from drinking water.
- Consumption of fluoride from the drinking of tea, particularly brick tea.
- In India, the most common cause of fluorosis is fluoride-laden water derived from deep bore wells.

Skeletal Fluorosis Phases

Osteosclerotic phase	Ash concentration (mgF/kg)	Symptoms and signs
Normal Bone	500–1,000	Normal
Preclinical Phase	3,500–5,500	Asymptomatic; slight radiographically-detectable increases in bone mass
Clinical Phase I	6,000–7,000	Stiffness of joints; Sporadic pain; osteosclerosis of pelvis and vertebral spine
Clinical Phase II	7,500–9,000	Arthritic symptoms; chronic joint pain; slight calcification of ligaments' increased osteosclerosis and cancellous bones; with/without osteoporosis of long bones
Phase III: Crippling Fluorosis	8,400	Limitation of joint movement; calcification of ligaments of neck vertebral column; crippling deformities of the spine and major joints; neurological defects/ compression of spinal cord; muscle wasting

When a concentration of 10 mg/L is exceeded, crippling fluorosis can ensue. It leads to permanent disability.

In general:

Concentration of fluorine	Manifestation
<1 ppm	Normal
>2 ppm	Dental mottling
>4 ppm	Skeletal fluorosis
>8 ppm	Osteosclerosis
>10 ppm	Growth disturbances

Genu Valgum

- This is a new type of fluorosis *usually seen in people whose staple was sorghum (Jowar) seen in some districts of Andhra Pradesh.*
- Studies showed that fluorides retention is far more when the diet based on sorghum than on rice.
- It is characterized by *genu valgum and osteoporosis.*

Investigations

Laboratory Findings

- Urinary fluorides level of 1.2–10 mg/24 h is indicative of endemic fluorosis.
- Serum fluoride level is elevated in endemic fluorosis.
- Anaemia is usually mild to moderate.
- Serum calcium, phosphorus, magnesium and glucose level remains unchanged.
- Total alkaline phosphatase and parathyroid hormone level may be mildly elevated.

Radiological Findings

- Bone appears chalky white.
- Ill-defined trabecular pattern.
- Dense cortices due to amorphous subperiosteal new bone formation.
- Osteosclerosis, osteophytosis and ossification of ligaments and fascial attachment.
- Calcification of interosseous membrane, para-articular and tendinous insertions.
- Osteophytosis of vertebral canal is the hallmark of the disease (Bamboo spine).

Management

- There is no specific treatment for this condition.
- Use new source of drinking water with lower fluoride content (0.5–0.8 mg/l).
- Chemically defluoridation of water by *Nalgonda technique* (Developed by *NEERI Nagpur*), technique for removing fluoride by addition of two chemicals (lime and alum) in sequence followed by flocculation, sedimentation and filtration.
- In endemic fluorosis, the use of fluoride toothpaste for children up to 6 years of age is not recommended.
- If there is evidence of osteomalacia and secondary hyperparathyroidism, this can be treated with calcium and vitamin D.
- *Magnesium metasilicate (serpentine):* In the doses of 50 mg, bd. ameliorated symptoms subjectively and also decreases the fluoride load. It makes the urine markedly alkaline and this too, facilitates fluoride excretion.
- Future trends: IV magnesium oxide and hydroxide are being evaluated as potential chelators of fluoride.

> **Q3. Discuss aetiology, pathology, clinical features, laboratory and radiological findings and management of rickets.**

Rickets is primarily a childhood disease of malnutrition, characterized by *abnormal mineralization, skeletal deformities, weakness and bone pain.*

It is a disease of *growing bone occurs before the epiphyses closure,* due to lack of *adequate mineralization,* resulting in *unmineralized matrix* at the growth plate.

Aetiology

Vitamin D disorders

- Nutritional deficiency
- Congenital vitamin D deficiency
- Secondary vitamin D deficiency
    - Malabsorption
    - Celiac disease
    - Hepatic osteodystrophy
- Reduced amount of sunlight
- Pigmented skin
- Increased degradation
- Decreases liver 25-hydroxylase
- Vitamin D-dependent type I and II
- CRF

Calcium Deficiencies

Low intake

- Premature infants (rickets of prematurity)
- Reduced dietary intake

Malabsorption

- Primary disease
- Dietary inhibitors of Ca absorption

Phosphorous Deficiency

Inadequate intake

- Prematurity
- Aluminium-containing antacids

Distal RTA (Renal Tubular Acidosis)

Disorders secondary to excess phosphatonin

Renal Loss

- X-linked hypophosphatemic rickets
- Autosomal dominant hypophosphatemic rickets
- Hereditary hypophosphatemic rickets with calciuria
- Fanconi syndrome

- Dent disease
- Overproduction of phosphatonin
  - Epidermal nevus syndrome
  - McCune-Albright syndrome
  - Neurofibromatosis
  - Tumour induced

Miscellaneous

- Anticonvulsant drugs (phenytoin, barbiturates)
- Hypophosphataemia

Metabolic Abnormality

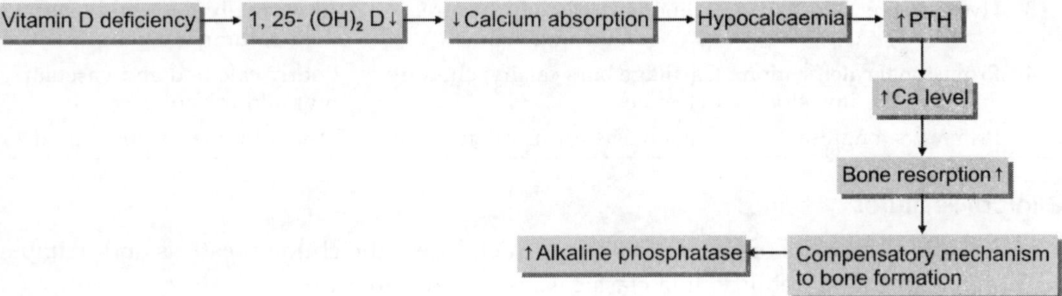

Pathology

Pommer in 1885 observed changes in the growth plate and described four distinct zones: During endochondral ossification, four distinct zones (From the epiphyses to diaphyses) seen at the light-microscope level are:

- *Zone of resting cartilage:* This zone contains normal, resting hyaline cartilage. The chondrocytes are of moderate size and are scattered throughout the intercellular space.
- *Zone of proliferation:* Consists of thin or wedge shapes cells stacked in column. In this zone, chondrocytes undergo rapid mitosis, forming distinctive looking stacks.
- *Zone of maturation / hypertrophy:* chondrocytes are still arranged in columns. It is during this zone that the chondrocytes undergo hypertrophy. Chondrocytes contain large amounts of glycogen and begin to secrete alkaline phosphatase.
- *Zone of calcification:* In this zone, chondrocytes are either dying or dead, leaving cavities that will invaded by osteoblastic cells.

Basic pathology: *unmineralized matrix or osteoid tissue* (calcium and phosphorus salt fails to deposit)

In active stage of disease:

- The orderly progression of the *enchondral ossification becomes irregular and interrupted.*
- Proliferation of the cartilage cells, palisade arrangement and formation of matrix proceeds in a normal manner but the *calcification is deficient (inadequate mineralization).*
- The cartilage cell columns proliferate 10–20 times the normal depth but in haphazard manner.
- In the metaphyses, thick layers of osteoid are laid down.
- Poor mineralization of the zone of calcification.

In the healed phase:
- Calcium salts are deposited in the zone of provisional calcification.
- Capillaries pass into the columns of proliferating chondrocytes and lay down the osteoid about the calcified cartilage.
- The osteoid promptly becomes calcified and is transformed to bone.

Histological Changes in Rickets

S. no.	Zones	Normal	Rickets
1.	Resting zone	Normal	Normal
2.	Proliferation	Active cell division, cells arranged in columns	Normal
3.	Hypertrophy	Ballooned cells which store glycogen arrangement	Abnormally thick and loose their columnar arrangement
4.	Provisional calcification and vascular invasion	Cartilage bars calcify, chondro cytes die	Poorly calcified and vascular invasion irregular
5.	Primary spongiosa	Osteoblasts forms calcified bone	Osteoid remains uncalcified

Clinical Features

It occurs after 6 months of life up to 3 years in children, the child is restless and irritable with signs of general debility. In a classical case the findings are:

General

- Failure to thrive
- Listlessness
- Protruding abdomen (Pot belly)
- Proximal muscle weakness
- Fractures

Head

- *Caput quadratum*: Frontal and parietal eminences with flat occiput and vertex leading to large head.
- *Craniotabes*: softening of the cranial bones; soft and compressible, sensation is similar to the feel of pressing into a ping-pong ball. It is the earliest manifestation.
- Frontal bossing
- Delayed fontanelle closure
- Delayed dentition caries
- Craniosynostosis

Chest

- *Rachitic rosary*: Widening of costochondral junctions results in *Rachitic rosary*.
- *Harrison groove or sulcus*: Horizontal depression along the lower anterior chest due to pulling of the softened ribs by the diaphragm during inspiration.
- *Pigeon chest*: Chest is narrow in transverse section and elongated in AP with angled manubrium sterni.

- Respiratory infections
- Atelectasis

Back

- Scoliosis
- Kyphosis
- Lordosis

Extremities

- Enlargement of wrists and ankles (due to widening of the growth plate).
- Valgus or varus deformities (Genu valgum or knock-knees; Genu varum or Bowlegs).
- Windswept deformity or tackle deformity (combination of valgus deformity in one leg with varus deformity of the other leg).
- Anterior bowing of the femur and tibia.
- Coxa vara with waddling gait with secondary ligamentous laxity.
- Leg pain.

Hypocalcemic Symptoms

- Tetany
- Seizures
- Stridor due to laryngeal spasm.

Miscellaneous

- Delayed dentition
- Delayed walking (poor tone of muscles)
- Skin pallor (Secondary anaemia)

Diagnosis and Investigations

Majority are diagnosed based on characteristic features on radiograph. It is further supported by history, examination and laboratory findings.

Laboratory Findings

Condition	Calcium	Phosphorus	PTH	$1,25-(OH)_2D$	Alkaline phosphatase	Urine calcium	Urine phosphorus
Vitamin D deficiency	N, ↓	↓	↑	↓, N, ↑	↑	↓	↑
Vitamin D dependent rickets/type I	N, ↓	↓	↑	↓	↑	↓	↑
Vitamin D dependent rickets/type II	N, ↓	↓	↑	↑↑	↑	↓	↑

Radiological Findings

- Widening and broadening of the epiphyseal plate.
- Fraying, splaying and cupping of the metaphyses.
- Ill-defined and indistinct cortex due to uncalcified subperiosteal osteoid.
- Rickets rosary: Cupping of the anterior end of the ribs.
- "Trumpeting" or Champagne glass appearance (widening and cupping of distal end of long bones)
- Development of scoliosis.
- In healing rickets, the zones of provisional calcification become denser than the diaphysis. A dense white line appears at epiphyses and metaphyseal junction.
- Impression of the sacrum and femora into the pelvis, leading to a triradiate configuration of the pelvis.
- Bowing and deformity of longs bone.

Treatment

Medical Treatment

Aim: To bring quick healing

Vitamin D and adequate nutritional intake of calcium and phosphorus.

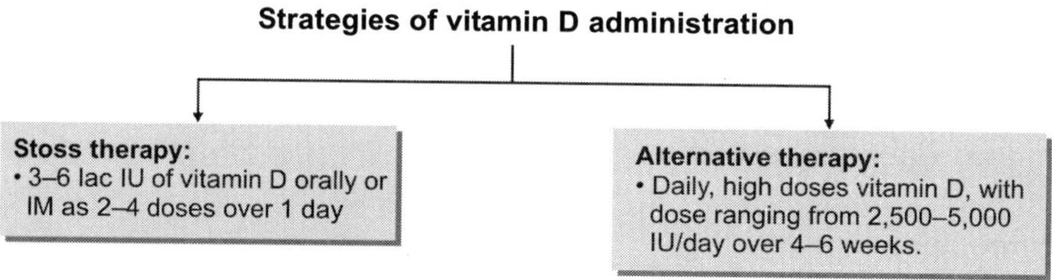

Orthopaedics Treatment

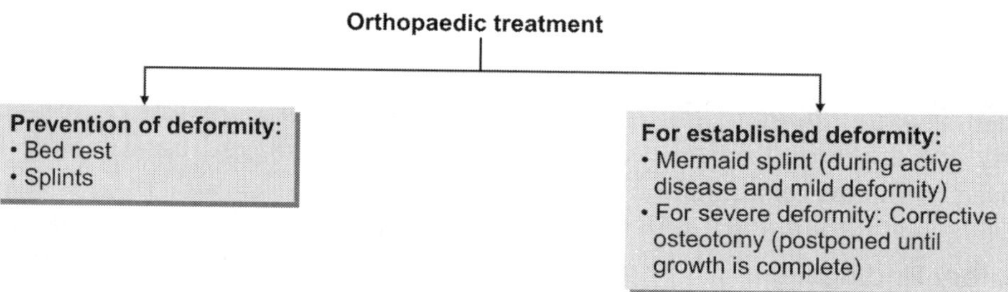

Prevention of Rickets

It can be prevented by universal administration of a multivitamin containing 200–400 IU of vitamin D to children who are breast-fed.

Q4. Discuss aetiology, pathology, clinical features, laboratory and radiological findings and management of osteomalacia.

Osteomalacia (mollities ossium) is a generalized bone disorder of adults characterized by softening of bone because of inadequate mineralization results in the accumulation of unmineralized osteoid.

Features are mainly because of softening of bone, since the epiphysis has fused deformities are not very severe, the usual cause is dietary insufficiency or poor exposure to sunlight.

Aetiology

- Vitamin D deficiency
- In western world, derangement of phosphate and vitamin D metabolism (either acquired or hereditary)

Pathogenesis

Intestine

Promotion of Ca absorption by gut.

Vitamin D Deficiency

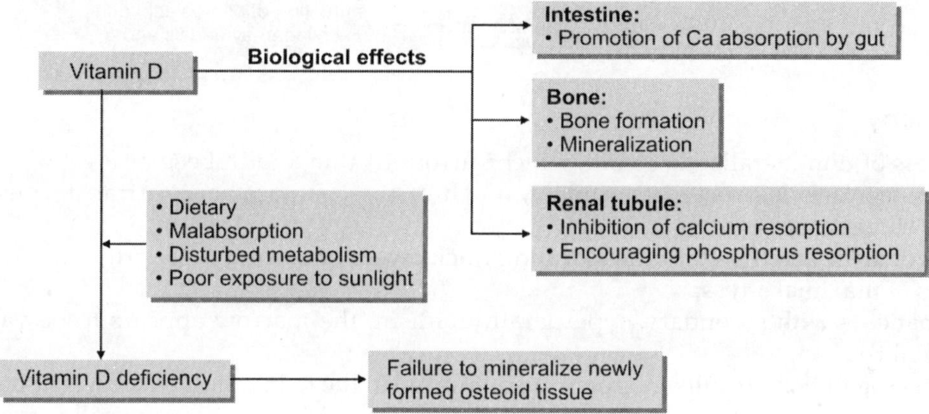

Inorganic Phosphate

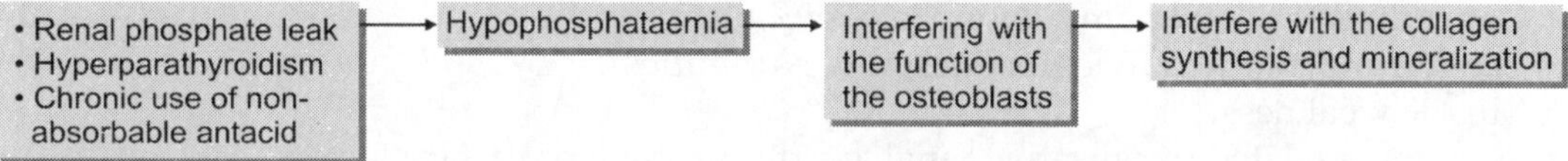

Chronic Acidosis

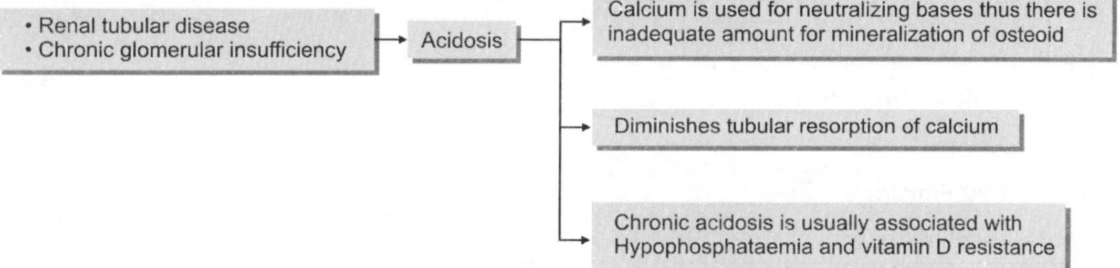

In general:

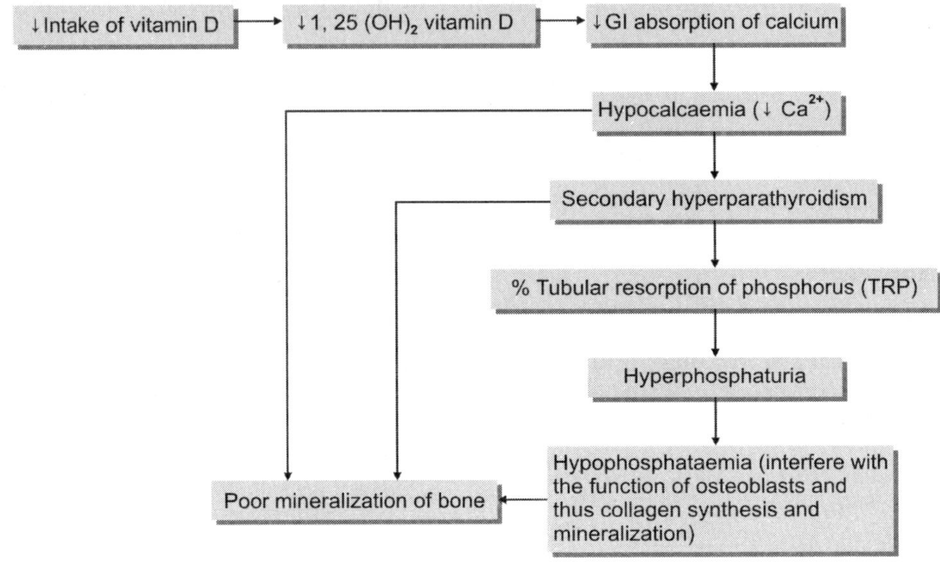

Pathology

- Excess of unmineralized osteoid, which surrounds thin, old trabeculae.
- As osteoclasis is proceeds normally, much of the compact bone is transformed into cancellous bone.
- Osteoblastic activity continues forming thick layers of osteoid most pronounced at the sites of maximal stress.
- In patients with secondary hyperparathyroidism, the marrow appears to be vascular and fibrous.
- Softening of bone results in grotesque deformities due to bending with weight-bearing.
- Fractures are usually multiple, heals well but union is delayed as the callus is chiefly consist of osteoid.

Clinical Features

- Generalized skeletal pains, anorexia, weight loss.
- Tenderness confined to lower back and extremities.
- Muscle weakness.
- Symptoms related to causative renal, gastrointestinal or dietary factors.
- Acute onset of pain and tenderness suggests pathological fracture.
- Deformities: particularly of weight-bearing structures:
  - Kyphotic and scoliotic deformities of the spine.
  - Coxa vara.
  - Protrusio acetabuli.
  - Bowing of thigh and leg.

Investigations

Laboratory Findings

- *Biochemical findings*:

Condition	Calcium	Phosphorus	Alkaline phosphatase	PTH
Osteomalacia	N or ↓	N or ↓	↑	↑

- *Metabolic studies* to rule out gastric and hepatorenal causative factors.
- *Bone biopsy:* decalcified specimen showing plenty of osteoid (poorly mineralized protein matrix) with increased osteoblastic activity. Segment taken from looser line or umbauzonen, milkman's pseudofracture is composed entirely of osteoid.

Radiological Findings

- Generalized demineralization, diffuse osteoporosis.
- Loss of transverse trabeculae.
- Diffusely rarefied and cortices are thin.
- No subperiosteal resorption of bone in contrast to hyperparathyroidism.
- Milkman syndrome (multiple, incomplete, transverse, symmetrical lines of rarefaction across the bones pseudo-fracture/looser zones).
- Pelvic deformity with protrusio acetabuli.
- Triradiate pelvis.
- Kyphoscoliotic spine due to wedge compression fractures.
- "Cod fish" spine
- Skull: basilar invagination

Treatment

Essentially conservative.

Medical Treatment

- High protein diet (3.5 g/kg for infants, down to 1.0 g/kg for adult).
- Diet rich in phosphorous, calcium and protein like meat, seafood and dairy products.
- Correction of gastrointestinal disorders that interfere with the absorption of vitamin D and calcium.
- Calcium lactate or gluconate (0.5–3 g) three times a day.
- Daily administration of about 10,000 units of vitamin D and as healing occurs the dose should be titrated to 800 units.

Orthopaedics Treatment

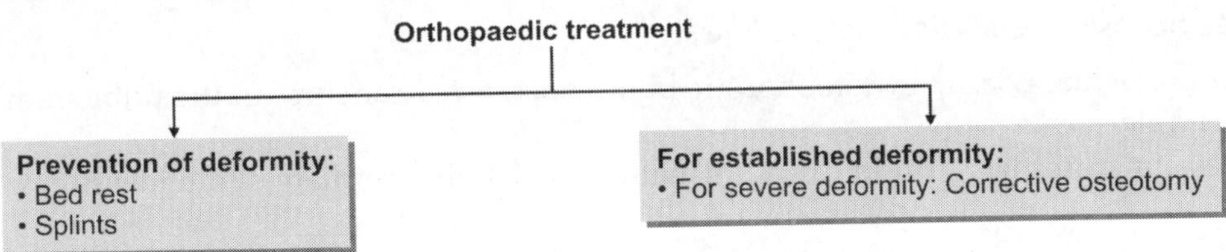

Q5. Write short note on looser zones or pseudofracture.

Looser zones or pseudofractures or Milkman's fracture are radiological hallmark of active osteomalacia. These are transverse, bilaterally symmetrical ribbon-like area of rarefaction often at right angles to long axis of the bone.

These are incomplete fractures or radiolucent areas in the bone that are composed of unmineralized osteoid. Typically, these fractures are one to several mm in thickness and are quite sharply defined.

Aetiology

- Old theory: They were in the sites of vascular channels (pulsating large vessels) that cause resorption of bone.
- New theory: Their position is most likely to be related to sites of stress in the skeleton.

Histology

It has shown that they consist of unmineralized fracture callus with a variable content of fibrous tissue.

Sites

- Axillary margins of the scapula immediately below the glenoid
- Ribs
- Pubic rami
- Proximal ends of the femur (medial portion of neck) and ulna
- Less common sites include metatarsals and metacarpals, the base of the acromium and the ilium.

Features

- It is pathognomonic feature of osteomalacia.
- Radiolucent lines those are perpendicular to the bone cortex.
- Bilaterally symmetrical.
- Incomplete do not extend across the entire bone shaft, and characteristically have a sclerotic margin.
- Most often occur on the concavity of bone.
- Lasts for months or years without regressing.

Differential Diagnosis

Paget disease: Fissure or incremental fractures:
- These multiple microfractures occur in the convexity (outer) of deformed bones.
- Typical features of Paget's disease (enlarged, disorganized trabecular pattern and sclerotic bone) serve as distinguishing radiological features.

Osteoporosis: Insufficiency Fractures

- These fractures occur in osteoporotic bones such as calcaneum, in the pubic rami and sacral ala.
- These fractures have florid callus formation, which differentiates from looser zone.

Treatment

These osteoid zones or looser zones invariably heal when the cause of the osteomalacia is identified and treatment is given.

> **Q6. Discuss aetiology, pathology, clinical features, laboratory and radiological findings of osteoporosis.**

WHO definition of osteoporosis:
- Bone mineral density (BMD) in a patient is related to peak bone mass and, subsequently, bone loss.

- The World Health Organization (WHO) has established the following definitions of osteoporosis based on BMD measurements:
  - *Normal*: BMD within 1 standard deviation (SD) of the mean bone density for young adult women (T-score at –1 and above)
  - *Low bone mass (osteopenia)*: BMD between 1–2.5 SD below the mean for young adult women (T-score between –1 and –2.5)
  - *Osteoporosis*: BMD 2.5 SD or more below the normal mean for young adult females (T-score at or below –2.5)
  - *Severe or "established" osteoporosis*: BMD 2.5 SD or more below the normal mean for young adult females (T-score at or below –2.5) in a patient who has already experienced 1 or more fractures.
- *T-score* is the bone density compared with the BMD of control subjects who are at their peak BMD
- *The Z-score* reflects a bone density compared with that of patients matched for age and sex

Aetiology and Clinical Features

Primary Osteoporosis

It occurs in patients, in whom a secondary cause of osteoporosis cannot be recognized, including:
- Juvenile osteoporosis
- Idiopathic osteoporosis
- Postmenopausal (type I)
- Age-associated or senile (type II) osteoporosis

Juvenile Osteoporosis

- It usually occurs in children or young adults of both sexes.
- These patients have normal gonadal function.
- The age of onset usually is 8–14 years.
- The hallmark characteristic of juvenile osteoporosis is abrupt bone pain and/or a fracture following trauma.

Idiopathic Osteoporosis

Type I osteoporosis (postmenopausal osteoporosis):
- It occurs in women aged 50–65 years.
- This type of osteoporosis is characterized by a phase of accelerated bone loss.
- This bone loss occurs primarily from trabecular bone.
- In this phase, fractures of the distal forearm and vertebral bodies are common.

Type II osteoporosis (age-associated or senile):

- It occurs in women and men >70 years.
- This form of osteoporosis represents bone loss associated with aging.
- Usually involves cortical bone.
- Fractures occur in trabecular and cortical bone.
- Besides wrist and vertebral fractures, hip fractures are often seen in these patients.

Secondary Osteoporosis

It occurs when an underlying disease, deficiency, or drug causes osteoporosis.

Genetic (congenital) causes of osteoporosis include the following:
- Cystic fibrosis
- Ehlers-Danlos syndrome
- Glycogen storage disease
- Gaucher disease
- Haemochromatosis
- Homocystinuria
- Hypophosphatasia
- Idiopathic hypercalciuria
- Marfan syndrome
- Menkes steely hair syndrome
- Osteogenesis imperfecta
- Porphyria
- Riley-Day syndrome
- Hypogonadal states

Hypogonadal states that can cause osteoporosis include the following:
- Androgen insensitivity
- Anorexia nervosa/bulimia nervosa
- Female athlete triad
- Hyperprolactinemia
- Panhypopituitarism
- Premature menopause
- Turner syndrome
- Klinefelter syndrome

Endocrine disorders that can cause osteoporosis include the following:
- Acromegaly
- Adrenal insufficiency
- Cushing syndrome
- Estrogen deficiency
- Diabetes mellitus
- Hyperparathyroidism
- Hyperthyroidism
- Hypogonadism
- Pregnancy
- Prolactinoma

Deficiency states that can cause osteoporosis include the following:
- Calcium deficiency
- Magnesium deficiency
- Protein deficiency
- Vitamin D deficiency
- Bariatric surgery
- Celiac disease
- Gastrectomy

- Malabsorption
- Malnutrition
- Parenteral nutrition
- Primary biliary cirrhosis

Inflammatory diseases that can cause osteoporosis include the following:

- Inflammatory bowel disease
- Ankylosing spondylitis
- Rheumatoid arthritis
- Systemic lupus erythematosus

Hematologic and neoplastic disorders that can cause osteoporosis include the following:

- Hemochromatosis
- Hemophilia
- Leukemia
- Lymphoma
- Multiple myeloma
- Sickle cell anaemia
- Systemic mastocytosis
- Thalassaemia
- Metastatic disease

Medications known to cause or accelerate bone loss include the following:

- *Anticonvulsants*: Phenytoin, barbiturates, carbamazepine (these agents are associated with treatment-induced vitamin D deficiency)
- Antipsychotic drugs
- Antiretroviral drugs
- *Aromatase inhibitors*: Exemestane, anastrozole
- *Chemotherapeutic/transplant drugs*: Cyclosporine, tacrolimus, platinum compounds, cyclophosphamide, ifosfamide, methotrexate
- Furosemide
- *Glucocorticoids and corticotropin*: Prednisone ($\geq$5 mg/day for $\geq$3 months)
- Heparin (long-term)
- *Hormonal/endocrine therapies*: Gonadotropin-releasing hormone (GnRH) agonists, luteinizing hormone-releasing hormone (LHRH) analogs, depo medroxyprogesterone, excessive thyroid supplementation
- Lithium
- Methotrexate
- Selective serotonin reuptake inhibitors
- Excessive Thyroxine

Miscellaneous causes of osteoporosis include the following:

- Alcoholism
- Amyloidosis
- Chronic metabolic acidosis
- Congestive heart failure
- Depression
- Emphysema
- Chronic or end-stage renal disease
- Chronic liver disease

- HIV disease/AIDS
- Idiopathic calciuria
- Idiopathic scoliosis
- Immobility
- Multiple sclerosis
- Ochronosis
- Organ transplantation
- Pregnancy/lactation
- Sarcoidosis
- Weightlessness

Risk factors for osteoporosis include the following:
- Advanced age (50 years or older)
- Female sex
- White or Asian ethnicity
- Genetic factors, such as a family history of osteoporosis
- Thin build or small stature
- Amenorrhoea
- Late menarche
- Early menopause
- Postmenopausal state
- Physical inactivity or immobilization
- Use of drugs: Anticonvulsants, systemic steroids, thyroid supplements, heparin, chemotherapeutic agents, insulin
- Alcohol and tobacco use
- Androgen or estrogen deficiency
- Calcium deficiency

Investigations

Following laboratory-finding help to assess the causes of osteoporosis:
- Complete blood count (CBC)
- Serum chemistries, including calcium, phosphate, creatinine, liver function tests, electrolytes (Levels of serum calcium, phosphate, and alkaline phosphatase are usually normal in persons with primary osteoporosis)
- Thyroid-stimulating hormone (TSH) level
- 25-Hydroxyvitamin D level

Other laboratory studies used to evaluate for secondary causes include the following:
- Twenty-four-hour urine calcium to assess for hypercalciuria
- Intact PTH level
- Thyrotropin (if on thyroid replacement) level
- Testosterone and gonadotropin levels
- Erythrocyte sedimentation rate (ESR) and C-reactive protein (CRP) value
- Urinary free cortisol and tests for adrenal hypersecretion
- Serum protein electrophoresis (SPEP) and urine protein electrophoresis (UPEP)
- Antigliadin and antiendomysial antibodies for celiac disease
- Serum tryptase, urine N-methylhistamine for mastocytosis
- Bone marrow biopsy if a hematologic disorder is suspected

- *Biochemical markers of bone metabolism in clinical use*: Primary use of biochemical markers is for monitoring the response to treatment.
    - Bone formation
        - Serum bone-specific alkaline phosphatase
        - Serum osteocalcin
        - Serum propeptide of type I pro-collagen
    - Bone resorption (better markers; prediction of fracture risk, independently of bone density)
        - Urine and serum cross-linked N-telopeptide
        - Urine and serum cross-linked C-telopeptide
        - Urine total free deoxypyridinoline

X-rays

- Generalized osteopenia (when 40% of the skeleton is lost)
- Ground glass appearance
- Fish mouth or cod fish vertebrae of Albright
- Prominent vertical trabeculae
- Resorption of horizontal trabeculae
- Pathological fracture
- *Singh index*: Singh et al. (1970) measured the femoral cortical thickness at the level of the isthmus of the right femur by the criteria below:
    - Grade VI: All normal groups of trabeculae are visible in the X-ray of upper end of femur.
    - Grade V: The secondary compression trabeculae are not clearly demarcated. Bone biopsy from these patients showed normal histology.
    - Grade IV: Secondary tensile is not clear, but the bone histology was normal among these patients.
    - Grade III: Principal tensile trabeculae seen only in the upper part not visible in lower part. This indicates *definite osteoporosis*.
    - Grade II: Principal tensile trabeculae are not seen even in the upper part indicating *advanced osteoporosis*.
    - Grade I: Even the principal trabeculae are not clearly visible. This shows a *severe degree of osteoporosis*.

Bone Biopsy

Tetracycline labeling of the skeleton allows determination of the rate of remodelling as well as evaluation

Bone Density (Measurement of Bone Mass)

Non-invasive techniques are now available for estimating skeletal mass or density. These include:

- *Dual-energy X-ray absorptiometry (DXA)*:
    - Two X-ray energies are used to estimate the area of mineralized tissue, and the mineral content is divided by the area
    - Measure the heel (calcaneus), forearm (radius and ulna), or finger (phalanges)
    - T-scores, which compare individual results to those in a young population that is matched for race and gender.

- Z-scores compare individual results to those of an age-matched population that is also matched for race and gender.
- A T-score below –2.5 in the lumbar spine, femoral neck, or total hip is taken as a diagnosis of osteoporosis
- *Single-energy X-ray absorptiometry (SXA)*
- *Quantitative CT:*
  - The technique is three-dimensional and can provide a true density (mass of bone tissue per unit volume).
  - Analyze trabecular bone and cortical bone content and volume separately
  - Expensive, involves greater radiation exposure, and is less reproducible than DXA
- *Ultrasound:*
  - Measure bone mass by calculating the attenuation of the signal as it passes through bone
  - Ultrasound assesses properties of bone other than mass (e.g. quality)
  - Relatively low cost and mobility, ultrasound is can be for use as a screening procedure

Q7. Discuss in brief the management of osteoporosis.

Treatment of the patient with osteoporosis frequently involves:
- Management of acute fractures
- Treatment of underlying disease
- Nutritional recommendations
- Exercise
- Pharmacologic therapies
- Nonpharmacologic approaches

I. Management of Acute Fractures

Treatment depends upon:
- General status of the patient
- Fracture:
  - Location
  - Type
  - Configuration
  - Condition of the neighbouring joint

Procedures

- Open reduction and internal fixation with screws and plates (locking)
- Hemiarthroplasties (with bone cement)
- Total arthroplasty (with bone cement)
- These procedure should be followed by intense rehabilitation
- Other fractures (e.g. vertebral, rib, and pelvic fractures) are usually managed with supportive care, requiring no specific orthopedic treatment (except in especial circumstances).

For vertebral compression fractures: Recently developed technique involves:
Percutaneous injection of artificial cement (polymethylmethacrylate) into the vertebral body (*vertebroplasty or kyphoplasty*).

II. Management of the Underlying Disease

Risk factor reduction:
- Patient should be educated to reduce the impact of modifiable risk factors associated with bone loss and falling.
- Thorough evaluation of patients on glucocorticoids/TSH therapy.
- Smoking cessation.
- Reducing risk factors for falling includes:
  - Alcohol abuse treatment
  - Review of medications that may be associated with orthostatic hypotension and/or sedation, including *hypnotics* and *anxiolytics*
  - Frequency of nocturia (common precipitant of a fall) should be reduced (by decreasing or modifying diuretic use)
  - Patient should be educated about the environmental safety with regard to eliminating exposed wires, curtain strings, slippery rugs, and mobile tables.
  - Treatment for impaired vision is recommended
  - Specialized supervision and care of elderly patients with neurologic impairment (e.g. stroke, Parkinson's disease, Alzheimer's disease)
  - *Important preventive measures:*
    - Avoiding stocking feet on wood/slippery floors
    - Checking carpet condition (particularly on stairs)
    - Providing good light in paths to bathrooms and outside the home are

III. Nutritional Recommendations

Calcium

Adequate calcium intake:

Life stage group	Estimated adequate daily calcium intake, mg/d
Young children (1–3 years)	500
Older children (4–8 years)	800
Adolescents and young adults (9–18 years)	1300
Men and women (19–50 years)	1000
Men and women (51 and older)	1200

- Preferred source of calcium is from dairy products (*milk, yogurt, and cheese*) and other foods, but many patients require calcium supplementation.
- Calcium supplements should be calculated based on the elemental calcium content of the supplement, not the weight of the calcium salt.
- Side effects/precaution:
  - Eructation and constipation (minimal; mostly with carbonate salts)
  - Patient with history of kidney stones should have a 24-hour urine calcium determination before starting calcium therapy.

Vitamin D

- Vitamin D is synthesized in skin under the influence of heat and ultraviolet light
- The Institute of Medicine recommends daily intakes of:
  - 200 IU for adults <50 years of age

– 400 IU for those from 50–70 years

– 600 IU for those >70 years

Other Nutrients

- Salt, high animal protein intakes, and caffeine may have modest effects on calcium excretion or absorption.
- Adequate *vitamin K* status is required for optimal carboxylation of osteocalcin.
- Magnesium supplementation may be warranted in patients with *inflammatory bowel disease, celiac disease, chemotherapy, severe diarrhea, malnutrition, or alcoholism.*

IV. Exercise

- Weight-bearing exercise prevents bone loss.
- Exercise also has beneficial effects on neuromuscular function, and it improves coordination, balance, and strength, thereby reducing the risk of falling.
- Exercise habits should be consistent, optimally at least three times a week.
- Depending on the patient's personal preference and general condition, recommend dancing, walking, racquet sports, cross-country skiing, and use of gym equipment.

V. Pharmacologic Therapies:

Agents

- Estrogen
- Progestin
- Selective estrogen response modulators (SERMs)
- Bisphosphonates
- Calcitonin
- PTH

Estrogens

Types of Estrogens

- Conjugated equine estrogens
- Estradiol
- Estrone
- Esterified estrogens
- Ethinyl estradiol
- Mestranol

Functions

- Reduce bone turnover
- Prevent bone loss
- Induce small increases in bone mass of the spine, hip, and total body

Mode of Action

- Acts through Two subtypes of ERs, α and β
- Estrogens may inhibit osteoclasts directly (controversial)

- Effects on bone resorption are mediated indirectly through paracrine factors produced by osteoblasts. These actions include:
    - Increasing IGF-I and TGF-β
    - Suppressing IL-1 (α and β), IL-6, TNF-α
    - Osteocalcin synthesis
- The indirect estrogen actions primarily decrease bone resorption.

Dose of Estrogen

For *oral estrogens*, the standard recommended doses:

- 0.3 mg/d for esterified estrogens
- 0.625 mg/d for conjugated equine estrogens
- 5 µg/d for ethinyl estradiol

For *transdermal* estrogen: 50 µg estradiol per day

Beneficial Effect

- 50% reduction, on average, of osteoporotic fractures, including hip fractures.
- 37% reduction in risk of colon cancer

Side effects

- Fatal and nonfatal myocardial infarction
- Stroke
- Venous thromboembolic disease
- Risk of breast cancer

Progestins

In women with a uterus, daily progestin or cyclical progestins (Medroxyprogesterone acetate and norethindrone acetate)at least 12 days per month are prescribed in combination with estrogens

SERMs

Agents

Two SERMs are currently being used in postmenopausal women:
- Raloxifene: approved for prevention and treatment of osteoporosis
- Tamoxifen: approved for the prevention and treatment of breast cancer

Functions (estrogenic effect on skeletal)

- Reduces bone turnover
- Reduces bone loss

Dose

Raloxifene (60 mg/d).

Mode of action

Mediates though ERs (ER α and β-subtypes)

Bisphosphonates

Agents approved for prevention and treatment of *postmenopausal osteoporosis*:
- Alendronate
- Risedronate
- Ibandronate

Agents approved for the treatment of *steroid-induced osteoporosis*:
• Risedronate
• Alendronate

Agents Approved for treatment of *osteoporosis in men*:
• Alendronate
• Risedronate
• Zoledronic acid
• Although it is not yet approved for use in osteoporosis, the data/trial suggest that it is highly effective in fracture risk reduction.

Mode of action

Impair osteoclast function and reduce osteoclast number, in part by the induction of apoptosis.

Dose

• Alendronate, 70 mg once weekly
• Risedronate 35 mg once weekly
• Ibandronate: 150 mg/month PO or 3 mg every 3 months IV
• Zoledronic acid: 5 mg as a single IV infusion annually

Precautions while oral preparation:
• It should be given with a full glass of water before breakfast, as bisphosphonates are poorly absorbed.
• The patients remain upright for at least 30 min after taking the medication to avoid oesophageal irritation.
• It is contraindicated in patients who have stricture or inadequate emptying of the oesophagus

Side effects

• Oesophagitis
• Oesophageal ulcer
• Oesophageal stricture
• Osteonecrosis of the jaw (ONJ) (especially with doses of zoledronic acid or pamidronate)

Calcitonin

Indications

• Paget's disease
• Hypercalcaemia
• Osteoporosis in women >5 years past menopause

Mode of action

Calcitonin suppresses osteoclast activity by direct action on the osteoclast calcitonin receptor.

Dose

• Nasal spray containing calcitonin (200 IU/d)
• It can also be administrated SC/orally (recently)

Side effects

Nausea and facial flushing (especially with injectable form).

Parathyroid Hormone

- Exogenous PTH analogue (1–34 hours PTH; teriparatide): now approved for the treatment of established osteoporosis in both men and women.
- Single daily injection given for a maximum of 2 years
- It is best administered as monotherapy and followed by an antiresorptive agent such as a bisphosphonate.

Mode of action

Direct actions on osteoblast activity by stimulating IGF-I and collagen production; stimulating replication, enhancing osteoblast recruitment, and inhibiting apoptosis

Side effects

- Muscle pain
- Weakness
- Dizziness
- Headache
- Nausea
- One case of osteosarcoma

Fluoride

- Potent stimulator of osteoprogenitor cells.
- Increments in bone mass of up to 10%

Strontium Ranelate

- It increases bone mass throughout the skeleton
- Strontium is incorporated into hydroxyapatite, replacing calcium, a feature that might explain some of its fracture benefits.

Side effects

- Venous thrombosis
- Seizures
- Abnormal cognition

Other Potential Anabolic Agents

Agent showing positive effects on skeletal mass:
- Growth hormone (GH), alone or in combination with other agents
- Anabolic steroids, mostly derivatives of testosterone
- Statin drugs (may be associated with increased bone mass and reduced fractures)

VI. Nonpharmacologic Approaches

- Kyphoplasty and vertebroplasty (for painful vertebral fractures; no long-term data available)
- *Kyphoplasty and Vertebroplasty* are safe and effective and has useful role in painful osteoporotic vertebral compression fractures that do not respond to conventional treatments.
- *Vertebroplasty*: It is a minimally invasive image-guided procedure involving the injection of bone cement (Polymethyl methacrylate (PMMA)) into a vertebral body fracture in an effort to improve pain and stability of the fracture.

- *Balloon kyphoplasty*: is a similar procedure that utilizes an inflatable balloon tamp, in an effort to reduce the fracture and create a space to theoretically allow safer injection of cement into the fractured vertebral body.
- Appliance (protective pads) around hip joint to prevents fracture.

Q8. Discuss in brief the function of parathyroid hormone and hormonal regulation of calcium and phosphorus metabolism.

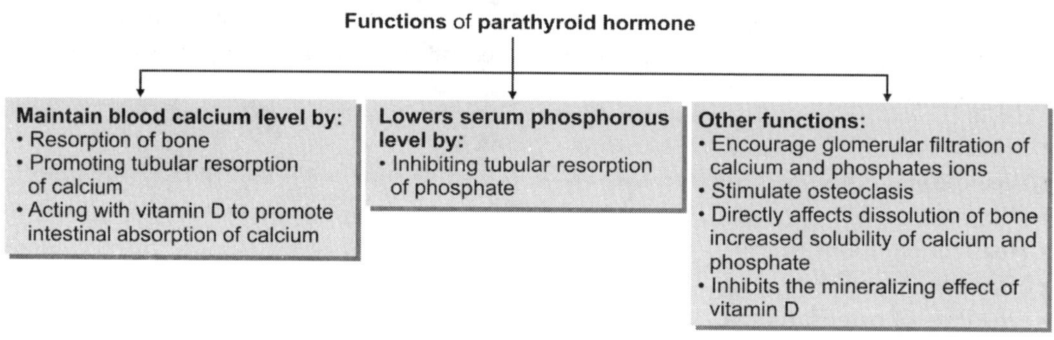

Regulation of calcium and phosphorus metabolism:

Hormones	Action as end organs			
	Intestine	*Kidney*	*Bone*	*Net effect*
Paratharmone	• No direct effect • Acts indirectly on bowel by increasing $1.25\,(OH)_2\,D$	• Converts $25(OH)D$ to $1.25\,(OH)_2\,D$	• Stimulate osteoclastic resorption of bone	• Stimulate recruitment of pro-osteoclasts
		• Increase absorption of calcium • Promotes excretion of phosphorus	• stimulates recruitment of pro-osteoclasts	• Decreased phosphorus level
$1,25(OH)_2D$	• Strongly stimulates intestinal absorption of calcium and phosphorus		• Strongly stimulate osteoclastic resorption of bone	• Increased calcium • Increased phosphorus level
Calcitonin	–	• Decreases tubular resorption as calcium	• Inhibits osteoclastic resorption of bone	• Decreased serum calcium level

Q9. Discuss in clinical features and management of primary hyperparathyroidism.

Hyperparathyroidism is a generalized disorder of calcium, phosphate, and bone metabolism characterized by excess production of PTH, is a common cause of hypercalcemia and is usually the result of autonomously functioning adenomas or hyperplasia.

Aetiology: (*Primary hyperparathyroidism is also known as von Recklinhaughsen's disease or osteitis fibrosa cystica*)

- Solitary adenomas (most common)
- Multiple endocrine neoplasia (MEN)

Clinical Features

- Asymptomatic (~50%)
- Mnemonic *"Painful bones, Renal stones, Abdominal groans, and Psychic moans,"* classically describe the presentation of hyperparathyroidism

Central Nervous System

Neuropsychiatric illness:
- Altered mental status
- Signs of mental depression
- Poor general health
- Low energy levels
- Decreased ability to complete routine work
- Decreased social interaction
- Pain, particularly in the legs

Cardiovascular System

- Increased risk of hypertension
- Left ventricular hypertrophy
- Vascular calcification and stiffness
- Deleterious myocardial events

Musculoskeletal System

- Bone/joint pain and tenderness
- Osteopenia/osteoporosis
- Increased fracture risk
- Cystic bone lesions (*osteitis fibrosa cystica*)
- Vertebral collapse
- Chondrocalcinosis and pseudogout

Neuromuscular Manifestations

- Proximal muscle weakness
- Easy fatigability
- Atrophy of muscles

GI System

- Anorexia
- Nausea
- Abdominal discomfort
- Constipation

- Pancreatitis
- Pancreatic calcification
- Peptic ulcer disease

Renal System

- Recurrent UTI
- Nephrolithiasis (calcium oxalate or calcium phosphate)
- Nephrocalcinosis (causes decreased renal function and phosphate retention)
- Uremia

Investigation

Laboratory Findings

- Elevated immunoreactive PTH level in a patient with asymptomatic hypercalcemia clinches the diagnosis
- Serum calcium increased
- Serum alkaline phosphatase increased
- Serum phosphate is usually low but may be normal, especially if renal failure has developed

Histologically characterized by:
- Giant multinucleated osteoclasts in scalloped areas on the surface of the bone
- Reduction in number of trabeculae
- Howship's lacunae
- Brown tumors (resorbed bone is replaced by fibrous tissue)

X-rays

- Resorption of the phalangeal tufts
- Replacement of the usually sharp cortical outline of the bone in the digits (middle phalanx) by an irregular outline (subperiosteal resorption: earliest sign) of middle and index finger (radial sites)
- Generalized osteopenia
- Pathological fracture
- Chondrocalcinosis
- Cod fish spine
- Salt and pepper skull
- Pin head stippling of skull
- Loss of lamina dura of teeth
- Arrow head distal phalanges

Bone Density

Cortical bone density is reduced:
- Dual-energy X-ray absorptiometry (DEXA) of the spine provides reproducible quantitative estimates (within a few percent) of spinal bone density.
- CT is a very sensitive technique for estimating spinal bone density, but reproducibility of standard CT is poor.

Treatment

Medical

The approach to medical treatment of hypercalcaemia varies with its severity:

Treatment	Advantages	Disadvantages
Hydration with saline Forced diuresis; saline plus loop diuretic	Rehydration Rapid action	Volume overload cardiac decompensation intensive monitoring electrolyte disturbance
Bisphosphonates 1st generation: Etidronate	Intermediate onset of action	Less effective than other bisphosphonates
2nd generation: Pamidronate	High potency; inter-mediate onset of action	Fever in 20% hypophosphataemia, hypocal-cemia, hypomagnesaemia
3rd generation: Zoledronate	High potency; rapid infusion; prolonged duration of action	Minor; fever, rarely hypocalcaemia or hypo-phosphatemia
Calcitonin	Rapid onset of action; useful as adjunct in severe hypercalcaemia	Rapid tachyphylaxis
Other therapies Phosphate (oral or IV) Glucocorticoids	Oral therapy, antitumour agent	Active only in certain malignancies; glucocorticoid side effects
Dialysis	Useful in renal failure; onset of effect inhours; can immediately reverse life threatening hyper-calcaemia	Complex procedure, reserved for extreme or special circumstances

Surgical

Successful parathyroidectomy induces normocalcaemia in 95–98% of patients with hyperparathyroidism, and 82% of patients have symptomatic improvement.

Guidelines for Parathyroid Surgery in Asymptomatic Primary Hyperparathyroidism:

Measurement	Guidelines, 1990	Guidelines, 2002
Serum calcium (above upper limit of normal)	0.3–0.4 mmol/L (1–1.5 mg/dl) above normal	0.3 mmol/L (1.0 mg/dl) above normal
24-hour urinary calcium	>400 mg	>400 mg
Creatinine clearance	Reduced by 30%	Reduced by 30%
Bone mineral density	Z-score ≤2.0 (forearm)	T-score ≤2.5 at any site
Age	<50	<50

Orthopaedics Management

- Prevention of deformity/pathological fracture: Rest, splints
- Deformity: Corrective osteotomies

Secondary Hyperparathyroidism

- Results from renal damage
- Serum phosphorus is high
- Normal or lowered serum calcium
- *Rugger jersy spine*: Sclerotic band just adjacent to the vertebral end plates.

13

Myopathy

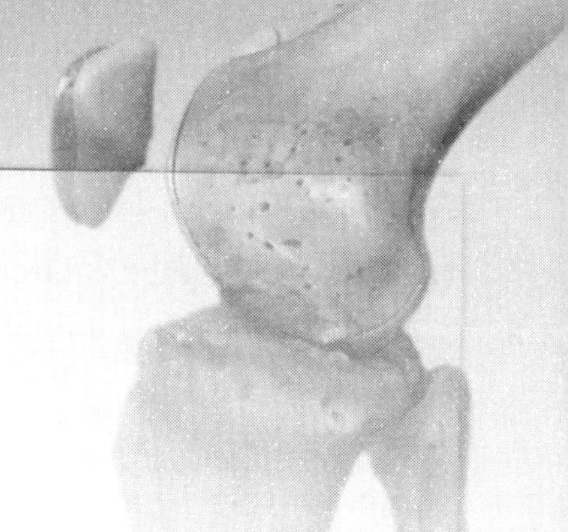

Q1. Write in brief about Duchenne muscular dystrophy.

Duchenne Muscular Dystrophy is a X-linked recessive disorder, sometimes also called *pseudohypertrophic muscular dystrophy*, has an incidence of ~30/100,000 live-born males is most common childhood muscular dystrophy.

Pathogenesis

- It is caused by a mutation of the gene that encodes *dystrophin*. It is localized to the short arm of the '*X*'-*chromosome at Xp21*. The most common gene mutation is a deletion.
- Dystrophin is a protein confined to the inner surface of the sarcolemma of the muscle fibre.
- The dystrophin-glycoprotein complex provides stability to the sarcolemma. If there is Deficiency of one member of the complex than it may cause abnormalities in other components. This deficiency weakens the sarcolemma causing membrane tears and a cascade of events that leads to muscle fibre necrosis.
- In Duchenne, dystrophy there is a primary deficiency of dystrophin, which may lead to secondary loss of the sarcoglycans and dystroglycan.

Clinical Features

- It is present since birth but disorder becomes apparent by the age of 3–5 years.
- Boys fall frequently and have difficulty in keeping pace with friends when playing.
- Jumping, running, and hopping are invariably abnormal.
- Muscle weakness is obvious by the age of 5 years.
- Gowers' manoeuvres present (Gowers' sign): On getting up from the ground, the patient uses his hands to climb up himself.
- By the age of 6 years the patient develop contracture of heel cord and iliotibial band that leads to toe walking and is associated with compensatory lordotic posture.
- There is progressive muscle loss, showing predilection for proximal limb muscle and flexors of neck; leg muscles are more severely involved than the arm muscles.
- By the age of 8–10 years patient may require braces.
- Prolonged sitting may leads to limitation of hip, knee, ankle, elbow and wrist movements and subsequently joint contractures.
- Patients are wheel chair dependent by the age of 12.
- In due course, the contracture becomes fixed; patient often develops scoliosis, which is progressive and associated with pain.
- Scoliosis further impairs the pulmonary function tests, which are already compromised due to muscle weakness.

- By age 16–18, patients are predisposed to serious pulmonary infections that sometimes proved fatal.
- Besides pulmonary infection, the causes of death are acute aspiration of food and acute gastric dilatation.
- Cardiomyopathy is present in almost all patients.
- There is nonprogressive intellectual impairment.

Laboratory Findings

- Serum CK levels are invariably elevated (20 and 100 times normal).
- EMG shows features typical of myopathy.
- Electrocardiogram (ECG) shows:
  - Increase net RS in lead V_1
  - Deep, narrow Q waves in the precordial leads
  - Tall right precordial R waves in V_1
- Muscle biopsy shows:
  - Muscle fibres of varying size
  - Small groups of necrotic and regenerating fibres.
  - Connective tissue and fat replace lost muscle fibres.
- Definitive diagnosis: deficiency of dystrophin (during mutation analysis on peripheral blood leukcocytes or in a biopsy of muscle tissue)

Treatment

- Glucocorticoids: prednisone in a dose of 0.75 mg/kg per day, significantly slow progression of Duchenne dystrophy for up to 3 years.
- Novel therapies: Replace the defective gene or missing protein.

> **Q2. Write in brief about: a. Landouzy–Dejerine dystrophy; b. Erb's dystrophy; c. Congenital myotonia; d. Myositis ossificans progressiva; e. Prussian disease; f. Arthrogryposis multiplex congenita**

a. Landouzy–Dejerine Dystrophy (Fascioscapulohumeral Muscular Dystrophy)

- Childhood to adult onset.
- Both sexes involved.
- Muscular pseudohypertrophy
- Contracture and skeletal deformities
- It has the characteristic cartoon 'Popeye' look, drooping eyelids, facial atrophy (myopathic face), thickened over-hanging upper lip (tapir lip), weak shoulder and arm (winging of scapula), no involvement of forearm muscles.

b. Erb's Dystrophy (Limb Girdle)

- Both sexes affected (2nd and 3rd decades)
- It involves shoulder and pelvic girdle muscle
- Face is not affected.
- Pseudohypertrophy is uncommon.

c. Congenital Myotonia (Thomsen's Disease)

This is a heredofamilial disease characterized by delayed muscular relaxation after a strong voluntary contraction.

Important Features

- Difficulty in activities of the child can be seen in early childhood.
- There is a surprising generalized muscular hypertrophy giving it a *Herculean appearance*.
- Characteristically, the first few attempts at movement are associated with painless stiffening contractions with slow relaxation, but subsequently the movements become easier.
- Affected patients have a typical *hatchet faced appearance* due to temporalis, masseter, and facial muscle atrophy and weakness.
- Cardiac disturbance occurs
- Other features associated include:
  - Intellectual impairment
  - Hypersomnia
  - Posterior subcapsular cataracts
  - Frontal baldness
  - Gonadal atrophy
  - Insulin resistance
  - Decreased oesophageal and colonic motility.

It is diagnosed by:

- A simple percussion test, which produces spasm followed by slow relaxation. An electrical stimulation of brief duration initiates a prolonged contraction and repeated electrical stimuli will abolish the phenomenon.
- Electromyography is diagnostic.
- The hypertrophic muscle has a greater ability to store creatine, with high urinary excretion of creatinine.

Treatment

- Quinine is specific and has to be continued indefinitely.
- Calcium is a useful adjunct.
- Newer drugs like procainamide in doses of 250 mg, thrice a day give excellent results.

d. Myositis Ossificans Progressiva

- Congenital condition (autosomal dominant)
- It appears within the first decade of life as spontaneous or injury-induced exacerbations.
- The lesions are characterized by painful swellings in soft connective tissue, including tendons, ligaments, fascia, and skeletal muscle.
- It is characterized by ossification of muscles, fascia and tendons, often starting in the paraspinal muscles and then subsequently all over.
- Two clinical features define classic fibrodysplasia ossificans progressiva: malformations of the great toes and progressive heterotopic ossification.

Investigation

- Blood shows elevated eosinophils count.
- serum alkaline phosphatase activity may be increased
- Urinary basic fibroblast growth factor levels may be elevated
- Radiologically sheets of ossified zones may be seen in the neck and cervicodorsal region, often obviously visible.

Treatment

- There is no known effective treatment.
- Treatment with biphosphonates may prevent progression.
- In the worst cases, movements are restricted and the patient is severely disabled.

e. Prussian Disease

- It is a type of myositis ossificans traumatica.
- This is usually seen in soldiers doing a lot of horse riding and develops ossification in the adductor muscle of the thigh which is constantly damaged by the saddle and the deltoids by carrying rifles hanging around the shoulders.

f. Arthrogryposis Multiplex Congenita

- This is a nonprogressive rare congenital disorder
- It is characterized by multiple joint contractures and can include muscle weakness and fibrosis. AMC is typically symmetrical and involves all four extremities

Types

There are two major types of arthrogryposis multiplex congenita (AMC):
- Amyoplasia (classic arthrogryposis): Multiple symmetric contractures occur in the limbs.
- Distal arthrogryposis: The hands and feet are involved, but the large joints are spared.

Clinical Features

- This is failure of development of skeletal muscles congenitally, resulting in deforming contracture of joins.
- The child is usually born with involvement of one or all limbs with fixed deformities.
- More common signs and symptoms are associated with the:
    - Shoulder (internal rotation)
    - Elbow (extension and pronation)
    - Wrist (volar and ulnar)
    - Hand (fingers in fixed flexion and thumb-in-palm)
    - Hip (flexed, abducted and externally rotated, often dislocated)
    - Knee (flexion)
    - Foot (clubfoot (equinovarus))
    - The head muscles are usually spared.
- There is no visceral abnormalities.
- Cognition and language are usually normal

Complications

- Scoliosis
- Lung hypoplasia
- Respiratory problems
- Growth retardation
- Midfacial hemangioma
- Facial and jaw variations
- Abdominal hernias

Diagnosis

- Clinical evaluation
- Testing for cause
- Evaluation should include a thorough assessment for associated abnormalities.
- Electromyography and muscle biopsy are useful to diagnose neuropathic and myopathic disorders.
- In classic AMC, muscle biopsy typically shows amyoplasia, with fatty and fibrous replacement of tissues.

Treatment

- It is basically aimed at stretching out the contractures and surgical treatment of various joint deformities.
- Physical and occupational therapies

Q3. Discuss the clinical features and management of Myasthenia gravis.

A disorder of neuromuscular transmission marked by fluctuating weakness and fatigue of certain voluntary muscles.

This is due to rapid depletion of acetylcholine receptors at the neuromuscular junction, characterized by involvement of bulbar innervated muscles, i.e. face, lips, eyes, tongue, throat, and neck.

Underlying Defect

Decrease in the number of available acetylcholine receptors at neuromuscular junctions (or at the postsynaptic muscle membrane) due to an antibody-mediated autoimmune attack.

Clinical Features

- Common in females
- 20–30 years of age
- Pronounced fatigue of following muscles:
  - Eyes: Ptosis and diplopia.
  - Oral: Dysarthria (*"mushy" quality* speech) and difficulty in swallowing.
- Facial weakness produces a "snarling" expression when the patient attempts to smile
- The limb weakness in myasthenia gravis is often proximal and may be asymmetric.
- Bulbar weakness is especially prominent in MuSK antibody–positive MG.
- Despite the muscle weakness, deep tendon reflexes are preserved.
- In about 65% the thymus is 'hyperplastic', with the presence of active germinal centres, while 10% of patients have thymic tumors (thymomas).

Diagnosis

History

- Diplopia, Ptosis
- Weakness in characteristic distribution
- Fluctuation and fatigue: worse with repeated activity, improved by rest

Physical Examination

- Ptosis, diplopia
- Motor power survey: Quantitative testing of muscle strength

- Forward arm abduction time (5 minutes)
- Vital capacity
- Absence of other neurologic signs

Laboratory testing

Anti-AChR radioimmunoassay

- Approximately 85% positive in generalized myasthenia gravis; 50% in ocular myasthenia gravis; definite diagnosis if positive
- Negative result does not exclude myasthenia gravis.
- Approximately 40% of AChR antibody-negative patients with generalized myasthenia gravis have anti-MuSK antibodies.
- Repetitive nerve stimulation; decrement of >15% at 3 Hz: highly probable
- Single-fibre electromyography: blocking and jitter, with normal fibre density; confirmatory, but not specific
- Edrophonium chloride (Tensilon) 2 mg + 8 mg IV; highly probable diagnosis if unequivocally positive
- For ocular or cranial MG: Exclude intracranial lesions by CT or MRI

Treatment

Prompt response with edrophonium chloride and neostigmine.

Medical

Anticholinesterase Drugs

- Neostigmine, pyridostigmine, edrophonium chloride
- Pyridostigmine is the most widely used anticholinesterase drug. Start with 30–60 mg three to four times daily. beneficial action of oral pyridostigmine begins within 15–30 min and lasts for 3–4 hours.

Steroids and other immunosuppressive drugs:

- Glucocorticoids, when used properly, produce improvement in myasthenic weakness in the great majority of patients. To minimize adverse side effects, prednisone should be administer in a single dose rather than in divided doses throughout the day.
- Mycophenolate mofetil, azathioprine, cyclosporine, tacrolimus, and occasionally cyclophosphamide are effective in many patients, either alone or in various combinations.

Plasmapheresis

A course of five exchanges (3–4 L per exchange) is generally administered over a 10–14 day period

Intravenous Immunoglobulins:

- The usual dose is 2 g/kg, administered over 5 days (400 mg/kg per day).
- If tolerated, the course of IV Ig can be shortened to administer the entire dose over a 3-day period.

Surgical

Beneficial results have been shown after thymectomy or irradiation of thymus (3000 R over 3–6 weeks).

Miscellaneous Diseases

Paget's disease (or osteodystrophia deformans) is an idiopathic chronic condition characterized by excessive resorption of bone by osteoclasts, followed by the replacement of normal marrow by vascular, fibrous connective tissue leading to bony thickening and deformity.

Aetiology

- Remains *unknown*, but evidence supports both *genetic and viral etiologies.*
- *Positive family history* (homozygous deletion of the TNFRSF11B gene, which encodes osteoprotegrin causes juvenile Paget's disease).
- Electron microscopy shows cytoplasmic and nuclear inclusions resembling *paramyxoviruses (respiratory syncytial virus and measles)* in pagetic osteoclasts suggestive of *viral aetiology.*
- Prevalence is greater in males and increases with age; rare under the age of 40 years.

Pathophysiology

- Basic abnormality in Paget's disease is the *increased number and over activity of osteoclasts.*
- Pathognomonic feature of Paget's disease is increased bone resorption accompanied by accelerated bone formation associated with hypervascularity and fibrosis.
- Resorption of the existing bone is brought about by osteoclasts and bone formation by osteoblasts.

The *pathogenesis* of Paget's disease is described in three stages that are:
- Osteoclastic activity
- Mixed osteoclastic-osteoblastic activity
- Exhaustive (burnt out) stage.

Causes of over activity of osteoclasts are:
- Hypersensitivity of osteoclastic precursors are to *1, 25(OH) $_2$D$_3$.*
- Decreased response of osteoclasts to *RANK ligand (RANKL)* (the osteoclast stimulatory factor).
- Increased *RANKL expression* in marrow stromal cells from pagetic lesions.
- *Overexpression of (IL) 6* in pagetic osteoclasts, which increases the recruitment of osteoclast precursor.
- Increased expression of the *proto-oncogene c-fos*, which increases osteoclastic activity.
- Overexpression of *antiapoptotic oncogene Bcl-2* in pagetic bone.

Skeleton sites of predilections: The *pelvic bones* are most commonly involved, followed by femur, skull, tibia, lumbosacral spine, dorsal spine, clavicles and ribs.

Clinical Features

- Most commonly, the disease *exits asymptomatically* and are often diagnosed accidentally by discovery of an elevated ALP level on routine blood chemistry testing or as an incidental finding on a skeletal radiograph obtained for another indication.
- *Pain* is the most important and common presenting symptom.

Presentation can be:

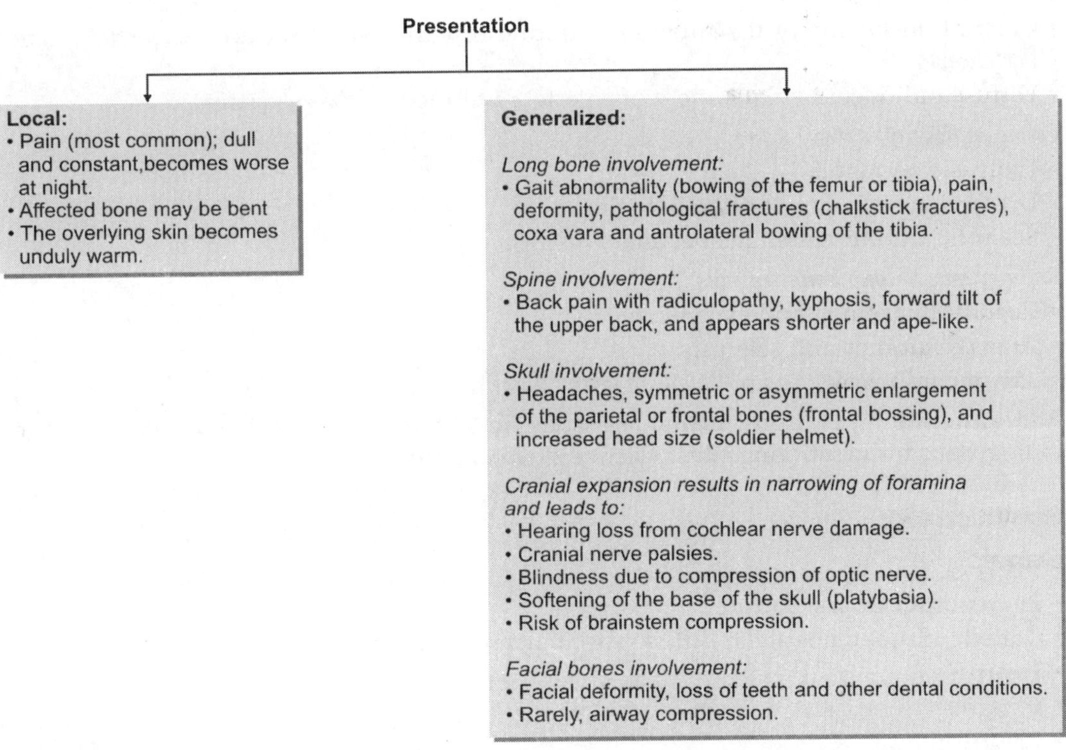

Investigations

It usually diagnosed from *radiologic and biochemical abnormalities*.

Biochemical Abnormalities

- Rise in *serum ALP (heat-labile Alkaline Phosphatase; 10 times the upper limit of normal)* and urinary hydroxyproline levels, markers of bone formation and resorption, respectively; confirm the fundamental pathological process of *bone formation and resorption in Paget's disease.*
- Urinary and serum *deoxypyridinoline, C-telopeptide, and N-telopeptide levels* are products of type I collagen degradation and are more specific for bone resorption than hydroxyproline
- Serum *calcium and phosphate levels* are normal.

Radiological Findings

- Enlargement or expansion of affected bone.
- The bone shows cortical thickening, deformity, coarsening of trabecular markings, and typical lytic and sclerotic changes.

Skull radiographs reveal:
- Regions of *"cotton wool,"* or *osteoporosis circumscripta*.
- Thickening of diploic areas.
- Enlargement and sclerosis of all or a portion of one or more skull bones (*soldier helmet*: cranium is so heavy that it becomes difficult for the patient to hold the head erect).

Vertebral involvement shows:
- Cortical thickening of the superior and inferior end plates produces a *"picture frame"* vertebra.
- Diffuse radiodense enlargement of a vertebra termed as *"ivory vertebra"*.

Pelvic radiographs may shows:
- Protrusio acetabuli.
- Disruption or fusion of sacroiliac joint.
- Sclerotic and thickened ileopectinal line (*Brim sign*).

Radiographs of long bones reveals:
- Cortical thickening and expansion
- Areas of lucency and sclerosis
- Advancing lytic wedge or *"blade of grass"* lesion.

Radionuclide ^{99m}Tc bone scans: less specific but are more sensitive than standard radiographs for identifying sites of active skeletal lesions.

Complications

General

- High output cardiac failure
- Calcific aortic stenosis and diffuse vascular calcification
- Deafness
- Blindness
- Paraplegia.

Local

- Fractures of long bones (femoral shaft and subtrochanteric regions).
- Osteosarcomas especially in along standing pagetic lesion.
- Osteoclast-rich benign giant cell tumors.

Treatment

Medical Management

Biphosphonates and calcitonin are the chief agent used to suppress the pathological process and all act by inhibiting the resorption.

Biphosphonate

- Etidronate 400 mg/d for 6 months fasting PO.
- Tiludronate (2nd generation biphosphonate) 400 mg/d for 3 months fasting PO.

- Pamidronate 30 mg/d for 3 doses or 60–90 mg once IV.
- Alendronate (2nd generation biphosphonate) 30 mg/d for 2 months fasting PO.
- Risedronate (2nd generation biphosphonate) 30 mg/d for 2 months fasting PO.
- Zoledronate 5 mg IV.
- In patients with high bone turnover, vitamin D (400–800 IU daily) and calcium (500 mg three times daily) administrated to prevent hypocalcaemia and secondary hyperparathyroidism.

Calcitonin: Calcitonin (Miacalcin) 100 U daily SC *(nasal spray is not approved for use in Paget disease). Dose titrated to 50 U/d three times weekly* after an initial favourable response.

Mithramycin

- It is a cytotoxic *DNA directed RNA inhibitor.*
- Lowers serum calcium, relieves bone pain, reduces serum ALP and urinary hydroxyproline and improves CCF.

Physiotherapy: To maintain joint mobility

Surgical Management

- Before any surgical procedure especially during the active stage of disease, *preoperative drug treatment is necessary to reduce the activity and vascularity of the disease.* A course of Calcitonin is preferred.
- *Fractures:* ORIF with compression plate or intramedullary rod is advisable.
- *Severe degenerative arthritis*: Joint replacement surgeries.
- *Deformities*: Corrective osteotomy.
- *Nerve entrapment*: Decompression.
- *Severe spinal stenosis*: Decompression.

Q2. Write short note on Infantile Cortical Hyperostosis or Caffey's disease or Caffey's-Silverman syndrome.

Infantile cortical hyperostosis is an idiopathic self-limited inflammatory disorder of infants under 6 month of age and characterized clinically by bone changes, tender subperiosteal swelling, hyperaesthesia and constitutional signs of fever, elevated ESR and leucocytosis.

Aetiology

- Unknown.
- Both sporadic and familial (autosomal dominant) forms occur.
- Genetics: associated with COL1A1.
- The condition is often confused with hypervitaminosis A.
- Constitutional sign such as fever leucocytosis suggest an *infection (viral) origin.*
- Inflammation of periosteum and adjacent soft tissue

Pathophysiology

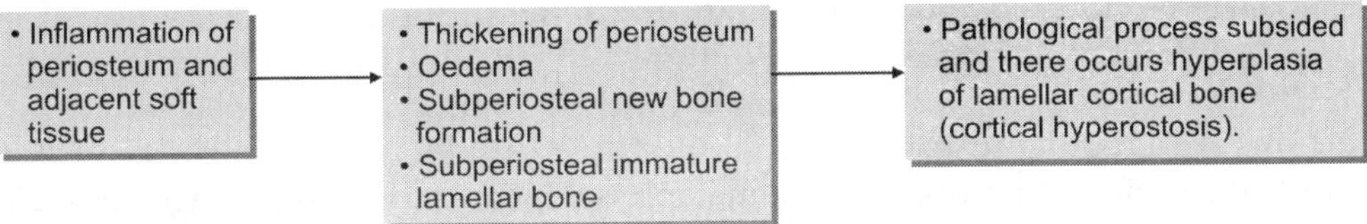

Clinical Features

- Onset is acute.
- Triad of *soft-tissue swelling, fever, and irritability.*
- Infant is fretful, irritable, crying and failure to thrive.
- Swelling due to subperiosteal ossification appears suddenly over the diaphysis of long bone especially the clavicle, ulna and sometimes scapula.
- *Bilateral mandibular swelling* is common and characteristic.
- Other affected bones include *tibia, ulna, clavicle, scapula, ribs, humerus, femur, fibula, skull, ilium, and metatarsals.*
- Swelling, although a soft tissue mass is deep, firm, and may be tender but not warm.
- Variable degree of fever is present.

Investigation

Laboratory Findings

- ESR is elevated
- ALP is raised
- Leukocytosis
- CRP is raised
- Anaemia.

X-rays Finding

- Periosteal new bone formation (onion peel appearance) *(subperiosteal hyperostosis).*
- Pronounced cortical thickening.
- Distribution is *asymmetric and patchy* but multifocal (mandible is invariable involved)
- Periosteal *'cloaking'* is confined to the diaphyses; sparing of epiphyses and metaphyses

Differential Diagnosis

Hypervitaminosis A

- Shows involvement after 1 year of age.
- Mandible is never involved.
- Fever is absent.
- Vitamin A level is raised.
- Discontinuing of vitamin A effects a cure within 1 week.

Scurvy

Ground glass, osteoporotic appearance with dense line (Wimberger's line) of all bone is characteristic.

Osteomyelitis

- Fever is high.
- Localized involvement and destruction of bone.
- Bacteria can be cultured and antibiotic are effective.

Child Abuse

- Fractures are a regular feature
- Periosteal reaction is predominantly metaphyseal, contrary to the images in Caffey's disease.

Ewing Sarcoma

- It is similar in appearance because of its typical onion-peel laminations and accompanying constitutional symptoms.
- Biopsy reveals the true nature of the lesion.

Syphilitic Hyperostosis

Treatment

- As this is a self limited disease treatment is unnecessary.
- Antibiotics should be given and vitamins are discontinued until the diagnosis is ascertained.

Q3. Discuss in brief: Vertebra plana or Calve disease.

Vertebra Plana is characterized by *rapid collapse and flattening of single vertebral body* with relatively preserved intervertebral disc space, which appear as *dense wafer in X-rays.*

Calve preferred the use of the term *"osteochondritis"* of the vertebral body with clinical aspects of Potts spine (Calve's disease of the spine) to this process. Buchman, however, suggested the name "vertebra plana".

However, recent biopsy study of similar lesions is in accord with the behaviour of eosinophilic granuloma, particularly in the rapidity of the destructive phase.

Aetiology

Osteochondritis, eosinophilic granuloma (most common), Hand-Schutiller-Christian disease, Hodgkin's disease, osteogenesis imperfecta, hyperparathyroidism, unidentified malignant disease, and injury in tetanus, Gaucher disease, TB, aneurysmal bone cyst, infection, etc.

Clinical Features

- Onset is insidious.
- Slight to moderate pain, night cries, fatigue and localized tenderness over the affected spinous process.
- Muscle spasm, limitation of motion of the back and spinal gibbus may be found.
- Gradually develops kyphosis or scoliosis.
- Symptoms subside over a period of 2–3 months but the deformity remains.

X-rays

Three stages can be distinguished.

Early stage

- Seen only in rare cases.
- The shape of the vertebra is intact, but the central part is transparent.
- The edges show minor irregular areas of densification.

Destructive stage

- An *extensive collapse of the vertebral body which is flat* and not wedge-shaped.
- The *intervertebral spaces are normal.*
- As it becomes progressively more compressed, it assumes greater density.

Regeneration: It is slow. Usually in the course of years the body height is moderately restored, but hardly ever recovers its normal shape.

Treatment

- Recumbency.
- Splinting and rest (Gradually, the lesion becomes less painful).
- Spinal brace.
- Irradiation, based on assumption that eosinophilic granuloma is present.

Prognosis

The vertebral body may re-ossify, with little loss of height and with strong bony trabeculation.

 Rule out tuberculosis in all such cases as confusion may occur with tuberculosis in the early stages. The discs are unaffected, the ESR is normal. Tuberculin test should be done. When in doubt, biopsy is indicated.

Q4. Discuss the clinical features and management of Eosinophilic granuloma.

Eosinophilic granuloma, also known as histiocytosis limited to bone is slowly progressing disease *benign, solitary, rarely multiple, bone destroying lesion* characterized by *histiocytic and eosinophilic leukocytes infiltrate* of unknown origin *with no extra skeletal involvement*. This differentiates eosinophilic granuloma from other forms of *Langerhans cell histiocytosis (Letterer-Siwe or Hand-Schüller-Christian variant)*.

Aetiology

- Unknown
- Proliferative disorder (involving a specialized types of histiocytes similar to Langerhans of epidermis) of unknown aetiology.
- Granulomatous histiocytic proliferation.
- Cause of this proliferation is obscure but a *viral infection* and an *immunological disorder* have been suggested.
- Male preponderance; peak age is between 5 and 15 years.

Area of Predilection

The lesion is usually *monostic* and *rarely polyostotic*.

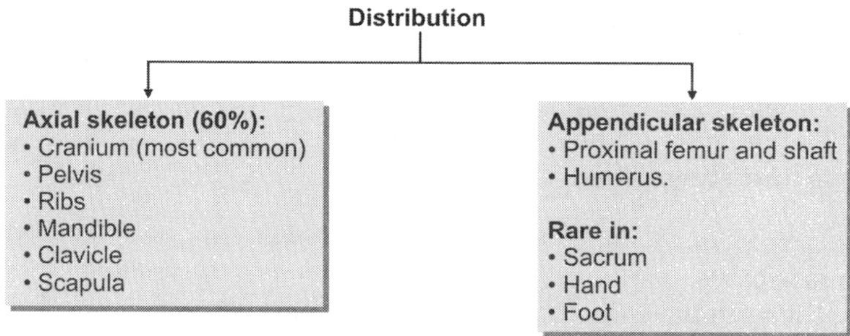

- In vertebrae, it generally affects the body.
- In the long bones, the favoured sites are the diaphyses and metaphyses with the sparing of epiphyses.

Pathology

- Predominance of histiocytes-like *Langerhans cells and eosinophils*.
- *Langerhans cells* have vesiculated, pale and often lobulated nuclei and *weekly eosinophilic cytoplasm*.

- Positive staining for langerhans cell *for S-100 protein and Bierbeck granules (Pathognomonic) and CD1a antigen* seen by electron microscopy are confirmatory.

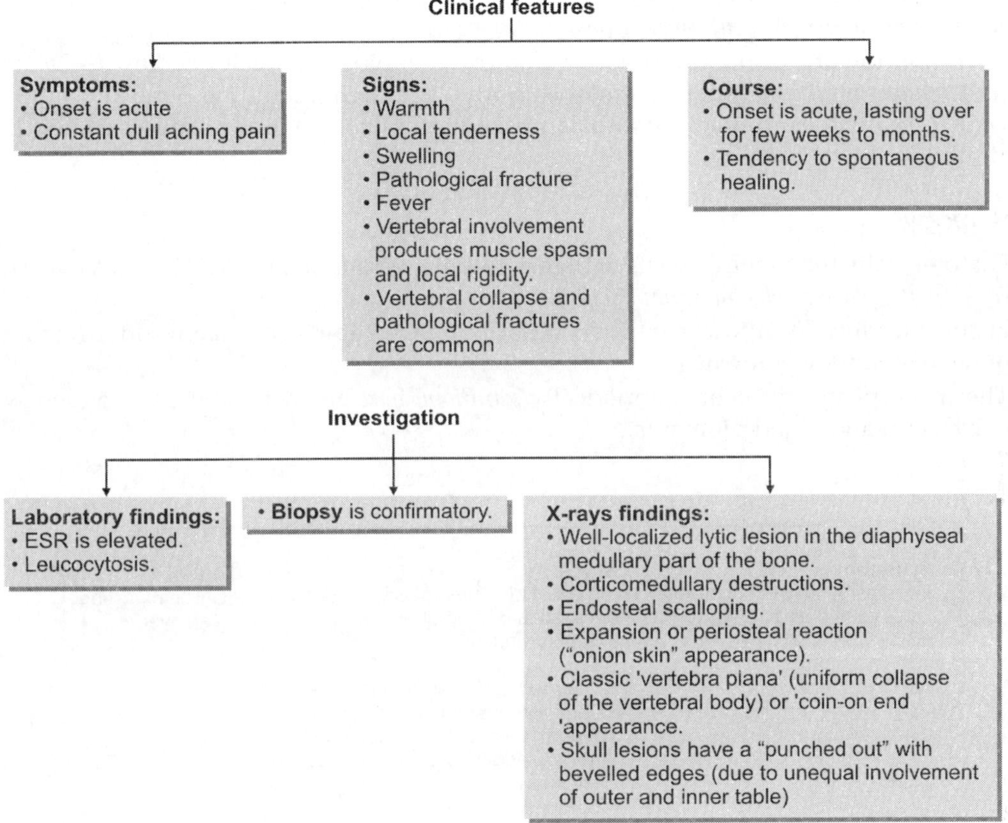

Treatment

Eosinophilic granuloma tends to *involutes spontaneously* without treatment; therefore, *treatment should be conservative.*

- In accessible site: *Curettage* of the lesion and packing the cavity with *bone grafts.*
- Ribs and clavicle lesions requires only *subperiosteal segmental resection.*
- As the lesion is *radiosensitive,* in inaccessible region like spine and pelvis a low dose radiation (10Gy or 500–1000 rads) can be considered.
- The use of anterior decompression and anterior fusion in patient with severe neurological symptoms.
- Chemotherapeutic agents are indicated; in cases with multiple lesions, not responding to the surgery or radiation therapy.

Q5. Write a short note on Hand-Schüller-Christian disease and Letterer-Siwe disease.

Eosinophilic granuloma, Letterer-Siwe and Hand Schüller Christian disease are regarded as manifestations of the same pathologic entity designated as *histiocytosis X*. The fundamental denominator is an *inflammatory histiocytosis.*

Hand-Schüller-Christian disease

The classic triad of Diabetes insipidus, exophthalmos, and punched-out lytic bone lesions (Hand-Schüller-Christian disease) are associated with granulomatous lesions visible on MRI, as well as a characteristic *axillary skin rash.*

It is subacute or chronic condition of unknown aetiology characterized by *disseminated granulomatous infiltration* of the reticuloenthothelial system including bone and multiple organs typically the pituitary, hypothalamus, lungs, mucocutaneous surfaces spleen, liver and orbit.

Pathology

- Histologically the tissue consists of highly cellular *reticuloenthothelial tissue, macrophages, eosinophils, plasma cells and lymphocytes.*
- Histiocytes form multinucleate giant cells containing lipids and haemosiderin in areas of necrosis and haemorrhage.
- The macrophages are characteristically *xanthoma foreign body giant cells* loaded with cholesterol and blood pigments.

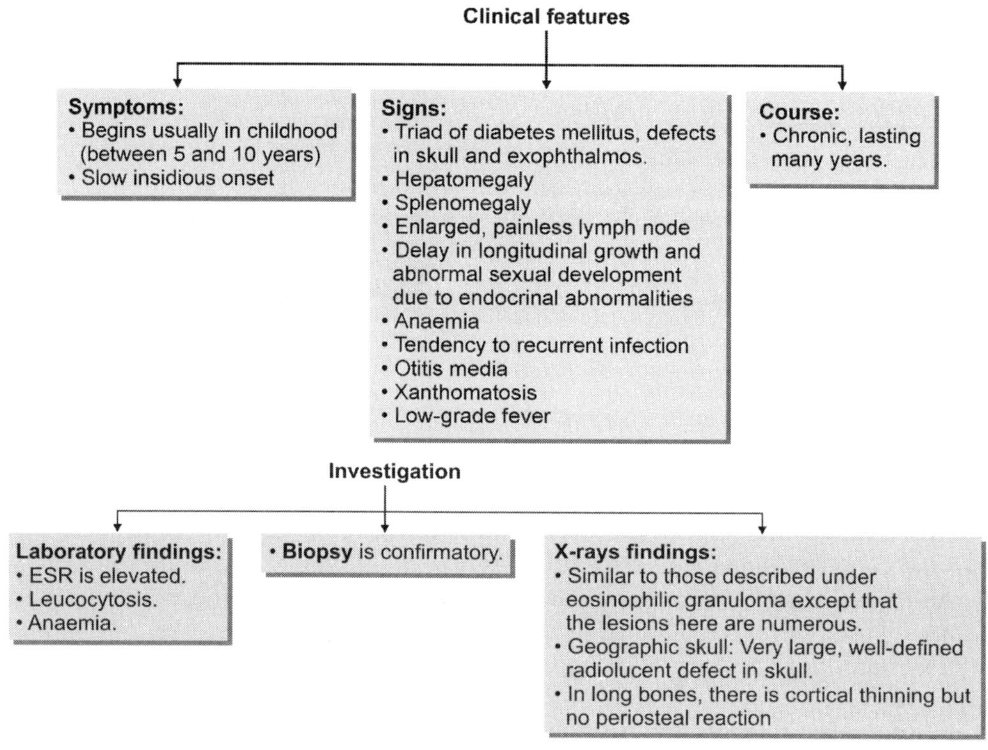

Treatment

- The *lesions are radiosensitive* following which the lesions may completely reossify.
- Surgical treatment by *curettage and packing with bone grafts or segmental subperiosteal resection.*
- Pathological fracture needs fixation plus medical treatment for generalized disease.
- Chemotherapeutic agent *vinblastin* is indicated in patient not responding to surgery or radiation or corticosteroids.

Letterer-Siwe disease

An acute *fulminating generalized reticuloenthothelial disease* of infants, invariable fatal. There is widespread histiocytic dissemination involving the red marrow of flat bones, vertebrae, skull and many organs.

Pathology

- Histologically the tissue consists of highly cellular *reticuloenthothelial tissue, macrophages, eosinophils, plasma cells and lymphocytes.*
- *The histiocytes are highly vacuolated but contain little or no lipoid; foam cells are rare (non-lipid histiocytosis).*

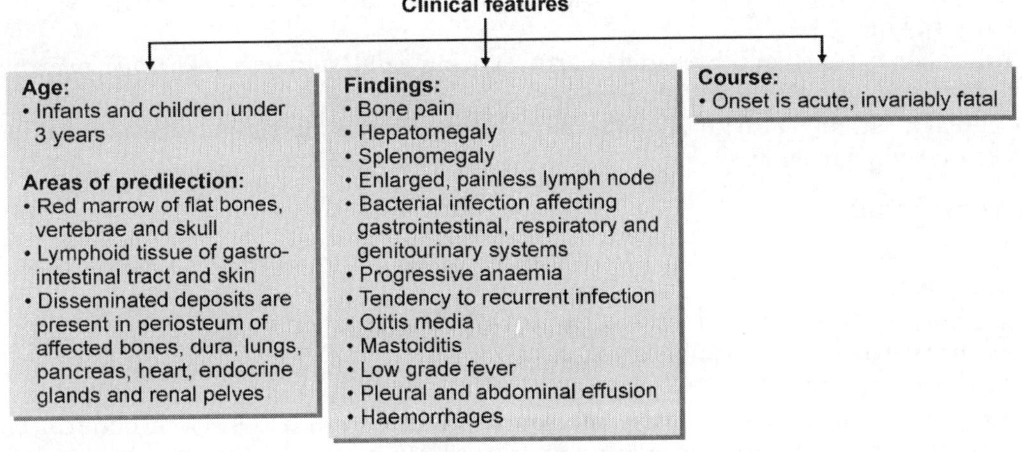

Treatment

- No treatment works.
- Prolonged survival and possible cure could be possible by using various antibiotics, radiation, and steroid.

Q6. Discuss the features and management of Gaucher's disease.

Gaucher disease is an autosomal recessive disorder that results from defective or decreased activity of *glycolipid degradation enzyme, acid α-glucosidase* (glucosylceramide α-glucosidase) resulting in storage of these cells in the bone, lymph nodes, spleen and liver.

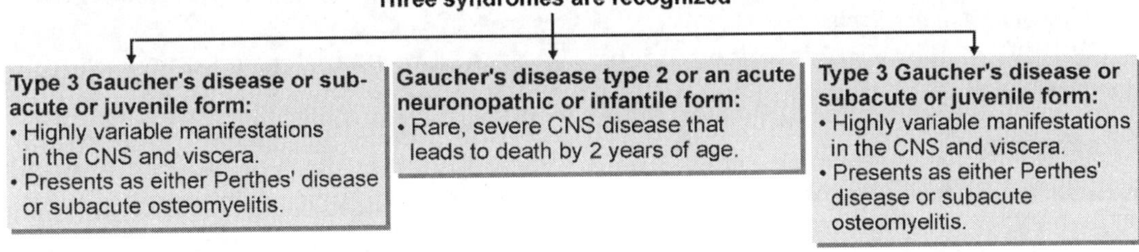

Aetiology

- Transmitted as an autosomal recessive disorder.
- The most common mutation in the Ashkenazi Jewish population (N370S) shares a 100% association with nonneuronopathic or type 1 Gaucher's disease.
- Both sexes are equally affected.

Pathophysiology

- The disease is due to defect in gene *lysosomal gluco-cerebrosidase* (also known as beta-glucosidase) on the first chromosome (1q21).
- This enzyme catalyses the breakdown of a complex lipid, a sphingolipid designated as *glucocerebroside*, a cell membrane *constituent of red and white blood cells.*
- The *macrophages* that clear these cells are unable to eliminate the waste product, which accumulates in fibrils, and turn into *Gaucher's cells (hallmark)*, resembling *crumpled silk or cigarette paper* on light microscopy.
- Wavy fibrillae are stained with *PAS or with Mallory trichrome's* connective tissue stain.
- Cytoplasm of these cells also demonstrates strong *acid phosphatase activity*. Increased amount of finely dispersed ferritin imparts a bluish hue of Gaucher cell when stained by Prussian blue.
- Infiltration of Gaucher cells lead to marrow packing with *subsequent ischaemia, infarction, necrosis, and cortical bone destruction.*
- Cellular infiltration also involves the *lungs, kidney, adrenal, thyroid and thymus and all sites where lymphoid tissue exists.*

Clinical Features

- *Type 1 Gaucher's disease or chronic non-neuronopathic type* is usually encountered by orthopaedic surgeon.
- *Hepatosplenomegaly* occurs in virtually all symptomatic patients
- *Splenic infarctions* can resemble an acute abdomen.
- *Pulmonary hypertension*
- Bone remodeling is defective, bone marrow involvement, with loss of total bone calcium leading to *avascular infarction, osteopenia, osteonecrosis, and vertebral compression fractures and spinal cord involvement.*
- *Avascular necrosis of the femoral head* is common symptomatic manifestation, as is fracture of the femoral neck.
- The femur may be typically involved showing *Erlenmeyer flask appearance (Fischer sign)* at the lower end of femur with generalized mottled appearance, increased breadth of the marrow cavity resulting in flaring of distal femur with thinning of the cortex.
- *"Bone crises"* are associated with localized, *excruciating pain, and occasionally with, local erythema, fever, and leukocytosis.*
- Softening and necrosis of bones produces *marked deformity and degenerative changes* about the hip and shoulder joint.
- Painful, acute onset, with fever, localized tenderness *simulating acute hematogenous osteomyelitis in children.*
- Multiple vertebral compression fracture in spine produces kyphotic and scoliotic deformity.

Investigations

- *Bone marrow smears*: presence of Gaucher's cell.
- *Serum acid phosphatase* level is markedly increased (King-Armstrong method).
- *Measurement of enzymatic activity*: Decreased acid α-glucosidase activity (0–20% of normal) in nucleated cells.
- *Anemia*, thrombocytopenia
- *X-rays*: shows mottled or diffuse translucencies, erosion and thinning of cortex, *Erlenmeyer flask appearance* of the distal femur, degenerative changes, changes of avascular necrosis, marked osteoporosis, multiple vertebral compression fractures.

- *Nuclear scans*: bone crises represent acute infarctions of bone, as evidenced in by localized absent uptake of pyrophosphate agents.

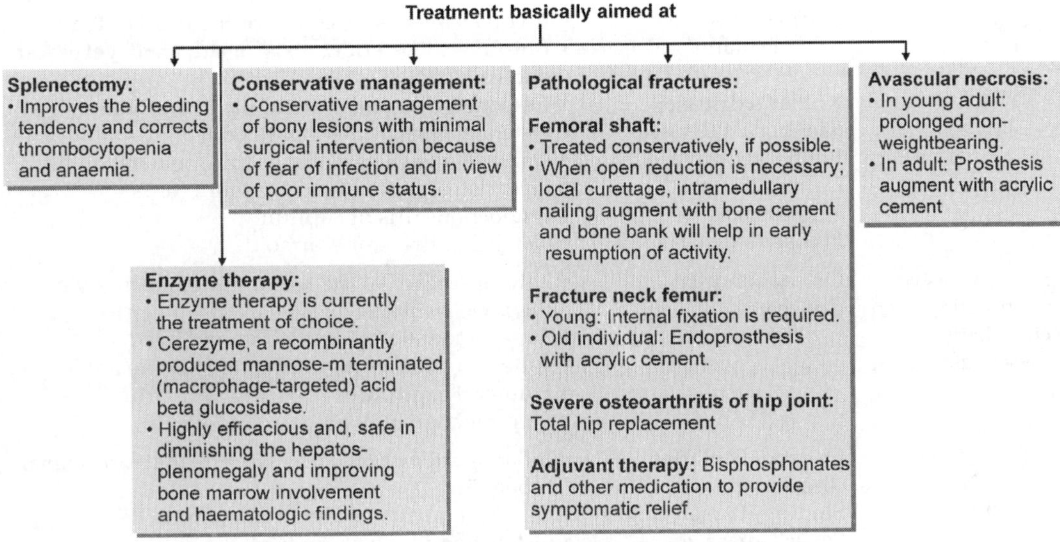

Q7. What is osteochondritis and enumerate different types of it.

Osteochondritis is a disease of unknown aetiology causing temporary softening of the ossific centres of a child leading to deformation under pressure and damaged growth subsequently.

The involve area shows increased vascularity and osteogenesis in response to death of cell in the osteoarticular fragment suggestive features of ischemic necrosis. It is common in adolescent and young adults, frequently during phases of increased physical activity.

Subdivision

Based on mechanism leading to avascular necrosis, it is, subdivided into:

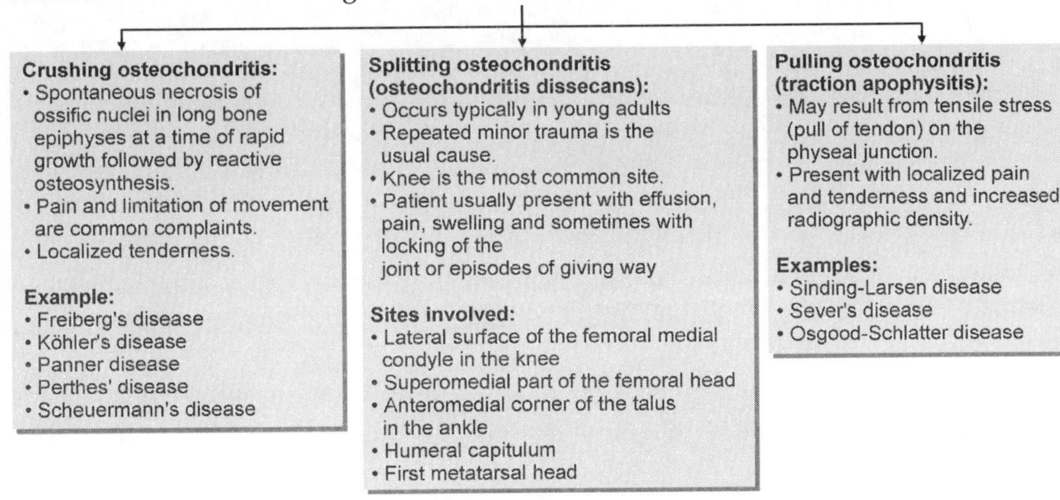

Classification and Types

Type	Condition	Bone affected
Crushing osteochondritis	Perthes' disease	• Involves the ossific centre of the head of femur
	Scheuermann's disease	• Epiphyseal osteonecrosis of adjacent vertebral bodies
	Köhler's disease	• Osteonecrosis of the tarsal navicular bone
	Kienböck's disease	• Osteonecrosis of the lunate bone
	Freiberg's disease	• Osteonecrosis of second or third metatarsal head
	Calve's disease	• Collapse of body of one vertebra (dorsal)
	Panner disease	• Osteochondritis of capitulum
	Preoser's disease	• Osteochondritis of scaphoid
Splitting osteochondritis (osteochondritis dissecans)	Osteochondritis dissecans	• Lateral surface of the femoral medial condyle in the knee • Superomedial part of the femoral head • Anteromedial corner of the talus in the ankle • Humeral capitulum • First metatarsal head
Pulling osteochondritis (traction apophysitis)	Osgood–Schlatter disease	• Inflammation of the growth centre that forms tibial tuberosity
	Sinding–Larsen disease	• Osteochondritis of lower pole of patella
	Sever's disease	• Osteochondrosis of the heel

15

Orthopaedic Neurology

Q1. Give classification of nerve injury.

Seddon's classification of nerve injuries: (*generally accepted but rarely used*):

I. Neuropraxia

- Minor contusion or compression of a peripheral nerve.
- Preservation of the axis-cylinder.
- Transmission of impulses is physiologically interrupted for a short time
- Recovery is complete in a few days or weeks.
- Tinel sign is absent.

II. Axonotmesis

- Significant injury with breakdown of the axon and distal Wallerian degeneration.
- Preservation of the Schwann cell and endoneurial tubes.
- Spontaneous regeneration with good functional recovery is expected.
- Tinel sign is present.

III. Neurotmesis

- More severe injury with complete anatomical transection of the nerve.
- Axon and the Schwann cell and endoneurial tubes are completely disrupted.
- Perineurium and epineurium also are disrupted to varying degrees.
- Significant spontaneous recovery cannot be expected.
- Tinel Sign is present.

Sunderland Classification (1951)

This classification is more readily applicable clinically

Classification of nerve injuries:

Degree of injury		Histopathological changes					Tinel Sign	
Sunderland	Seddon	Myelin	Axon	Endo-neurium	Perineu-rium	Epineu-rium	Present distally	Pro-gresses
I	Neurapraxia	±					−	−
II	Axonotmesis	+	+				+	+
III		+	+	+			+	+
IV		+	+	+	+		+	−
V	Neurotmesis	+	+	+	+	+	+	−

Q2. What is Wallerian degeneration?

Any part of a neuron detached from its nucleus degenerates and is destroyed by the process of phagocytosis. This process of degeneration distal to a point of injury is called *secondary, or Wallerian degeneration.*

The reaction proximal to the point of detachment is called *primary, traumatic,* or *retrograde degeneration.*

Q3. Discuss the diagnosis, management, and prognosis of peripheral nerve injuries.

Diagnosis

I. Electrodiagnostic Studies

- Electrophysiological studies have been used for several decades to diagnose and also to prognosticate various neuromuscular disorders.
- Most common electrodiagnostic methods used to study nerve injuries are nerve conduction velocity (NCV) and electromyography (EMG).
- These tests provide vital information regarding:
  - Nerve conductivity
  - Axon or myelin involvement
  - Muscle recruitment capability

Nerve Conduction Velocity

- Recording of the electrical response of a muscle to stimulation of its motor nerve at two or more points along its course permits conduction velocity to be determined in the fastest-conducting motor fibres between the points of stimulation.
- It is a measure of the conduction velocity of impulse in a nerve.
- An electrode is placed on the skin overlying the nerve.
- The nerve is stimulated proximal to, distal to, and across the level of injury.
- Stimulation of a peripheral nerve readily evokes a response from the muscle innervated by that nerve and this response can be seen, palpated, and measured.
- The velocity of the conduction of the impulse between any two points of the nerve can be calculated.
- Immediately after injury: Stimulation elicits a normal response.
- As Wallerian degeneration ensues (within 5–10 days):
- There is progressive reduction in the amplitude and alterations in the configuration of the evoked potential.
- If there is neurapraxia: Conductivity distal to the lesion seems to be normal even after 10 days, and this has a considerably more favourable outcome.

Electromyography (EMG)

- In electromyography, the study of the electrical activity of contracting muscle gives crucial information regarding the structure and function of the motor units.
- This may make it possible not only to localize the site of pathology affecting either muscle or its innervations but also it frequently provides evidence regarding the nature of the pathological process.
- EMG is much more sensitive in detecting more subtle neurological injury.

Advantages

- Detect the presence or absence of injury.
- If present then it helps to detect whether complete or incomplete.
- Any regeneration is taking place or not.

Disadvantage

- No idea about the severity of injury.
- No idea about the level of injury.

EMG

- Positive sharp wave consistent with denervation 10–14 days after injury.
- Spontaneous denervation fibrillation potentials present within 14–18 days after injury.

There are four classification of the spontaneous activity:

- Fibrillation activity.
- Positive sharp waves.
- Fasciculation potentials.
- Repetitive discharges

Fibrillation Potential

Fibrillation potential is seen in the denervated muscle as they give spontaneous discharges because they are hypersensitive to circulating acetylcholine (ACh). Classically, it is seen in lower motor neuron disorders such as:

- Anterior horn lesions.
- Radiculopathies.
- Peripheral nerve lesions
- Polyneuropathies with axonal degeneration, it is seen in myopathic disease like:
    - Dermatomyositis
    - Polymyositis and
    - Muscular dystrophy.
    - Myasthenia gravis.

Positive Sharp Waves

- It is a form of *electrical potential associated with fibrillating muscle* fibres, which are recorded as a biphasic, positive negative action potential initiated by needle movement, and recurring in uniform patterns.
- Positive sharp wave is *seen in primary muscle disease* like muscular dystrophy, polymyositis but sometimes, it is also seen in upper motor neuron lesions.
- These waves are characteristic features of denervated muscle.

Fasciculations

- A *random spontaneous twitching of muscle fibres* or a group may be visible through skin.
- This is seen in irritation or degeneration of anterior horn cell.
    - *Muscle spasm or cramps*
    - *Motor neuron disease*
    - *Nerve root compression*
    - *Pathology of spinal cord*
    - *Pathology of root level.*

Repetitive Discharges

- These are also known as bizarre *high frequency discharge*.
- The potential of repetitive discharge represents various forms. The characteristic features of the repetitive discharges are:
  - Amplitude: 50–1 mV
  - Frequency: 5–100 per sec

Strength Duration Curve

- The threshold for activation of a fibre depends not only on stimulus strength, but also on the duration of the stimulus.
- The relationship between the strength of a stimulus and its duration for producing minimal excitation is expressed by the strength-duration (S-D) curve.
- The strength-duration curve for a typical neural membrane is similar, but differs in that the curve clearly flattens out with long stimulus durations, reaching an asymptote called the **Rheobase**.
- *Rheobase* is *minimum current or voltage, which can produce minimal muscle excitation when a large duration impulse is applied*
- When the stimulus strength is below the Rheobase, stimulation is ineffective even when stimulus duration is very long.
- Given that two nerves have the same Rheobase, the **Chronaxie** (*the stimulus duration in millisecond corresponding to twice the Rheobase*) can give an indication of their relative excitabilities

SD Curves Characteristic

- Right hand part of the curve—for denervation
- Left hand part of the curve—for innervations
- Kink is at point where both the curves meet.
- If large denervated fibres: The curve rises steeply and kink toward right
- If large innervated fibres: The curve lowers and flattened and kink will be towards left
- Progressive innervated: The kink will appear and the curve will move down and towards left
- Progressive denervation: The kink will appear with an increase in slope and the curve shifts to right.

Uses of Curves

- It demonstrates the presence of innervated fibres in the muscle being tested.
- It demonstrate the changes in the innervations by means of successive graphs.
- It indicates the value of Rheobase, Chronaxie and utilization time.

Tinel's Sign

This sign provides a useful guide to the presence of growing sensory axon tips and their progress down the nerve.

How to elicit Tinel sign?

- Gentle percussion by a finger along the course of an injured nerve.
- Transient tingling sensation appreciated by the patient in the distribution of the injured nerve rather than at the area percussed.
- Tingling sensation persist for several seconds after stimulation.

Interpretation

- Positive Tinel sign is presumptive evidence that regenerating axonal sprouts but not obtained complete myelinization are progressing along the endoneurial tube.
- Positive response fades as myelinization take place.

Sweat Test

Basis

Presence of sweating within the autonomous zone of an injured peripheral nerve indicates that complete interruption of the nerve has not occurred

Different tests of assessing sweat patterns in the hand:

- Observing beads of sweat through the +20 lens of an ophthalmoscope as pointed out by Kahn.
- *Iodine starch test*: In the denervated area, powder remains dry and light gray and assumes a deep purple colour throughout the area of normal sweating.
- *Ninhydrin print test (Aschan and Moberg)*

Skin Resistance Test

- Richter dermometer is used to test skin resistance to flow of current.
- Autonomous zone with absence of sweating shows an increased resistance to the passage of electrical current
- Adjacent innervated areas have a normal resistance.

Electrical Stimulation

- *Faradic stimulation* is of little value because even normally innervated muscles may fail to respond to this current.
- *Galvanic stimulation* is useful in determining chronaxy and the strength-duration curve. These parameters give early evidence of denervation following nerve injury.

Management

Guidelines for management of peripheral nerve injuries:

If nerve cut and exposed: Repair the nerve:

- **Primary** if wound clean and fresh.
- **Secondary** or delayed if wound potentially contaminated.

If wound closed: Wait and watch for 3–6 weeks

If no recovery by the end of 3–6 weeks do:

- EMG and nerve conduction velocity
- Explore and repair the nerve if:
    - If there is no motor or sensory response
    - EMG shows no voluntary motor Potential
    - Positive sharp waves and Fibrillation potentials
- Wait and watch as the nerve is on its way to recovery if:
    - EMG shows positive sharp waves,
    - Fibrillations potentials and a few voluntary muscle potentials

Types of Repair

- *Primary*: 6–8 hours after injury and wound is clean.
- *Delayed primary*: 7–18 days after injury or when the wound is contaminated
- *Secondary repair*: 18 days after injury or when present late or there is failure of conservative method or in complete injury

Techniques of nerve repair

- Endoneurolysis (Internal Neurolysis): Freeing of the nerve entrapped within scar tissue.
- Partial Neurorrhaphy (Perineurial (fascicular) or epineurial): Partial severance of the larger nerves
- Neurorrhaphy and nerve grafting: When a nerve has been completely severed

Methods of Closing Gaps between Nerve Ends:

There are several methods of closing gaps between nerve ends. These are:
- Mobilization of nerve from soft tissues proximally and distally.
- Nerve transposition
- Transportation of nerve subcutaneously.
- Flexing the joints, positioning of extremity.
- Bone resection.
- Nerve grafting (the most commonly used donor is sural nerve).
- Nerve crossing (pedicle grafting)

Tendon Transfer

Considered after 18 month of injury if:
- There is no functional improvement even after repair of nerve
- Patient present very late

Arthrodesis

Consider if:
- No tendons are available for transfer
- Future recovery is not possible

Treatment—Specific

Type of injury

Closed injury: If associated with *fracture with neurological deficit*:
- Treat conservatively with analgesic, gabapentin and methylcobalamine.
- Reduce fracture
- Wait for recovery.

If associated with *fracture and injury after manipulation*: Explore immediately.

Open injuries: If clean cut incised wound then primary repair is done.

If clean, cut wound but delayed presentation then delayed primary repair is done after 5–7 days.

If crush/contaminated wound:
- Debridement of wound
- Secondary repair during the intervening period

- Treat by splintage
- Passive movements of all joints.

Prognosis

- *Motor or sensory component*: Purely motor or purely sensory nerves recover better that mixed nerve because there is less likelihood axonal confusion. Radial has best prognosis while ulnar has worst.
- *Age*: Neurorrhaphy are more successful in children than in adults and are more likely to fail in elderly patients.
- *Nature of injury*: sharp cut end has better prognosis the gap can be overcome easily.
- *Delay between time of injury and repair*: Delay of neurorrhaphy affects motor recovery more profoundly than sensory recovery.
- *Level of injury*: more proximal the levels of injury, the more incomplete the overall return of motor and sensory function, especially in the more distal structures.

> **Q4. Write short note on: a. Radial nerve injury and its management; b. Ulnar nerve injury and its management; c. Median nerve injury and its management; D. Intrinsic plus and minus hand; e. Foot drop**

a. Radial Nerve Injury

Anatomy

Radial nerve is a branch from the posterior cord of the brachial plexus:

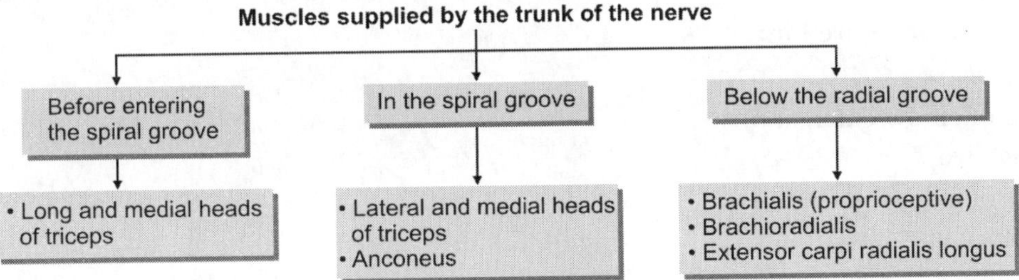

The radial nerve ends by dividing into terminal branches:

- The superficial nerve
- Deep or posterior interosseous nerve

Motor and sensory supply by the branches of radial nerve:

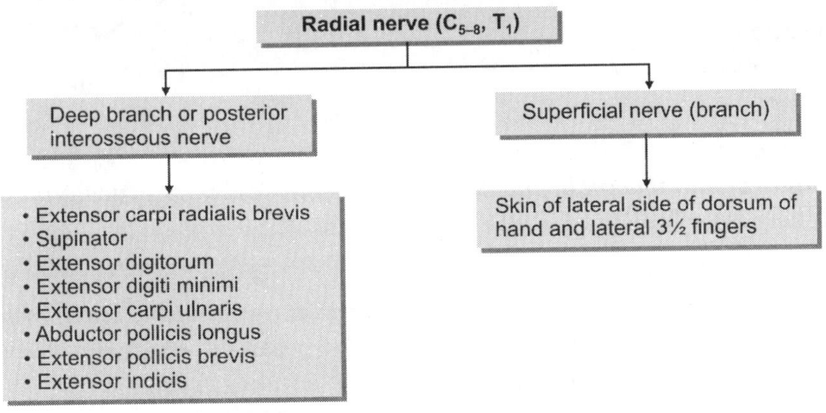

Injury to radial nerve (levels of lesion):

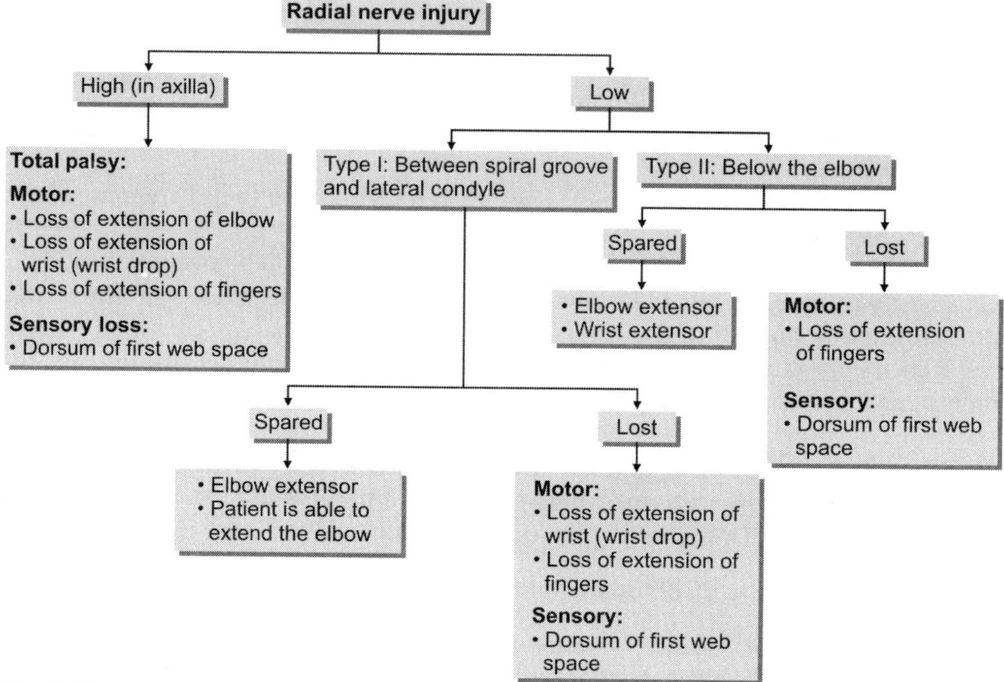

In Nutshell:

If radial nerve injured in:

Axilla:

- Loss of elbow extension
- Wrist drop
- Loss of finger extension
- Sensory loss

Between spiral groove and the lateral epicondyle:
- Wrist drop
- Loss of finger extension
- Sensory loss

Below elbow:
- No wrist drop
- Loss of finer extension
- Sensory loss

Always keep in mind:

If there, is *injury of radial nerve below the elbow or is there is injury of posterior interosseus nerve* than there is *no "WRIST DROP."*

Why?

Reason is simple: In these cases, the nerve supply to the *supinator, brachioradialis and extensor carpi radialis longus* will be *undamaged,* and because the latter muscle is powerful it will keep the wrist joint extended, and *wrist drop will not occur.*

Management

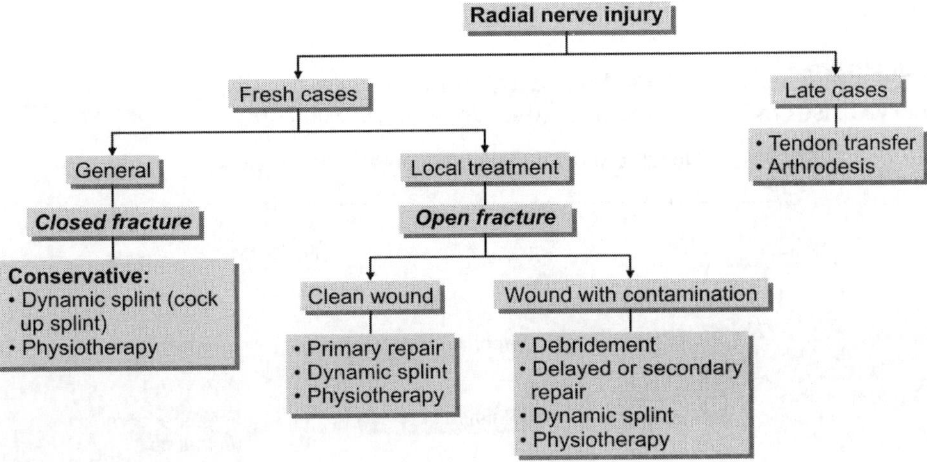

Late Presenting Cases

Tendon transfer

Choice of tendon:

- Flexor carpi ulnaris
- Pronators teres
- Flexor digitorum superficialis

Tendon transfer for radial nerve palsy:

High palsy or Low type I

For:

- *Wrist extension*: Pronators teres transfer
- Finger extension: Flexor carpi ulnaris to extensor digitorum communis (modified Jones)
- Thumb extension: Palmaris longus or flexor digitorum superficialis (ring finger)

Low type II: Wrist extensors are spared so here we have to think about finger and thumb extensors.

For:

- *Finger extension*: Flexor carpi ulnaris to extensor digitorum communis (modified Jones)
- *Thumb extension*: Palmaris longus or flexor digitorum superficialis (ring finger)

Omer's technique

It comprises of splitting of *flexor carpi ulnaris* into five slips and rerouting into all the five fingers instead of four.

Boyes

It comprises of using *flexor digitorum superficialis* of middle and ring finger to bring about extension of fingers.

Rehabilitation

- A/E splint or cast
- Elbow in flexion (90°), forearm pronated, and wrist in extension (30°)

- Thumb is in extension and abduction
- After 4 weeks mobilization encouraged.

b. Ulnar Nerve

This nerve arises from the medial cord of brachial plexus comprising of C_8 and T_1.

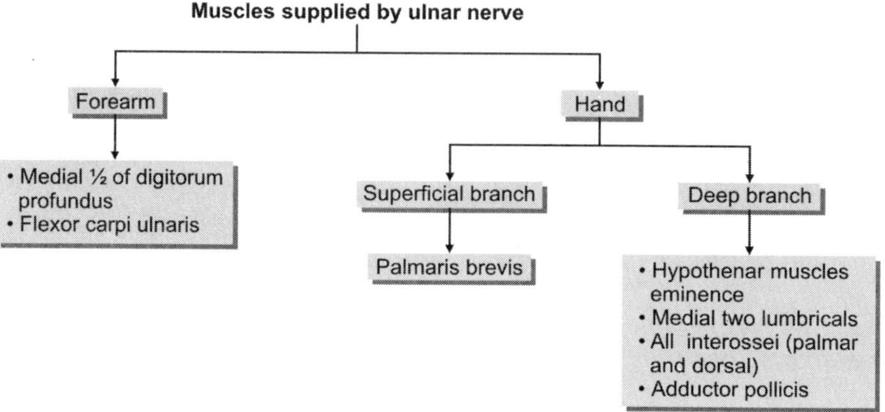

Since a violinist uses most of the intrinsic muscles of hand, the ulnar nerve is the musician's nerve.

Causes

- Supracondylar fracture (malunited with cubitus valgus)
- Dislocation of elbow
- Osteoarthritis overgrowths
- Lacerations
- Leprosy (leads to palsy).

Manifestation of Injury to Ulnar Nerve:

Cubital tunnel syndrome (behind median epicondyle):

- On attempting to flex the wrist, the hand is abducted, due to unopposed action of flexor carpi radialis.
- Medial four fingers cannot be abducted or adducted due to paralysis of dorsal and palmar interossei.
- Due to paralysis of interossei the fingers are extended at their Metacarpophalangeal joint by the action of common digital extensors and this result in passive flexion of the interphalangeal joint (Medial two fingers) – *Claw hand*
- The thumb cannot be adducted due to paralysis of adductor pollicis.
- Wasting of hypothenar eminence muscles.
- Loss of sensation over the anterior and posterior surfaces of medial third of the hand and the medial 1½ finger.

At or below the wrist (Guyon's canal):

- **Abduction and adduction** of the wrist is **not affected** (as flexor carpi ulnaris is spared).
- The **condition of claw hand is much more obvious in wrist lesion** because the flexor digitorum profundus muscle is not paralyzed, and marked flexion (active) of the terminal phalanges *(ulnar paradox)*.

- Loss of sensation over the anterior and posterior surfaces of medial third of the hand and the medial 1½ fingers.

Note:

The *small muscles of the hand* will be paralyzed and show wasting except for the muscles of the thenar eminence and the first two lumbricals (Lateral) which are supplied by *median nerve.*

How to test an ulnar nerve injury?

Froment's sign or book sign or Jeanne's sign	*CARD test*	*Egawa's test*	*Wartenberg's sign*
Basis: • Three muscle (first pulmar interossei, adductor pollicis and flexor pollicis longus) and required to hold a book between the thumb and other fingers **In ulnar nerve palsy:** • The first two muscles are paralyzed • Now to hold the book, the patient has to depend only on flexor pollicis longus, which flexes the thumb permanently	**Basis:** • *Palmar interossei are responsible for adduction of medical fingers* *"Tip : Mn : Paid"* – In ulnar nerve palsy: • The patient is unable to hold a card or paper in-between fingers due to loss of adduction by the palmar interossei	**Basis:** • Dorsal interosseo are abductors "Tip : Mn : Diabetes" PI : Palmar Interossei Abductors • With palm flat on the table, the patient is asked to move the middle finger sideways. This is a test for the dorsal interossei of the middle finger	• Abduction of the small finger due to the third palmar • DI: Dorsal Interossei
Positive Froment's sign (reliable sign for ulnar nerve palsy)	Positive card test		

Management

Cascade for the general treatment will remain the same as discussed above.

For correction of *claw hand deformity*, consider tendon transfers:

Criteria	Technique	Tendon consider for transfer
• Finger flexor are strong • Wrist flexors and extensors are strong • No habitual flexion of the wrist	Modified Stiles–Bunnell procedure	Flexor digitorum superficialis
• Flexion of the wrist becomes habitual • Flexion contracture of the wrist	Riordan's procedure (in order to spare the wrist flexors)	Flexor carpi radialis + brachioradialis graft
• Finger flexor are week • Wrist flexor are week • Wrist extensor are strong	Brand's procedure	Extensor carpi radialis longus or brevis + free tendon graft
• Finger flexors, wrist extensors and wrist flexors are not available	Fowler's technique	Extensor digitorium longus of the index and ring finger

When tendon is selected, it is passed through the lumbrical canal and is attached to the dorsal digital expansion, which then brings about the lost function of the intrinsic muscles.

When no tendon is available for transfer then consider:

- If joints are, supple: *Capsulodesis or tenodesis*
- If joints are not supple: *Arthrodesis in functional position.*

c. Median Nerve

Anatomy

- This nerve arises by two roots, one from the lateral cord (C_{5-7}) and the other from the medial cord (C_8 and T_1) of the brachial plexus
- *Median nerve is called the* **labourers nerve,** *since it supplies most of the large flexor muscle of the forearm.*

Summary of Distribution of Median Nerve

Summary of distribution of median nerve (C_{5-8}, T_1) ventral rami:

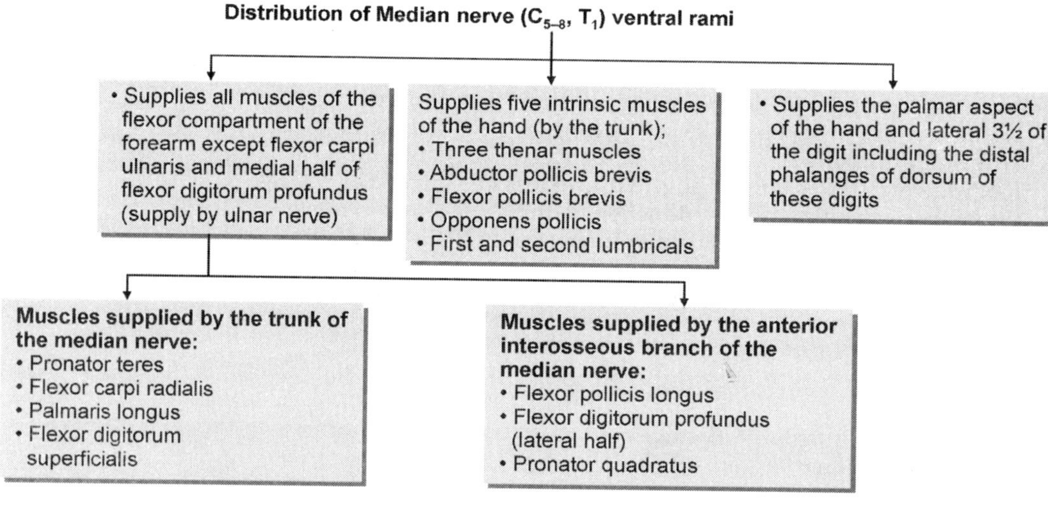

Causes

- Fracture of humerus
- Supracondylar fracture
- Posterior dislocation of elbow
- Compression neuropathy at the wrist due to carpal tunnel syndrome
- Volkmann's ischaemia

Manifestation of an Injury to Median Nerve

At the elbow:

- Loss of flexion of second phalanges of all digits due to paralysis of flexor digitorum superficialis
- Loss of flexion of terminal phalanges of index and middle fingers because of paralysis of lateral half of flexor digitorum profundus
- Flexor of terminal phalanx of thumb is lost because of paralysis of flexor pollicis longus.
- Thumb remains adducted and extended.

- Wasting and paralysis of thenar muscles (APE-like hand)
- Loss of sensation over palmar three and half lateral digits and nail beds

At the middle of the forearm: The branch of the flexor digitorum superficialis to the index finger may be involved (occasionally middle finger). This may be associated with weakness of index finger and the unopposed exoticism of that finger is manifested by—*pointing index finger (Benediction sign)*.

Carpal Tunnel Syndrome

- Flattening of thenar eminence (**ape like hand)**
- **Partial clawing** of index and middle fingers due to paralysis of 1st and 2nd lumbricals
- Loss of sensation over 3½ lateral digits and nail beds
- **No loss** of sensation over the **thenar eminence**

How to test Median nerve?

Pen test	Pointing index or Oschner's clasp test	Benediction test
• Patient is unable to touch the pen due to loss of action of abductor pollicis brevis	• Oschner's clasp test • When both the hands are clasped together, index and middle fingers, fail to flex due to loss of action of long finger flexors of the index and middle fingers supplied by median nerve	• For the same reason mentioned in pointing index, the patient is unable to flex the index and middle finger on lifting the hand. (This is the position a clergyman uses to bless the couple during marriage hence called the benediction test)

Management

Cascade for the general treatment will remain the same as discussed above.

If after nerve repair, there is no functional recovery then tendon transfer is done.

Opponensplasty

- Bunnell procedure: Flexor digitorum superficialis of ring finger through a pulley of flexor carpi ulnaris to opponens.
- *Camitz procedure*: Palmaris longus extended by a strip of palmar fascia to APB.
- *Burkhalter procedure*: Extensor indicis proprius is used as a donor to restore opponens.
- *Huber*: Abductor digiti minimi is the donor.

Arthrodesis

If available muscle power is unable to stabilize the metacarpophalangeal joint of thumb: Arthrodesis (15° of flexion and slight internal rotation) is necessary.

d. Intrinsic Plus and Minus Hand

Impairment can be due to *intrinsic palsy (intrinsic minus hand) or intrinsic contracture (intrinsic plus hand)*. Trauma is the most frequent cause besides nerve injuries (isolated ulnar or median nerve injuries or a combination of both).

Loss of intrinsic muscle contraction results in impairment of the metacarpo-phalangeal (MCP) joint flexion and interphalangeal joint extension, leading to an metacarpo-phalangeal (MCP) hyperextension and interphalangeal joints flexion of the fourth and fifth fingers

(Duchenne sign). This posture is known as the ***intrinsic minus or claw posture***. Abduction and adduction of finger is lost, the thumb cannot be adducted or opposed across the palm. There is flattening of carpal and metacarpal arches. It is due to the involvement of ulnar and sometimes ulnar and medial nerve.

The intrinsic plus hand occurs most commonly secondary to the spasticity of the intrinsic muscles, leading to flexion of the metacarpo-phalangeal (MCP) joints and extension of the interphalangeal joints. The thumb is similarly involved and is adducted into the palm. This is due to contracture of intrinsic muscles, collagen diseases, and lumbrical over activity following severance of long flexor tendons distal to the origin of lumbrical muscle, ischaemic hand injuries.

Evaluation

- Thorough physical examinations
- Electrodiagnostic tests
- High-resolution ultrasound and MRI are useful diagnostic tools.

Management

Intrinsic plus hand: Distal intrinsic release:
- The goal is to decrease the tension on the proximal interphalangeal joint without affecting the MCP joint.
- It is used to treat tightness that involves the proximal interphalangeal joint
- This consists of resecting the intrinsic tendon distal to the transverse fibres.
- Therapeutic options include: Proximal intrinsic release, intrinsic muscle slide, botulinum toxin type-A injections, and ulnar nerve motor branch neurectomy.

Proximal intrinsic release:
- It is indicated in cases with fibrotic intrinsic muscles with no movement
- By releasing the transverse and oblique fibres of the intrinsic mechanism proximal to the MCP joint, the action of the intrinsic muscles is eliminated.

Intrinsic muscle slide:
- It is indicated in cases with spasticity.
- It consists of a subperiosteal elevation of the intrinsic muscles, thus allowing the interosseus muscles to slide distally while MCP joints are extended.

Ulnar neurectomy:
It is indicated in cases with spasticity. However, it is not effective if there is a fixed contracture of the MCP joint.

Intrinsic minus hand:
- Acute ulnar nerve injury: Immediate exploration and primary neurorrhaphy
- Contaminated wound: delayed manner ideally <72 hours, but up to seven days without any detriment to the outcomes.
- In cases with simple clawing, tendon transfers correct the metacarpo-phalangeal (MCP) joint hyperextension whereas, in complex clawing transfer, the active proximal interphalangeal (IP) extension should also be provided.
- Passive palliative procedures: Preventing MCP hyperextension to allow the extensor communis tendon to extend the interphalangeal joints.
- Active palliative procedures are not only intended to correct the claw deformity, but also to restore some function to the intrinsic muscles.

e. Foot Drop

Foot drop, or drop foot refers to a weakening of the muscles that allow one to flex the ankle and toes, causing the individual to drag the front of the foot while walking and to compensate for this scuffle by bending the knee to lift the foot higher than usual.

Foot drop could be either *complete* (as in *sciatic nerve or lateral popliteal or common peroneal nerve* injury) or *incomplete* (as in injury to either *superficial or deep peroneal nerve*).

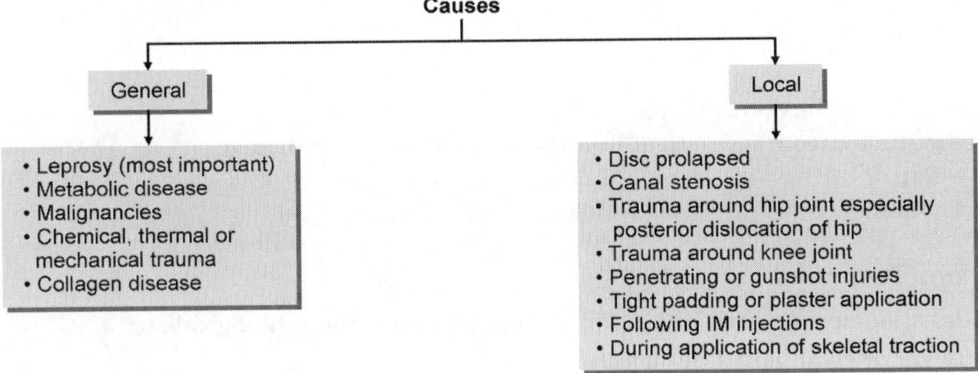

Muscles Commonly Affected

Affects the muscles responsible for dorsiflexion and inversion, specifically the anterior tibialis, extensor hallucis longus and extensor digitorum longus

Level of lesion

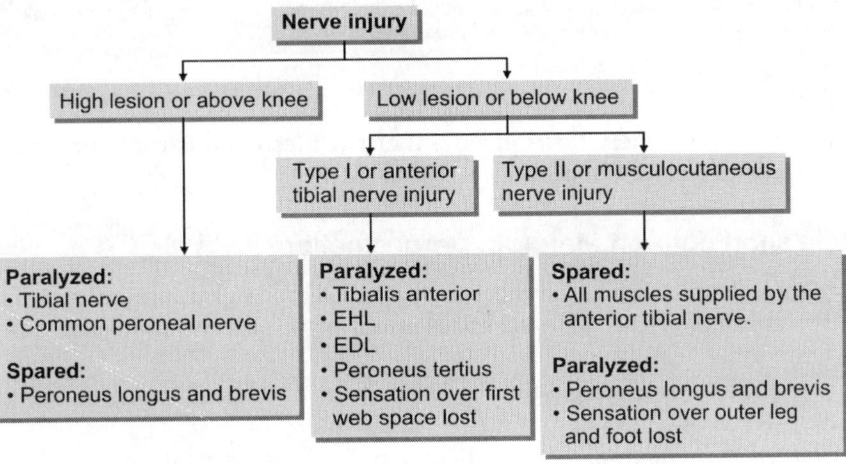

Symptoms

- Unable to dorsiflex ankle
- High steppage gait (most common symptom): High steppage gait is associated with one of the following:
    - Dragging of the foot and toes
    - Scraping of the toes across the ground
    - Uncontrolled slapping of the toes against the ground.
- Unable to stand on heels.

- An exaggerated, swinging hip motion.
- Limp foot
- Tingling, numbness and slight pain in the foot.
- Muscle atrophy in the leg
- Sensory loss along the distribution of the nerve.

Treatment

Conservative for early foot drop.

Splintage:

- knee in 20° of flexion and ankle in 90° for the night-time
- In day-time encourage patient to walk with foot-drop appliance:
    - Static or
    - Dynamic

General Treatment

Besides splintage, provide general treatment to correct the aetiological factor.

If > 1 year or established deformity:

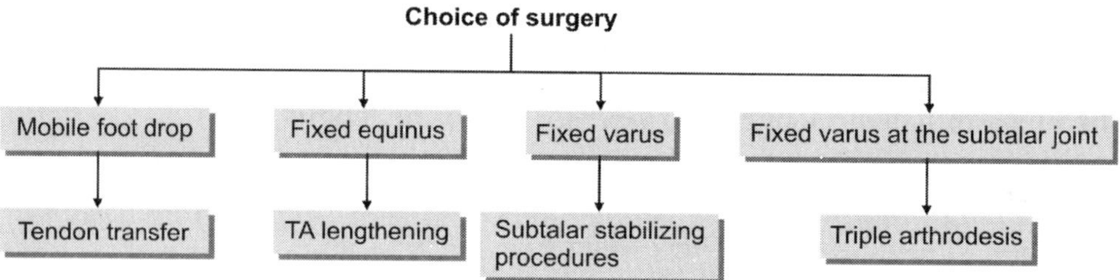

Tendon Transfer

Tibialis posterior is routinely transferred either by interosseous route or by circumtibial route (preferred) to dorsum of foot

Q5. Write short note on Meralgia paraesthetica.

Meralgia paraesthetica painful mononeuropathy of the lateral femoral cutaneous nerve (LFCN), it is commonly due to focal entrapment of this nerve as it passes through the inguinal ligament.

Roth coined the term meralgia paraesthetica from the Greek words *meros* (thigh) and *algos* (pain).

The *lateral femoral cutaneous nerve* is responsible for the sensation of the anterolateral aspect of the thigh. It is a purely sensory nerve and has no motor component.

Aetiology

- Idiopathic
- Direct trauma
- Stretch injury
- Ischaemia
- Iatrogenic (during bone grafting, pelvic procedures or prone position for different surgeries)

- Pregnancy, tight clothing, and obesity
- more common in diabetics

Lateral femoral cutaneous neuropathies are most common during middle age. However, they have been reported in all age groups.

Clinical Features

- Paresthesias and numbness of the upper anterolateral aspect of thigh region are the presenting symptoms.
- Symptoms are typically unilateral.
- Walking or standing may aggravate the symptoms; sitting tends to relieve them.

Diagnosis

- It is based on history and examination.
- NCV studies are used to verify the presence of the neuropathy and rule out other causes for the symptoms.
- If there is relief in symptoms following injection of local anaesthetic, the diagnosis is certain.

Treatment

Conservative

- Use of NSAIDs, tricyclic antidepressants ([TCAs]; e.g. amitriptyline and anticonvulsant agents (e.g. gabapentin) may be helpful in providing some degree of symptomatic relief.
- Local injections using steroid and local anaesthetic preparations may reduce symptoms

Surgical Procedures

- If pain persists even after medication then decompression should be planned.
- Decompression of the compressive forces, nerve spontaneously heals if the compression is relieved.
- Neurolysis, neurolysis with transposition, and transection are the most commonly performed surgical procedures.
- Transection may be the only alternative if the nerve has been severely damaged or if multiple branches are affected.

Q6. Describe the anatomy of brachial plexus and discuss in brief the clinical features and management of brachial plexus injury.

Anatomy

- The brachial plexus lies in the lower part of the posterior triangle of neck, behind the clavicle, and in upper part of axilla.
- It is formed by anterior rami of C_5 to T_1 nerves; the first thoracic ganglion connects with T1 ramus which carries sympathetic fibres.
- The plexus consists of *roots, trunks, division, cords and branches.*

Roots

These are constituted by the anterior primary rami of spinal nerves C_{5-8} and T_1, with contribution from the anterior primary rami of C_4 and T_2.

Trunks

- *Upper trunk* is formed by C_5 and C_6 roots
- *Middle trunk* is formed by C_7 root
- *Lower trunk* is formed by C_8 and T_1 roots

Each trunk divides into *ventral and dorsal divisions*.

Cords

- *Lateral cord*: It is formed by the union of the ventral division of the upper and middle trunks.
- *Medial cord*: It is formed by the ventral division of the lower trunk.
- *Posterior cord*: It is formed by the union of the dorsal division of all the three trunks.

Branches of the Cords

- *Lateral cords gives off*:
    - Lateral pectoral
    - Musculocutaneous
    - Lateral root of median nerve
- *Medial cord gives off*:
    - Medial pectoral
    - Median cutaneous nerve of arm
    - Median cutaneous nerve of forearm
    - Ulnar nerve
    - Medial root of median nerve
- Posterior cords gives off:
    - Upper subscapular
    - Nerve to latissimus dorsi
    - Lower subscapular
    - Axillary
    - Radial nerve

Mechanism of Injury

- *Traction*: Head fall and lateral stretching of neck, birth trauma, and breech delivery
- *Compression*: Fracture clavicle, infection in the neck
- *Penetrating injury*: Gunshot/ stab injury in the neck

Types of injuries and assessment of injuries:

Preganglionic lesions: These lesions represent root avulsions from the spinal cord.

Categories

- Central avulsions: Nerves are avulsed directly from the spinal cord
- Intradural ruptures: Rootlets are ruptured proximal to the dorsal root ganglion

Prognosis

These injuries have limited spontaneous recovery.

Findings seen with preganglionic lesions include:

- Anaesthesia above the clavicle
- Horner's syndrome
  - It is caused by avulsion of the T1 root resulting in interruption of the T1 sympathetic ganglion
  - Results in interruption of sympathetic nerve supply to the eye
  - Causes *Miosis (constriction of pupil), Ptosis (dropping of upper eyelid), Enophthalmos (sinking of the orbit), and Anhidrosis (dry eyes)*
- Abnormal axonal reflex
- Winging of scapula (serratus anterior)
- Weak levator scapula and rhomboids
- Elevated hemidiaphragm (X-rays)

Postganglionic Injuries

- No Horner's syndrome
- Better prognosis
- Patient is able to elevate the scapula
- In late stages, Tinel's sign is present

Distinguishing features between the pre- and postganglionic injuries:

Features	Preganglionic (root avulsion) injury	Postganglionic
• Tinel's sign	Present in some cases	Present in C_5/or C_6 nerve injury
• Fracture of the transverse process of the cervical spine and first rib	Present in most cases	Absent
• Horner's syndrome	Present in association with T_1 nerve root avulsion	Absent or transient
• Arterial injury	Often present in subclavian artery injury	Present usually in axillary artery injury
• Denervation in the area of the posterior ramus of the spinal nerves	Present if detected denervation potentials in the paravertebral muscles	Absent
• Axon reflex	Present	Present if a negative response of axon reflex test. False-positive response in some cases
• Recording of sensory nerve evoked potential	Present	Not detected
• Cervical myelography and CT myelography	Present if dural defect and pseudo-meningocele and no rootlets configuration	Normal or slight abnormality of the dura with rootlets configuration in majority of cases
• MRI of cervical spine	Dural injury or CSF outflow from the dura and signal changes in the spinal cord	Signal changes in the brachial plexus but no change in the spinal cord
• Electrodiagnosis during exploration	Absent in the response of somato-sensory evoked potential (SEPs) and evoked Spinal cord potentials (ESCPs)	Present in the response of somatosensory evoked potential (SEPs) and evoked Spinal cord potentials (ESCPs)

(Contd.)

Features	Preganglionic (root avulsion) injury	Postganglionic
• **Histological examination of the root**	Denervation and decreased acetyl-cholinesterase activity	Preservation of the axons and good acetylcholines-terase activity
• **Prognosis**	Poor	Better

Investigations

- *X-rays*: To rule out any cervical fractures
- *CT scan*: Helps to study the cross-sectional anatomy
- *MRI*: Soft tissue damages
- *Myelogram*: Show meningocele
- Electrodiagnostic studies including EMG, NCV, SEP (somatosensory evoked potential), PES, etc.

Treatment

Early cases

- Maintain full passive range of movement
- Maintain extensibility of soft tissue structures
- Restore function through splinting and advise on one-armed activities
- Prevent contractures
- Prevent damage to aesthetic arm
- Restore social skills and regeneration into normal life
- Passive range of motions in order to prevent contractures and deformity
- *Splinting*: Flail arm splint provides:
    - Shoulder support: Allows some abduction but prevents subluxation of the joint
    - Elbow lock device with five alternative position of flexion
    - A forearm to wrist support
    - Relieve of pain: Transcutaneous electrical nerve stimulation is best method of pain relief for avulsion pain of the brachial plexus.

Recent Trend

- The current trend is for an early repair.
- Patient should be observed up to 8–10 weeks for spontaneous recovery.
- After 4 weeks a baseline electromyography and CTM/MR myelography should be performed.
- Patients with avulsion injury (Completely flail and anaesthetic limb, severe deafferentation pain, Horner's syndrome and pseudomeningoceles on imaging) can be operated at this time.
- Other patients should be followed for another 6–8 weeks for spontaneous recovery

Repair can be done using:
- Nerve grafts
- Nerve allograft
- Fibrin glue in nerve repair
- Nerve conduits
- Nerve transfers

Surgical Measures Especially for Late Cases (>2 years)

Reconstructive surgery: Surgeries are planned according to the residual paralysis:

For shoulder function:

- Improvement of abduction: Transfer of trapezius to the neck of humerus.
- Arthrodesis of shoulder joint in functional position

For elbow function:

Steindler's flexorplasty: Transfer of pectoralis major or latissimus dorsi to biceps.

For wrist and finger extension:

- Wrist extension: Pronators teres transfer
- Finger extension: Flexor carpi ulnaris to extensor digitorum communis (modified Jones)
- Thumb extension: Palmaris longus or flexor digitorum superficialis (ring finger)
- Re-education of transplanted muscle

Erb and Klumpke's Paralysis

Upper Cord Type (Erb–Duchenne Paralysis C_{5-6})

Upper cord injury may occur due to:

- Obstetrical injury
- Traction injury
- Fall on shoulder joint

Clinical Features

- It involves injury to C_5–C_6 nerve roots.
- Muscles affected are deltoid, the biceps, brachialis, brachioradialis and supinator
- Deformity: Affected limb becomes internally rotated, extended at the elbow and pronated in the well-known position of *'Policeman taking a tip'*.
- There may be sensory loss over the outer side of the arm and upper part of the lateral aspect of the forearm.

Treatment

Wait and watch, recovery takes 2–3 years.

Early:
- Splintage, hand to occiput position.
- Passive range of motions in order to prevent contractures and deformity.

Late:
- If recovery is not complete, explore and repair the roots of brachial plexus.
- Tendon and nerve transfers with shoulder arthrodesis should be done if hand functions are spared.

Lower Cord Type (Klumpke's Paralysis C_8–T_1)

- Such injury occurs due to *forceful abduction* of the shoulder, which may occur during *breech presentation* with arms above the head.
- In adult this injury may occur when a *falling person clutches at an object* or a person failing to obtain a foothold on a passing bus may forcefully hyper abduct his arm.
- The C_8 and T_1, nerve roots may be affected though T_1 is more often involved.

Clinical Features

Deformity: Claw hand (paralysis of the intrinsic muscles of the hand and features of combined median and ulnar nerve palsy) with anaesthesia of the inner-side of the forearm, head and inner 1½ finger

Horner's syndrome

- Ptosis
- Miosis
- Enophthalmos
- Anhidrosis
- Loss of spinocilliary reflex

Prognosis

Poor

Treatment

Same as that of Erb's paralysis.

Q7. What are the principles and criteria for tendon transfer?

Tendon transfer is indicated when dynamic muscle imbalance results in deformity that interferes with the normal function of the extremity or ambulation.

Timing of Surgery

Tendon transfer procedures should be delayed until a maximum return of expected muscle strength in the involved muscle has been achieved.

Objectives

- To provide active motor power replacing the function of paralyzed muscle.
- To eliminate the deformity effect of muscle when its antagonist is paralyzed.
- To improve stability of the muscle imbalance.

Important Principles

- The transfer should not significantly decrease the remaining function of the hand.
- The transfer should not create a deformity if significant return of function occurs following a nerve repair.
- The transfer should be phasic or capable of phase conservation.

Criteria

The donor tendon should have the following criteria:
- It should have a power grade V preferably. If it is not feasible then should have at least IV because it loses its power grade by one following transfer.
- It should have same phasic activity.
- It would be about of same size in cross section and equal strength.
- It should have its own blood and nerve supply.
- Synergistic group should be preferred so that the post surgery rehabilitation would be easier.

- The tendon should be routed in a straight line and it must be ensured to have adequate padding to prevent wear and tear.
- It should be sutures under moderate tension.
- Any contractures, joint stiffness or deformity should be corrected before tendon transfer.
- Minimum age of the patient should be 5 years (re-education of muscle strength and rehabilitation would be easier)
- Any infection of bone and adjacent joints should be controlled before tendon transfer.
- There should be fair range of passive movements available at the joints.
- It could be placed in proper relationship to the axis of the joint.

Q8. Write short note on: a. Cerebral palsy; b. Poliomyelitis.

a. Cerebral Palsy (Little's Disease)

Cerebral palsy is due to cerebral hypoxia during pregnancy, labour or immediately after birth, causing a variety of neuromuscular in coordination with or without mental retardation. In cerebral palsy with mental retardation (MR), the child is grossly handicapped; recovery and prognosis is very poor.

"Cerebral palsy is a non-progressive, non-hereditary encephalopathy that occurs in the prenatal or perinatal period and is characterized by altered motor, sensory, and, often, intellectual function"

Three distinctive features common to all patients:
- Some degree of motor impairment
- An insult to the developing brain (Injury to the developing brain can occur anytime from gestation to early childhood and typically is categorized as prenatal, perinatal, or postnatal.)
- A neurological deficit usually permanent and non-progressive

Risk factors for cerebral palsy:

In prenatal period:
- Factors inherent to the fetus (the most common *genetic disorders*)
- Factors inherent to the mother (*seizure disorders, mental retardation, and previous pregnancy loss*)
- Factors inherent to the pregnancy itself (*Rh incompatibility, polyhydramnios, placental rupture, and drug or alcohol exposure*)
- External factors, such as TORCH (*toxoplasmosis, other agents, rubella, cytomegalovirus, herpes simplex*)

In the perinatal period, from birth until a few days after birth:
- Asphyxia
- Trauma
- Oxytocin augmentation
- Umbilical cord prolapse
- Breech presentation

In the post-natal period:
- Hypoxic–ischaemic encephalopathy
- Meconium aspiration and persistent foetal circulation with true ischaemia are the most common causes of hypoxic-ischemic encephalopathy
- Infections such as encephalitis and meningitis, mc caused by group B *Streptococcus* and herpes
- Traumatic brain injury (accidents or child abuse)

Increases incidence in:

- Low-birth-weight infants
- Pregnancies involving multiple births

Associated conditions in patients with cerebral palsy are:

- Mental impairment or learning disability (40%)
- Seizures (30%)
- Complex movement disorders (20%)
- Visual impairment (16%)
- Malnutrition and related conditions, such as gastroesophageal reflux, obesity
- Undernutrition (15%)
- Hydrocephalus (14%)

Geographical Classification

Monoplegia

One extremity involved, usually lower

Hemiplegia

- Both extremities on same side involved.
- Usually upper extremity involved more than lower extremity

Paraplegia

Both lower extremities equally involved

Diplegia

- Most common anatomical type of cerebral palsy,
- Lower extremities more involved than upper extremities
- Fine-motor/sensory abnormalities in upper extremity

Quadriplegia

- All extremities involved equally
- Normal head/neck control

Double Hemiplegia

All extremities involved, upper more than lower

Whole body or Total body

- All extremities severely involved
- No head/neck control

Physiological Classification

- Spastic type (affects the cortico-spinal (pyramidal) tracts)
- Extra-pyramidal type (affects the other regions of the developing brain). Extra-pyramidal types of cerebral palsy include:
- Athetoid

- Choreiform
- Ataxic
- Rigid
- Hypotonic

Spastic Type

- Most common type
- Spasticity resulting from an injury to the pyramidal tracts (cerebral cortex) in the immature brain
- Increase in muscle tone
- An exaggerated stretch reflex is pathognomonic of spasticity
- In an exaggerated stretch reflex, resistance is felt as a sudden passive movement of the muscle, followed by relaxation of the muscle.
- This tightening and relaxation may become cyclical, with a fast passive stretch of the muscle resulting in clonus.
- Fatigue
- Loss of dexterity and coordination
- Balance difficulties
- Joint contractures subluxation, and degeneration

Athetoid Cerebral Palsy

- Second most common clinical type
- injury to the extra-pyramidal tracts
- Athetosis is a type of dyskinesia (abnormal movement or purposeless movements caused by an extra-pyramidal brain lesion).
- The movement disorder is one of continuous motion,
- Dystonia, characterized by increased overall tone and distorted positioning in response to voluntary movements, or hypotonia also can occur with athetoid cerebral
- Joint contractures are not common in this type of cerebral palsy.
- It is further subdivided into five groups, each characterized by a type of abnormal posture movement:
    - Tension athetosis
    - Dystonia
    - Choreiform
    - Ballismus
    - Rigidity

Choreiform

Purposeless movements of the patient's wrists, fingers, toes, and ankle.

Rigid

- Most hypertonic
- Absence of hyper-reflexia, spasticity, and clonus
- *"Cogwheel"* or *"lead pipe"* muscle stiffness

Ataxic

- Very rare
- Result of an injury to the developing cerebellum

- Disturbance of coordinated movement, most commonly walking
- Hypotonic
- Weakness
- Low muscle tone
- Normal deep tendon reflexes
- Difficulties with sitting balance, head positioning, and communication
- It can progress to spastic or ataxic cerebral palsy

Mixed

Show signs of pyramidal and extra-pyramidal deficits.

Clinical Features

- The child has abnormal looks and gestures with clumsy movements.
- Delayed milestones
- Scissoring of legs (scissor gait)
- All the jerks are exaggerated with ankle clonus and extensor plantar reflex.
- Mentally retarded child has:
    - Abnormal facial expression
    - Dribbling saliva
    - Unable to sit up
    - Stand or walk
    - Incontinence of urine, faeces
    - Aphonia

Treatment

It is a multidisciplinary team approaches—including:
- Physical, occupational, and speech therapy
- Orthotics
- Nutrition
- Social work
- Orthopaedics
- General paediatrics

Aims of Treatment

Rehabilitate the child depending on his IQ level so as to make him, self sufficient for daily activities and bread earning.

Modes

- Physiotherapy
- Speech therapy
- Occupational therapy
- **Nonoperative:**
    - *Medication* (most common are diazepam and baclofen (act centrally) and dantrolene (level of skeletal muscle))

- *Botulinum toxin:*
    - Botulinum toxin type A (BTX-A) used to weaken muscles selectively in patients with cerebral palsy

        ↓

    - Injected directly into the muscle acts at the level of the motor end plate

        ↓

    - Blocking the release of the neurotransmitter acetylcholine

        ↓

    - Inhibiting muscle contraction
    - Contraindications to BTX-A therapy include:
        - Known resistance or antibodies
        - Fixed deformity or contracture
        - Concurrent use of aminoglycoside antibiotics
        - Failure of previous response
        - Myasthenia gravis
- *Splinting and bracing :*
    - To prevent or slow progression of deformity
    - Most commonly used braces for the treatment of cerebral palsy include *ankle-foot orthoses, hip abduction braces, hand and wrist splints, and spinal braces or jackets*
- *Physical therapy:*
    - Has a very vital role in all aspects of care
    - Helps in strengthening of weakened muscles, contracture prevention, and gait and balance training; for severely affected individuals, goals are improvements in sitting balance, hygiene
- **Operative**:
- *Indications*:
    - Contractures or deformities that:
        - Decrease function
        - Cause pain
        - Interfere with activities of daily living

Procedures Aiming

- Correct static or dynamic deformity:
    - Corrected with:
        - Muscle-tendon lengthening procedure (tenotomy or Z-Plasty)
        - Capsulotomies
        - Osteotomies
- Balance muscle power across a joint: tendon transfer
- Reduce spasticity (neurectomy): mechanical and chemical methods
- Stabilize uncontrollable joints:
    - For mild to moderate joint destruction: osteotomies combined with soft-tissue releases
    - For severe joint destruction: arthrodesis and resection arthroplasty
    - In patients with end-stage arthritis: Joint replacement

Neurosurgical Intervention

- Selective dorsal root rhizotomy: Division of dorsal roots (L_1–S_2) can theoretically result in loss of inhibition from higher centers; restore balance and lessen muscle tone.

- Indicated in child 3–8 years old with:
  - Spastic diplegia
  - Voluntary motor and trunk control
  - Pure spasticity
  - No fixed contractures

Complications:
- Hip subluxation and dislocation
- Lumbar hyperlordosis (especially in patients with >60° of lordosis preoperatively)
- Spondylolysis
- Spondylolisthesis
- Plano-valgus foot deformities (~50%)

b. Poliomyelitis

It is a viral infection caused by echovirus of three types *(Leon, Lancing and Burnhilde)* localized in the anterior horn cells of the spinal cord and certain brainstem motor nuclei.

Pathophysiology

- Initial invasion by the virus occurs through the GI and respiratory tracts (oropharyngeal route) and spreads to the CNS through a haematogenous route.
- The poliovirus causes damage to brain stem and anterior horn cells of spinal cord.
- Incubation period is 6–20 days.
- There is LMN type of paralysis (flaccid type) with normal sensation.
- It involves mainly the antigravity group of muscles.
- Muscles innervated by the cervical and lumbar spinal segments are most often affected
- *Paralysis*: Lower extremity muscles >> upper extremity muscles.
- In the lower extremity, the most commonly affected muscles are the:
  - Quadriceps
  - Glutei
  - Anterior tibial
  - Medial hamstrings
  - Hip flexors
- In the upper extremity the most commonly affected muscles are the:
  - Deltoid
  - Triceps
  - Pectoralis major

Clinical Course

Three stages:
- Acute
- Convalescent
- Chronic

Acute

- Lasts 7–10 days
- Symptoms range from mild malaise to generalized encephalomyelitis with widespread paralysis

- Listlessness
- Sore throat
- Slight temperature elevation
- Hyperesthesia or paraesthesia in the extremities
- Severe headache
- Vomiting
- Nuchal rigidity
- Back pain
- Limitation of straight leg raising
- Characteristic asymmetrical paralysis
- Muscular pain
- Arthralgia
- Superficial reflexes usually are absent first, and deep tendon reflexes disappear when the muscle group is paralyzed
- Injection or exercise may precipitate the stage of paralysis.
- In bulbar paralysis, respiratory failure occurs.

Treatment

- Rest
- Proper positioning (to prevent flexion posturing and contractures)
- Warm moist packs
- Analgesics
- Gentle physiotherapy
- Respiratory assistance

Convalescent Stage

- Begins 2 days after the temperature returns to normal and continues for 2 years
- Muscle power improves spontaneously

Treatment

- Similar to that during the acute stage
- Assessment of muscle strength monthly for 6 months and then every 3 months
- Physical therapy

Chronic

- Usually begins 24 months after the acute illness
- Causes of deformities are:
    - Muscle imbalance
    - Faulty positioning during recovery
    - Gravity
    - Contracture of fascia/capsule
    - Growth disturbance due to uneven growth of epiphyseal plate

Principles of Treatment

- Prevention of deformities
- Re-establishment of muscle power by tendon transfer, muscle transplant

- Stabilization of loose/flail joints by arthrodesis/braces/calipers.
- Release of contractures-fascia, ligaments, capsule, etc.
- Correction of deformity by tendon lengthening and osteotomy.
- Limb length discrepancy by shoe raise, Ilizarov lengthening.

Surgical Management

Upper Limb

- Deltoid paralysis: Shoulder arthrodesis in 60° abduction and 30° of flexion.
- To restore elbow flexion: Steindler's flexorplasty
- Wrist drop: Arthrodesis of the wrist to improve hand functions.
- Thumb opposition: Bunnell's transfer of FDS of ring finger to the 1st metacarpal

Lower limb

Hip:
- Fixed Flexion: Soutter's release
- Fixed abduction contracture: Yount's procedure, division of iliotibial tract and fascia lata.
- Associated pelvic/knee deformity: Yount's release of fascia lata.

Knee:
- Strong quadriceps and poor hamstrings results in *genu recurvatum*: Corrected by supracondylar posterior wedge osteotomy of the femur.
- Strong hamstrings and poor quadriceps results in flexion contracture: corrected by hamstring release, hamstring to quadriceps transfer or supracondylar anterior wedge osteotomy.
- Biceps dominance causes *triple deformity* (*flexion, external rotation, posterior subluxation*) treated by soft tissue release.

Ankle:
- Poor dorsiflexion and strong tendo-Achilles results in *equinus* which is treated by tendo-Achilles release, calipers (below knee with toe raising device). Tibialis post-transfer anteriorly and arthrodesis for flail ankle.
- Poor gastrocnemius results in *Calcaneo cavus* deformity treated by transfer of tibialis anterior to tendo-Achilles.

Subtalar: Varus/valgus treated by subtalar Grice extra-articular arthrodesis and Dunn's triple arthrodesis.

Flail foot: This is treated by pantalar arthrodesis.

Spine: Kyphoscoliosis treated by anterior/posterior spinal fusion, spinal braces.

Regional Orthopaedics

Q1. Write short note on: a. Cervical Spondylosis; b. Torticollis; c. Thoracic Outlet Syndrome (Cervical Rib); d. Kyphosis and Lordosis

a. Cervical Spondylosis

It is a type of osteoarthritis involving the spine of the body due to degeneration of intervertebral disc (most common C_5-C_7) and the posterior facet joints leading to local pain, spasm, radiculopathy and vertigo.

Clinical Features

Patient may present with:

- Neck stiffness
- Neck pain
- Severe radicular pain along the neck, may radiate to the occiput shoulder, arm and forearm extending to the hand
- It may be associated with paraesthesia, numbness, weakness and clumsiness of arm and hand.
- Muscle spasm
- Vertigo
- Neck movements are painfully restricted
- Rule out diabetes, if the changes are too advanced for the age of the patient

Nerve root compression shows sensory, motor and reflex changes in dermatomal pattern:

Root involved	Motor	Reflex	Sensory
C_5 (C_{4-5})	Deltoid (weakness of shoulder abduction)	Sluggish bicep reflex	Numbness in the deltoid region
C_6 (C_{5-6})	Weakness of wrist extension	Sluggish brachio-radialis reflex	Numbness in the dorsolateral aspect of the thumb and index finger
C_7 (C_{6-7})	Weakness of wrist flexion	Sluggish triceps reflex	Numbness in the index, middle and dorsum of hand
C_8 (C_{7-8})	Weakness of finger flexion	—	Numbness in ring and little finger and medial border of forearm

Radiographic Evaluation

Cervical spine AP and lateral view:
- Osteophyte or spur (lipping) formation
- Reduction of canal space/intervertebral disc space
- Loss of normal lordotic spinal curvature

MRI

More sensitive for showing compression of nerve roots.

Management

Conservative:
- Hot moist fomentation
- Cervical collar (restricting neck movements)
- Traction
- Drugs like: anti-inflammatory drugs muscle relaxants, injection B_1, B_6, B_{12}
- Cervical exercises (mobilization and strengthening exercise)

Surgical

For root or cord compression: Discectomy and fusion by anterior approach.

b. Congenital Muscular Torticollis

Congenital muscular torticollis, also called wryneck, is caused by fibromatosis within the sternocleidomastoid muscle. A palpable mass is usually discovered at birth or becomes so, usually in the first 2 weeks of life. The infant keeps his or her head tilted to one side and has difficulty turning the head to the opposite side.

Aetiology

- Malposition of the fetus *in utero*
- Birth trauma
- Infection
- Vascular injury

Associated musculoskeletal disorders:
- Metatarsus adductus
- Developmental dysplasia of the hip
- Talipes equinovarus

Features

- Right side is involved 75% of the time
- More often, it is localized near the clavicular attachment of the muscle
- Usually, it diminishes and disappears within 1 year
- If it fails to disappear, the muscle becomes permanently fibrotic and contracted

Pathophysiology

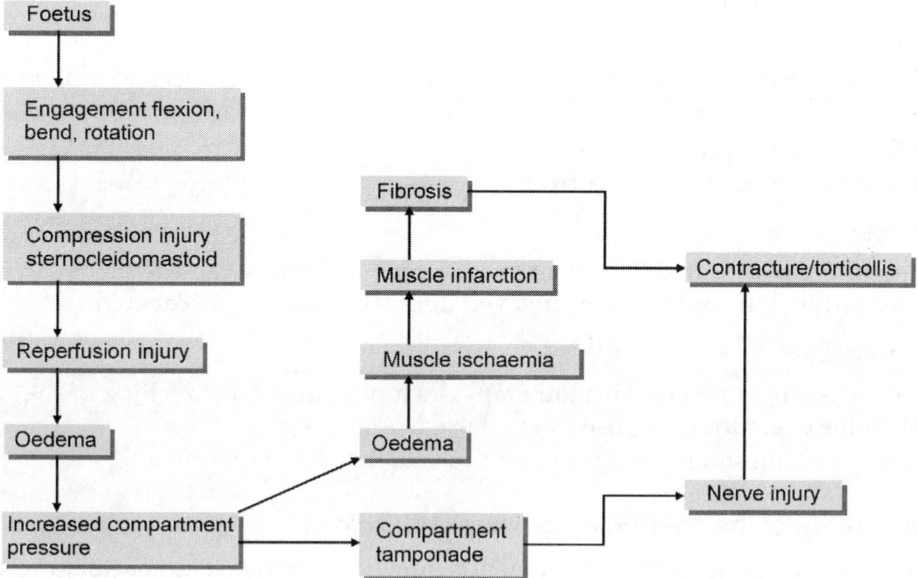

Clinical Features

- Deformity
- Taut sternocleidomastoid muscle
- Head becomes inclined toward the affected side
- Face turned toward the opposite side
- Ipsilateral shoulder becomes elevated
- Fronto-occipital diameter of the skull may become less than normal
- Measurement from the outer canthus of the eye to the angle of mouth is smaller
- Eyebrow is less arched
- Nose is less flattened
- Cheek is less full than on the sound side
- Sometimes Ocular problems like compensatory squint develops

Management

- 90% will respond to passive stretching within the first year of life
- During infancy, only conservative treatment is indicated in form of stretching of the sternocleidomastoid muscle by manipulating the infant's head manually
- CMT did not resolve spontaneously if it persisted beyond the age of 1 year and therefore need some surgical intervention.
- Surgery is delayed until evolution of the fibromatosis is complete, and then, if necessary, the muscle can be released at one (unipolar) or both ends (bipolar).
- An exercise program is likely to be successful if the restriction of motion <30° and there is no facial asymmetry.

Unipolar release

Resection of 2.5 cm inferior ends of tendons of the sternal and clavicular attachments of the sternocleidomastoid muscle.

Drawbacks

Unipolar release is followed by:

- Tethering of the scar to the deep structures
- Reattachment of the clavicular head or the sternal head of the sternocleidomastoid muscle
- Loss of contour of the muscle
- Failure to correct the tilt of the head
- Failure of facial asymmetry to correct

Recommendation

Tethering of the scar to the deep structures is common before the age of 1 year, so it is recommended that the operation be delayed until the child is 1–4 years old.

After treatment

- At 1 week postoperatively, physiotherapy, including manual stretching of the neck to maintain the overcorrected position, is started.
- Manual stretching should be continued thrice daily for 3–6 months

Bipolar Release of the Sternocleidomastoid Muscle

In bipolar release, clavicular and mastoid attachments of sternocleidomastoid muscle are cut, and Z-plasty is performed on sternal origin (Ferkel et al. modified bipolar release and Z-plasty of the muscle).

Indication

- Children with severe deformity
- After failed operation
- Patient between 3–5 years who do not respond to nonoperative treatment

After treatment

- Head-halter traction or a cervical collar during the first 6–12 weeks after surgery
- During early postoperative period:
- Physical therapy consisting of stretching, muscle strengthening
- Active range-of-motion exercises

c. Thoracic outlet Syndrome (Cervical Rib):

Compression of the lower trunk of the brachial plexus (C_8 and T_1) and subclavian vessels between the clavicle and the first rib produces characteristic neurological and vascular symptoms and signs in the upper limb.

Incidence

Young female ~30 years (often long-necked).

Aetiology

- Cervical rib
- Scalenus anticus muscle
- Costoclavicular syndrome
- Pectoralis minor syndrome

- Wide first thoracic rib
- Fracture of the first rib or clavicle
- Pancoast tumor

Pathology

Compression of the brachial plexus or subclavian artery and/or vein in the region near the thoracic outlet.

Clinical Features

Local

- Weakness of the muscle of the shoulder girdle
- Sagging or drooping of the shoulder girdle with the advent of puberty
- Hard and fixed lump in the posterior triangle of the neck (cervical rib)
- Localized tenderness

Neurogenic

Sensory

- Tingling
- Numbness
- Pain along the medial side of forearm and hand

Motor

- Loss of power of hand
- Wasting of the thenar and hypothenar eminence
- Claw hand deformity

Vasomotor

- Excessive sweating
- Circulatory impairment leads to gangrene

Vascular

- Pain, which get worse with exercise
- Hand becomes cold (compare to opposite side)
- On elevation hand, look pale and in prolonged dependent position becomes cyanotic
- Feeble radial pulse on the affected side

Worsening of Symptoms

- At night
- Bracing the shoulders
- Working with arms above shoulder height

Clinical Tests

Adson's test

- Patient neck extended
- Turned toward the affected side and ask the patient to breath deeply

- This manoeuvre compresses the interscalene space and causes paraesthesia and obliteration of the radial pulse.

Wright's Test

- On hyper-abduction and external rotation of arm.
- Recurrence of symptoms and disappearance of pulse on the affected side.

Roose's Test

- Asked the patient to hold his /her arms high above the head, then rapidly open, and close the fingers.
- This manoeuvre may cause cramping pain on the affected side.

Investigations

- *X-rays:*
  - Neck: To exclude cervical rib
  - Lung: To exclude pancoast tumor/apical tumor
  - Shoulder: To exclude any painful etiology
- *Angiography/venography*: reserved for patient with vascular symptoms
- *Electrodiagnostic test* (EMG/NCV): to exclude any peripheral nerve lesions

Treatment

Conservative treatment

- Counseling
- Exercise
- Postural training
- Ways of preventing drooping of shoulder and muscle fatigue
- NSAIDs

Operative

Indications

- Severe pain not responding to the conservative therapy
- Severe muscle wasting
- Vascular disturbances

Procedure

Decompression of the space by removing the first rib (or cervical rib)

d. Kyphosis and Lordosis

Kyphosis is an exaggeration of the normal spinal primary curves (dorsolumbar).
- Forward bending of spine
- Increased dorsal convexity
- It is also known as round back or hump back.

Causes

- Postural
- Compensatory (in FFD hip; CDH; Lumbar lordosis)

- Congenital
- *Developmental*: Scheuermann's disease
- *Metabolic*: Rickets, osteoporosis
- Degenerative: Osteoarthritis
- *Traumatic*: Wedge compression
- *Neoplastic*: Primary (osteoclastoma, eosinophilic granuloma), secondary (from gut, breast).

Types

- *Knuckle*: this is due to:
  - Trauma: Collapse of *single* vertebrae (prominence of single spine)
  - Tuberculosis of spine
- *Angular*: This is due to:
  - Fracture: collapse of the *two or three* vertebral body,
  - Late stages of tuberculosis of spine
  - Secondaries
- *Round or gentle curve*: This is due to developmental or degenerative causes
  - Postural:
    - Usually associated with:
      - Flat foot
      - Seen in girls approaching puberty
      - Women after childbirth or with obesity
  - Scheuermann's disease:
    - Osteochondritis affecting the epiphyseal plates of the vertebrae
    - Usually seen in teenagers
    - The most common complaint is backache
    - X-rays:
      - Thoracic 6th–10th vertebrae are usually involved and wedged shaped
      - Epiphyseal plate appear fragmented especially anteriorly and contain small translucent areas (*Schmorl's nodes*)
  - Senile osteoporosis

Treatment

Mild Cases

- Observation
- Anterior hyperextension brace

Severe cases

Surgical decompression and stabilization

Lordosis

This is an exaggerated *lumbar curve*.

Types

- *Primary*: This is due to:
  - Advanced pregnancy
  - Potbelly seen in rickets/cretinism
  - Spondylolisthesis: Osteochondrosis of the vertebral epiphysis in children

- *Secondary*: This is compensatory type; due to:
  - Kyphosis
  - Flexion contracture of hip
  - CDH, coxa vara
  - Bilateral short tendo-Achilles

Q2. Discuss clinical features and management of scoliosis.

Scoliosis is defined as lateral deviation of the spine, causing deformity, disfigurement and displacement of viscera.

The causes may be non-structural (postural, compensatory) or structural (idiopathic, congenital, neuromuscular, post-traumatic, mesenchymal disorders, etc.)

Types

Non-structural or Mobile Scoliosis

- Curves are flexible
- Readily correctable with side bending

It may be:

a. Postural:

- This is usually seen in young girls with a mild curve usually convex to the left side.
- The important diagnostic feature is that on forward bending the spine straightens completely.
- Recovery is spontaneous.

b. Compensatory:

- This is usually because of obvious deforming reasons like:
  - Limb length discrepancy
  - Fixed flexion deformity of hip
  - Short sternomastoid
  - Ocular disorders
  - Empyema

c. Sciatic:

This is a lateral tilt of the spine associated with lumbar disc prolapse and paraspinal spasm.

Structural Scoliosis

- Non-flexible
- Curves are fixed and fail to correct with side bending

It may be:

- Idiopathic (most common)
- Congenital
- Paralytic

a. Congenital:

- It is caused by the presence of vertebral anomalies that result in an imbalance of the longitudinal growth of the spine.
- Often is rigid and correction is difficult

- Causes/classification:
  - Failure of formation:
    - Partial failure of formation (wedge vertebra)
    - Complete failure of formation (hemivertebra)
  - Failure of segmentation :
    - Unilateral failure of segmentation (unilateral unsegmented bar)
    - Bilateral failure of segmentation (block vertebra)
  - Miscellaneous
- Progressive
- Require *fusion* on both the convex and concave side of the curve

b. Paralytic:
- Loss of muscle strength or voluntary muscle control and loss of sensory abilities, such as proprioception may result in neuromuscular scoliosis
- Causes/classification:
  - Neuropathic
    - Upper motor neuron
      - Cerebral palsy
      - Spinocerebellar degeneration
      - Friedreich ataxia
      - Charcot-Marie-Tooth
      - Roussy-Levy
      - Syringomyelia
      - Spinal cord tumor
      - Spinal cord trauma
    - Lower motor neuron
      - Poliomyelitis
      - Other viral myelitides
      - Traumatic spinal muscle atrophy
      - Werdnig-Hoffmann
      - Kugelberg-Welander
      - Dysautonomia (Riley-Day syndrome)
    - Myopathic
      - Arthrogryposis
      - Muscular dystrophy(Duchenne, Limb-girdle, Facioscapulohumeral)
      - Fibre-type disproportion
      - Congenital hypotonia
      - Myotonia dystrophica
- Many neuromuscular spinal deformities require *operative intervention*

Idiopathic Scoliosis

This accounts for 75% of the cases, generally females undergoing rapid precocious growth.

It may appear in the following types:

1. *Infantile type*:
- It occurs during the first 3 years of life (most common)
- Male predominance

- Having a left thoracic curve
- Invariably resolving spontaneously

2. *Juvenile type*:
- It occurs between 3 and 10 years of age
- With right thoracic curve
- Equally involving both sexes

3. *Adolescent type*:
- It occurs between 10 and 15 years of age
- With right thoracic and thoracolumbar curves
- Female preponderance
- First occurs during growth spurt and usually progressive.
- The younger the child, the worse the outlook

Curves Patterns

- *Simple curve*: When a single spinal deviation occurs.
- *Compound curve*: When displacement occurs in both left and right direction.
- *Primary curve*: The one, which develops first.
- *Secondary curve*: The one, which develops in response to balance the primary curve. When the curve is flexible and corrects by bending towards the convex side it is *non-structural curve*, when it fails to correct by side bending it is a *structural curve*, implying changes in the vertebrae in soft tissues, which have already occurred.
- *Major curve* is the one with significant structural change and is the main curve of greatest degree.
- *Compensatory curves* occur in opposite direction to the major curve in an effort to balance it.
- *Apical vertebrae*: Most deviated vertebra from the vertical axis of the patient.
- *End vertebrae*: Uppermost vertebra whose superior surface maximally tilts toward the concavity of the curve; lowermost vertebra whose inferior surface maximally tilts towards the concavity of the curve.

Clinical Features

Initial evaluation of the patient should include a thorough history, complete physical and neurological examinations, and radiographs of the spine

- Pain symptoms include mechanical back pain, buttock pain, and occasionally radiculopathy or neurogenic claudication
- Patient is usually a young girl with obvious deformity of the spine and ribs called the *razorback* involving the thoracic region with secondary curve in the lumbar region. Deformity increases on forward bending.
- One should always look for associated:
  - Skin pigmentation
  - Muscle weakness
  - Neurological disorder
  - Limb length discrepancy
  - Cardiothoracic diseases
- An assessment of pulmonary function is always beneficial.

Investigations

Plain radiography

View:
- PA view of spine
- Lateral view of spine
- Right and left bending view of spine
- Oblique view of spine

Radiological Parameters

To assess maturity:

When the stage of maturity is reached, the rate of spinal growth is minimum and thereby reducing the progress of deformity. The maturation is assessed by:
- Assessment of bone age at the hand and wrist
- Development of the iliac apophysis (Risser sign)
- Maturation of the vertebral ring apophysis

Risser Sign

- Uses ossification of iliac apophysis to grade the skeletal maturity
- Completion of ossification of iliac apophysis anterior to posterior (from lateral to medial)
- Grading:
    - Grade I: Ossification of lateral 25%
    - Grade II: Ossification of lateral 50%
    - Grade III: Ossification of lateral 75%
    - Grade IV: Ossification of lateral 100%
    - Grade V: Fusion of ilium
- Importance: Completion of skeletal growth (maturity) can be assessed radiologically which suggests no progression of the curve.

Measurement of Curve

It is done by following methods:

Cobb Method

The vertebrae, with wedges on the concave side are considered, horizontal line is drawn at the superior border of the top vertebrae, and another line along the inferior border of lower vertebrae is drawn, perpendicular lines are then drawn directed from these horizontal lines and the intersecting angle is measured.

Risser–Fergusson Method

- A small dot is placed at the centre of upper and lower vertebrae and the centre of apical vertebrae.
- Straight lines are then drawn to join these dots and the intersecting angle is measured.

Vertebral Rotation

The two most commonly used methods:
- Nash and Moe
- Perdriolle and Vidal

In the method of *Nash and Moe*:

- If the pedicles are equidistant from the sides of the vertebral bodies, no vertebral rotation is present (0 rotation).
- The grades progress to grade IV rotation, in which the pedicle is past the center of the vertebral body

Perdriolle and vidal: The Perdriolle torsion meter is a template that measures the amount of vertebral rotation on a spinal radiograph

Rib vertebral angle of Mehta:

- *Rib vertebral angle*: intersection of line perpendicular to the apical vertebrae end-plate and line drawn to the mid-neck to the mid-head of the corresponding rib.
- Rib vertebral angle difference (RVAD): It is the difference of RVA between the convex and concave side of the apical vertebrae.
- If RVAD <20°: Progression is unlikely
- If RVAD >20°: Show progression

Factors Related to Progression of Adolescent Idiopathic Scoliosis:

- Girls > boys
- Premenarchal
- Risser sign of 0
- Double curves > single curves
- Thoracic curves > lumbar curves
- More severe curves

Management

Observation

- Young patients with mild curves of < 20°—examined every 6–12 months
- Adolescents with larger degrees of curvature—examined every 3–4 months
- Skeletally mature patients with curves of <20°—generally do not require further evaluation
- Skeletally immature patients curve of >20°—more frequent examination, usually every 3 to 4 months, with standing PA radiographs
- If progression of the curve (an increase of 5° during 6 months) beyond 25°—orthotic treatment is considered.
- For curves of 30–40° in a skeletally immature patient—orthotic treatment is advised at the initial evaluation.
- For curves of 30–40° in a skeletally mature patient—generally do not require treatment but require close observation because there is potential for progression in adult life (yearly standing PA radiographs for 2–3 years after skeletal maturity, then every 5 years throughout life.)

Orthotic Treatment

Indications

- Flexible curve of 20–30° in a growing child (skeletally immature) with documented progression of ≥5°.
- Curves in the 30–40° range in growing children (initial evaluation).
- Cosmetically acceptable double major curve of 40 to 45° (usually surgery is indicated).

Time of Bracing

- If the curve is <35° and does not show significant vertebral wedging—part-time brace wear (≤16 hours)
- If significant progression of the curvature is noted during use of the part-time protocol, full-time bracing (23 hours)

Brace

Charleston bending brace:
- Low-profile, anterior-opening, lightweight, thermoplastic orthosis
- Worn only during nighttime sleeping hours
- Used mostly for single curves

Boston Brace

It is more effective than the Charleston brace in both preventing curve progression and avoiding the need for surgery

Complications of Bracing

- Poor compliance
- Excessive sweating
- Allergic dermatitis
- Increased gastric pressure and GERD

Operative

Indications

- Increasing curve in growing child
- Severe deformity (>50°) with asymmetry of trunk in adolescent
- Pain uncontrolled by nonoperative treatment
- Thoracic lordosis
- Significant cosmetic deformity

Goals of Surgery

- Correct or to improve the deformity
- To maintain sagittal balance
- To preserve or to improve pulmonary function
- To minimize morbidity or pain
- To maximize postoperative function
- To improve or at least not to harm the function of the lumbar spine

Procedures

- Anterior, posterior, or combined anterior and posterior procedures
- Anterior spinal fusion
- Posterior spinal fusion
- Posterior spinal instrumentation:
  - Harrington rod
  - Dwyer's instrumentation

– Cotrel-Dubousset (CD) system
– Pedicle screw instrumentation

Crankshaft Phenomenon

- *"Despite solid posterior fusion, continued anterior growth causes increase in deformity"*
- Spinal fusion stopped the longitudinal growth in the posterior elements, but the vertebral bodies continued to grow anteriorly.
- The anterior growth causes the vertebral bodies and discs to bulge laterally toward the convexity and to pivot on the posterior fusion, causing:
- Loss of correction
- Increase in vertebral rotation
- Recurrence of the rib hump
- A combined *anterior and posterior* procedure should be considered if the patient is deemed at *risk for the crankshaft phenomenon*

In general:

Idiopathic Scoliosis in Nutshell:

	Infantile	*Juvenile*	*Adolescent*
Age at presentation	Birth–3 years	4–9 years	10–20 years
Male: female	1:1 to 2:1	<6 years: 1:3 >6 years: 1:6	1:6
Curve types	Left thoracic L:R (2:1) Left thoracic/right lumbar	Right thoracic R:L (6:1)	Right thoracic R:L (8:1)
Associated findings	Mental deficiency, CDH, plagiocephaly, congenital heart defects	None	None
Risk of cardiopulmonary compromise	High	Intermediate	Low
Risk of curve progression	<6 mo: low >1 year: high	67%	23%
Rate of curve progression	Gradual progression: 2–3°/year Malignant progression: 10°/year	Progression at puberty: 6°/year Malignant progression: 10°/year	1–2°/month during puberty
Curve resolution	<1 year: 90% >1 year: 20%	20%	Rare
Curve magnitude and maturity	Gradual progression: 70–90° Malignant progression: >90°	Progression at puberty: 50–90° Malignant progression: >90°	Curves >90° are rare
Orthotic management	Effective at delaying and slowing rate of progression Ultimate progression: 100%	Decreases rate of progression until puberty (failure rate: 30–80%)	Effectively controls curves <40° (success rate: 75–80%)

(Contd.)

	Infantile	*Juvenile*	*Adolescent*
Surgical treatment	Instrumentation without fusion <8 years After 8 years: ASF (anterior spinal fusion)-PSF (posterior spinal fusion) After 11 years: PSF	Instrumentation without fusion <8 years after 8 years: ASF-PSD Arfter 11 years PSF	PSF with instrumentation ASF if <11 years with open triradiate cartilage
Risk of crankshaft	High	High	Low

Congenital Scoliosis

Conservative

Indications:
- Long, flexible curves
- Curves that could be corrected either in traction or on side bending
- Curves with a mixture of anomalous and non-anomalous vertebrae

Procedures

Bracing:
- Lumbar curves: TLSO
- Thoracic curves: Milwaukee brace

Operative treatment of congenital curves:
- Posterior fusion without instrumentation
- Posterior fusion with instrumentation
- Combined anterior and posterior fusion
- Combined anterior and posterior convex hemi-epiphysiodesis
- Hemivertebra excision
- Vertebrectomy
- Instrumentation without fusion

Q3. Discuss the aetiology and management of backache.

Backache is a pain in the back caused by degenerative changes, injury, swelling or rarely, cancer/metastatic. Usually the lower part of the back is involved and the pain worsens when a person bends forward. The pain can be acute (sudden and severe) or chronic if it has lasted more than three months.

This is perhaps the price we pay for being erect and a large number of causes are responsible for it. They may be broadly grouped as under:
- Vertebral (10%)
  - *Congenital*: Spina bifida
  - *Developmental*: Spondylolisthesis
  - *Inflammatory*: Tubercular, pyogenic spondylitis
  - *Degenerative*: Osteoarthritis of the lumbar vertebrae
  - *Tumors*: Primary, secondary deposits
  - *Trauma*: Causing fracture and ligament injuries
- Lumbar disc degeneration and subsequent prolapse (85%).
- Sacroiliac joint: Strain, degeneration, infections

- Myofascial inflammation and strain
- *Metabolic*: Osteomalacia, senile osteoporosis
- Diabetes mellitus, Paget's disease, rheumatoid, ankylosing spondylitis
- Peripheral neuropathy, compression radiculopathy (disc prolapse)
- Psychosocial and occupational: In labourers and industrial workers
- Spinal canal stenosis
- Referred: Renal, colon, tubo-ovarian, paraspinal abscess

Approach to Patient

- Detailed history, thorough clinical examination.
- Imaging like X-ray, CT scan, myelography, MRI, bone scan, etc. to reach the appropriate diagnosis.
- Haematological investigations: complete blood picture, ESR, CRP to rule out any infective/inflammatory pathology.
- Blood sugar (fasting, PP), serum creatinine and urea
- Alkaline phosphatase, acid phosphatase to rule out any metastatic deposits.
- Specialized test: Serum electrophoresis (for multiple myeloma), HLA typing (for ankylosing spondylosis)

Treatment

Conservative therapy is the mainstay of treatment
It is directed at rest and relief of pain by:
- Managing the basic cause
- Rest and sleep lying on a firm, flat surface, if possible.
- Avoid stooping, bending, lifting and sitting on low chairs.
- Spinal strengthening exercises, spinal braces, physical therapy.
- *Pharmacotherapy*: Goal of pharmacotherapy is to reduce pain and inflammation. Analgesics, muscle relaxants, local steroid and analgesic injections
- Chemotherapy (ATT or any other specific regime if necessary)
- *Patient education*: Patient education focuses on prevention and includes the following:
  - Promoting weight loss where indicated
  - Performing back strengthening exercises
  - Teaching proper lifting technique
  - Increasing overall physical conditioning
- *Surgery:* (Decompression and stabilization) for the following conditions:
  - Infection: Tubercular, pyogenic
  - Instability: Due to trauma, spondylolisthesis degenerative
  - Compression: Disc prolapse, tumours
- Early return to work on light duty or restricted activity lead to better long-term outcomes.

Q4. Discuss classification, clinical features and management of spondylo-listhesis.

Spondylolisthesis is forward slipping of the proximal part of the vertebral column on the subjacent lower vertebrae, commonly associated with a defect in the pars inter-articularis, invariably appearing between L_4 and L_5 and at times between L_5 and S_1. *Spondyloptosis* is a state when the entire body of L_5 on a lateral standing radiograph is totally below the top of S_1.

Normally the laminae and facet form a locking mechanism, which prevents vertebral slipping.

Classification

Wiltse, Newman, and Macnab's Classification:

Type I, dysplastic	• Congenital abnormalities of the upper sacral facets or inferior facets of the fifth lumbar vertebra that allow slipping of L_5 on S_1 • No pars inter-articularis defect is present in this type.
Type II, isthmic	• Defect in the pars inter-articularis that allows forward slipping of L_5 on S_1 Three types of isthmic spondylolisthesis are recognized: – Lytica stress fracture of the pars interarticularis – Elongated but intact pars interarticularis – Acute fracture of the pars interarticularis
Type III, degenerative	• Results from inter-segmental instability of a long duration with subsequent remodeling of the articular processes at the level of involvement
Type IV, traumatic	• Results from fractures in the area of the bony hook other than the pars interarticularis, such as the pedicle, lamina, or facet
Type V, pathological	• Results from generalized or localized bone disease and structural weakness of the bone, such as osteogenesis imperfecta

Marchetti-Bartolozzi Classification:

Developmental	Acquired
High dysplastic	Traumatic
With lysis	Acute fracture
With elongation	Stress fracture
Low dysplastic	Post-surgery
With lysis	Direct surgery
With elongation	Indirect surgery
	Pathological
	– Local pathology
	– Systemic pathology
	Degenerative
	– Primary
	– Secondary

Clinical Features

Characteristics	True spondylolisthesis (isthmic)	Congenital	Degenerative
Presentation	• Low backache • Pain: buttock, thighs, legs or feet History of trauma	• Usually cause no symptoms in children • Postural deformity or gait abnormality	• Also known as pseudospondylo-listhesis • Commonly seen in elderly • More common in females

(Contd.)

Characteristics	True spondylolisthesis (isthmic)	Congenital	Degenerative
Physical findings	• Increased lumber lordosis • Step-off or slip at the lumbosacral junction • Scoliosis is relatively common in younger patients and is of three types: sciatic, olisthetic, or idiopathic • Sacrum becomes more vertical • The buttocks appear heart shaped (because of the sacral prominence) • Abdomen protrudes forward • With increased severity, trunk becomes shortened and often leads to complete absence of the waistline • On SLR, tightness of hamstrings • L_5 spinous process may be prominent	• Children walk with a peculiar spastic gait, (pelvic waddl) because of the hamstring tightness and the lumbosacral kyphosis • Buttocks are flat • Stiffness of spine • Tight hamstring sometimes the only physical finding	
Neurology	Motor weakness, reflex change, or sensory deficit due to nerve root involvement (L_5)	Seldom have objective signs of nerve root compression	Neurological claudication may be present L_{3-4} involvement is common

Investigations

X-rays

- *Views*: Include AP views, standing lateral views, Ferguson coronal view and an oblique view
- Oblique view: A defect in the pars interarticularis but no slipping (*"Scottish dog sign"* or *collar around the dog's neck picture*)

Meyerding radiographic grading system for Spondylolisthesis (most common):
- The slip grade is calculated by determining the ratio between the AP diameter of the top of the first S_1 and the distance the L_5 vertebra has slipped anteriorly
- Grading:
  - Grade I : Displacement of 25% or less
  - Grade II : Between 25 and 50%
  - Grade III: Between 50 and 75%
  - Grade IV: >75%

Bone Scan

- Especially in children in whom an acquired pars defect is believed to be present but cannot be confirmed by plain films.
- Detect the stress reaction stage before the fracture occurs
- A *single-photon emission computed tomography (SPECT)* bone scan is necessary to show whether uptake is increased in the pars, if increased uptake is confirmed, a CT scan is advised

CT Scan

To evaluate whether:
- There are thickened cortices consistent with a stress reaction
- There is an acute stress fracture

Management

Conservative:
- Rest
- Hot moist fomentation
- Lumbo-sacral belt
- Correction of posture
- NSAIDs, muscle relaxants
- Elimination of stressful activities
- Changing of occupation
- Exercise to strengthens the trunk and hamstring muscles

Surgical

Indications
- Failure of conservative treatment (9 months–1 year)
- Development of a neurological deficit
- Progression of the slip
- Gd III/IV spondylolisthesis
- Persistent tight hamstrings
- Abnormal gait
- Severe pelvic trunk deformity

Procedure
- Spinal decompression
- Reposition of displaced vertebrae
- Posterior spinal fixation by pedicle screws
- Fusion by bone grafts
- In high dysplastic spondylolisthesis: Reduction and fusion with internal fixation

Q5. Discuss clinical features and management of spinal canal stenosis.

Lumber canal stenosis is *cauda equina compression syndrome* where lateral or AP diameter of the canal is narrow with or without alternation in cross sectional area. There may be narrowing of the nerve root canal and intervertebral foramina.

Acquired forms of spinal stenosis usually are degenerative. The L_{4-5} level is the most commonly involved, followed by L_5–S_1 and L_{3-4}.

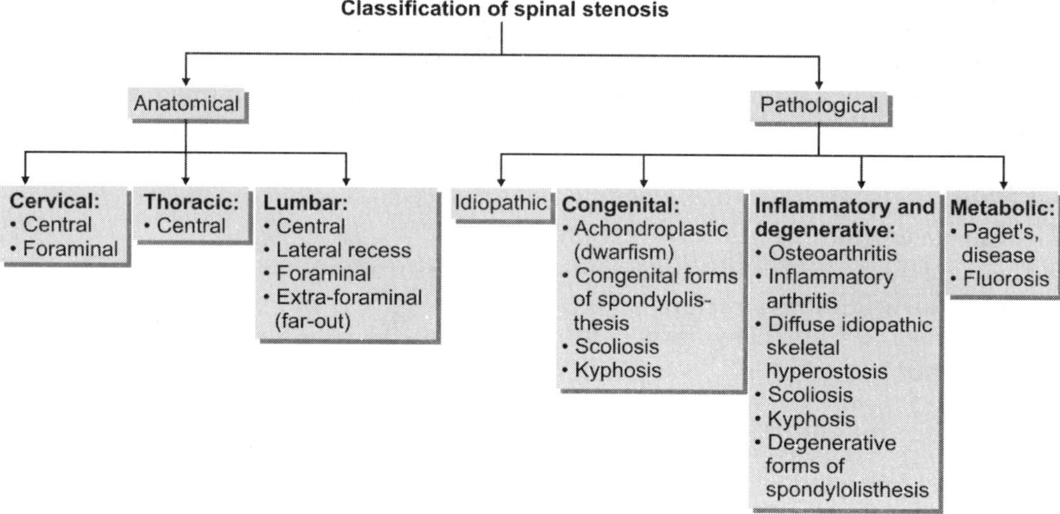

Clinical Features

- Insidious onset of deformity, pain and paresthesia involving the L_5 root invariable and at times L_4/S_1
- Back pain
- Sciatica
- Claudication
- Patients reports:
  - Claudication improves with trunk flexion, stooping, or lying
  - Better endurance walking uphill or up steps
  - Tolerate riding a bicycle better than walking on a treadmill because of the flexed or stooped posture that occurs
- Sensory disturbance in the legs
- Motor weakness was present
- Voiding disturbance
- Central spinal stenosis:
  - Symptoms usually are bilateral
  - Involve the buttocks and posterior thighs in a non-dermatomal distribution.
- With lateral recess stenosis:
  - Symptoms usually are dermatomal because these are related to a compression of specific nerve.
  - More pain during rest and at night
  - More walking tolerance than patients with central stenosis

Differentiation of symptoms of vascular and neurogenic claudication:

Characteristic	Vascular	Neurogenic
• **Walking distance**	Fixed	Variable
• **Provocative factors**	Walking	Walking/standing
• **Palliative factors**	Standing	Sitting/bending

(Contd.)

Characteristic	Vascular	Neurogenic
• **Walking uphill**	Painful	Painless
• **Bicycle test**	Positive (painful)	Negative
• **Pulses**	Absent	Present
• **Skin**	Loss of hair; shiny	Normal
• **Weakness**	Rarely	Occasionally
• **Back pain**	Occasionally	Commonly
• **Back motion**	Normal	Limited
• **Pain character**	Cramping—distal to proximal	Numbness, aching—proximal to distal
• **Muscle atrophy**	Uncommon	Occasional

Investigations

Plain radiography shows:
- Short pedicles on the lateral view
- Narrowing between the pedicles on the anteroposterior view
- Ligament ossification
- Narrowing of the foramen
- Hypertrophy of the posterior articular facets

CT Scan and MRI

For early noninvasive diagnosis of lumbar canal stenosis.

Electrodiagnostic Studies

For assessment of nerve damage.

Tests

Stoop test:
- It is positive in lumbar canal stenosis.
- Patient walk briskly → develop pain → stooped posture → symptoms disappears
- Stooped posture increases the length of canal and thus decreasing the pain

Bicycle test: Patient pedals stationary cycle → develop pain → attained forward flexion posture → symptoms disappears and he pedals more.

Walking test: Patient walks on even surface → develop pain → attained forward flexion posture → symptoms disappears and he walks more.

Management

Acute stage

Conservative

It is successful in most patients

It includes:
- Rest not exceeding 2 days
- Sedative, hot fomentation
- Pain management with anti-inflammatory medications or acetaminophen
- Trunk-stabilization exercise program
- Shortwave diathermy in the lumbar region
- Pelvic traction

Corticosteroid

- Corticosteroids are potent anti-inflammatory medications and result in inhibition of cytokines, a decrease in leucocyte migration, and membrane stabilization
- One course of oral corticosteroids on a 7-day tapered schedule

Epidural injection

Indications: Acute radicular symptoms or neurogenic claudication unresponsive to traditional analgesics and rest, with significant impairment in activities of daily living

Complications

It includes:
- Hypercorticism
- Epidural haematoma
- Temporary paralysis
- Retinal haemorrhage
- Epidural abscess
- Chemical meningitis
- Intracranial air

After the pain is relieved:
- Maintain lumbar corset and spinal exercises.
- Working habits and lifestyle should be changed

Operative

Indications.

Absolute

- Failure of a good conservative treatment regimen
- Increasing pain that is resistant to conservative measures
- Deterioration of neurology

Relative

Inability to tolerate the restricted lifestyle.

Prognostic factors include better results with:
- Disc herniation
- Stenosis at a single level
- Weakness of <6 weeks' duration
- Monoradiculopathy
- Age <65 years

Procedure

- Decompression by laminectomy or a fenestration
- Fusion indicated in:
    - Unstable spine
    - Isthmic or degenerative spondylolisthesis
    - Scoliosis
    - Kyphosis

Q6. Give anatomy of normal disc and aetiology of disc prolapse.

There are *23 discs* in the human spine: *6 in the cervical region, 12 in the thoracic region, and 5 in the lumbar region.*

The disc is composed of three distinct areas:
- The *nucleus pulposus*:
  - Developed from the notochord
  - Semi-gelatinous
  - A water rich gel in the center of the disc due to proteoglycan aggrecan (white glistening mucoid material), which trap and hold water within the disc.
  - Both the disc and annulus are comprised mainly of water, i.e. the nucleus is 80% water, and the annulus is 65% water.
- The *annulus fibrosis*:
  - Thick peripheral ring of lamellated fibrous tissue
  - The fibrous outer portions of the disc that is made up of type I collagen.
- The *vertebral end-plates*:
  - It separate above two structures from the body of the adjacent vertebrae.
  - Cartilaginous plates that attach the discs to the vertebrae and supply food (nutrients) to the inner 2/3rd of the annulus and entire nucleus pulposus.

Functions

Fluctuant shock absorbers.

Aetiology

Multi-factoral aetiology
- Heavy lifting on the job
- Tall men
- Heavy women
- Individuals with a small spinal canal
- Cigarette smoking
- Frequent diving from a board
- Use of vibrating equipment
- Internal disc derangement
- Significant trauma
- Obesity
- Stressful occupations (doctors, police)
- Improper posture while doing work
- Multigravida

Q7. Discuss clinical features and management of prolapsed intervertebral disc.

Natural History of Disc Degeneration

Degenerative process divided into three separate stages:

I. Dysfunction
- Usually seen in individuals 15–45 years old.

- It is characterized by:
  - Circumferential and radial tears in the disc anulus
  - Localized synovitis of the facet joints

II. Instability

- Found in 35–70-year-old patients
- It is characterized by:
  - Internal disruption of the disc
  - Progressive disc resorption
  - Degeneration of the facet joints with capsular laxity
  - Subluxation
  - Joint erosion

III. Stabilization

- Present in patients older than 60 years
- Segmental stiffening or frank ankylosis due to development of hypertrophic bone around the disc and facet joints

Types of Disc Herniation

Normal bulge/desiccation:
- In this stage, age-related changes in the collagen that forms the nucleus pulposus cause the disc to lose water and weaken, without rupture.
- At this stage, there are most likely annular fissures or tears that disrupt the integrity of the annulus, and the disc may appear to bulge on imaging studies

Protrusion or Prolapse

In this stage, the nucleus pushes through layers of the annulus, but remains contained by the outermost layers, causing a localized deformity of the disc, which may project into the spinal canal.

Extrusion

Here the gel-like nucleus pulposus escapes the surrounding annulus fibrosus

Sequestration

At this stage, the extruded gel-like material loses contact with its disc of origin and is sequestered in the spinal canal.

Presentation

These are best separated into symptoms related to the *spine itself, symptoms related to nerve root compression, and symptoms of myelopathy.*

Radicular pain is the most common symptom. Radicular pain is frequently described as a sharp, lancinating, radiating pain, often shooting from the low back down into the lower limb(s) in a radicular distribution

Cervical

- Complaints of neck pain, medial scapular pain, and shoulder pain.
- Pain radiating into the arm or chest with numbness in the fingers and motor weakness.

- Occasionally sharp pain or generalized tingling sometimes may be associated with neck extension similar to *Lhermitte sign* in multiple sclerosis.
- Cervical paraspinal spasm.
- Limitation of neck motion.

Sensory, motor deficit and reflex change as level of disc prolapse:

Disc prolapse	Sensory deficit	Motor weakness	Reflex change
• C_{4-5} disc rupture or other pathological condition at that level (C_5 nerve root compression)	• Upper lateral arm • Elbow	• Deltoid • Biceps (variable)	• Biceps (variable)
• C_{5-6} disc herniation or other local pathological condition at that level (C_6 nerve root compression)	• Lateral forearm thumb, and index finger	• Biceps • Extensor carpi radialis longus and brevis	• Biceps • Brachioradialis
• C_{6-7} disc rupture or other pathological condition at that level (C_7 nerve root compression)	• Middle finger (variable because of overlap)	• Triceps • Wrist flexors (flexor carpi radialis) • Finger extensors (variable)	• Triceps
• C_7–T_1 disc rupture or other pathological condition at that level (C_8 nerve root compression)	• Ring finger • little finger • Ulnar border of palm	• Interossei • Finger flexors (variable) • Flexor carpi ulnaris (variable)	• None
• T_{1-2} disc rupture or other pathological condition at that level (T_1 nerve root compression)	• Medial aspect of elbow	• Interossei	• None

Thoracic Disc Disease

- Least common location for disc pathology
- Pain is the most common presenting feature (axial, and the other is band-like radicular pain along the course of the intercostal nerve (most commonly T_{10}))
- Associated sensory changes of paraesthesias and dysesthesia in a dermatomal distribution also occur
- High thoracic discs (T_2 to T_5) can manifest in a similar fashion as cervical disc disease with upper arm pain, paresthesias, radiculopathy, and Horner syndrome.
- Myelopathy also may occur (*Sustained clonus, a positive Babinski sign, and wide-based and spastic gait*)
- Complaints of generalized weakness, by the patient, typically involving both lower extremities occur in the form of mild paraparesis.
- Bowel and bladder dysfunction occur (15–20%)

Lumbar Disc Disease

- Repetitive lower back and buttock pain.
- Pain can be decreased by rest, especially in the semi-Fowler position, and can be exacerbated by straining, sneezing, or coughing.

- Weakness and paresthesias.
- Stretch of the sciatic nerve at the knee produces buttock, thigh, and leg pain.
- A Lasègue sign usually is positive on the involved side.
- Contralateral leg pain produced by straight leg raising (SLR) should be regarded as pathognomonic of a herniated intervertebral.
- Cauda equina syndrome (if herniation or fragment is large).
- Cauda equina syndrome includes numbness and weakness in legs, rectal pain, numbness in the perineum, and paralysis of the sphincters.

Disc prolapse	Sensory deficit	Motor weakness	Reflex change
• L_{3-4} disc herniation or pathological condition localized to L_4 foramen (L_4 Root compression)	• Postero-lateral thigh, anterior knee, and medial leg	• Quadriceps (variable) • Hip adductors (variable)	• Patellar tendon (Westphal's sign) • Anterior tibial tendon (variable)
• L_{4-5} disc herniation or pathological condition localized to L_5 foramen L_5 Root compression	• Anterolateral leg, dorsum of the foot, and great toe	• Extensor hallucis longus • Gluteus medius • Extensor digitorum longus and brevis	• Usually none
• L_5–S_1 disc herniation or pathological condition localized to the S_1 foramen S_1 Root Compression	• Lateral malleolus • Lateral foot • Heel • Web of fourth and fifth toes	• Peroneus longus and brevis • Gastrocnemius-soleus complex · Gluteus maximus	• Achilles tendon (gastrocnemius-soleus complex)

Sensory motor deficit and reflex change as level of disc prolapse.

Various Clinical Tests

- *Lasègue sign or straight leg raise test*: With the patient supine, the straight leg at the involved side is flexed at the hip joint. It is significant if <70°.
- *Bragaard's sign*: Dorsiflexion of the ankle with SLR in line with internal rotation at the hip, indicative of a positive test of root or neural irritation.
- *Valleix's points*: Pressure on certain points along the course of the sciatic nerve or its branches may cause or exacerbate radicular pain.
- *Bowstring sign*: SLR → pain appears → flexion of knee → pain disappear → pressure on nerve in popliteal nerve → reproduce radicular pain → test is positive and negative if pain occurs only in popliteal fossa.
- *Sicard's test or Roch's test*: Forced plantar flexion (Sicard's test) or forced dorsiflexion of the foot (Roch's test) may exacerbate the radiated pain.
- *Crossed straight leg-raising or well leg raising test or Fajersztajn's sign test*: SLR on the painless or asymptomatic leg produces pain in the contralateral leg this may correlate with the central disc herniation.
- *Femoral stretch test or reverse SLR*: Patient prone, knee flexed and the limb is extended form the hip, stretching of femoral nerve elicit pain.

Investigations

X-rays

- Plain radiographs do not reveal disk herniation; They are usually advised to exclude other conditions (e.g. fracture, isthmic defect, cancer, infection).

- AP, lateral and oblique views
- Reveals indirect findings of disk degeneration in the form of:
  - Loss of height of the intervertebral disk (reduction of disc space)
  - Vacuum phenomenon in the form of gas in the disk
  - Endplate osteophytes

Myelography

- A myelogram requires introduction of radiographic contrast media (dye) into the sac (dura) surrounding the spinal cord and nerves.
- It is helpful in spinal stenosis, intraspinal lesions, incomplete decompression.
- Side effects include headache, nausea and vomiting. In view of its side-effects and equal in efficacy with noninvasive modalities (CT, MRI) it should be avoided as a first-line investigation.

Discography

Discography is an invasive procedure involving the injection of contrast media or saline into the disc nucleus, aiming to reproduce the patient's pain. It can be combined with plain X-rays or a CT scan.

CT Scan

- Useful noninvasive test
- It shows a soft-tissue mass with effacement of the epidural fat and displacement of the thecal sac. It May demonstrate calcification or, less commonly, gas in the herniation.

MRI

- Useful noninvasive test.
- It is the investigation of choice. Delineates herniated nucleus pulposus (HNP) and its relationship with adjacent soft tissues.

Management

Aim

- Relieve pain
- Restoration of normal movements
- Prevention of recurrence

Conservative: It is normal to allow 6 weeks to 3 month to elapse before considering surgery.

Acute Attack

- Absolute bed rest (at least for 2 days)
- Rest in semi-Fowler position (i.e. on the side with the hips and knees flexed) with a pillow between the legs (relieve most pressure on the disc and nerve roots).
- Ice fomentation/massage, muscle relaxants to manage muscle spasm.
- Pain relief and anti-inflammatory effect can be achieved with NSAIDs.
- Skin or pelvic traction in bed.
- Back braces or corsets in some patients.
- Physical therapy like USG, diathermy, IFT, etc.

As the pain diminishes: Patient should be encouraged to:
- Begin isometric abdominal and lower extremity exercises (Any exercise that increases pain should be discontinued.)
- If pain is relieved with passive extension, extension exercises should be advised and if pain is relieved with passive flexion, flexion exercises should be advised.
- Walking within the limits of comfort

Patient should be discouraged:
- Sitting, especially riding in a car
- Lifting heavy weight

Patient should be taught: Correct body posture.

Epidural Steroids

Indications

Lumbar disease:
- Lumbosacral disk herniation.
- Spinal stenosis with radicular pain (central canal stenosis, foraminal and lateral recess stenosis).
- Compression fracture of the lumbar spine with radicular pain.
- Facet or nerve root cyst with radicular pain.

Cervical disease:
- Pain associated with acute disk herniation and radiculopathy
- Post-laminectomy cervical pain
- Cervical strain syndromes with associated myofascial pain
- Post-herpetic neuralgia

Thoracic disease:
- Acute thoracic disk pathology
- Thoracic radicular pain secondary to disk herniations
- Post-herpetic neuralgia
- Trauma
- Diabetic neuropathy
- Degenerative scoliosis
- Idiopathic thoracic neuralgia
- Thoracic compression fracture

Agent used: Methylprednisolone

Frequency: 3–4 injections for acute radicular pain syndromes with an interval of 2 weeks.

Complication

- Backache, postural punctures headache, nausea, vomiting, dizziness, and vasovagal reaction.
- Bleeding along the trajectory of the injection, including in proximity to the nerve roots and/or the spinal cord (epidural hematoma), is a rare but potentially serious complication.
- Infection is more common in immunocompromised patients and can include epidural abscess and meningitis.
- Nerve root injury
- Other rare complications include anterior cord syndrome, presumably resulting from the injection of particulate steroid into the artery of Adamkiewicz.

Operative

Indications

- Unilateral leg pain extending below the knee persisting for at least 6 weeks , initially responded to conservative modality and then returned to the initial levels after a minimum of 6–8 weeks of conservative care
- Failure of conservative treatment
- Deterioration of neurology during the course of treatment
- Progressive neurological deficit
- Cauda equina syndrome

Procedures

- Laminectomy and disc excision.
- *Spinal fusion*: This is a surgical procedure in which, disc tissue is removed and bone is placed between the vertebral bodies. The goal of this surgery is to fuse the vertebra around the disc that is causing pain.
- *'Fenestration and discectomy' or 'minidiscectomy'* (procedures are undertaken under direct vision or with the aid of magnification).
- *Microdiscectomy*: In a microdiscectomy, an operating microscope is used to provide illumination and magnification through a very small incision (MISS: Minimal Invasive Spinal Surgery).
- *Percutaneous discectomy*: Percutaneous discectomy involves removal of the disc nucleus through a cannula which has be en placed in the disc nucleus under radiological control.
- *Chemonucleolysis*: Chemonucleolysis involves chemical destruction of the disc nucleus. The disc nucleus is cannulated under radiological control and an enzyme, chymopapain or collagenase is injected. The enzyme breaks down the protein component of the nucleus (not effective if there are free fragments or sequestration of the disc).
- *Total disc replacement:*
  - Artificial disc replacement has been used as an alternative to spinal fusion, with the goal of pain reduction or elimination, while still permitting motion throughout the spine.
  - Artificial discs are usually made of metal or plastic-like (biopolymer) materials, or a combination of the two.
  - Usually nucleus replacement devices are made of plastic-like (biopolymer) materials. One such material is hydrogel. This material expands as it absorbs water. The device is placed into the nuclear cavity of the disc and hydrates to expand and fill the cavity.
  - The device is compressible and by this means, allows motion, much like a normal disc nucleus. Another design consists of a piece of a plastic-like material that coils around to fill the nuclear cavity.

Prevention of Recurrence

- Change of lifestyle
- Back education
- Proper posture training (learn correct posture and body mechanics)
- Standard exercise training: The exercise programme included passive lumbar flexion, pelvic tilt, strengthening of flexor muscles, strengthening of extensor muscles, spine mobilization and stretching exercise.
- Always better to avoid sport-specific activities

Q8. Discuss in brief: a. Painful arc syndrome and rotator cuff tears; b. Tennis elbow; c. Frozen shoulder; d. Madelung's deformity.

a. Painful Arc Syndrome or Impingement Syndrome

Incidence

- Patients <40 years: Usually glenohumeral instability, and acromioclavicular joint disease/injury.
- Patients >40 years: Consider glenohumeral impingement syndrome/rotator cuff disease and glenohumeral joint degenerative disease.
- Male preponderance.
- High-risk occupation:
  - Laborers and those working in jobs that require repetitive and excessive overhead activity
  - Athletic event (e.g. swimming, throwing sports, tennis, volleyball)

Pathology

Developmental stages of Impingement syndrome (Neer's):

Stage 1: Edema and haemorrhage
- Typical age of patient: <25 years old
- Clinical course: Reversible
- Treatment: Conservative

Stage 2: Fibrosis and tendinitis
- Typical age of patient: 25–40 years old
- Clinical course: Recurrent pain with activity
- Treatment—consider bursectomy or division of coraco-acromial ligament

Stage 3: Bone spurs and tendon rupture
- Typical age of patient: >40 years old
- Clinical course: Progressive disability
- Treatment: Anterior acromioplasty, rotator cuff repair

Types of impingement syndrome (Neer):
- Primary impingement (most common).
- Secondary impingement: It is secondary to instability of the glenohumeral joint or abutment of structures against the coraco-acromial arch.
- Subcoracoid impingement: Caused by a prominent coracoid (idiopathic and iatrogenic conditions).
- Internal impingement: Internal contact of the rotator cuff occurs with the posterosuperior aspect of the glenoid when the arm is abducted, extended, and externally rotated.

Clinical Presentation

- Sudden onset of sharp pain in the shoulder with tearing sensation (suggestive of a rotator cuff tear) or Gradual increase in shoulder pain with overhead activities (suggestive of an impingement problem)
- Swelling
- Muscle wasting (shoulder girdle)
- Tenderness
- Limitation of range of motion

- Painful arc (40°–120°) of motion may be experienced with elevation above the shoulder level in patient specially with impingement syndrome

Special Tests

- *Neer test:* Forcefully elevate an internally rotated arm in the scapular plane, causing the supraspinatus tendon to impinge against the anterior inferior acromion. Pain and a grimacing facial expression indicate impingement of the supraspinatus tendon, indicating a positive Neer impingement test.
- *Hawkins-Kennedy test:* Forcefully internally rotate a 90° forwardly flexed arm, causing the supraspinatus tendon to impinge against the coraco-acromial ligamentous arch. Pain and a grimacing facial expression indicate impingement of the supraspinatus tendon, indicating a positive Hawkins impingement sign.
- *Impingement test:* Inject 10 ml of 1% lidocaine solution into the subacromial space. Repeat testing for an impingement sign. Elimination or significant reduction of pain constitutes a positive impingement test.
- *Drop arm test:* The patient places the arm in maximum elevation in the scapular plane and then lowers it slowly (the test can be repeated following subacromial injection of lidocaine). Sudden dropping of the arm suggests a rotator cuff tear.
- *Supraspinatus isolation test/empty can test or Jobe test:* The supraspinatus may be isolated by having the patient rotate the upper limb so that the thumbs are pointing to the floor and apply resistance with the arms in 30° of forward flexion and 90° of abduction (the position assimilates emptying a can). This test is positive when weakness is present (compared to the unaffected side), suggesting weakness or insufficiency of the supraspinatus tendon.

Investigation

X-rays

- Anterior-posterior (AP) view of the glenohumeral joint.
- Internal rotation view of the humerus with 20° upward angulation: to show acromio-clavicular joint
- *Axillary view*: To rule out subtle signs of instability (e.g. glenoid avulsion, Hill-Sachs lesion) and to visualize presence of an os acromiale.
- Supraspinatus outlet view: to assess the supraspinatus outlet space. If the space is <7 mm, then an increased risk for impingement syndrome exists

MRI

- Gold standard and investigation of choice.
- Detect intrasubstance tendon degeneration or partial rotator cuff tears.
- Detect inflammation, edema, haemorrhage, or scarring.
- Use of gadolinium increase the sensitivity to detect partial rotator cuff tears.

Arthrography

- To assess the integrity of the glenohumeral joint.
- Helps in evaluating rotator cuff tears.

Treatment

Conservative Treatment

- Physiotherapy (aiming stretching for full shoulder motion and strengthening the rotator cuff)

- Anti-inflammatory medications
- One or at most two subacromial cortisone injections

Operative

- Patient fails to respond after 3–4 months of conservative therapy
- Arthroscopic or open acromioplasty
  - Principles of acromioplasty:
    - Release (but not resection) of the coraco-acromial ligament
    - Removal of the anterior lip of the acromion
    - Removal of part of the acromion anterior to the anterior border of the clavicle
    - Removal of the distal 1–1.5 cm of clavicle if significant degenerative changes are found

Rotator Cuff Tears

Rotator cuff muscles (*subscapularis, supraspinatus, infraspinatus, and teres minor*) activity have been shown to stiffen the capsule and decrease glenohumeral translation.

Types

Loss of continuity of the rotator cuff can be:
- Acute and chronic
- Partial or full thickness
- Traumatic or degenerative

Partial tendon tears:
- <50% of the depth of the tendon
- >50% of the depth of the tendon

Full-thickness rotator cuff tears (Cofield et al.):
- < 1 cm: small tears
- 1–<3 cm: medium tears
- 3–<5 cm: large tears
- 5 cm or larger: massive tears

Chronic tears can be (based on fatty degeneration on MRI or CT):
- Stage 0: Corresponds to a completely normal muscle, without any fatty streak
- Stage 1: The muscle contains some fatty streaks
- Stage 2: The fatty infiltration is important, but there is still more muscle than fat
- Stage 3: There is as much fat as muscle
- Stage 4: More fat than muscle is present

Ellman Classification

- Location (articular, bursal, and interstitial)
- Grade (grade 1, <3 mm deep; grade 2, 3–6 mm deep; grade 3, >6 mm deep)
- Tear area (in mm)

Presentation

Most patients with a pathological condition of the rotator cuff have:
- Many patients with full-thickness rotator cuff tears are asymptomatic
- Insidious onset of progressive pain and weakness

- Pain usually is present at night and may be referred to the area of the deltoid insertion
- Concomitant loss of active motion

Investigation
MRI

- Gold standard
- It shows detailed anatomical information, including the size of rotator cuff tears and the status of the rotator cuff muscles

Treatment
Partial-thickness tears

Nonoperative:
- Activity modification
- Stretching and strengthening exercises
- Anti-inflammatory medication

Operative Management

Goal:
- Pain relief
- Improvement of function

Indication

If conservative management fails.

Procedures

- Debridement or repair of tendon.
- <50% of cuff thickness: Acromioplasty and debridement.
- If tear is longer or thicker: excision of the diseased tendon and suturing to a trough in bone.

Massive and Irreparable Tears

For irreparable rotator cuff tears:
- Tendon transfer: It involve transfer of rotator cuff tendons or other muscle-tendon units.
- For anterosuperior tears involving the subscapularis and the supraspinatus: transfer of the pectoralis major is considered.
- For posterosuperior tears involving the infraspinatus and supraspinatus: transfer of the latissimus dorsi (Gerber et al.) is considered.

For deficient rotator cuff tendon: The deficiency is replace by free grafts (autologous or autogenous), such as the intrinsic portion of the biceps and fascia lata, or synthetics
For massive tears without possibility for repair even in abduction: Decompression and debridement Arthroscopically or open (*Rockwood*).

b. Tennis Elbow

Lateral epicondylitis (tennis elbow) is an overuse injury involving the extensor muscles (usually extensor carpi radialis brevis (ECRB)) that originate on the lateral epicondylar region of the distal humerus. Runge made the first description of lateral epicondylitis (tennis elbow) in 1873 and it was termed "tennis elbow" by Major. Despite the misnomer of lateral epicondylitis (tennis elbow), the histology of lesions shows neither acute nor chronic inflammatory cell infiltrate. It is believed to be a degenerative disorder.

Incidence

It occurs more frequently in non-athletes than athletes, with a peak incidence in the early fifth decade and a nearly equal gender incidence

Aetiology

- Activities involving wrist extension and/or supination can be associated with overuse of the muscles originating at the lateral epicondyle.
- Tennis has been the activity most commonly associated with the disorder. In tennis player, factors associated with tennis elbow are improper technique, size of racquet handle, and racquet weight, bad backhand and forehand strokes, incorrect grip size, string tension and underlying weak muscles of the shoulder, elbow and arm.
- Besides, in tennis players it also occurs in non-tennis players like (95% of tennis elbow occurs in non-tennis players):
  - Cricketers (Sachin Tendulkar)
  - Swimmers
  - Carpentry, plumbing, textile workers
  - Activities like twisting a screw driver, lifting heavy luggage with the palm down
  - House wives (while making chapattis and washing clothes)

Pathophysiology

- Inflammatory processes of the synovium, radial humeral bursa, periosteum, and the annular ligament.
- Overuse and repetitive trauma in this area causes fibrosis and micro tears in the involved tissues.
- Microscopic tearing with formation of reparative tissue (i.e. angiofibroblastic hyperplasia) in the origin of the extensor carpi radialis brevis (ECRB) muscle usually following strain of the extensors (widely accepted theory).
- Besides ECRB, pathology can involve the tendons of the extensor carpi radialis longus and the extensor digitorum communis

Progressive Stages

Nirschl defined the following:
- Stage 1: Inflammatory changes that are reversible
- Stage 2: Nonreversible pathologic changes to origin of the extensor carpi radialis brevis (ECRB) muscle
- Stage 3: Rupture of ECRB muscle origin
- Stage 4: Secondary changes such as fibrosis or calcification

Presentation

- Pain over lateral condyle (approximately 5 mm distal and anterior to the midpoint of the condyle)

- Pain with resisted wrist extension, finger extension and resisted radial deviation.
- Point tenderness over or just distal to the lateral humeral epicondyle, which radiates down the forearm and incapacitates the person even to lift small objects.
- *Special tests*:
  - *Cozen's test*: Dorsiflexion of the wrist against resistance with the elbow in extension will elicits pain over the lateral condyle.
  - *Mill's test*: While palpating the lateral epicondyle, the examiner pronates the patient's forearm, and flexes the wrist fully and extends the elbow. A positive test is indicated by pain over the lateral epicondyle of humerus.
  - *Maudsley's test*: The examiner resists extension of the 3rd digit or middle finger of the hand, stressing the extensor digitorum muscle and tendon. A positive test is indicated by pain over the lateral epicondyle of the humerus.

Imaging

- Radiographs: AP and Lateral views to rule out disorders or concomitant intra-articular pathology (e.g. osteochondral loose body, posterior osteophytes) or Calcification
- MRI is the most appropriate imaging study to confirm the presence of degenerative tissue in the ECRB muscle origin.
- Sometimes, electromyography (EMG) or NCV to rule out any neural component.

Management

Conservative Treatment

- It is the mainstay (95% of patients) of care for patients with lateral epicondylitis (tennis elbow).
- Elimination of activities those are painful
- Rest
- Hot fomentation, ultrasonic iontophoric therapies or electrical stimulation.
- Use of a counterforce brace or cock up wrist splinting.
- *Pharmacology*: NSAIDs, local steroid injections.
- Autologous blood injections for lateral epicondylitis shows benefits in some patients.
- Low-level laser therapy appears to provide short-term pain relief.
- Use of extracorporeal shockwave therapy.
- Injection of botulinum toxin at the extensor origin showed a significant decrease in pain scores in patients with lateral epicondylitis.
- When the patient is free of pain through a full range of motion, begin strengthening therapy.
- Patient education: Before resumption of activity (e.g. correct technique or address equipment concerns in athletes who participate in racquet sports, modify jobs or activities in patients who are not athletes).

Mills Manoeuvre

- Manipulation under anesthesia: It is indicated in patients with concomitant flexion contractures.
- The manoeuvre involves sudden, forcible, full extension of the elbow with the wrist and fingers flexed and the forearm pronated.

Surgery

In recalcitrant cases, surgery is the choice.

- Boyd and McLeod: Excision of the proximal portion of the annular ligament, release of the entire extensor origin, excision of an adventitious bursa (Osgood), and resection of hypertrophic synovium in the radiocapitellar articulation
- Baumgard and Schwartz: Percutaneous lateral release

In cases of persistent pain: Epicondylar resection and anconeus muscle transfer

Arthroscopic Release

Advantages

- Allows intra-articular examination for other pathology
- Shorter postoperative rehabilitation period
- Earlier return to work

c. Frozen Shoulder

Periarthritis scapula-humerale or frozen shoulder or adhesive capsulitis is a clinical syndrome that causes the painful restriction of active and passive glenohumeral and periscapular shoulder range of motion.

Incidence

- Usually affects patients aged 40–70 years
- Females' preponderance
- No predilection for race
- Higher incidence exists among patients with diabetes (10–20%)

Aetiology

There are various triggers that may predispose patients to this problem appear to exist. A few reported etiologic agents include the following:
- Trauma
- Surgery
- Inflammatory disease
- Diabetes
- Regional conditions
- Others: Hyperthyroidism, ischemic heart disease, and cervical spondylosis

Classification

- Primary or idiopathic (no inciting agent).
- Secondary (factors preceded shoulder symptomatology, such as trauma or surgery to the affected upper extremity).

Pathology

Chronic inflammatory response with fibroblastic proliferation due to prolonged and repeated overhead activities.

Phases

Primary frozen shoulder symptomology have been divided into 3 phases:

The painful phase or freezing phase:
- There is gradual onset of diffuse shoulder pain lasting from weeks to months.
- The pain at times disturbs the patient's sleep.

The stiffening phase or frozen phase:
- It is characterized by a progressive loss of range of motion that may last up to 1 year.
- Majority lose glenohumeral external rotation, internal rotation, and abduction during this phase.
- The patient is unable to lift up the arm or brush his back or females

The thawing phase: It is measured in weeks to months and constitutes a period of gradual motion improvement.

Presentation

- Pain
- Decrease range of motion of shoulder joint both active and passive (*cardinal sign of frozen shoulder is loss of external rotation*)
- Patients complain of difficulty reaching up their back (undoing a brassier for women and putting on a suit coat or putting their hands in their back pockets for men).

Imaging Evaluation

- *X-rays*: following views to rule out any pathology:
    - Anteroposterior (AP) view of the glenohumeral joint in neutral rotation
    - Supraspinatus outlet view
    - Axillary lateral view (if possible)
- *MRI*: To rule out a possible rotator cuff tear or intra-articular pathology

Treatment

Early

- Hot fomentation or shortwave diathermy
- Analgesics
- Physiotherapy

Late

Treated with intra-articular steroid injections and mobilization of shoulder.

In refractory or recalcitrant frozen shoulder: Invasive techniques (e.g. *manipulation, distention arthrography, open surgical release or arthroscopic release of the rotator interval*) may be required.

d. Madelung's Deformity

Madelung deformity is an abnormality (growth disturbance) of the palmar ulnar part of the distal radial physis that results in a volar and ulnar tilted distal radial articular surface, volar translation of the hand and wrist, and *dorsal subluxation of the distal ulna*. Malgaigne probably first described the deformity in 1855 and later by Madelung in 1878.

Incidence

- It occurs predominantly in adolescent females (aged 10–14 years)
- More commonly bilateral and affects girls more frequently than boys

Aetiology

Vender and Watson classified Madelung and Madelung-like deformities into four different aetiologic groups, as follows:

- Posttraumatic
- Dysplastic (include dyschondrosteosis (most common form of mesomelic dwarfism), multiple hereditary osteochondromatosis, Ollier disease, achondroplasia, multiple epiphysial dysplasias, and the mucopolysaccharidoses (e.g. Hurler and Morquio syndromes))
- Chromosomal (Turner syndrome) or genetic (transmitted in an autosomal dominant pattern)
- Idiopathic or primary
- *Others*: Abnormal ligament "ligament of Vickers" impede the growth of the ulnopalmar aspect of the distal radius

Presentation

- It usually manifests in late childhood or early adolescence, with decreased range of motion and minimal pain.
- It worsens as growth occurs.
- Deformity typically consists of:
  - Volar subluxation of the hand
  - Prominence of the distal ulna
  - Volar and ulnar angulation of the distal radius
- On physical examination:
  - hand is translated volarly to the long axis of the forearm
  - The ulna, being relatively unaffected, abuts the carpus and becomes prominent dorsally
  - Range of motion is decreased, with a limitation of supination, dorsiflexion, and radial deviation.
  - Pronation and flexion usually are normal.

Radiographic Evaluation

Diagnosis is confirmed radiographically with PA and lateral views of the forearm and wrist.

Dannenberg et al. described elements of radiographic diagnostic criteria including:

- Lateral and dorsal curvature of the radius
- Widened interosseous space
- True shortening of the total length of the radius
- Premature fusion of the ulnar half of the distal radial physis
- Focal osteopenia in the area of the ulnar portion of the distal radius
- Exostosis at the distal ulnar border of the radius
- Triangularization of the distal radial epiphysis
- Ulnar and palmar facing distal radial articular surface
- Relative dorsal subluxation of the ulna

- Increased radiodensity of the ulnar head
- The overall length of the ulna is decreased
- Carpal wedging with the lunate at the apex of the wedge
- An arched curvature of the carpal bones in direct continuation of the dorsal bowing of the radius on the lateral radiograph

CT Scan

Better delineation of deformity, physeal and articular morphology.

Treatment

Conservative approach: if
- Minimal pain and excellent function
- Splintage/POP cast
- NSAIDs

Surgery

Surgical decision is based on following factors:
- Patient's age and the growth remaining in the distal radius
- Severity of the deformity
- Severity of the symptoms (persistent pain)
- Clinical and radiographic findings

Procedure

Early Presentation

When the deformity is noticed early and significant growth remains: Excision of the ligament of Vickers (Vickers physiolysis).

Late Presentation

In skeletally immature patients:
- Distal radial osteotomy with ulnar shortening (Milch recession) is a preferred treatment
- In skeletally mature patients: Osteotomy combined with a judicious Darrach excision of the distal ulnar head may be used.

> **Q9. Write short note on: a. Carpal tunnel syndrome; b. deQuervain's tenosynovitis; c. Ganglion; d. Dupuytren's contracture.**

a. Carpal Tunnel Syndrome

Most common entrapment neuropathy described in 1854 by Paget, *carpal tunnel syndrome* (tardy median palsy) is the result of compression of the median nerve within the carpal tunnel.

Boundaries of carpal tunnel:
The carpal tunnel is bounded by:
- *Dorsally*: Transverse arch of the carpal bones
- *Medially*: The hook of the hamate, triquetrum, and pisiform
- *Laterally*: The scaphoid, trapezium, and fibro-osseous flexor carpi radialis sheath.

- *Ventral (palmar) aspect, or "roof,"* :flexor retinaculum, consisting of the deep forearm fascia proximally, the transverse carpal ligament over the wrist, and the aponeurosis between the thenar and hypothenar muscles distally.

Important Contents

- The most ventral (palmar) structure in the carpal tunnel is the *median nerve.*
- Lying dorsal (deep) to the median nerve in the carpal tunnel are the *nine flexor tendons* to the fingers and thumb

Incidence

- It occurs most often in patients 30–60 years old.
- It is 2–3 times more common in women than in men.

Aetiology

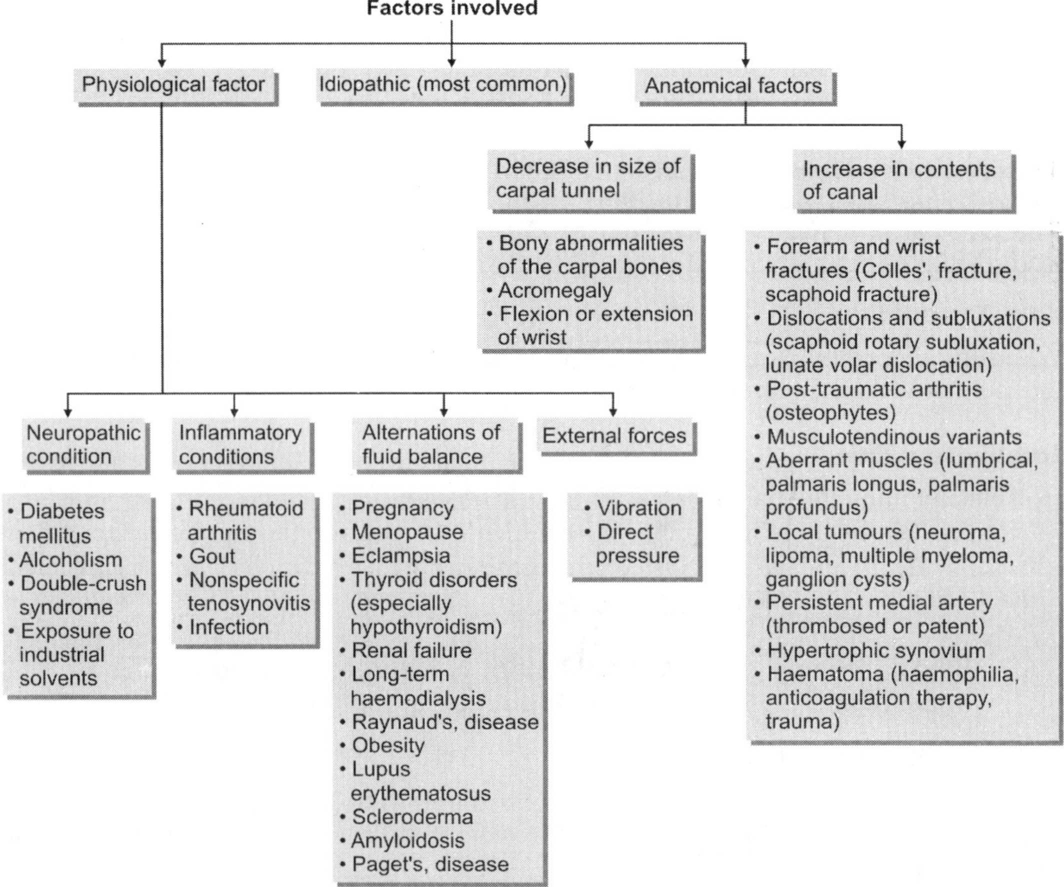

Pathogenesis

Elevation of tunnel pressures > 20–30 mm Hg impedes epineurial blood flow, and nerve function is impaired

Clinical Features

- Paraesthesia over the sensory distribution of the median nerve is the most frequent symptom (palmar aspect of the first three digits and radial ½ of the fourth digit).
- Nighttime symptoms (burning and numbness of the hand) that wake the individual are more specific to carpal tunnel syndrome, especially if the patient relieves symptoms by shaking the hand/wrist.
- Atrophy to some degree of the median-innervated hand muscles (*first and second lumbricals, opponens pollicis, abductor pollicis brevis, flexor pollicis brevis*)
- *Hoffmann-Tinel sign* is positive: Percussing the median nerve at the wrist elicits tingling in the nerve's distribution.
- *Phalen test* is positive: Acute flexion of the wrist for 60 seconds in some, but not all, patients or strenuous use of the hand increases the paresthesia.
- **Carpal compression test** (*Durkan*) is positive: This test involves applying firm pressure directly over the carpal tunnel, usually with the thumbs, for up to 30 seconds to reproduce symptoms.
- The *square wrist sign*: The ratio of the wrist thickness to the wrist width is > 0.7.
- Static 2-point discrimination: Failure to determine separation of at least 5 mm.
- Moving 2-point discrimination: Failure to determine separation at least 4 mm

Imaging Evaluation

- *Electrophysiologic studies*: Electromyography (EMG) and nerve conductions studies (NCS). A distal motor latency of > 4.5 ms and a sensory latency of > 3.5 ms are considered abnormal
- *Magnetic resonance imaging (MRI)*: It is particularly useful preoperatively if a space-occupying lesion in the carpal tunnel is suspected.
- *USG* potentially can pick up some space-occupying lesions or presence of any effusion in the carpal tunnel
- *Vibrometry*: Vibrometer placed on palmar side of digit, amplitude at 120 Hz, increased to threshold of perception, compare median and ulnar bilaterally. Asymmetry compared with contralateral hand or median to ulnar in ipsilateral hand.

Treatment

If mild symptoms have been present, and there is no thenar muscle atrophy:
- Use of night splints (usually in neutral position)
- Injection of cortisone preparations into the carpal tunnel
- Analgesics (NSAIDs)

Patients with intermediate and advanced (chronic) syndromes, failed conservative treatment: Division of the deep transverse carpal ligament is indicated (*open or endoscopic*)

Factors causing recurrence post surgery:
- Incomplete release of the transverse carpal ligament
- Reformation of the flexor retinaculum
- Scarring in the carpal tunnel
- Median or palmar cutaneous neuroma
- Palmar cutaneous nerve entrapment
- Recurrent granulomatous or inflammatory tenosynovitis
- Hypertrophic scar in the skin

b. deQuervain's Tenosynovitis

Incidence

- It occurs typically in adults 30–50 years old.
- Women are affected six to 10 times more frequently than men.

Aetiology

- Related to overuse, either in the home or at work
- Associated with rheumatoid arthritis

Pathology

Stenosing tenosynovitis (inflammation of the common sheath) of the *abductor pollicis longus* and *extensor pollicis brevis tendons*.

Clinical Feature

- Pain at the wrist
- Swelling
- Tenderness at the radial styloid
- Thickening of the fibrous sheath is palpable
- *Finkelstein test* is positive: "on grasping the patient's thumb and quickly abducting the hand ulnarward, the pain over the styloid tip is excruciating (*most pathognomonic objective sign*)
- *Eichoff's maneuver:* exacerbation of pain by passive wrist ulnar deviation while the thumb is flexed and the fingers curled around it.

Treatment

Conservative

- Rest on a splint
- Analgesics
- Ultrasonic radiation
- Injection of a steroid preparation
- Injections of steroids and local anesthetic into the tendon sheath

Surgery

- When pain persists despite conservative treatment then surgery is the treatment of choice.
- With the thumb abducted and the wrist flexed, identify and lift the abductor pollicis longus and extensor pollicis brevis from their groove, slitting and excision of common tendon sheath done.
- If there is any difficulty in releasing them, look for additional "aberrant" tendons and separate compartments
- Take precautions to avoid damage to the superficial branch of radial nerve.

c. Ganglion

Ganglions are the most common cause of focal masses in the hand and characteristically arise from synovial lining of a joint or tendon as a cystic lesion, where they may cause snapping or trigger fingers.

Aetiology

- Unknown
- History of acute or recurrent chronic injury, possibly occupational
- Theories include:
- Mucoid degeneration
- Trauma

Incidence

- Female preponderance
- Most ganglions occur in persons aged 10–40 years, with a range from childhood to the ninth decade of life.

Site

- Dorsal scapholunate ligament (most frequent site)
- Volar just radial to the flexor carpi radialis tendon (second frequent site)
- Volar retinaculum between the A1 and A2 pulleys
- Mucous cysts occur over the dorsal digit at the DIP joint level.
- Other sites include the:
    - Carpometacarpal (CMC) joint
    - Extensor tendons (especially associated with the first dorsal compartment)
    - Carpal tunnel
    - Guyon's canal

Pathophysiology

Several hypotheses have been proposed. These include the following:
- Synovial herniation or rupture through the tendon sheath (Eller, 1746)
- Synovial dermoid or rest due to "arthrogenesis blastoma cell nests" or embryonic periarticular tissue (Hoeftman, 1876)
- New growths from synovial membranes (Henle, 1847)
- Modifications of bursae or degenerative cysts (Vogt, 1881)
- Theory of mucoid degeneration offered by Ledderhose in 1893 was widely accepted
- Microtrauma and hyaluronic acid production (the most recent theory)

Presentation

- Usually asymptomatic or minimally symptomatic.
- Masses are round and hard and often tender to firm pressure.
- Appears as a small peanut size swelling which is tense and gradually increases in size, fixed to the deeper structures, smooth surface with free overlying skin.
- Associated with aching or a feeling of weakness.
- Pain is continuous and aggravates with joint movements and strain.
- Depending upon their location produces myriad of symptoms like dull aching pain, change in size, spontaneous drainage, and sensory nerve dysfunction or, less commonly, motor nerve dysfunction.
- Some ganglions can exert a mass effect on nearby structures, such as *arteries, veins, tendons, and nerves*. The impingement of such structures can cause *pain, triggering of tendons, and vascular compromise.*

Imaging Evaluation

- Standard PA, lateral, and oblique views (interosseous or juxtaosseous).
- MRI or ultrasonography can be used when the diagnosis is in doubt.
- Bone scans: It is indicated if intraosseous masses are metabolically active and capable of causing pain.

Histological Findings (FNAC)

Fluid evacuated from ganglion cysts consists of Mucin composed of:
- Glucosamine
- Albumin
- Globulin
- Hyaluronic acid

Histologic sections of the cyst reveal:
- Compressed collagen fibres and a few flattened cells without any evidence of epithelial or synovial lining.
- Multiple clefts may be present off the main cystic duct.
- No inflammatory or mitotic activity is seen

Management

Medical

- Observation, simple splint immobilization and NSAIDs
- Closed rupture (associated with high recurrence rate)
- Aspiration with or without injection of corticosteroid or other sclerotic agent
- Multiple punctures with a needle (18G) preceded by the administration of a local anesthetic (associated with a 13% cure rate)
- Suturing (nylon or non-absorbable suture) the lesion externally (The main aim is to re-epithelize the track) is associated with a 95% 6-month cure rate but an unacceptable rate of infection

Surgical Treatment

Indication:
- Intractable pain
- Cosmetic
- Pressure effect

Procedure

Most accepted surgical treatment for ganglion cyst involves *removal of the masses with adequate stalk resection with an open surgical technique*

Complication

Recurrence (most common) secondary to inadequate or incomplete resection.

d. Dupuytren's Contracture

Dupuytren's disease is a proliferative fibroplasia of the subcutaneous palmar tissue occurring in the form of nodules and cords that may result in slowly progressive thickening and shortening of the palmar fascia and irreversible flexion contractures of the finger joints

Aetiology

- Exact cause is unknown
- Probably genetic in origin (autosomal dominant with variable penetrance)
- Additional risk factors include:
  - Manual labor with vibration exposure
  - Prior hand trauma
  - Alcoholism
  - Smokers
  - Diabetes mellitus
  - Hyperlipidemia
  - Peyronie disease
  - Complex regional pain syndrome (CPRS)

Conditions possibly related to *Dupuytren's contracture* include the following:

- Diabetes mellitus
- Alcohol abuse
- HIV infection
- Epilepsy
- Trauma
- Manual labour with vibratory exposure
- Cigarette smoking

Incidence

- Most common in whites of Northern European descent
- Male predominance (expression of androgen receptors in Dupuytren's fascia)
- Usually a middle aged man
- Incidence of Dupuytren's increases with age
- Involvement, although often bilateral (45%), rarely is symmetrical

Pathophysiology

Essential problem is fibroblast proliferation and collagen deposition leading to contractures of the palmar fascia.

Dupuytren's disease occurs in the following three stages:

- *Proliferative phase*: Proliferation of fibroblast and development of a nodule
- *Involutional phase*: Contracture develops with associated nodular thickening of the palmar fascia. Myofibroblasts are predominant during this phase and align themselves along tension lines within the nodule.
- *Residual phase*: Myofibroblasts disappeared. A joint contracture is present with diffuse thickening of the palmar fascia. The nodular tissue tends to regress during this stage. Type III collagen replaces the normal type I collagen

Clinical Features

- Usually begins in line with the *ring finger* (most commonly involved) at the distal palmar crease and progresses to involve the ring and little fingers. The index finger and the thumb are typically spared.
- On physical examination:
  - Firm nodules that may be tender to palpation
  - Painless cords proximal to the nodules

- Skin blanching upon active finger extension
- Atrophic grooves or pits in the skin
- Tender knuckle pads over the dorsal aspect of the PIPs (*Garrod nodes*): It suggest more aggressive disease.
- Plantar fascia involvement, known as *Ledderhose disease* (6–31%): This can indicate more severe disease.
- Presence of MCP and PIP joint contractures
- Hueston table-top test: If the patient is unable to lay the palm flat on a tabletop, the test is considered positive.

Imaging Evaluation

- No routine radiographs are necessary.
- USG can demonstrate thickening of the palmar fascia as well as the presence of a nodule.
- A histologic staging system: Luck described 3 progressive stages. In all stages, a core of type I collagen is surrounded by type III collagen.
  - Proliferative stage
  - Involution stage
  - Residual stage

Treatment

Medical

- Observation (*in cases of mild disease with minimal contractures*)
- Intralesional *corticosteroid* injection
- Splinting: This is most helpful postoperatively or post-injection
- *Recent*:
  - Use of calcium channel blockers nifedipine locally early in the course and use of collagenase in advanced cases. Collagenase *Clostridium histolyticum (Xiaflex)* for the treatment of Dupuytren's contracture. Injected collagenase extracted from *C. histolyticum* weakens and dissolves the Dupuytren's cords.
  - *Ilomastat*: Ilomastat is an investigational medication that functions as an MMP inhibitor (MMP play a role in cell-mediated collagen production and the transition from type I to type III collagen).
  - Intralesional injection of *ó interferon* provides symptomatic relief.

Surgery

Indications:
- MCP Flexion contracture >30°
- PIP flexion contracture >15°

Five surgical procedures commonly used:
- Subcutaneous fasciotomy
- Partial (selective) fasciectomy
- Complete fasciectomy
- Fasciectomy with skin grafting
- Amputation

The appropriate procedure depends on the:
- Degree of contracture
- Nutritional status of the palmar skin
- Presence or absence of bony deformities
- Patient's age
- Patient's occupation
- Patient's general health

Complications

Intraoperative complications include digital nerve and arterial injury.

Postoperative complications occur in 17–20% of patients. They include:
- Loss of motion
- Skin sloughing
- Haematoma formation
- Infection
- Swelling
- CPRS (CPRS occurs more often in patients with extensive surgery)

Q10. Discuss the clinical features and management of Perthes disease or coxa plana.

Legg-Calve-Perthes disease (LCPD) is avascular necrosis and disordered enchondral ossification of the proximal femoral head resulting from compromise of the tenuous blood supply to this area.

Incidence

- Legg-Calvé-Perthes disease usually occurs in children aged 4–10 years, with a mean age of 7 years.
- Male-to-female ratio of 4:1
- The condition is rare, occurring in approximately 4 of 100,000 children.
- Insidious onset
- Usually unilateral. Both hips are involved in less than 10% of cases
- High incidence in underprivileged communities.

Predisposing Factors

The cause unknown, but children with Legg-Calvé-Perthes disease (LCPD) have:
- Delayed bone age
- Disproportionate growth
- Mildly shortened stature

Legg-Calvé-Perthes disease (LCPD) may be idiopathic, or it may result from:
- Slipped capital femoral epiphysis
- Trauma
- Steroid use
- Sickle-cell crisis
- Deficiencies of antithrombotic factor
- Inherited thrombophilia

- Toxic synovitis
- Congenital dislocation of the hip

Pathophysiology

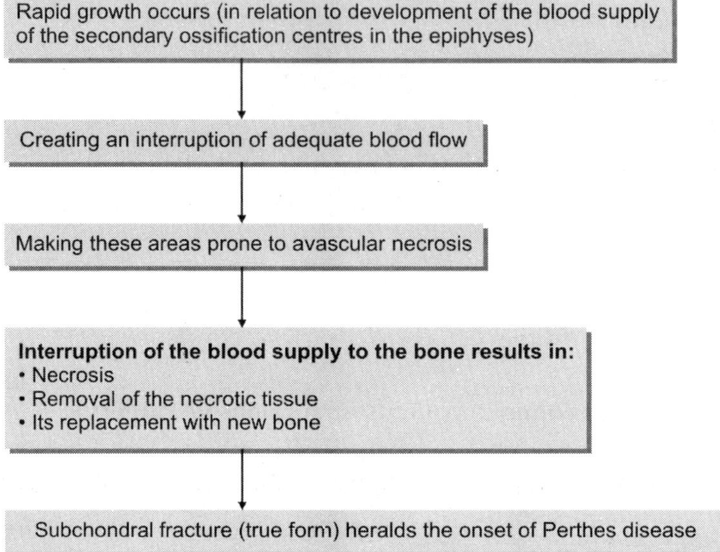

Clinical Features

- Usually common in 4–10-year-old age group
- Intermittent limp (abductor lurch; earliest sign)
- Painless limp (classical presentation)
- Mild or intermittent pain in the anterior part of the thigh

On Examination

- Antalgic gait
- Spasm of muscles
- Wasting of proximal thigh muscle
- Short stature
- Trendelenburg gait resulting from pain in the gluteus medius muscle
- Thomas test reveals fixed flexion deformity
- Limitation of abduction and internal rotation

Classification

Caterall et al. classified patients into groups according to the amount of involvement of the capital femoral epiphysis:
- Group I: partial head or <½ head involvement
- Groups II and III: >½ head involvement and sequestrum formation
- Group IV: involvement of the entire epiphysis

"Head at Risk" Signs

- Lateral subluxation of the femoral head from the acetabulum
- Speckled calcification lateral to the capital epiphysis
- Diffuse metaphyseal reaction (metaphyseal cysts)
- A horizontal physis
- *Gage sign*, a radiolucent V-shaped defect in the lateral epiphysis and adjacent metaphysis

These head at risk signs are correlated positively with poor results, especially in patients in groups II, III, and IV.

Salter and Thompson Classification

Type A

- If the extent of the fracture (line) is <50% of the superior dome of the femoral head, the involvement is considered
- Good prognosis

Type B

- If the extent of the fracture is >50% of the dome
- Fair or poor prognosis

This classification is simple and accurate and can be applied early in the course of the disease to determine management

Herring et al. classification based on the height of the lateral pillar
- Group A: No involvement of the lateral pillar (uniformly good outcomes)
- Group B: At least 50% of lateral pillar height maintained (<9 years good outcomes, but patients >9 years had less favorable results)
- Group C: <50% of lateral pillar height maintained (worst results)

Advantage of herring classification:
- It can be applied easily during the active stages of the disease
- The high correlation between the lateral pillar height and the amount of femoral head flattening at skeletal maturity allows accurate prediction of the natural history and treatment methods

Stulberg Classification

- Grade I: Round head, normal hip
- Grade II: Round head coxa magna
- Grade III: Oval or mushroom-shaped head, coxa magna
- Grade IV: Flat head, congruent with acetabulum
- Grade V: Flat head, in congruent

Radiographic Evaluation

Plain X-ray

X-ray shows a wide range of changes depending on the stage of the disease.

Early
- Increased joint space (*Waldenstrom sign*) with slight lateral subluxation.
- Failure of the ossification centre to increase.

- Subchondral fracture (Salter sign) or crescent sign on lateral radiograph
- A convex, rounded enlargement of superior margin of the femoral neck (*Gage's sign*), segmental fracture of the superolateral aspect of the head.

Late

- Avascular necrosis and anterolateral segmental collapse of the femoral head.
- Entire ossific centre becomes necrotic, fragmented, deformed, flattened, mushroomed, broadened etc.
- The neck becomes short and wide with rarefaction of the metaphysis below the growth plate.
- Early osteoarthritic changes of the hip and symmetrical adaptive changes in the acetabulum occur depending on the deformity of the head.

Initial radiographs can be normal, but radiographic changes can be divided into five distinct stages representing a continuum of the disease process.
- *Stage 1* reveals cessation of femoral epiphyseal growth.
- *Stage 2* is a subchondral fracture.
- *Stage 3* shows resorption.
- *Stage 4* demonstrates reossification
- *Stage 5* is the healed or residual stage

Salter Extrusion Angle

- To assess the extrusion of femoral head.
- Horizontal line at bottom of acetabular 'teardrops' and perpendicular lines at lateral ossified margin of acetabulum drawn. Lines from intersections of these lines, through midpoint of physis, give angle.
- Normal is $\geq 50°$.

Bone Scan

Establish the diagnosis much earlier.

MRI: Better Delineated

- The extent and location of Legg-Calvé-Perthes disease involvement
- Infarction and contour (sphericity) of femoral head

Treatment

Goal

Treatment goals include:
- Eliminating hip irritability
- Restoring and maintaining good range of motion in the hip
- Preventing femoral epiphyseal collapse
- Attaining a spherical femoral head when the hip heals

Nonoperative:

To maintain containment:
- Bed rest
- Skin traction in wide abduction (to avoid subluxation) until hip irritability decreased
- Weight-relieving caliper (ischial weight-bearing brace)

- Physiotherapy including active and active-assisted range-of-motion, abduction exercises and muscle stretching exercises to the hip and knee

If already subluxated/dislocated: CR under GA and percutaneous adductor longus tenotomy, followed by an ambulatory abduction cast (Petrie) for 6 weeks or more.

Containment Methods

Non-operative:
- Abduction spica casts
- Abduction brace

Operative:

Indications for reconstructive surgery in Legg-Calvé-Perthes disease are:
- Hinged abduction, for which *valgus subtrochanteric osteotomy* is indicated
- Malformed femoral head in late Catterall group III or residual group IV, for which *Garceau cheilectomy* can be used
- Coxa magna, for which a *shelf augmentation* would provide coverage
- Large malformed femoral head with subluxation laterally, for which *pelvic osteotomy* may be considered
- Capital femoral physeal arrest, for which trochanteric advancement or arrest can be performed

Innominate Osteotomy

Advantages

- Anterolateral coverage of the femoral head
- Lengthening of the extremity (possibly shortened by the avascular process)
- Avoidance of a second operation for plate removal

Disadvantages

- Inability sometimes to obtain proper containment of the femoral head, especially in older children
- An increase in acetabular and hip joint pressure that may cause further avascular changes in the femoral head
- An increase in leg length on the operated side compared with the normal side that may cause a relative adduction of the hip and uncover the femoral head

Lateral Shelf Procedure

For older children who are not candidates for femoral osteotomy because of:
- Insufficient remodelling capacity
- Shortening of the femur would cause a persistent limp

Varus Derotational Osteotomy

Indication

- When containment of the femoral head is necessary but failed to achieved with a brace for psychosocial or other reasons
- When the child is 8–10 years old and without leg-length inequality
- When on arthrogram or MRI most of the femoral head is uncovered and the angle of Wiberg is decreased
- When there is a significant amount of femoral anteversion

Advantages

- The ability to obtain maximal coverage of the femoral head, especially in an older child
- The ability to correct excessive femoral anteversion

Disadvantage

- Excessive varus angulation that may not correct with growth (especially in an older child)
- Further shortening of an already shortened extremity
- Gluteus lurch
- Nonunion of the osteotomy
- Requirement of a second operation to remove the internal fixation

Lateral opening wedge osteotomy: For children 5 years of age and younger

Arthrodiastasis

Rationale

Distraction or diastasis *(Hinged external fixator (Orthofix))* of the joint not only widens, but also:

- Unloads the joint space
- Reduces the pressure on the femoral head
- Allows fibrous repair of articular cartilage defects
- Preserves congruency of the femoral head

Reconstructive Surgery in Legg-Calvé-Perthes disease

Valgus extension osteotomy: Indicated for malformed femoral heads with hinge abduction

Valgus Flexion Internal Rotation Osteotomy

The combined procedure:
- Corrects the functional coxa vara and hinge abduction (valgus osteotomy)
- Establishes a more normal articulation between the posteromedial portion of the true femoral head and the acetabulum
- Corrects external rotation deformity of the distal limb (internal rotation osteotomy)
- Improves joint congruity and anterolateral femoral head containment in hips with associated acetabular dysplasia

Cheilectomy

A cheilectomy can be used for lateral protuberance of the head outside the acetabulum.

Chiari Osteotomy

It is indicated when the head is mushroom-shaped, as in coxa plana, and subluxating from the acetabulum, and when the hip is painful.

> **Q11. Discuss the aetiology clinical features and management of Slipped Capital Femoral Epiphysis.**

The femoral epiphysis along with the head of femur gradually slips backwards and ultimately separates.

Incidence

- Age 10–16 years (in the rapid growth phase)
- Obese children (chubby boys)
- Twice as common in boys as in girls
- Twice as often in black children as in white children
- Left hip is affected twice as often as the right
- Bilateral involvement is reported to occur in 25–40% of children

Aetiological Factors

- Local trauma
- Mechanical factors (especially obesity, growth spurts, and puberty)
- Inflammatory conditions
- Endocrine disorders (e.g. hypothyroidism, hypopituitarism, and chronic renal disease)
- Genetic factors
- Down syndrome and seasonal variations

Clinical Presentation

- Insidious in onset
- Pain in the groin, medial thigh or knee
- Gradually progressive limping
- On examination:
  - Abduction, external rotation deformity
  - True shortening
  - Positive Trendelenburg sign (slip is of a moderate degree)
  - Limitation of hip motion, especially internal rotation
  - In bilateral involvement a typical waddling gait

Radiographic Evaluation

X-rays

- AP view of the hip will show that the *Klein's line* (along the upper border of the neck of femur) passing above the head of femur, due to the slip (*Trethowan's sign*). Normally, it cuts through the upper third of the head of femur.
- "Frog-leg" lateral view best shows subtle slipping
- Cross-table, or true, lateral view : determine the extent of posterior displacement of the epiphysis

CT Scan

It may help confirm the diagnosis in patients with early, mild slipping that is not apparent on radiographs.

Ultrasonography and MRI

- These have been used for diagnosis and evaluation of SCFE.
- Although MRI may not show the slip, it may reveal edema around the physis on T_2-weighted images, (sign that a slip is present)

Traditional Classification

It is based on duration of symptoms and the severity of the slip.

Acute Slips

- These are those with a sudden onset of severe symptoms
- Usually present for <2 weeks.
- Radiographs show the epiphyseal displacement with no evidence of bone healing or remodelling.

Chronic Slips

- These are characterized by gradual onset and symptoms
- Usually >2 weeks duration
- Some bony healing and remodeling along the posterior and medial femoral neck usually are visible on radiographs.

Treatment

Goal

- Prevent additional slipping of the epiphysis
- Stimulate early physeal closure
- Avoiding the complications of osteonecrosis, chondrolysis, and osteoarthritis

Nonoperative Treatment

- Traction and spica cast immobilization (12 weeks)
- Rarely used today because of complications

Operative Treatment

Choice of treatment must be individualized for each child, depending on age, type of slip, and severity of displacement.

- Percutaneous and open in situ pinning (single cannulated screw fixation)
- Open reduction and internal fixation
- Epiphysiodesis
- Osteotomy
- Reconstruction by arthroplasty
- Arthrodesis
- Cheilectomy

Early stage: Fixation by pins

Late cases: Wedge correction osteotomy of the neck of femur

Complications

- Osteonecrosis (10–15%)
- Chondrolysis (joint space <3 mm wide (normal 4–6 mm) and a decreased range of motion of the hip joint)
- Femoral neck fracture (infrequent)
- Continued slipping

Q12. Discuss causes of: a. Painful knee and b. Painful foot

a. Painful knee

Chondromalacia Patellae

Chondromalacia (sick cartilage) is an affliction of the *patellofemoral joint's hyaline cartilage. Lateral positioning of the patella in the patella-femoral joint, tight lateral retinaculum or a lateral synovial plica, an abnormal Q angle* is often the causes. This is commonest cause of anterior knee pain in young women (attributed to increased Q angles in women) usually following prolonged sitting. On clinical examination, there is medial retro-patellar tenderness, obvious patellar lesion and loose body can be seen on X-ray and arthroscopy. Medical management comprises of patella stabilizing braces, physical therapy for quadriceps strengthening, orthotics which decrease pronation of the foot, and NSAIDs medication. In cases failure to respond to medical management it is treated by arthroscopic shaving of the damaged patellar cartilage and if necessary removal of the loose body.

Recurrent Subluxation of Patella

This is due to the tight lateral retinaculum causing the patella to subluxates laterally in flexion, causing severe pain and discomfort in young girls with mild knee valgus, a high riding patella or hypotrophic lateral femoral condyle.

Treatment

a. Campbell's procedure (lateral retinacular release with medial double breasting).
b. Shifting of the insertion of ligamentum patellae proximally

Fat-pad Syndrome

Hoffa's (infrapatellar) fat pad (HFP) is an intracapsular, extra-synovial structure that fills the anterior knee compartment, and is richly vascularized and innervated and, therefore, a source of anterior knee pain. Repetitive local micro-traumas, impingement, and surgery causing local bleeding and inflammation are the most frequent causes of pain. MRI is the investigation of choice. Managed by physical therapy, taping, gait training, intralesional injection of local anaesthetic plus corticosteroids and IFP ablation with ultrasound guided alcohol injections have promising results. Refractory cases will require surgical intervention.

Loose Bodies in the Knee

Patient presents with features of acute pain, effusion and recurrent locking. The loose bodies may be (a) few as in cases of intra-articular chip fracture, chondromalacia patellae, osteoarthritis or may be (b) multiple as in case of synovial osteochondromatosis/villonodular synovitis and neuropathic joint. X-ray shows multiple loose bodies like a bunch of grapes or solitary one. Keep in mind *"fabella". This is an ossification in the lateral head of gastrocnemius.* Arthroscopic removal of loose bodies has favourable outcome.

Osgood–Schlatter Disease

This is apophysitis involving the tibial tuberosity, common in young boys of adolescent age, preventing with pain and progressive swelling in the area of insertion of the ligamentum patellae (as shown below), X-ray shows avulsion and fragmentation of the tuberosity in different stages, the condition is self limiting and need assurance, rest and limitation of outdoor sports. A knee immobilizer and analgesics often helps. In advanced cases surgical excision of the fragments and fixation of the tuberosity may be required.

b. Forefoot pain

This is usually due to:
- Hallux valgus
- Hallux rigidus
- Hammer-toes
- Splayed foot
- In-growing toenail
- Paronychia
- Plantar corns

Metatarsal Pain

- After a stress fracture of 2/3rd metatarsal
- *Morton's metatarsalgia* (neuritis involving digital nerves between 3/4 toes)
- *Freiberg's disease* (crushing osteochondritis of 2nd/3rd metatarsal head)

Midfoot

- Pes cavus
- Flat-foot
- Plantar fascitis
- Varicose veins

Hindfoot

- Calcaneal spur (heel pad)
- Tendo Achilles bursitis is usually due to gout, diabetic tendonitis.

Q13. Write short note on: a. Painful Heel/Plantar fasciitis; b. Hallux valgus.

a. Painful Heel/Plantar Fasciitis

Pain at the heel is due to inflammation of the plantar fascia due to *overweight, faulty footwear, long hours of standing or diabetes mellitus.*

Skiagram may show calcaneal spur.

Management

Usually conservative
- Alternate hot/cold dip (contrast fomentation)
- Ultrasonography
- Padded heel in the footwear
- Local hydrocortisone injection

b. Hallux Valgus

Hallux valgus (lateral deviation of the great toe) is a complex deformity of the first ray . It is most commonly encountered valgus deformity of the metatarsophalangeal joint of forefoot.

It is characterized by lateral deviation of the first toe and, usually, by medial deviation of the first metatarsal. The first metatarsal is in varus position while the proximal phalanx deviates laterally.

Aetiology

- Faulty footwear
- Arthritic/metabolic conditions
  - Gouty arthritis
  - Rheumatoid arthritis
  - Psoriatic arthritis
- Connective tissue disorders such as Ehlers-Danlos syndrome, Marfan syndrome, Down syndrome, and ligamentous laxity
- Neuromuscular disease
- Multiple sclerosis
- Charcot-Marie-Tooth disease
- Cerebral palsy
- Traumatic compromise
- Mal-unions
- Intra-articular damage
- Soft tissue sprains
- Dislocations

Staging

Root et al. described the patho-mechanical development of hallux valgus in following four. stages.

- *Stage 1*: Excessive pronation causes hypermobility of the first ray, causing the tibial sesamoid ligament to be stretched and the fibular sesamoid ligament to contract, and lateral subluxation of the proximal phalanx occurs.
- *Stage 2*: Hallux abduction progresses, with the flexor hallucis longus and flexor hallucis brevis gaining lateral mechanical advantage.
- *Stage 3*: Further subluxation occurs at the first metatarsophalangeal joint, with formation of metatarsus primus adductus.
- *Stage 4*: The first metatarsophalangeal joint finally dislocates.

Clinical Features

- Dull aching pain in the metatarsal head secondary to shoe irritation that is relieved when the shoes are removed.
- Deformity
- Varus deformity of the first metatarsal
- Valgus of the great toe
- Bunion formation: The head of the first metatarsal becoming prominent with overlying skin and soft tissue developing recurrent bursitis (Bunion)
- Sometimes tingling in the dorsal aspect of the bunion, which indicates entrapment neuritis of the medial dorsal cutaneous nerve
- Corns
- Calluses

- Metatarsalgia (pain)
- Arthritis of the first metatarsophalangeal joint
- Hammer toe of one or more toes
- Limitation of motion and pain at the MTP joint of the great toe

X-rays

- Standing dorso-planar, lateral view
- Non-standing lateral oblique view
- Axial View

Classification

Based on **Hallux Valgus angle (HV angle):** It is created by the bisection of the longitudinal axis of the hallux and longitudinal axis of the first metatarsal.

IMT angle (Intermetatarsal angle): Determined by the bisection of the longitudinal axes of the first and second metatarsal

	HV angle	IMT angle	Incongruent MTPJ
Normal	<15°	<9°	No
Mild	15–20°	9–11°	No
Moderate	20–40°	11–18°	Yes
Severe	>40°	>18°	No

Treatment

Conservative

- Adequate padding with a number of different materials (e.g. felt) to reduce pressure on the painful prominence of the bunion.
- Splints (foot orthotics).
- Physical therapy can be used to help with the symptoms and improve the range of motion.
- Passive stretching of the abductors of the toes.

Surgical

Indications: Absolute indications are:
- Pain (not responding to conservative modality)
- Cosmetic

Surgical Procedures

Bump removal surgery:
- Silver
- McBride

Head osteotomy: Austin/Chevron.

Shaft osteotomy: Mitchell procedure.

Procedure proximal first netatarsal: Lepidius.

Joint Destructive Procedures

- First metatarsophalengeal joint arthodesis.
- Keller's procedure (combines resection hemiarthroplasty of the first MTPh joint with removal of the medial eminence of the first MT)

Digital Procedure

Akin procedure: Types of surgical procedure based on severity of deformity:

Mild deformity:

- Mild-to-moderate deformity (IM angle ranges 9–13°)
- Soft tissue procedure (modified McBride procedure) or distal osteotomy (Chevron or Mitchell type)

Moderate deformity: Moderate-to-severe deformities (13–20°) is best treated with soft tissue release and proximal MT osteotomy.

Prominent medial eminence: consider a concomitant silver procedure.

Severe deformity:

- Hallux valgus deformity >30° and IM angle >12° consider distal soft tissue release with proximal osteotomy
- MTP joint arthrodesis
- Lepidus procedure: Indicated for severe deformity + hypermobile 1st ray

In young patients:

- *Simmonds' procedure*: Requires osteotomy of first metatarsal and wedge resection of the medial side of the first metatarsal head.
- *Wilson's operation*: Oblique osteotomy through the distal third of the metatarsal.

In adults:

- Beveling of the medial prominence of the metatarsal head.
- *Keller's operation*: Excision of proximal third of the phalanx and prominent portion of the metatarsal head, combined with proximal metatarsal osteotomy.
- *Mayo's operation*: Excision of metatarsal head and prominent part of proximal phalanx.
- *Arthrodesis*: Surgical refashioning of the deformed joint and fusion

Q14. Discuss in brief: a. Pes cavus; b. Pes planus.

a. Pes Cavus

A *cavus foot* is one with an abnormally *high longitudinal arch (medial)*; usually accompanies spectrum of deformities.

Multiple Deformities

- Hyperextension of the toes at the metatarsophalangeal joints
- Hyperflexion at the interphalangeal joints
- Pronation and adduction of the forefoot (forefoot valgus)
- A 'bony' dorsum of the mid-foot with wrinkled skin folds on the medial plantar aspect
- Lengthened lateral border of the foot and shortened medial border
- Calluses beneath the metatarsal heads
- Stiffness of the subtalar joint
- Fixed or flexible varus deformity of the heel
- Tightness of the Achilles tendon with or without an equinus contracture

Aetiology

- Idiopathic
- Skeletally mature patients:
  - Neuromuscular disease:
    - Charcot-Marie-Tooth disease
    - Poliomyelitis
    - May result in cavus deformity if not treated before skeletal maturity
      - Spinal dysraphism
      - Cerebral palsy
      - Primary cerebellar disease
      - Arthrogryposis
      - Severe clubfeet
  - *Trauma*: Deep posterior compartment syndrome (fracture of the tibia or fibula or malunion of mid-foot fractures or fracture-dislocations).

Clinical Features

- Usually present at the age of 8–10 years.
- Pain while walking
- Reduced walking tolerance
- High longitudinal arch (medial)
- Adducted and pronated forefoot
- Plantar flexed first ray
- Mid-foot equinus
- Heel varus
- Clawing of toes
- Painful callosities
- Contracted plantar fascia
- Sensory/neurological deficit or findings (as per neuromuscular pathology)

Investigation

Radiographic Findings

Standing lateral view and standing AP views:
- To assess the contribution of the hindfoot (talus and calcaneus), mid-foot (navicular and cuboid-cuneiform), and forefoot (Lisfranc) to the cavus deformity.
- To determine the severity of the fixed deformity.
- Assessing first and second metatarsal plantar flexion.
- To calculate (on lateral view) "calcaneal pitch" and "Meary's angle":
  - In normal foot the calcaneal pitch is between 10 and 30° whereas Meary's angle, formed by the axes of the talus and first metatarsal, is 0°, i.e. these axes are parallel.
- Other radiographic findings that may be helpful include:
  - Degenerative changes, in the tibiotalar, subtalar, or midtarsal Lisfranc joints
  - Rotation of the talus in the ankle mortise (caused by talar dorsiflexion and varus at the subtalar joint)
  - Dystrophic ossification in soft tissue suggesting tendon or ligament injury on the oblique view

Investigations (besides detailed physical examination) that helps to land on aetiology:
- Electromyography
- Neurological studies
- MRI
- Myelography
- Arteriography
- Genetic studies

Treatment

Non-surgical: For mild deformity
- Counselling
- Daily manipulation
- Anterior arch bar
- Night splint

Surgical: For moderate-to-severe/neglected deformities.
Aim: To provide a pain-free, plantigrade, supple but stable foot.
Cavus foot requires correction of the separate components within the foot and ankle.

Claw Toes

For fixed contractures at the metatarsophalangeal and interphalangeal joints, the following
are recommended:
- Lengthening of the extensor hallucis longus and extensor digitorum longus
- Tenotomy of the extensor digitorum brevis and the extensor hallucis brevis
- Dorsal capsulotomy of the metatarsophalangeal joints
- Resection of the head and neck of the proximal phalanges
- Release of the plantar fascia, if indicated
- Arthrodesis of the interphalangeal joint of the hallux.

Forefoot Equinus

- Double plantar fasciotomies
- Closing wedge greenstick dorsal proximal metatarsal osteotomies
- Jones procedure: Tendon suspension of the first metatarsal and interphalangeal joint
  arthrodesis
- Jahss procedure: Tarsometatarsal truncated-wedge arthrodesis

Midfoot Cavus

- Anterior tarsal wedge osteotomy (Coles' procedure)
- V-Osteotomy of the Tarsus (Japas procedure)
- Combined cavus (Calcaneo-cavus deformity):
    - Crescentic calcaneal osteotomy (Samilson)
    - Osteotomy of the calcaneus (Dwyer)

*Calcaneocavovarus and Cavovarus Deformity Associated with Arthritic Changes of the
Subtalar and Midtarsal Joints:*
Triple Arthrodesis.

b. Pes planus

Pes planus (or flat foot) refers to loss of the normal medial longitudinal arch as a result the medial border of the foot is in contact with the ground.

Other Anatomical Abnormalities

- Valgus posture of the heel
- Subluxation (mild) of the subtalar joint
- Head of the talus tilts medially and plantar-ward
- Eversion of the calcaneus at the subtalar joint
- Lateral angulation (abduction) at the midtarsal joint (talonavicular and calcaneo-cuboid joints)
- Supination of the forefoot relative to the hindfoot
- Shortened Achilles tendon

Aetiology

- Congenital
- Acquired

Types

Flexible

- Appear as normal in toddlers and disappears when medial arch development is complete
- Occasionally persist in adult: On non-weight bearing or on simply dorsiflexing the great toe, the arch can be restored.

Rigid

- The deformity is fixed and cannot be corrected passively.
- Two most common example of fixed/rigid pes planus are *congenital vertical talus and tarsal coalition*

Clinical Features

- Symptoms usually depends upon the age of presentation (babies, children or in adults)
- Flattened arch
- Valgus heel
- Fore-foot adducted and pronated

Treatment

For flexible pes planus:

Children 2 years old: No treatment.

Child from walking age to 3 years:
- Counsel the parents
- Shoe modifications and inserts (Thomas heels, medial heel wedges (1/8–3/16 inch), and navicular pads)

3–9-year-old child:
- Asymptomatic: counsel the parents

- Symptomatic:
  - Arch support is placed in a leather shoe with:
  - Firm heel counter
  - Extended medial counter
  - Steel shank
  - Thomas heel
  - Medial heel wedge

Symptomatic resulting from severe pes planus deformity: Custom orthosis is recommended

10–14-year-old patient:

- *Asymptomatic*: No specific treatment
- *Symptomatic*:
  - Moulded orthosis (*raises the heel and reduces heel valgus*), usually polypropylene, is made from a positive mould (cast), in which the foot has been placed in the corrected position (a neutral heel and forefoot position, plantar flexion of the first ray, and restitution of the medial longitudinal arch
  - Excision of the accessory navicular (pre-hallux) may relieve:
    - a painful bursa
    - posterior tibial tendinitis
    - synchondritis (between the accessory and main navicular bone)
- *If calcaneo-navicular coalition*: Excising the area of coalition

Surgical Treatment

- Durham pes planus plasty (Caldwell; Coleman) (advancement of the posterior tibial tendon and osteo-periosteal flap with arthrodesis of the navicular-1st cuneiform joint)
- Plantar flexion osteotomy of medial cuneiform (Hirose and Johnson)
- Triple arthrodesis (triplane)
- Posterior calcaneal displacement osteotomy (Koutsogiannis)
- Anterior calcaneal lengthening-distraction wedge osteotomy (Mosca)

Rigid Pes Planus

Rigid pes planus usually are symptomatic; frequently require an operative procedure.

Tarsal Coalition

Conservative treatment:

- Reduced activity
- 4–6 weeks in a short leg walking cast
- Use of a molded, firm arch support

If not responding then:

- Resection of the calcaneo-navicular bar with interposition of muscle or fat at the site of resection
- Resection of the fibrous or bony talocalcaneal bar
- Subtalar arthrodesis
- Triple arthrodesis

Congenital Vertical Foot

- Open reduction of talonavicular joint usually is necessary.
- *Children 1–4 years old*: Open reduction and realignment of the talonavicular and subtalar joints.
- *Children 3 years old or older with severe deformity*: Navicular excision is required at the time of open reduction.
- *Children 4–8 years old*: Open reduction and soft-tissue procedures combined with extra-articular subtalar arthrodesis
- *Children 12 years old or older*: Triple arthrodesis

17

Bone Tumours

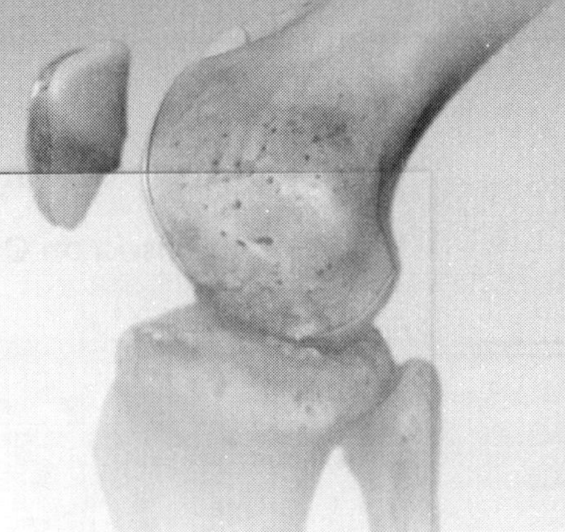

Enneking system can be applied to both bone and soft tissue tumours. Broadly, it is based on the assessment of *two basic parameters: Biologic aggressiveness and local extent of the disease based on compartment concept of bone and soft tissue.*

The surgical staging system, as described by Enneking et al. is dependent on the GTM classification: *grade (G), location (T) and lymph node involvement and metastases (M).*

Grade (G): the grade is an assessment of the biological behaviour of the lesions. It is further categories into following:

- *G0*: Benign
- *G1*: Low-grade or locally aggressive tumour with low probability of metastases (e.g. *Giant cell tumour, low-grade intraosseous osteosarcoma, parosteal osteosarcoma or grade I or grade II chondrosarcoma*)
- *G2*: High-grade or aggressive tumour with high metastatic potentials (*e.g. high-grade conventional osteosarcoma, Ewing's sarcoma, Gd3 chondrosarcoma, or malignant fibrous histiocytoma*)

Site of lesion (T): Represents the location or site, whether intracompartmental or extra-compartmental.

- *T1*: Intracompartmental (an individual bone with its medullary cavity is a single compartment)
- *T2*: Extracompartmental (extension of tumour beyond the cortex into adjacent soft tissue, joint or another bone)

Suffixes used to show compartmental involvement: *A (Intracompartmental) and B (Extra-compartmental)*

Metastases (M): Lymphatic spread is a sign of widespread dissemination. Regional lymphatic involvement is equated with distant metastases.

- *M0*: Absence of any metastases
- *M1*: Metastases

Surgical staging system (Enneking's):

Stage	Grade	Site (location)	Treatment planned
IA	Low (G1)	Intracompartmental (T1)	Wide excision
IB	Low (G1)	Extracompartmental (T2)	Radical excision
IIA	High (G2)	Intracompartmental (T1)	Wide amputation
IIB	High (G2)	Extracompartmental (T2)	Radical amputation
III	Any G	Any (T)	Chemotherapy/radiotherapy
	Regional or distant metastasis		

Q2. Give classification of tumour based on cell of origin.

Classification Based on Cell of Origin

Primary

Cell of origin	Benign	Malignant
A. Osseous		
a. Cartilage	Osteochondroma Chondroma Chondroblastoma Chondromyxoid fibroma	Chondrosarcoma
b. Osteoid	Osteoma Osteoid osteoma Periosteal fibroma	Osteogenic sarcoma
c. Resorptive bone cysts	Fibrous dysplasia Giant cell tumour	Giant cell tumour
B. Non-osseous		
a. Marrow	Solitary plasmacytoma Reticuloendotheliosis Xanthoma	Leucaemia Multiple myeloma Reticulum cell sarcoma Ewing's sarcoma
b. Muscle	Myoma	Myosarcoma
c. Inclusion	Chordoma Fibroma Angioma Synovioma Adamantinoma	 Fibrosarcoma Angiosarcoma Synovial cell sarcoma Squamous cell carcinoma

Secondary

- *Osteoblastic*: Brain, bronchus, breast, bowel, bladder, prostrate
- *Osteolytic*: Colon, thyroid, kidney, etc.

Q3. Discuss the WHO classification of the musculoskeletal tumours.

WHO classification of primary bone tumours and tumour-like lesions:

I. Bone-forming Tumours

A. Benign

1. Osteoma
2. Osteoid osteoma
3. Osteoblastoma

B. Malignant

1. Osteosarcoma (osteogenic sarcoma)
2. Juxtacortical osteosarcoma (periosteal osteosarcoma)

II. Cartilage Forming Tumours

A. Benign

1. Chondroma
2. Osteochondroma (osteocartilaginous exostosis)
3. Chondroblastoma
4. Chondromyxoid fibroma

B. Malignant

1. Chondrosarcoma
2. Juxtacortical chondrosarcoma
3. Mesenchymal chondrosarcoma

III. Giant cell tumour (Osteoclastoma)

IV. Marrow tumours

1. Ewing's sarcoma
2. Reticulosarcoma of bone
3. Lymphosarcoma of bone
4. Myeloma

V. Vascular tumours

A. Benign

1. Haemangioma
2. Lymphangioma
3. Glomus tumour (glomangioma)

B. Intermediate or indeterminate

1. Haemangioendothelioma
2. Haemangiopericytoma

C. Malignant

1. Angiosarcoma

VI. Other connective tissue tumours

A. Benign

1. Desmoplastic fibroma
2. Lipoma

B. Malignant

1. Fibrosarcoma
2. Liposarcoma
3. Malignant mesenchymoma
4. Undifferentiated sarcoma

VII. Other tumours

1. Chordoma
2. Adamantinoma
3. Neurilemmoma
4. Neurofibroma

VIII. Unclassified tumours

IX. Tumour like lesions

1. Solitary bone cyst
2. Aneurysmal bone cyst
3. Juxta-articular bone cyst
4. Metaphyseal fibrous defect
5. Eosinophilic granuloma
6. Fibrous dysplasia
7. Myositis ossificans
8. 'Brown tumour' of hyperparathyroidism

Primary bone tumours account for only 2% of total body tumours, 98% of all tumours metastasize in the bone.

Q4. Write in brief about the TNM classification of tumour.

AJCC *(American Joint Committee on Cancer)* system is based on the *four-part TNMG designation*:

- *T: Extent of tumour*
- *N: Nodal status*
- *M: Distant metastasis*
- *G: Grade*

Primary Tumour (T)

Tumour Extent	Definition
TX	Primary tumour cannot be assessed
T0	No evidence of primary tumour
T1	Tumour (maximum dimension) 8 cm at time of diagnosis
T2	Tumour (maximum dimension) >8 cm at time of diagnosis
T3	Skip metastasis—two discontinuous tumours in the same bone with no other distant metastases

Regional lymph nodes (N)

Nodal status	Definition
NX	Regional lymph node cannot be assessed
N0	No regional lymph node metastasis
N1	Regional lymph node metastasis to be considered equivalent to distant metastatic disease

Distant metastasis (M)

Metastasis	Definition
MX	Distant metastasis cannot be assessed
M0	No distant metastasis
M1	Distant metastasis
M1a	Lungs-only metastases
M1b	All other distant metastases including lymph nodes

Grade: *It represents the histologic grade of a lesion.*

In the most commonly used three-tiered classification:

- Grade I: low grade
- Grade 2 and 3: High grade

In less commonly used four-tiered classification:

- Grade 1, 2: low grade
- Grade 3, 4: high grade

Stage Grouping:

Stage	Grade	Tumour	Node	Metastasis
IA	G1,2	T1	N0	M0
IB	G1,2	T2	N0	M0
IIA	G3,4	T1	N0	M0
IIB	G3,4	T2	N0	M0
III	Any G	T3	N0	M0
IVA	Any G	Any T	Any N	M1a
IVB	Any G	Any T	N0/N1	M1b

Q5. How will you investigate a case of tumour?

General Approach to Musculoskeletal Neoplasms

History

- An adequate history and physical examination are the first and most important steps in evaluating a patient with a musculoskeletal tumour.
- Patients may present to the orthopaedic oncologist with
- **Pain**, patients with bone tumours most frequently present with pain.
- The pain initially may be activity related, but the patient with a malignancy of bone often complains of progressive pain at rest and at night.
- Other benign lesions, most notably osteoid osteoma, may initially cause night pain.
- **Swelling**
- **Pathological fracture**
- **Abnormal radiographic** finding detected during the evaluation of an unrelated problem.

Investigations

Non-invasive

Blood and Urine Tests

- If serum albumin <3.5 g/dl or total lymphocyte count <1500/ml then there is increased risk of wound-healing problems and infection
- A complete blood count may be helpful to rule out infection and leukemia.
- ESR usually is elevated in infection, metastatic carcinoma, and small "blue cell" tumours such as Ewing's sarcoma, lymphoma, histiocytosis, and leukemia.
- A *serum protein electrophoresis* should be ordered if multiple myeloma is part of the differential diagnosis.
- A *prostate-specific antigen (PSA)* should be ordered if prostate carcinoma is a possibility.
- *Hypercalcemia* may be present with metastatic disease, multiple myeloma, and hyperparathyroidism.

- *Alkaline phosphatase* may be elevated in metabolic bone disease, metastatic disease, osteosarcoma, Ewing's sarcoma, or lymphoma.
- *Blood urea nitrogen (BUN)* and *creatinine* may be elevated with renal tumours, and a urinalysis may reveal haematuria in this setting.
- Evaluation of *Serum calcium* and *parathyroid hormone* levels helps in differentiating Brown tumours of hyperparathyroidism from giant cell tumours.
- *Serum alkaline phosphatase* and *urinary pyridinium* cross-links helps in evaluation of Paget's disease.

Plain Roentgenograms

Compared with any other test, conventional roentgenography provides useful information. Often, the patient's age and plain roentgenographic findings are sufficient to arrive at a specific diagnosis.

- An *epiphyseal lesion* in a skeletally mature patient is likely to be a giant cell tumour, whereas an epiphyseal lesion in a skeletally immature patient is likely to be a chondroblastoma.
- *Diaphyseal lesions* include Ewing's sarcoma, lymphoma, histiocytosis, fibrous dysplasia, and Adamantinoma (especially in the tibia).
- Most vertebral lesions in adult patients are metastases, myelomas, or hemangioma.
- In the sacrum, chordoma is at the top of the list of differential diagnoses.
- In younger patients with a vertebral body lesion, the most likely diagnosis is histiocytosis; if the lesion is in the posterior elements, the differential diagnoses include *aneurysmal bone cyst, osteoblastoma, and osteoid osteoma.*
- Inactive lesions usually are well marginated, often with a surrounding rim of reactive bone formation.
- Aggressive lesions usually have a less well-defined zone of transition between the lesion and the host bone.
- Cortical expansion can be seen with aggressive benign lesions, but if there is frank cortical destruction then it is a sign of malignancy.
- Periosteal reactive new bone formation results when the tumour destroys cortex and may take the form of a Codman's triangle, "onion-skinning," or a "sunburst" pattern. It usually is a sign of malignancy but may be present with infection or histiocytosis.

Chest Radiograph

To search for evidence of metastatic disease or a primary focus from which a metastasis may have arisen.

Computed tomography (CT)

- It is most helpful in assessing *ossification and calcification* and in evaluating the integrity of the cortex.
- It also is the best imaging study:
    - To localize the nidus of an osteoid osteoma
    - To detect a thin rim of reactive bone around an aneurysmal bone cyst,
    - To evaluate calcification in a suspected cartilaginous lesion
    - To evaluate endosteal cortical erosion in a suspected chondrosarcoma.
    - *CT of the lungs* also is the most effective study *to detect pulmonary metastases.*

Technetium Bone Scans

These are indicated:

- To detect skeletal metastases
- To determine the presence of multiple lesions in such entities as osteochondroma, enchondroma, fibrous dysplasia, and histiocytosis.
- Bone scans frequently are falsely negative in multiple myeloma.
- With the exception of myeloma, however, virtually all malignant neoplasms of bone demonstrate increased uptake on technetium bone scans.
- Gallium scans are the most sensitive tests for locating nonpulmonary metastases.

Angiography

- Angiography previously was used to determine the relationship of a neoplasm to the vessels, has been supplanted by MRI.
- In centres where CT and MRI facilities are not available, the angiography plays an important role in management by:
  - Delineating the soft tissue extent
  - Involvement of the adjacent important structures
  - Demonstrating the tumour vascular anatomy
  - Indicating the best site for taking the biopsy
  - Discloses the abnormal vessels and displaced vessels
- To rule out non-neoplastic conditions such as:
  - Pseudoaneurysms or arteriovenous malformations
  - For preoperative embolization of highly vascular lesions, such as renal cell carcinoma and aneurysmal bone cysts.

Magnetic Resonance Imaging (MRI)

- It is the best study of choice to determine the size, extent, and anatomical relationships of both bone and soft tissue tumours.
- It is the most accurate technique for determining the limits or extent of disease both within and outside bone.
- MRI may yield a specific diagnosis with tumours such as lipoma, haemangioma, haematomas, or pigmented villonodular synovitis, all of which have very characteristic appearances.

Ultrasonography

It is useful for distinguishing cystic from solid soft tissue lesions.

Invasive

Biopsy

- It should be planned as carefully as the definitive procedure.
- *Biopsy should be planned only after noninvasive evaluations (clinical, laboratory, and roentgenographic examinations) are complete.*
- A biopsy can be done by:
  - *Fine needle aspiration (FNAC)*:
    - Fine needle aspiration yields 90% of accurate result at determining malignancy.

- Disadvantage:
    - Specificity is less
    - The absence of malignant cells on FNAC is less reassuring than a negative incisional biopsy.
  - *Core needle biopsy:*
    - Core needle biopsy can provide an accurate diagnosis in up to 90% of cases.
    - Disadvantage: The limited amount of tissue obtained may not be adequate for accurate grading or for any additional studies that may decide subsequent treatment.
  - *Open incisional procedure:*
    - Specific less chances of sampling error
    - It provides the most tissue for additional diagnostic studies such as cytogenetics and flow cytometry.
    - Disadvantage:
        - Complications are greater with incisional biopsy,

Differential Diagnosis of Lesion Based on Location

Differential diagnosis for epiphyseal lesions:
- Chondroblastoma (age 10–25)
- Giant cell tumour (age 20–40)
- Clear cell chondrosarcoma (rare)

Differential diagnosis for epiphyseal lesions:
- Ewing sarcoma (age 5–25)
- Lymphoma (adult)
- Fibrous dysplasia (age 5–30)
- Adamantinoma (consider in the tibia)
- Histiocytosis (age 5–30)

Differential diagnosis for lesions of the spine:
- *Older than 40 years:*
    - Metastases
    - Multiple myeloma
    - Haemangioma
    - Chordoma (in sacrum)
- *Younger than 30 years:*
    - Vertebral Body
    - Histiocytosis
    - Haemangioma
- *Posterior elements:*
    - Osteoid osteoma
    - Osteoblastoma
    - Aneurysmal bone cyst
- *Differential diagnosis for multiple lesions:*
    - Histiocytosis
    - Enchondroma
    - Osteochondroma
    - Fibrous dysplasia

– Multiple myeloma
– Metastases
– Haemangioma
– Infection
– Hyperparathyroidism

If there is metastases of unknown origin then:

- In patient >40 years, painful bone lesion suggests multiple myeloma and metastatic carcinoma
- Most common primary sources for bone metastases: Prostate cancer and breast cancer
- If a patient has no known primary tumour, then the most likely sources are lung cancer and renal cell carcinoma for bone metastases.
- History of any previous malignancies, past or remote.
- Physical examination includes not only the involved extremity, but also the lungs, thyroid, abdomen, prostate in men, and breasts in women
- Laboratory analysis should include:
  - Complete blood count
  - Erythrocyte sedimentation rate
  - Electrolytes
  - Liver enzymes
  - Alkaline phosphatase
  - Serum protein electrophoresis
  - Prostate-specific antigen
- Plain radiographs of the involved bone and the chest should be obtained.
- A whole body bone scan should be obtained to evaluate other possible areas of skeletal involvement, and a CT scan of the chest, abdomen, and pelvis should be obtained for further evaluation.

Q6. What is Lodwick's classification of patterns of bone destruction?

Bone destruction is usually the first radiographic sign of disease and sometimes the only evidence of progressive pathology. Analysis of the transition zone between the host and tumour bone is a good indicator of the growth rate in the lesion. The rapid the growth, the more *"aggressive"* the pattern of destruction and wider the transition zone between the host and tumour bone.

The American radiologist, *Gwilym Lodwick*, described *three patterns of bone destruction* associated with tumour and tumour-like lesions.

Type I: Geographic Bone Destruction

- Large solitary or occasionally multiple large osteolytic defects occur within bone.
- Least aggressive pattern of bone destruction.
- Slow growing lesion (indolent growth).
- Lesion will appear well marginated with a thin zone of transition between the normal and tumour bone.

Subdivision: It may be further subdivided into IA, IB and IC based on the appearance of the margin and the effect on the cortex.

Type IA

- Slowest growing
- Least aggressive
- Typified by a sclerotic margin.
- Majority are benign, e.g. *Enchondroma, non-ossifying bone fibroma, osteoid osteoma.*

Type IB

- Lesion is well demarcated (ragged and irregular) and without the sclerotic margin.
- Growth is relatively low than type IA lesion.
- Majority are benign however, some malignancies show this pattern, e.g. *giant cell tumour, chondroblastoma, juvenile bone cyst, osteoblastoma, chondromyxoid fibroma, aneurysmal bone cyst.*

Type IC

- Poorly defined margins.
- More aggressive pattern.
- Few benign lesions exhibit a type IC pattern, e.g. *Chondrosarcoma, Aneurysmal bone cyst.*

Type II: Moth Eaten

- Multiple small holes of lysis of varying size, ranging from 2 to 5 mm in diameter are noted.
- This type of pattern is usually appreciated in both the cortical and cancellous bone.
- Increasingly aggressive nature of the lesions.
- Poorly defined or demarcated lesion margin.
- Longer zone of transition from host to tumour bone.
- Destruction typically begins on the endosteal surface and erodes outward to produce cortical destruction, e.g. *malignant bone tumours and osteomyelitis shows moth eaten pattern of bone destruction.*

Type III: Permeative Pattern

- Countless numbers of extremely small diameter (≤ 1 mm) oval to elongated linear holes of destructions displays "streak like "character.
- Best visualized in cortical bone.
- Most aggressive osseous destructive pattern with rapid growth potential.
- Poorly defined margins and are without sclerosis.
- Its true dimensions are larger than that evident on the skiagram.
- Zone of transition is very long, e.g. *Ewing sarcoma, osteosarcoma.*

Q7. Write in brief about the periosteal response to adjacent tumour.

Tumours can produce widely differing *periosteal reaction* in a pathologic process that involves the formation of new bone.

Once the periosteum has been stimulated to produce new bone by some stimulus, a lag occurs in the time it takes for the appearance of mineralization of the radiograph. It can take about 10–21 days after the initiating stimulus for periosteal mineralization even with vigorous periosteal activity.

The rate of mineralization varies with the age, the younger the patient, the more rapid the appearance of the radiographic change, and *vise versa*.

The appearance of periosteal reaction in a diseased process is variable; it is rarely associated with tumours such as *fibrosarcoma* and *chondrosarcoma*, whereas it is typically present with *osteosarcoma, Ewing's sarcoma* and *solitary metastasis*.

Ragsdale et al. divided the periosteal reactions into three categories: *Continuous, interrupted and complex.*

Periosteum	Cortical bone	Appearance	Typical lesions
Continuous	Intact	Solid	Chronic osteomyelitis, Langerhans cell histiocytosis, osteoid osteoma
		Single lamellae	Chronic osteomyelitis, Langerhans cell histiocytosis
		Onion skin, spicule (radial)	Acute osteomyelitis, Ewing's sarcoma
	Destroyed	Single bowl	Aneurysmal bone cyst, enchondroma, chondroblastoma
		Lobulated bowl	Chondromyxoid fibroma, fibrous dysplasia, giant cell tumour
		Ragged bowl	Chondrosarcoma, plasmacytoma, metastases
Interrupted or discontinuous	Intact	Wedge-shaped	Aneurysmal bone cyst, giant cell tumour, chondromyxoid fibroma
		Codman triangle, interrupted onion skin radial	Aneurysmal bone cyst, osteosarcoma, Ewing's sarcoma, chondrosarcoma
Complex or combined	Destroyed	Combination of Codman triangle, interrupted onion skin, divergent rays	Osteosarcoma

Combined or Complex Periosteal Reaction

- More than one pattern of reaction may be manifest in the same case reflecting the varying rate of growth rate at different sites in same lesion.
- The divergent spiculated periosteal reaction also known as *"sun-ray"* or *"sun-burst"* appearance is a typical example of a complex pattern and is suggestive of osteosarcoma.

Q8. What is Enneking's staging of benign tumours.

Stages of Benign Tumour

Stage	Features
Latent	Well defines margins
	Grows slowly and then stop
	Remain static
	Heals spontaneously, e.g. osteoid osteoma
Active	Progressive growth limited by natural barriers
	Not self limiting, show a tendency to recur, e.g. aneurysmal bone cyst
Aggressive	Growth which is not limited by natural barriers, e.g. giant cell tumour

Q9. What is Mirel's scoring system of prophylactic internal fixation of bones in cases of metastatic disease and What are Bauer's criteria for assessing prognosis?

For evaluation of *fracture risk,* and need for *prophylactic internal fixation in a metastatic bone disease Mirel* devised a scoring system. It act as a guide as to whether the pathological fracture due to metastatic disease should be fixed or not.

Mirels combined four different features of bone lesions in an attempt to create a more reliable risk assessment.

Score	*1*	*2*	*3*
Site	Upper limb	Lower limb	Peritrochanteric
Size (as seen on X-ray, maximum destruction of cortex in any view)	<1/3	1/3–2/3	>2/3
Lesion	Blastic	Mixed	Lytic
Pain	Mild	Moderate	Functional

A *score of ≥8* indicates high risk and a need for internal fixation to be carried out prior to radiotherapy. *Maximum possible score is 12.*

Bauer's has suggested useful criteria for assessing prognosis. In his series of patients, he found survivorship at 1 year as follows:

- Of patients with 4 or 5 of Bauer's criteria 50% were alive.
- Of patients with 2 or 3 of Bauer's criteria 25% were alive.
- Of patients with only 1 or none of the Bauer's criteria, the majority survived for < 6 month and none were alive at 1 year.

Bauer's Five Positive Criteria for Survival

- No pathological fracture
- No visceral metastases
- A solitary skeletal metastases
- Primary tumour breast, kidney, lymphoma or myeloma.
- No primary lung cancer

Q10. Discuss the principles for biopsy of musculoskeletal tumours.

Biopsy is a key step in the diagnosis of a musculoskeletal tumour. It should be planned as carefully as the definitive procedure. Biopsy should be done only after clinical, laboratory, and Roentgenographic examinations are complete.

Principles for Biopsy

- Incision in-line with resection incision.
- Longitudinal incision in extremities.
- Transverse incisions should be avoided since they are extremely difficult or impossible to excise with the specimen and also they require a wider soft-tissue resection at the time of definitive surgery.
- Intramuscular (to bury haematoma).
- No skin or muscle flaps.
- The deep incision should go through a single muscle compartment rather than through an intermuscular plane.
- Avoid neurovascular structures and joints.
- Approach through soft tissue mass or weakened area of bone.
- Biopsy should be taken from the periphery of the lesion, which contains the most viable tissue.

- Exploring with the finger should be avoided.
- Biopsy track must be excised en bloc with the tumour.
- A frozen section should be sent intraoperatively to ensure the presence of representative tumour material in the specimen.
- Meticulous haemostasis.
- Tight closure.
- Drains should not be used routinely. If a drain is used, it should exit in line with the incision so that the drain track can also be excised en bloc with the tumour.
- The biopsy should be done by the surgeon who ultimately will be responsible for the definitive surgical treatment of the patient.

Q11. What are common benign bone-forming tumours? Discuss osteoid osteoma in brief.

Common benign bone-forming tumours include an *osteoma, osteoid osteoma* and *osteoblastoma*.

Osteoid Osteoma

Introduction

- It is a benign tumour.
- It consists of well-defined osteoblastic mass called nidus, surrounded by distinct zone of sclerosis (reactive bone).
- Zone of sclerosis represents a secondary reversible change that gradually weans off after removal of the nidus.
- Nidus is usually less than 1 cm in diameter.

Incidence

It accounts 10–20% of all benign bone lesions.

Age

- It occurs in teenagers and young adult; more than 80% of patients are between 5 and 25 years.
- Peak incidence: 2nd decade of life.
- Male: Female: 3:1 (2.2:1)

Site

- 50% occur in long bones of lower extremity.
- Femoral neck is the single most frequent anatomic site.
- Less frequent in bones of upper extremity, if it occurs then elbow is the most frequent site.
- Often present in small bones of hands and feet.
- Rare in axial skeleton, but if present are usually found in lumber region of spine.
- In vertebrae occurs exclusively in the posterior arch; rare in vertebral body.
- Very rare in flat bones and almost never occur in craniofacial bones.

Clinical Features

Most diagnostic symptoms:
- Pain of increasing severity that is relieved by *aspirin* and *other NSAIDs.*
- Occurs in more than 80% of cases.
- Pain is frequently worse at night and sometimes referred to the adjacent joints (usually non-radiating).

Cause of Pain

- *Old theory:* presence of nerves within the nidus *(evidenced by axonal silver stain and electron microscopy).*
- *Recent theory:* High levels of *prostaglandins* E_2 and *prostacyclins* released from the nidus that is responsible for pain, reactive sclerosis, and nonspecific inflammatory changes of soft tissue.

Other symptoms: Depend upon the location of tumour.

Location of tumour	*Symptoms*
Proximity of joint	Symptoms of arthritis (painful movements)
Involved bone is superficial especially in small hands and feet	Painful swelling of the adjacent soft tissue
Vertebral involvement	Painful scoliosis (due to unilateral muscle spasm)
Young patient with open growth plate	Significant limb-length discrepancy
Neglected cases	Severe dysfunction of the extremity, muscle atrophy

Radiological Features

- Reliable, characteristic and diagnostic tool.
- Well-demarcated lytic lesion (nidus) surrounded by a distinct zone of sclerosis.
- Edge of the nidus is always smooth; irregular is suggestive of infection.
- In cases of vertebral location: increased density of the pedicle, loss of distinct contour. When nidus is not visible on conventional radiographs, additional imaging techniques such as CT, radioisotope scanning, and MRI may be necessary. Radionuclide scanning shows intense uptake, which is useful for localization at surgery using a hand, held detector.

Biopsy

It is necessary for confirmation.

Pathology

Gross

- Well circumscribed, oval or round, reddish area (due to high vascularity and minimal bony tissue).
- Variable in consistency (friable, soft and granular to sclerotic).
- Surrounded by zone of sclerosis.

   Preoperative tetracycline labelling *(using tetracycline at a dosage of 4 mg/kg, four times daily, 2 days preoperatively, the nidus will have a golden yellow fluorescence)* or intraoperative scintillation probes after the administration of a radioisotope may be used to confirm identification.

Histology

- Nidus consists of an interlacing network of thin and uniformly distributed bone trabeculae that are variably mineralized.
- Osteoblasts rim the osteoid trabeculae and accompanied by numerous osteoclast like multinucleated giant cell.
- Central portion is heavily ossified, less cellular than the peripheral zone.
- Intertrabecular tissue is vascular.
- As a rule, cartilage is not an integral component of the nidus.
- Prominent large vessel may be present in the stromal tissue surrounding the nidus.
- Adjacent synovium may be thickened with chronic inflammatory cell infiltrate (that have lymphofollicular features).

Differential Diagnosis

- Osteoblastoma (indistinguishable; arbitrarily, a lesion that is smaller than 1.5 cm is considered as osteoid osteoma and that >1.5 cm is osteoblastoma).
- Chronic and acute osteomyelitis
- Bone abscess
- Brodie's abscess
- Intracortical haemangioma
- Bone islands (enostosis)
- Stress fracture
- Ewing's sarcoma
- Intracortical osteosarcoma
- Intracortical metastases from carcinoma especially from lung.

Treatment

- Pain may be relieved by *aspirin or other NSAIDs.*
- *En-bloc excision* after precise localization is the preferred treatment.
- *Curettage and bone grafting* is planned where en-bloc excision is not possible. This procedure has risk of recurrence (4.5%) due to incomplete removal.
- Alternative approach: *Percutaneous ablation by radiofrequency* especially for inaccessible site.
- Recent report: *Prolonged anti-inflammatory treatment* (30–40 mn) can induce permanent relief of symptoms and regression of the nidus may be seen on radiographs.

Q12. Discuss osteoblastoma and how can you distinguish it from osteoid osteoma.

Osteoblastoma is an uncommon benign progressively growing osteoid tissue-forming primary neoplasm of the bone.

It has clinical and histologic features similar to those of osteoid osteoma; therefore, *Dahlin and Johnson* consider the two tumours to be variants of the same disease with osteoblastoma representing a *giant osteoid osteoma.*

The problem of similarity of osteoblastoma to osteoid osteoma has been resolved by arbitrarily designating all lesions as osteoblastoma when the nidus is >1.5 cm in diameter.

Benign osteoblastoma has become the most widely accepted designation for the tumour and it was proposed Jaffes.

Incidence

It is Less than 1% of all primary bone tumours and around 3.5% of all benign tumours of bone.

Age

- Most patients are in between 5 and 45 years.
- The younger age group was predominantly affected and >90% of the patient are in first three decade of life.
- Peak incidence: 2nd decade of life.
- M:F:1.9:1 (male preponderance)

Sites

- The lesion shows a distinct predilection for axial skeleton in general and the *vertebral column* in particular (mostly the *posterior elements* including the arch and spinous process).
- Approximately 30–40% are localized in the spine and sacrum.
- Jaw-bone (cementoblastoma 29%) followed by craniofacial bones (14%) is the second most frequent site.
- Remaining, distributed throughout the appendicular skeleton with predilection for the *femur (lower extremity) and humerus (upper extremity)*.
- Occasionally in talus (dorsal aspects of the anterior portion).
- Rarely in ribs and flat bones.

Clinical Features

- These are not as characteristic as that of osteoid osteoma.
- Patient presents with dull, localized pain often progressive of several months' duration. In contrast to the pain associated with osteoid osteoma, the pain of osteoblastoma is *less intense, usually not worsening at night, and not relieved readily with aspirin and other NSAIDS*.
- Local swelling, tenderness, warmth, and gait disturbances.
- If the lesion is superficial, the patient may have localized *swelling and tenderness*.
- Spinal lesions can cause *painful scoliosis* (less common than osteoid osteoma).
- Sometimes lesions may mechanically interfere with the spinal cord or nerve roots, producing *neurologic deficits (ranging from muscle weakness to paraplegia) or radiculopathy*.
- Extremity lesions may present with limp and muscular wasting.
- Very rarely osteoblastoma may be associated with *osteomalacia*.

Radiological Features

Following radiographic patterns are usually encountered:

1. Well-circumscribed lytic lesion surrounded by the zone of reactive sclerosis (lesion is >1.5 cm in diameter) (most common pattern).
2. The second, an expansile lesion with multiple small calcifications and a peripheral sclerotic rim is the most common appearance of spinal osteoblastoma.
3. Third pattern has aggressive appearance, consisting of bone expansion (usually eccentric), osseous destruction, infiltration of the surrounding soft tissue and intermixed matrix calcification.

   In 20% of cases, the cortex is thinned out, focally destroyed with or without new bone formation (mimicking malignancy).

Bone Scintigraphy

It demonstrates marked radionuclide uptake (hot area).

CT Scan

- It is particularly useful for spinal lesions, which may be difficult to assess on routine skiagram.
- Lesions shows areas of mineralization, expansile remodelling of bone, sclerosis or thin osseous rim about its margin.
- It is valuable for determining the extent of the lesion and also to interpret the degree of intra-lesional bone formation has occurred.

Biopsy

It is necessary for confirmation.

Pathology

Gross

- It is same as that of osteoid osteoma.
- The tumour is Reddish brown, haemorrhagic, gritty, friable and granular neoplasm.
- There may be evidence of haemorrhages and cystic degeneration with blood filled space characterization of secondary aneurysmal bone cyst (ABC).

Histology

- Anastomosing bony trabeculae are rimmed with a single layer of osteoblasts.
- Intertrabecular spaces are loosely arranged, and occasionally contain spindle cell and capillaries.
- Osteoid trabeculae merge gradually with the adjacent normal bone.
- Varying degree of mineralization of osteoid can be seen.
- Secondary ABC like changes may be seen.

Differential Diagnosis

- Osteoid osteoma
- Osteosarcoma
- Bone abscess (Brodie's abscess)
- Aneurysmal bone cyst
- Giant cell tumour

Treatment

- Preferred treatment: *en-bloc excision and bone grafting*.
- In the posterior elements of the spine is usually inaccessible for complete excision and recurrence (10%) may be as high as 25% after surgery.
- Neurological deficit resulting from intraspinal compressions requires decompression laminectomy.
- Rapidly growing or recurrent lesions may be controlled with *radiotherapy*. However, it may be ineffective and may be associated with complications like *malignant transformation, spinal cord necrosis,* and *aggravation of spinal cord compression*.

- Recent studies shows that *chemotherapy* including *high dose methotrexate* and *doxorubicin* slow down the growth of aggressive osteoblastoma that are inaccessible to surgical removal.

Prognosis

- With complete surgical removal, prognosis is excellent with a low rate of recurrence.
- Malignant transformation of osteoblastomas is considered rare.

Clinical differentiation: Osteoid osteoma and osteoblastoma

Features	Osteoid osteoma	Osteoblastoma
Age	87% ≤30 years	91% ≤30 years
Incidence	Relatively common	Rare
Sex ratio	2.2:1	1.9:1
Duration until diagnosis	≤11.3 months (average)	≤12.3 (average)
Pain	Moderate/marked Nocturnal worsening Relieved by aspirin and other NSAIDs	Mild, dull localized pain. Poor response to aspirin or other NSAIDs
Location	Femur and tibia	Spine (usually posterior elements; rarely body)
Size of lesion	<1 cm	>1.5–2 cm (range 1.0–15 cm; average 3.6 cm)
X-ray findings	Typical appearance Lytic (nidus) is surrounded by sclerosis	Variable appearance Reactive peripheral sclerosis may be minimal or absent Erosive, expansile
Clinical course	Static (spontaneous regression) Limited growth if any	Higher growth potential No regression reported
Recurrence	4.5%	>10%

Q13. Describe the clinical features, histopathological and radiological features of Osteosarcoma.

Osteosarcoma is the most common primary malignant bone tumour. This disease is thought to arise from primitive mesenchymal osteoblastic cells, and its histologic hallmark is the production of neoplastic osteoid.

Incidence

Age

- The incidence increases steadily with age, increasing more dramatically in adolescence, corresponding with the adolescent growth spurt.
- Bimodal age distribution.
- Common in second decade (10–20 years).
- >75% of cases seen are <25 years.
- ~10% arises in patients > 60 years.

Sex

- Male preponderance (1.6:1)
- Girls develop tumour at an early age

Location

Metaphyseal region.

Site

The most common sites are the:
- Femur (42%, 75% of which are in the distal femur)
- Tibia (19%, 80% of which are in the proximal tibia)
- Humerus (10%, 90% of which are in the proximal humerus)

Other significant locations are the:
- Skull and jaw (8%)
- Pelvis (8%)

Risk Factors

- Rapid bone growth
- Environmental factors:
    - Exposure to radiation (>2000 rads)
    - Exposure to chemicals (20 methylcholanthrene, beryllium compounds)
- Genetic predisposition:
    - Bone dysplasias, including Paget's disease, fibrous dysplasia, enchondromatosis, and hereditary multiple exostoses and retinoblastoma (germ-line form) are risk factors.
    - Mutation of the RB gene (germline retinoblastoma) and radiation therapy is associated with a high risk of developing osteosarcoma
    - Li-Fraumeni syndrome (germline p53 mutation)
    - Rothmund-Thomson syndrome (autosomal recessive association of *congenital bone defects, hair and skin dysplasias, hypogonadism, and cataracts*).
- Virus: (these viruses known to produce tumour in animals)
    - DNA virus: Polyoma and SV 40
    - RNA virus: Harvey and Moloney mouse sarcoma virus

Classification/Subtypes of Osteosarcoma

Based on:
- Predominant histologic pattern
- Anatomic location
- Sometimes by its histologic grade

Osteosarcoma Types by Predominant Histological Pattern and Grading

Central:
- High-grade
    - Conventional (most common)
    - Telangiectatic
    - Small cell
    - Epithelioid
    - Osteoblastoma-like
    - Chondroblastoma-like
    - Fibrohistiocytic
    - Giant cell–rich

- Low-grade:
  - Low-grade central
  - Fibrous dysplasia–like
  - Desmoplastic fibroma–like

Surface

- Low-grade
  - Parosteal
- Intermediate-grade
  - Periosteal
- High-grade
  - Dedifferentiated parosteal
  - High-grade surface

Intracortical

Gnathic

Extraskeletal:

- High-grade
- Low-grade

Osteosarcoma by Anatomic Site:

Osseous:

- Central
- Surface
- Gnathic
- Multifocal

Soft tissue:

- Intramuscular
- Other

Prognostic Classification (Dahlin's)

- Osteoblastic: Poor 5-years survival rate
- Fibroblastic: 5-years survival rate 2 times more than osteoblastic type
- Chondroblast: 5-years survival rate 3 times more than osteoblastic type

Best Accepted Classification

Primary or Idiopathic

- Conventional
- Telangiectatic
- Small cell
- Fibrohistocytic
- Low-grade intramedullary
- Multicentric

Secondary

- Paget's disease
- Radiation
- Associated conditions (multiple hereditary exostosis, polyostotic fibrous dysplasia, multiple osteochondroma, diaphyseal aclasia)

Juxtacortical

- Parosteal
- Periosteal
- High-grade surface
- Dedifferentiated parosteal

Clinical Features

- Pain (most common), particularly pain with activity
- History of trauma (often)
- Limp
- Swelling at first minimal but become prominent in due course. It is usually has Fusiform eccentric configuration and variegated consistency (varies from soft to hard).
- Skin over the swelling: Stretched, shiny, warm and with dilated vein.
- Systemic symptoms, such as fever and night sweats, are rare.
- Pathologic fractures (most common with telangiectatic type)
- Respiratory symptoms and signs: Usually indicates extensive lung involvement (most common site of metastasis is lung)
- Decreased range of motion of adjacent joints
- Lymphadenopathy (local or regional)
- Examination of distal neurovascular status

Investigations

Laboratory Findings

Important laboratory studies include the following:
- LDH
- ALP (prognostic significance): It is consistently elevated as the lesion is composed of neoplastic osteoblasts. Patients with an elevated ALP at diagnosis are more likely to have pulmonary metastases
- Blood tests with prognostic significance are lactic dehydrogenase (LDH) and alkaline phosphatase (ALP).
- Complete blood cell (CBC) count, including differential
- Platelet count
- Liver function tests: Aspartate aminotransferase (AST), alanine aminotransferase (ALT), bilirubin, and albumin
- Electrolyte levels: Sodium, potassium, chloride, bicarbonate, calcium, magnesium, phosphorus
- Renal function tests: Blood urea nitrogen (BUN), creatinine
- Urinalysis

Imaging

X-rays

- Plain radiography (AP and lateral view) of the involved bone, including the joint above and the joint below the affected region and of chest (to rule out pulmonary metastasis)
- Feature are those of an aggressive, permeative, destructive lesion having osteoblastic activity
- >90% case the lesion is in metaphyseal region with encroachment on diaphysis.
- Lesions can be purely osteolytic (~30% of cases), purely osteoblastic (~ 45% of cases), or a mixture of both.
- Telangiectatic variety is often very cystic and can be mistaken for an aneurysmal bone cyst.
- Soft tissue mass.

Characteristic Features

Codman's Triangle

- Near the junction of the healthy bone with the tumour, there is a reactive new bone formation beneath the periosteum.
- At the edge of the tumour, this layer of new bone ends abruptly and gives a characteristic appearance
- Not specific; can be seen in Ewing's sarcoma, osteomyelitis, haemophilic Pseudotumour etc

Sunburst appearance (approximately 60% of cases):
- Usually seen along the Codman's triangle
- Spicules of tumourous bone are perpendicular to the long axis of bone, along with blood vessels elevated by periosteum

Longitudinal Laminations

Periosteal laminations follow the course of intramedullary lesion.

CT Scan

- CT scan of the primary lesion and of the chest
- Helps in:
    - Delineating the location and extent of the tumour
    - Identify accurately area of cortical break through
    - Soft tissue extension
    - Medullary spread
    - In long bones to identify, skip lesions
    - Preoperative planning especially for reconstructive surgery
- CT scanning of the chest is more sensitive than is plain film radiography for assessing pulmonary metastases.

MRI

- Method of choice to assess the extent of intramedullary disease as well as associated soft-tissue masses and skip lesions.
- Helps study for accurate surgical staging of the lesion with use of the Enneking staging system.

Radionuclide bone scanning with ^{99m}Tc): Methylene diphosphonate (MDP/MDI): It is important to evaluate for the presence of metastatic or multifocal disease Soft tissue extension.

Angiography

Accurate method of detecting and measuring the extent of occult.

Biopsy

Gross

- Metaphyseal region
- Large tumour with destruction of inner cortex.
- Consistency is variable from soft, fluctuant to firm to bony hard.
- Variegated—bluish white (cartilaginous), white (fibrous) or yellowish white (osteoblastic)
- Necrotic foci, cavitation and hemorrhage at the site of rapid growth
- The bone end is expanded and a resected bone sarcoma specimen's looks like the *"Leg of mutton appearance"*

Histopathological Findings

- The characteristic feature of osteosarcoma is the *presence of osteoid* in the lesion and sarcomatous stroma.
- Stromal cells may be spindle-shaped and atypical, with irregularly shaped nuclei.
- Stromal cells are large resembling osteoblast and exhibits malignant behaviours shown by: anisocystosis, poikilocytosis, nuclear pyknosis, pleomorphism and frequent mitotic figures.
- Conventional osteosarcoma based on the predominant features of the cells can be osteoblastic, chondroblastic, or fibroblastic.
- Telangiectatic type contains large, blood-filled spaces.

Depending on the predominant type of extracellular matrix, conventional osteosarcoma can be:
- Osteoblastic
- Chondroblastic
- Fibroblastic subtypes
- Telangiectatic osteosarcoma
- Small cell osteosarcoma

Staging

The key components to the staging system are the:
- Histologic grade of the tumour (low grade vs. high grade)
- Anatomic location of the tumour (intracompartmental vs. extracompartmental)
- Absence or presence of metastatic disease

The staging system is typically depicted as follows:
- Low-grade tumour, intracompartmental: IA
- Low-grade tumour, extracompartmental: IB
- High-grade tumour, intracompartmental: IIA
- High-grade tumour, extracompartmental: IIB
- Any tumour with evidence of metastasis: III

Q14. Discuss the management of osteosarcoma.

Osteosarcoma is the most common primary malignant tumour of bone, excluding plasma cell myeloma. The high recurrence rate indicates that most patients have micrometastatic disease at the time of diagnosis. Therefore, the use of adjuvant systemic chemotherapy is critical for the treatment of patients with osteosarcoma.

It is treated by a combination of *surgical excision and chemotherapy*. Combination of radical ablation, radiotherapy, chemotherapy and resection of pulmonary lesion vastly improved the prognosis.

General Principles

- Early radical ablation of primary tumour and/or reconstructive surgery
- Prevention of metastasis or control (if it already occurred) by neoadjuvant therapy (irradiation, chemotherapy or both).
- Resection of large pulmonary met.

General Treatment Recommendation

Stages IA–IB (Low Grade)

Primary treatment for patients with low-grade osteogenic sarcoma includes wide excision, with chemotherapy prior to excision; postoperative chemotherapy is also recommended [1, 2].

Stages IIA–IIB (High Grade)

- Chemotherapy is warranted for all stages of high-grade osteogenic sarcomas
- For non-metastatic osteosarcoma, 2–3 cycles of chemotherapy are typically given preoperatively; 3–4 cycles of chemotherapy are given postoperatively.

Role of Chemotherapy

- Chemotherapy is usually employed in the neoadjuvant or adjuvant situation.
- Improved survival is seen in patients who show a complete response to neoadjuvant chemotherapy.

Benefits of neoadjuvant therapy:
- Eliminates micro- or macrometastasis
- Necrosis of tumour
- Reduce tumour size/bulk and neovascularity
- Widens tumour-free surgical margins
- Facilitates placement of custom made prosthesis
- Prevent local recurrence

Effective Agent

Four major standard single agents are:
- Cisplatin
- Doxorubicin
- Ifosfamide
- High dose methotrexate
- Besides these, the combination of bleomycin, cyclophosphamide and dactinomycin has been effective.

Recommended Regimen

I. Doxorubicin and Cisplatin

- Doxorubicin 90 mg/m^2 IV 96 hours continuous infusion
- Cisplatin 120 mg/m^2 intra-arterially (for primary tumour) or IV on day 6
- Repeat every 4 weeks
- Three to four cycles must be administered preoperatively. Adjuvant therapy depends on the response of the primary tumour.
- It there is >90% of tumour necrosis, continue same regime for 3–6 postoperative courses.

II. MAP (high-dose Methotrexate, Cisplatin, and doxorubicin)

Requires administration of 15 mg leucovorin every 6 hours for 10 doses, starting 24 hours after initiation of high-dose methotrexate.

Neoadjuvant Setting

High-dose methotrexate 12 g/m^2 IV given over 4 hours on weeks 0, 1, 5, 6, 13, 14, 18, 19, 23, 24, 37, and 38, alternating with cisplatin 60 mg/m^2 IV + doxorubicin 37.5 mg/m^2/day IV for 2 days each on weeks 2, 7, 25, and 28.

Adjuvant Setting

- High-dose methotrexate 12 g/m^2 IV given over 4 hours on weeks 3, 4, 8, 9, 13, 14, 18, 19, 23, 24, 37, and 38, alternating with cisplatin 60 mg/m^2 IV + doxorubicin 37.5 mg/m^2/day IV for 2 days each on weeks 5, 10, 25, and 28
- 2 cycles are given preoperatively, and 4 cycles are usually given postoperatively.

III. After Primary Chemotherapy

If there is <90% of tumour necrosis switches to alterative regime:
- I: High dose methotrexate 12g/m^2 IV every 2 weeks for 8 weeks with leucovorin.
- II: Three week later, administer ifosfamide 2 g/m^2 IV over 2 hours for 5 consecutive days with Mensa 1200 mg/m^2 IV in 3 divided doses each day.
- III: Three to four weeks later, repeat the entire cycle of four courses of methotrexate and two courses of ifosfamide-doxorubicin.

Recurrence and Treatment of Refractory Disease

- Patient refractory to combination of doxorubicin and Cisplatin may respond to high dose methotrexate
- Patient refractory to high dose methotrexate may respond to combination of doxorubicin and Cisplatin
- Patient refractory to both may respond to ifosfamide or BCD (bleomycin, cyclophosphamide or dactinomycin)

Radiation Therapy

- Not very successful
- Give about 1000 rad in hope that it will reduce the viability of cells and thus inhibiting its dissemination.

Surgery

Ablative Surgeries

- Early and radical ablation is the procedure of choice
- Principle is to provide a normal cuff of tissue in all dimension
- Level of ablation depends upon imaging findings, leg length sonogram and bone scans.

Salvage Surgeries

- In early stages tumour excision and Endoprosthesis (modular or custom made) showing a better outcome. a number of options exist for limb-salvage reconstruction based on individual considerations, as follows:
- Autologous bone graft (vascularized or non-vascularized)
- Allograft
- Prosthesis
- Rotationplasty

Immunological Approach

Improving the immunological status by administer specific antibiotics, BCG vaccine, interferon therapy, allogenic sarcoma vaccine for 2 years in an attempt to manage the dreadful metastasis.

Pulmonary Metastasis

Surgical resection (most often by wedge resection) remains the only viable secondary therapy.

Q15. Describe the clinical features, histopathological, radiological and management of giant cell tumour or osteoclastoma.

Definition

Giant cell tumour of bone is a distinct, osteolytic, locally aggressive tumour composed of plump or oval, spindle mononuclear cells and uniformly distributed multinucleated giant cells.

These neoplasm are dominated by multinucleated osteoclast-type giant cells, hence the synonym osteoclastoma.

In 1818, Astley Cooper first described it and emphasizing its benign nature. In 1853, Paget called it 'brown or myeloid tumour'.

Incidence

- It is relatively uncommon; accounts for ~ 5% of all primary bone tumour.
- There is an unusually high prevalence in China and southern India (state of Andhra Pradesh).

Age

- Most patients are between 2 and 40 years of age.
- Peak incidence is in third decade.
- More than 70% of patients are diagnosed between of 20 and 45 years.
- On rare occasion seen in patients younger than 20 years or older than 45 years.
- There is a slight female predominance.

Sites/Location

- Most often in the epiphyseal end of the long bones.
- One theory suggests that these tumours are *originates in the metaphysis and later after the closure of the physis extend into the epiphysis.*
- In decreasing order of frequency: *Distal femur, proximal tibia, and distal end of the radius* are the most frequent sites.
- Uncommon in short tubular bones of hand and feet.
- Extremely rare in vertebral bodies.
- Sacrum is the most common site in axial skeleton.
- Osteoclastoma occurring at the distal end of the radius is often more whitish in colour and is termed as "white giant cell tumour or osteoclastoma alba."

In skeletally mature individuals, it most frequently involves the end of long bones. Although rare in skeletally immature patients, in this setting giant cell tumours arise in the metaphysis.

Clinical Features

- Pain was the most common complaint varying from a few months to two years duration.
- Vague discomfort with a swelling near the end of the bone.
- Approximately 50% of patients gave a history of trauma.
- Swelling is free from skin and soft tissue and it is bony swelling.
- Surface is usually smooth, no dilated veins.
- Temperature over the swelling is usually normal.
- Moderate-to-severe tenderness is present over the involved area.
- On palpation the paper-thin cortex may give the sensation of *"egg-shell cracking"*, or there may be a firm fibrous doughy consistency.
- Patient may present with pathological fracture in 10–30% of cases.
- Limitation of joint movements is not seen, it rarely involves the joint.

Radiological Finding

Radiographic findings often are diagnostic:

- Well-defined, eccentric, lytic subchondral lucency in the epiphyseal region of a mature skeleton.
- The tumour is almost abutting against the articular cartilage (subchondral bone).
- Overlying cortex is frequently expanded and focally destroyed.
- No new bone formation around the tumour.
- Sharp line of demarcation between the tumour and unaffected shaft.
- As there is irregular destruction of bone, the tumour is traversed by remnants of the original bone, which looks like heavily trabeculated, producing a typical *"Soap- bubble appearance"*.
- Pathological fracture at the junctional zone, with the diaphysis is seen in 5–10% of patient.
- Callus may be seen after pathological fracture occurring at the junctional zone.
- Intra-articular extension is rare.

Campanaccis' Radiographic Grading

Grade I

- Quiescent form of giant cell tumour, which is located in the cancellous bone.
- Cortical involvement is minimal, if any.

- 10–15% belongs to this grade.
- It can even be asymptomatic.

Grade 2

- This active grade shows extensive cortical thinning and bulging, sometimes similar to ABC.
- They even encroached the subchondral bone.

Grade 3

- This aggressive grade lesion breach the cortex and have soft tissue component covered by pseudo-capsule and periosteum.
- Rarely, the tumour extends its barrier, the articular cartilage, and enters the joint or invades the adjacent bone.

Pathology

Gross

- Large, soft, friable, fleshy, lobulated, grey to reddish brown in colour with cystic degeneration.
- Usually occupies an eccentric position in the epiphyseal end of long bone.
- Evidence of haemorrhages, cyst formation and necrosis.
- Areas of yellow discolouration indicating the presence of foam cells.
- No evidence of new bone formation.
- May be evidence of pathological fracture.

Microscopic/Histological Finding

Tumour shows the proliferation of two cell population *mononuclear or stromal cells and multinucleated giant cells.*

Stromal or Mononuclear Cell

- The stromal cells predominate
- These are of two types: Rounded and spindle
- The cytoplasm is moderately dark, slightly bluish and poorly delineation.
- Uniformly distributed with multinucleated giant cells
- Mitotic activity is often seen in these cells.
- These cells are the real culprit.

Multinucleated Giant Cell

- These are osteoclast-type of giant cell.
- The giant cells are large, 50–100 µ in diameter and there are, characteristically, 20–30 per low-power field.
- Their cytoplasm is slightly more acidophilic than that of the stromal cells and is often ill defined.
- They may contain from 3–200 nuclei of the stromal-cell type.
- These cells contain acid phosphatase only.

Histological Grading

Jaffe and Lichtenstein devise a histologic grading system, which would predict prognosis in giant cell tumour. They divided giant cell tumour of bone into:

Grade 1

- No appreciable atypism of the stromal cells
- Mitoses are few, and none abnormal
- Giant cell plenty

Grade 2

- Stromal cells may be slightly or strikingly atypical but not sufficiently to diagnose frank malignancy
- Abnormal mitotic figures may be found
- Giant cell decrease

Grade 3

- Stroma sarcomatous
- Frankly and obviously malignant with capacity to metastasize

Enneking Staging for giant cell tumour

Characteristic	Stage I (latent)	Stage II (active)	Stage III (aggressive)
Pt%	10–15%	~70%	10–15%
Symptoms	Asymptomatic	Pathological fracture pain	Pathological fracture pain
Radiograph	Sclerotic rim	Expanded cortex	Cortical perforation
Histology	Benign	Benign	Benign

Investigations

Chest Radiographs

Required at the time of diagnosis to stage the lesion.

CT Scan and MRI

- Important tool in diagnosing the neoplasm in early stage.
- Help in assessing the size and extent of soft tissue involvement.

MRI

- It is useful to determine the extent of the lesion within the bone and in the soft tissue.
- The lesion usually is dark on T1-weighted images and bright on T2-weighted images.
- It may reveal fluid-fluid levels typical of a secondary aneurysmal bone cyst, which occurs in 20% of patients.

Angiography

- Neovascularity with intense, inhomogeneous capillary blush.
- Intra and extraosseous extent.

Radionuclides Scan

It shows increased uptake by the tumour.

Biopsy

It is necessary for confirmation.

Treatment

- Simple curettage
- Simple curettage/intralesional excision and bone grafting,
- Extended curettage with adjuvant like cryotherapy, phenol application, insertion of methylmethacrylate, insertion of hydroxyapatite or other bone substitutes
- En-block excision
- Resection followed by reconstruction: Arthrodesis (turn-o-plasty, intercalary dual fibular grafts with intramedullary K-wires, long interlocking intramedullary nail) or arthroplasty (custom-made endoprosthesis).

Simple Curettage

- Create a cortical window of size at least as large as the lesion to prevent leaving residual tumour cells "around the corner" on the undersurface of the near cortex.
- The bulk of the tumour is scooped out with large curettes.
- Enlarge the cavity 1–2 cm in each direction with a power burr.
- Copious irrigation of wound and the cavity to remove any debris and tumour cells.

Disadvantage

Recurrence rates were as high as 50%.

Simple Curettage/Intralesional Excision and Bone Grafting

- Create a cortical window of size at least as large as the lesion to prevent leaving residual tumour cells "around the corner" on the undersurface of the near cortex.
- The bulk of the tumour is scooped out with large curettes.
- Enlarge the cavity 1–2 cm in each direction with a power burr.
- Copious irrigation of wound and the cavity to remove any debris and tumour cells.
- Fill the cavity with autogenous cortico-cancellous bone graft.

Advantage

- Recurrence rate is less.
- Bone graft supports the subchondral bone and preserve the joint thus permit early mobilization.
- Provides most rapid and most reliable healing rate.
- Osteogenic, osteoinductive, and osteoconductive.

Disadvantage

- Associated with additional morbidity at the harvest site.
- Insufficient amount to fill the large sized cavity.

Extended Curettage

"Extended" curettage includes the use of adjuvant, such as *liquid nitrogen, polymethyl-methacrylate, phenol, or thermal cautery* to extend destruction of tumour cells.

Advantage

The recurrence rate after *extended curettage* is now approximately 10%.

Adjuvants

Liquid nitrogen (cryotherapy)

- *Rationale:* The aim is to destroy any residual tumour at the margins by process of repetitive freezing and thawing.
- *Method: "direct pour" technique:* Three sprayed freeze/thaw cycle of liquid nitrogen is poured directly into the cavity through *funnel method* or a *double lumen probe* with circulating liquid nitrogen is used.

Advantage

- Greatly reduce the recurrence rate and reduces the rate of malignant transformation to 1.9% from 15%.
- It is Superior to methacrylate and phenol at creating a rim of necrotic bone ($\leq$14 mm).

Complication

- Skin necrosis
- Infection
- Skin blistering
- Neuropraxia
- Pathological fracture
- Delayed healing

Bone Graft (or Artificial Substitute)

Advantages

- Osteoconductive, are easy to use, and are readily available.
- Restoring normal biomechanics to the joint surface to prevent future degenerative joint disease
- Restoring bone stock, this may help if future procedures are necessary.
- Used alone or in combination with autogenous bone graft, bone marrow aspirates, or demineralized bone matrix.

Disadvantages

- To prevent a pathological fracture the joint must be protected for a long time.
- Tumour recurrence often is difficult to distinguish from graft resorption.

Bone-cement (Polymethylmethacrylate)

Rationale: The aim is to kill the residual tumour cell by the heat of polymerization.

Advantages

- Provides immediate structural support to the joint.
- Preserve the articular cartilage
- Quicker rehabilitation (allow full and early mobility)
- Lessens the risk of pathological fracture.
- It facilitates easier detection of recurrence, which is evident as radiolucency adjacent to the cement mantle.
- Theoretically it reduces the risk of recurrence.

Disadvantages

- Difficulty in removing it when revision is needed.
- Osteoarthritis (secondary to biomechanical alteration of the subchondral bone)
- Infection
- Pathological fracture

Thermal Cautery (Argon Beam Coagulator)

- Depth of necrosis in cancellous bone treated with argon beam coagulation to be ~ 4 mm.
- Easy to use, effective, and associated with few complications.

En-block Excision

- It is the initial procedure of choice in view of its *aggressiveness and potential for malignant transformation.*
- It is indicated especially when the *neoplasm eroded the cortex* and *extended into the surrounding soft tissues.*
- En-bloc excision of tumour with its surrounding bone shell and periosteum and a variable amount of soft tissue.
- A large defect following en-bloc resection requires *Arthrodesis, cancellous bone graft, Freeze-dried allograft or prosthetic replacement.*

Excision with Reconstruction or Limb Salvage Procedures

Fused Joint or Arthrodesis

- ***Turn-o-plasty:*** this procedure is especially indicated in case of tumour of distal end of femur or proximal end of tibia. After en-bloc excision of the tumour the other normal bone (either femur or tibia, as the condition may be), splits into two halves and one-half of it is turned upside down to bridge the gap and is fixed to the stump.
- Intercalary dual fibular grafts with intramedullary K-wires.
- Long interlocking intramedullary nail.

Mobile Joint or Arthroplasty

Most reconstructions involve preserving a mobile joint, for which three general options are available:
- Osteoarticular allograft reconstruction
- Endoprosthetic reconstruction
- Allograft-prosthesis composite reconstruction

Osteoarticular Allograft Reconstruction

Advantages

- Ability to replace ligaments, tendons, and intra-articular structures.
- It may have a role as a *temporary measure to preserve an adjacent physis in an immature patient* especially when the alternatives include amputation or sacrifice of both physes.
- In an *immature patient* in an attempt to *preserve the distal femoral physis*, a proximal tibial osteoarticular allograft could be used until skeletal maturity.

Disadvantages

High rate of complications, including:
- Nonunion at the graft-host junction

- Fatigue fracture
- Articular collapse
- Dislocation
- Degenerative joint disease
- Failure of ligament and tendon attachments

Endoprosthetic Reconstruction

Advantages

- Provides immediate stability, allows for quicker rehabilitation with immediate full weight bearing.
- Most endoprostheses are modular, provide facility for incremental limb lengthening as an immature patient grows.

Disadvantages

- Polyethylene wear
- Fatigue fracture
- Extraction of the remaining stem can be extremely difficult.

Allograft-prosthesis Composites

- Avoids complications of degenerative joint disease and articular collapse.
- Associated with fatigue fracture, infection, and nonunion at the graft-host junction.

Irradiation Therapy

- It has been shown to increase the rate of malignant transformation (high-grade sarcoma).
- It is permissible only for inaccessible sites like sacrum, spine and pelvis and those lesions, which are not amenable for surgery.
- Dosage ranges between 1500 and 5000 rad over a 5–6 weeks period.

Amputation or Limb Ablative Surgery

Indicated in:
- Widespread aggressive tumour with invasion of the soft tissue.
- Repeated recurrence.
- Malignant transformation.

In general:

Site	Treatment
Around knee	Excision and hemicondylar osteoarticular allograft reconstruction or a rotating hinge endoprosthesis
Distal end of femur	Excision with turn-o-plasty
Proximal end tibia	Excision with turn-o-plasty
Aggressive lesions of the distal radius	Primary resection and reconstruction with a proximal fibular autograft
Inoperable lesions in the spine or pelvis	Radiation or embolization (or both) may be used
Patients with pulmonary metastases	Resection should be attempted
Widespread aggressive tumour with invasion of the soft tissue	Amputation
Repeated recurrence	
Malignant transformation	

Follow-up

At minimum, patients should have radiographs of the primary tumour site and the chest at 3–4-month intervals for 2 years, at 6-month intervals for the following year, and annually thereafter.

Q16. Describe the clinical features, histopathological, radiological and management of Ewing sarcoma.

Ewing sarcoma is a primary malignant small round-cell tumour of bone. It is the fourth most common primary malignancy of bone, but follows osteosarcoma in patients younger than 30 years of age and the most common in patients younger than 10 years of age.

Current evidence indicates that both Ewing's and primitive neuroectodermal tumours (PNET) have a similar neural phenotype and as they share common chromosomal translocation these are sometimes grouped together in a category known as the Ewing family of tumours.

Aetiology

- Genetic: Chromosomal translocation.
- Ewing sarcoma is the result of a translocation between chromosomes 11 and 22 [t (11; 22) (q 24; q 12)], which fuses the EWS gene of chromosome 22 to the FLI1 gene of chromosome 11 Acts as a dominant oncogene.
- Other translocations: t (21; 22) (q 22; q 12) in 5–10% of cases, t (7; 22)(q 22; q 12) in less than 1% of cases.

Incidence

- Less than 1 per 1 million per year.
- Accounting for about 9% of primary malignancies of bone.

Age

- Most occur in patients 5–25 years old.
- ~80% are younger than 20 years of age.
- There is a slightly higher incidence in males.
- Significantly prominent in whites.

Sites/Location

- Most common locations include the diaphysis or metaphyses (often with extension into the diaphysis) of long bones (femur, tibia, fibula and humerus) and the flat bones of the shoulder and pelvic girdles.
- Rarely, it occurs in the spine or in the small bones of the feet or hands.

Clinical Features

- Pain is an almost universal complaint. Onset is insidious, worse at night and the pain may be of long duration.
- Skin is oedematous, reddened and contains dilated veins.
- Affected site is erythematosus frequently tender, warm and swollen.
- Weight loss, fatigue, fever may be present.
- Some patients have systemic findings, including fever, anemia, elevated ESR, an elevated C-reactive protein and leucocytosis mimicking infection and are often associated with fulminating course.
- ~10% of patient may present with pathological fracture.

Course

- Periods of remission and exacerbation with decreased and increased size of tumour respectively.
- Metastasizes to other bone particularly skull, vertebrae and ribs *(bone tumour that metastasize to bone)*.
- May metastasizes to lungs, causing hemoptysis and chest pain.

Investigations

Radiological Findings

- Permeative lytic lesion with periosteal reaction forming multiple thin layers parallel with the surface of the shaft called "onion peel appearance".
- Corticomedullary destruction of diaphysis (moth-eaten or cracked eye appearance).

Triad of Finding on Imaging

- Diaphyseal location
- Permeative or round cell appearance
- Large or an obvious soft tissue mass associated with the tumour.

MRI

It is best guide to *preoperative planning for biopsy and for the appropriate surgical resection.*
- To assess the extent of medullary osseous involvement.
- To assess the extent of soft tissue extension of the tumour.
- To study the relationship of tumour with major nerve and vessels.

CT

It helps in assessing the extent and degree of cortical destruction.

Whole body scan and CT chest: To assess the metastasis, in view of that 15–20% of children with Ewing sarcoma will present with metastatic disease.

Biopsy

For confirmation of diagnosis.

Pathology

Gross

- Tan-white or greyish white tumour.
- Firm and encapsulated by fibrous tissue.
- Usually vascular and frequently contains hemorrhage and necrosis.
- Usually spreading through the Haversian canal and in due course the cortex is destroyed.

Microscopy/Histology

- Compactly arranged *sheets of uniform small, polyhedral or round blue cells with ill-defined margins.*
- Cells are slightly larger than lymphocytes, have clear, scanty and *glycogen rich cytoplasm*.
- The nucleus is oval or round and possesses scattered chromatin.
- No or minimal interstitial stoma.
- Mitoses are rare.

- Flexner type *rosettes* (composed of tumour cells encircling or surrounding a central lumen) are rare and *Homer-Wright pseudorosettes* (composed of tumour cells surrounding a central pink fibrillary space).
- Show microscopic resemblance with reticulum cell sarcoma. These two can be distinguished by staining with PAS. Ewing sarcoma shows *diastase sensitive glycogen positivity by PAS* while glycogen is absent in reticulum cell sarcoma.

Cytogenetic or Immunohistochemical

t (11;22)(q24;q12) is the most common translocation diagnostic of Ewing sarcoma and is present >90% of cases

Prognostic Factors

Worst Prognostic Factors

- Presence of distant metastases.
- Fever, anemia, and elevation of laboratory values (erythrocyte sedimentation rate, white blood cell count, and lactate dehydrogenase) suggesting more extensive disease and a worse prognosis.
- Older age at presentation.
- Male gender.
- As all Ewing sarcomas are considered high grade, histological grade is of no prognostic significance.
- Pelvic bone if involved.

Treatment

- Tumour is invariably fatal. When diagnosed, tumour is well spread all over the body.
- Standard treatment for Ewing sarcoma is surgical resection after neoadjuvant chemotherapy followed by adjuvant chemotherapy and radiation therapy.
- Local treatment of the primary lesion is more controversial. Local treatment includes *surgery or radiation therapy, or both.*

Surgery

Radical surgery, by removing the major bulk of tumour either by *local excision extensively* or *ablation by amputation* of the full length of bone combined with radio and chemotherapy will increase the five-year survival rate.

Chemotherapy

- *Standard Chemotherapy comprises of drugs like doxorubicin, vincristine, cyclophosphamide, and dactinomycin.*
- Addition of the drugs *iphosphamide and etoposide* to standard chemotherapy significantly improved five-year survival in patients whose disease had not spread to other organs (non-metastatic tumour).

Radiation Therapy

- *Radiation responsiveness* was one of the cardinal features of the tumour described by Ewing. It *melts like an ice* only to appear again.
- Excellent local control for doses between 45 and 60 Gy.
- Dose <40 Gy have unacceptable local failures.
- In general, doses of 45 and 55.8 Gy are administered for microscopic and gross disease respectively.

Q17. Describe the clinical features, histopathological, radiological and management of multiple myeloma or plasmacytoma.

Multiple myeloma is disseminated malignancy of plasma cells. The tumour, its proteins and the patient response to it leads to organ dysfunctions and symptoms of bone pain or fracture, renal failure, anemia, hypercalcaemia, and occasionally clotting abnormalities, susceptibility to infection, neurologic symptoms, and manifestations of hyperviscosity.

Aetiology

- Exact cause of myeloma is *unknown*.
- Exposure to *nuclear radiations*.
- It is seen more often among *farmers, wood workers, leather workers, and those exposed to petroleum products.*
- Though there is controversy, *Interleukin (IL) 6* may play a role in driving myeloma cell proliferation.
- Genetic factor may have a role: 13q14 deletions, 17p13 deletions, and 11q abnormalities predominate. The most common translocations *are t (11; 14) (q13; q32) and t (4; 14) (p16; q32).*
- In some cases, there is *overexpression of myc or ras genes.*

Incidence

- It is most common primary malignancy of bone, representing >40% of primary bone cancers
- Myeloma accounts for ≤1% of all malignancies in whites and 2% in blacks; 13% of all haematologic cancers in Whites and 33% in Blacks.

Age

- The median age at diagnosis is 68 years; it is uncommon <40.
- peak incidence is in the fifth to seventh decades.
- Male preponderance.

Sites

- Bone in the axial skeleton is affected more often.
- The following distribution was found in a large series of cases: Vertebral column (66%), ribs (44%), skull (41%), pelvis (28%), femur (24%), clavicle (10%) and scapula (10%).

Pathology

Gross

- Osseous and extraosseous tumours are friable, variably red, tan or grey and have consistency ranging from fleshy to gelatinous.
- Bony lesions are well distinct from the surrounding tissues.
- The tumour erodes and extends beyond the cortex.
- Moderate enlargement of the lymph nodes, liver, and spleen is occasionally observed.
- Kidneys are often contracted in size.

Microscopic examination and immunohistochemistry:

- The microscopic hallmark of the multiple myeloma in bone marrow is nodular aggregated or sheets of plasma cells.
- Increased number of plasma cells which usually constitute >30% of the marrow cellularity.
- Diffuse infiltration of plasma cells or in sheet-like masses that completely replace the normal haematopoietic tissues.

- Neoplastic plasma cells small, round blue cells with "clock face" nuclei and abundant cytoplasm with a perinuclear clearing or "halo."
- Other cytologic variants includes flame cells, with fiery red cytoplasm; Motts cells having multiple blue grape like cytoplasmic droplets; and cells containing a variety of inclusions, such as fibrils, crystalline rods, and globules, sometimes Russell bodies (cytoplasmic) or Dutcher bodies (nuclear).
- With disease progression, plasma cell infiltration can be encountered in the kidney, liver, lungs, spleen, lymph nodes, or other soft tissues.
- Myeloma cells usually stain positive for the natural killer antigen CD56, whereas reactive plasma cells usually do not.

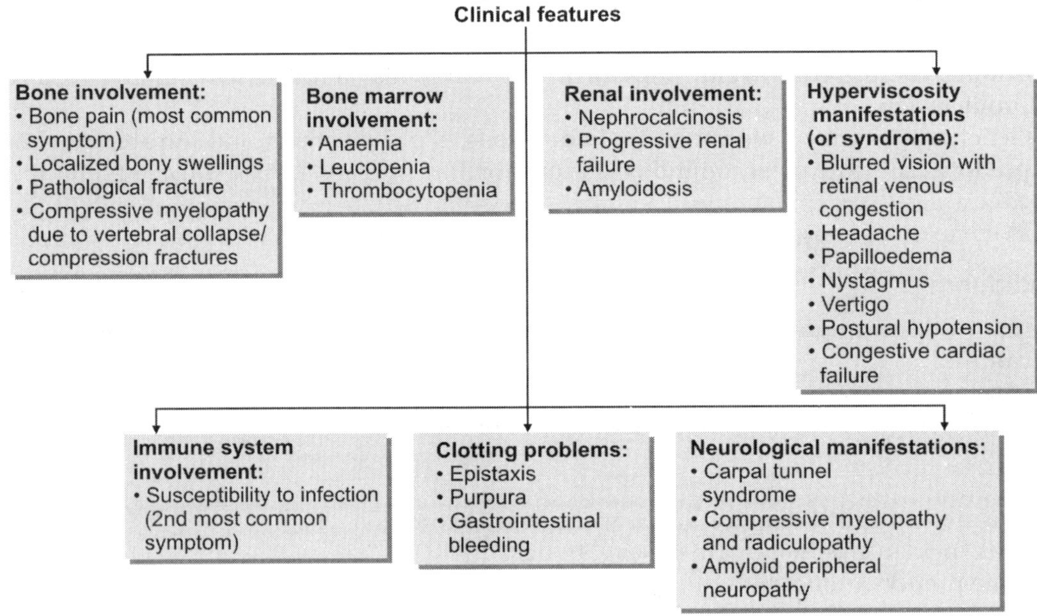

Investigations

Laboratory Findings

- *Anaemia*: usually normocytic and normochromic
- *Erythrocyte sedimentation rate* is elevated.
- In 2% of cases may have *plasma cell leukemia* with >2000 plasma cells/IL.
- Serum calcium, urea nitrogen, creatinine, and uric acid levels may be elevated.
- *Protein electrophoresis and measurement of serum immunoglobulins* and free light chains: For detecting and characterizing M spike/component, (serum M component will be IgG in 53% of patients, IgA in 25%, and IgD in 1%)
- *Immunoelectrophoresis:* it is sensitive for identifying even low concentrations of M component that is non-detectable by simple protein electrophoresis.
- *Serum Alkaline Phosphatase*: it is usually normal even with extensive bone involvement because thee is no osteoblastic activity.
- *Urine:* Will show Bence-Jones protein (light chain proteins) in 50% of the patients (on boiling, a white precipitate appears at about 50°C, which disappears on further boiling and reappears on cooling).
- *Marrow biopsy:* Bone marrow smear will show typical cartwheel myeloma cells in the marrow.

- *Serum β₂-microglobulin* is the single most powerful predictor of survival. Patients with β₂-microglobulin levels <0.004 g/L have a median survival of 43 months while those with levels >0.004 g/L have only 12 months.

Imaging

- Chest and bone skiagram may reveal *lytic lesions or diffuse osteopenia.*
- Bone lesions appear radiographically as *punched-out defects (classic lesions),* usually 1–4 cm in diameter.
- In solitary type, it may show a solitary *punched out lesion* in one bone with multilocular expansion.
- In the generalized variety *multiple punched out defects in the skull,* pelvis, long bone and vertebral involvement is seen as biconcave vertebrae and collapse with extensive rarefaction giving it a disappearing vertebrae picture, without any marginal new bone formation.
- Occasionally, myeloma is characterized by marked bone expansion, giving rise to a "ballooned" appearance.
- MRI offers a sensitive tool to evaluate extent of bone marrow infiltration and cord or root compression in patients with pain syndromes.

Diagnosis and Staging

- The diagnosis usually can be confirmed by serum immunoelectrophoresis, which shows a monoclonal gammopathy.
- The *classic triad* of myeloma is *marrow plasmacytosis (>10%), lytic bone lesions, and a serum and/or urine M component.*
- Bone marrow plasma cells are CD138+ and monoclonal.

Diagnostic criteria for multiple myeloma and its variant: **Durie-Salmon** staging system is based on the *hemoglobin, calcium, M component, and degree of skeletal involvement.*

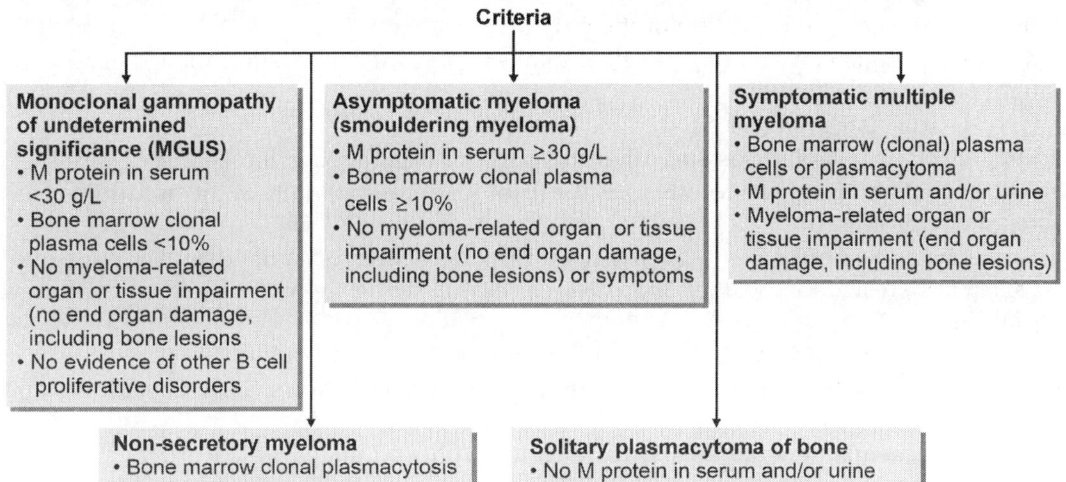

Multiple Myeloma Staging System

Durie-Salmon staging system:

Stage	Criteria	Estimated tumour burden × 10^{12} cells/m^2

I	All of the following:
	1. Normal bone X-ray or solitary lesion
	2. Haemoglobin >100 g/l (>10 g/dl)
	3. Serum calcium <3 mmol/L (<12 mg/dl)
	4. Low M-component production
	   a. IgG level <50 g/L (<5 g/dl)
	   b. IgA level <30 g/L (<3 g/dl)
	   c. Urine light chain <4 g/24 hours
		<0.6 (low)

II	Fitting neither I nor III	0.6–1.20 (intermediate)

III	One or more of the following:
	1. Advanced lytic bone lesions
	2. Haemoglobin <85 g/L (<8.5 g/dl)
	3. Serum calcium >3 mmol/L (>12 mg/dl)
	4. High M-component production
	   a. IgG level >70 g/l (>7 g/dl)
	   b. IgA level >50 g/l (>5 g/dl)
	   c. Urine light chains >12 g/24 hours
		>1.20 (high)

Treatment

Aim

- *Supportive care*: To prevent the serious morbidity from complication of the disease.
- *Systemic chemotherapy*: To control the disease progression.

General measures or supportive care:

- Improve the general condition of the patient.
- Maintain adequate hydration, high fluid intake to prevent dehydration and to help excrete light chains and calcium.
- Give appropriate analgesics to reduce bone pain.
- Oral antibiotic prophylaxis and other measures to fight against infections.
- Sodium bicarbonate given orally to make urine alkaline especially in those patients with renal compromised.
- Renal failure should be treated promptly; medically or with dialysis if needed (plasmapheresis is ~10 times more effective at clearing light chains than peritoneal dialysis).
- Skilled physiotherapy may significantly improve the quality of life.
- Anemia may respond to erythropoietin along with haematinics (iron, cobalamin, and folate).
- Hypercalacaemia generally responds well to bisphosphonates, glucocorticoid therapy, hydration, and natriuresis.
- Bisphosphonates (e.g. pamidronate 90 mg or zoledronate 4 mg once a month) reduce osteoclastic bone resorption, decrease bone-related complications, and may also have antitumour effects.
- Plasmapheresis is the therapy of choice for hyperviscosity syndromes.
- Prophylactic administration of IV γ globulin preparations is used in cases of recurrent serious infections.

The main options for therapy include:
- Chemotherapy
- Immune modulating treatments such as thalidomide, lenalidomide, and bortezomib (a proteasome inhibitor).
- Corticosteroids such as prednisone or dexamethasone.
- Stem cell (bone marrow) transplantation

Chemotherapy

Patients who are transplant candidates:
- *Melphalan* should be avoided since they damage stem cells.
- High-dose pulsed glucocorticoids have been used either alone (*dexamethasone 40 mg for 4 days every 2 weeks*) or in combination VAD chemotherapy (*vincristine, 0.4 mg/day in a 4-day continuous infusion; doxorubicin, 9 mg/m^2 per day in a 4-day continuous infusion dexamethasone, 40 mg/day for 4 days per week for 3 weeks*) for initial cytoreduction.

Patient who are not transplant candidates:
- Intermittent pulses of an alkylating agent, *L-phenylalanine mustard (L-PAM, Melphalan) and prednisone* administered for 4–7 days every 4–6 weeks.
- Usual doses of Melphalan/prednisone (MP) are Melphalan, 8 mg/m^2 per day, and prednisone, 25–60 mg/m^2 per day for 4 days.
- In patients >65 years, combining thalidomide with Melphalan and prednisolone (MPT) obtains higher response as well as overall survival rates than MP alone, and it (MPT) is the standard therapy for patients who are not transplant candidates

Maintenance therapy

IFN-α has allowed modest benefit but has significant side effects (under trial).

Radiotherapy

Patients with extramedullary plasmacytomas and solitary bone plasmacytomas may be expected to enjoy prolonged disease-free survival after local radiation therapy of around 40 Gy.

Autologous Stem Cell Transplant

There are three types of transplantation, based on the source of the stem cells:
- Autologous transplantation (most common): the stem cells are obtained from the individual with multiple myeloma.
- Allogeneic transplantation: the bone marrow or stem cells are obtained from a donor with a tissue type matching that of the patient. This type of transplantation carries very high risks and usually not recommended for most individuals with multiple myeloma.
- Syngeneic transplantation: the stem cells or bone marrow are obtained from an identical twin of the individual.

Relapsed Myeloma

- It can be treated with novel agents including *lenalidomide and/or bortezomib*.
- The combination of *bortezomib* and *liposomal doxorubicin* is active in relapsed myeloma.
- High-dose Melphalan and stem cell transplant, if not used earlier, also have activity in patients with refractory disease

Surgery

- **Pathological fractures:** Treat impending or actual pathological fractures of the spine, acetabulum, proximal femur, or proximal humerus using internal fixation augmented with methacrylate or cemented total joint arthroplasty or hemiarthroplasty.
- **Vertebral compressions:** Vertebroplasty, laminectomy, instability requires spinal fusion but seldom necessary.

Prognosis

- Median overall survival of patients with multiple myeloma is 5–6 years, with subsets of patients surviving over 10 years.
- The major causes of death are progressive myeloma, sepsis, renal failure, or therapy-related acute leukaemia or myelodysplasia.
- Poor prognostic factors:
    - Serum β_2-microglobulin(those with levels >0.004 g/L have a median survival of only 12 months)
    - Elevated levels of IL-6
    - High labeling index
    - High levels of lactate dehydrogenase
    - Hemoglobin <85 g/L (<8.5 g/dL)
    - Serum calcium >3 mmol/L (>12 mg/dL)
    - Advanced lytic bone lesions

Q18. Name the benign cartilage-forming tumours and discuss the clinical features, histopathological, radiological and management of: a. Chondroblastoma or Write short note on Codman tumour; b. Osteochondroma (exostosis)

Common Benign Cartilage-forming Tumours

- Chondroma
- Osteochondroma (osteocartilaginous exostosis)
- Chondroblastoma
- Chondromyxoid fibroma

a. Chondroblastoma or Codman tumour

Chondroblastoma is a rare, benign bone tumour of *immature cartilage* that arises in the epiphysis of long bones in skeletally immature patients. It is composed of *chondroblasts, giant cells with 'chicken-wire' pattern of ossification.* Codman first described it and thus it is termed as *"Codman tumour"*.

Incidence

- Tumour represents 1% of all bone tumours
- Typically occurs in patients 10–25 years old
- Males are affected twice than females

Location

Epiphyseal region of long bones.

Site

- Most common locations are in lower extremity (70%)
- 50% occur around knee
- The distal femur, proximal humerus, and proximal tibia are the most common sites of occurrence
- About 10% occur in the small bones of the hands and feet
- May also occur in apophyses
- Most common tumour of patella

Clinical Findings

- Progressive pain
- Redness
- Swelling
- Wasting of muscles
- Limitation of motion
- Pathological fracture (rarely)

Imaging Findings

Plain Radiographs

In children, a *well-circumscribed epiphyseal lesion* that crosses an open growth plate is diagnostic of chondroblastoma.
- Conventional radiographs are usually diagnostic
- Geographic lytic lesion arising in the epiphysis of a child
- May have scalloping or expansion of epiphyseal cortex
- May extend to adjacent metaphysis
- Eccentric
- Up to half may have internal calcifications (punctate or streky)
- Well-defined sclerotic margin

CT Scan

- Extent of involvement of epiphysis
- Proximity of lesion to articular cartilage

MRI

- Low signal intensity on T_1
- High or variable intensity on T_2

Biopsy: to confirm the diagnosis

Pathology

Gross

- Well-delineated lesion
- Dark red, haemorrhagic and friable tissue
- Scattered yellow zones of calcification, bluish white translucent zones of cartilage and spicule of necrotic bone.

Microscopic

- Occasional scattered collections of giant cells
- Sheets and islands of chondroblasts usually with a background of chondroid matrix (*pavement appearance*)
- Multinucleated giant cells are abundant, and secondary ABCs are present in 20% of patients
- Island of chondroblast
- Usually polyhedral, though may be spindle elements
- Cell membrane thick and sharply defined
- Nuclei:
  - Vary in shape from round to indented and lobulated
  - Some resemble those of Langerhans' cells
  - Mitoses exceptional
- Intracytoplasmic glycogen granules
- Reticulin fibres surround each individual cell
- Small zones of focal calcification:
  - Distinctive
  - Range from network of thin lines (*'chicken wire' or picket fence*) to obvious deposits surrounded by giant cell

Special Stains and Immunohistochemistry

Cells of chondroblastoma:
- Co-express:
  - Vimentin
  - S-100 protein
- May be immune-reactive for:
  - Neuron-specific enolase
  - Muscle-specific actin
  - Low-molecular-weight keratins

Treatment

- Extended curettage and packing with allograft or autograft bone chips or methylmethacrylate.
  - It is a preferred treatment
  - It provides local control in >80%
- In cases of recurrence or when chondroblastoma is associated with ABC: Curettage followed by cryosurgery gives better result.
- *Complicated cases*: Radiotherapy (should not be used for uncomplicated case in view of its potential hazard of inducing malignant transformation)

Complications

- High rate of recurrence (10–20%)
- Most common locations for recurrence to occur are proximal femur and pelvis
- Pathologic fractures (very rare)

Malignant transformation

- Extremely rare
- Pulmonary metastases or local invasion are possible, even with "benign" tumours

Prognosis

Excellent.

b. Osteochondroma (Osteocartilaginous Exostosis)

Osteochondromas are most common benign bone tumour. They probably are developmental malformations rather than true neoplasms and are thought to originate within the periosteum as small cartilaginous nodules.

It is a mushroom-like protrusion in then metaphyseal zone growing away from the growth plate, the growth of this tumour stop, once the patient attains skeletal maturity.

Incidence

Account for ~35% of benign bone tumours and 9% of all bone tumours.

Age/Sex

- Usually seen during the period of rapid skeletal growth. Their growth usually ceases when skeletal maturity is reached.
- Most are found in patients <20 years
- Male: female: 2:1

Location

- Metaphysis of a long bone near the physis.
- Most commonly involves distal femur, the proximal tibia, and the proximal humerus.
- In axial skeleton: Ilium (most common)

Types

- Pedunculated (most common)
- Broad-based or sessile
- Any definite stalk is move away from the physis/growth plate adjacent to which it takes its origin.
- The projecting part of the lesion has *cortical and cancellous components*, both of which are continuous with corresponding components of the parent bone (*the medullary canal of the stalk and the bone are in continuity*).
- A *cartilaginous cap* that often is irregular and usually cannot be appreciated on radiographs covers the lesion; occasionally, calcification within the cap may be seen.

Presentation

- Usually asymptomatic and are discovered incidentally.
- Bony hard swelling (palpable mass)
- Overlying skin is freely mobile
- Pain due to:
    - Irritation of surrounding structures
    - Bursitis/tendinitis
    - Osteonecrosis of the cap
    - Neural compression (pressure effect)
    - False aneurysms of major lower extremity vessels (pressure effect)
    - Fracture through the stalk
    - Malignant transformation

Investigations

- Plain radiographs (well-defined exostosis emerging from metaphysis) usually are sufficient to make a diagnosis.
- CT (especially when in pelvis and the scapula) or MRI (assess the thickness of cap: malignant transformation) sometimes is needed.
- Rarely biopsy is required : to confirm the diagnosis:
  - Gross: The stalk is contiguous with the intramedullary marrow
  - Microscopic:
    - Perichondrium covers the cartilage cap.
    - The cap merges into the underlying spongiosa, where the chondrocytes are arranged according to an epiphyseal growth plate.
    - Spongiosa of the stalk is continuous with the underlying cancellous bone

Treatment

Operative (once the longitudinal growth is completed).

Indications

- Pain
- Fracture of the stem
- Pressure symptoms
- Interference with joint function
- Cosmetic excision especially in females only after completion of longitudinal growth
- Malignancy (imaging features)

Procedures

- *Surgical resection* (en-bloc) requires excision of the lesion with an intact perichondrium, as recurrence of tumour growth may arise from perichondrium left behind.
- Patients with multiple hereditary exostoses: osteotomies to correct deformity.

Malignant Transformation

- Incidence of malignant degeneration is thought to be about 1% for *solitary osteochondromas* and from 5–25% in cases of *hereditary multiple exostoses*.
- Malignant transformation is best evaluated by CT or MRI
- Features suggestive of *malignant transformation*:
  - Previously quiescent lesion in an adult grows rapidly
  - If the cartilaginous cap is >1 cm
  - If the cartilaginous cap shows snowstorm appearance or calcification
  - Destruction of subchondral bone
  - Inhomogeneous appearance
  - Loss of distinctive bony margin and adjacent soft tissue mass.

Multiple Hereditary Exostoses

- Constitute an *autosomal dominant* condition with variable penetrance.
- Mutations in the EXT1 and EXT2 genes cause hereditary multiple exostoses
- In this disease, osteochondromas of many bones are caused by an anomaly of skeletal development.

- More common in males
- The most striking feature is the presence of multiple exostoses.
- Disturbances in growth also occur, such as:
  - Abnormal tubulation of bones, producing:
    - Broad and blunt metaphyses
    - Bowing of the radius
    - Shortening of the ulna, producing ulnar deviation of the hand
- Most dreaded complication: malignant transformation (chondrosarcoma).
- ***Diaphyseal achalasia***: triad of *multiple osteochondroma, wide deformed trumpet shaped metaphysis and stunted growth.*

Q19. Describe a Chondroma or Enchondroma.

Chondromas are benign, purely hyaline to myxoid mass of cartilaginous origin. They usually arise in the medullary canal, where they are referred to as *"enchondromas."*

Rarely, they arise on the surface of the bone, where they are referred to as *"Juxtacortical Chondromas or "Periosteal Chondromas".*

Incidence

- Most common tumour of the small bones of the hands and feet
- It affects the patient of 10–50 years of age.
- Both sexes are equally affected.

Location

- It may be centrally or subperiosteally.
- Diaphyseal areas is most frequently involved
- Phalanges of the hand are the most common location.
- Femur, humerus , ribs and innominate bone are less commonly involved.

Clinical Features/Presentation

- These usually are asymptomatic and frequently are discovered incidentally during an unrelated radiographic examination
- Pathological fracture
- Multiple enchondromatosis may occur in three distinct disorders:
  - *Ollier disease:*
    - Nonhereditary disorder
    - Cartilaginous tumours appear in the large and small tubular bones and in the flat bones
    - These are due to failure of normal endochondral ossification
    - Usually located in the epiphysis and the adjacent parts of the metaphysis and shaft, and many bones may be affected
    - Predilection for unilateral distribution
    - Deformities resulting from the tumours include:
    - Shortening caused by lack of epiphyseal growth
    - Broadening of the metaphyses
    - Bowing of the long bones
    - Considerable disability

- When associated with *haemangiomas* of the overlying soft tissues, the condition is known as *Maffucci's syndrome*
- Significant risk of malignant transformation in Ollier's disease (25%) and Maffucci's syndrome

Maffucci's Syndrome

- Non-hereditary and is less common than Ollier disease.
- This syndrome results in *multiple haemangiomas* in addition to *enchondromas.*

Metachondromatosis

- It consists of multiple enchondromas and osteochondromas.
- It is the only one that is hereditary, which is by autosomal dominant transmission

Radiological Finding

- Benign-appearing tumours with intralesional calcification
- Calcification is irregular; described as *"stippled," "punctate," or "popcorn."*
- Erosion and expansion of the overlying cortex
- *Endosteal erosion* (2/3rd of the thickness of the cortex) frequently indicates a chondrosarcoma
- Any associated soft-tissue mass always indicates a chondrosarcoma
- Juxtacortical chondromas:
  - Usually are small (<3 cm)
  - Well-defined lesions that appear to fit in a saucer-shaped defect on the surface of the bone.
  - Underlying cortex appears sclerotic
  - Edges of the lesion appear to be buttressed by a thick ring of cortical bone.

CT Scan

CT is best to evaluate endosteal erosion that helps in diagnosing the chondrosarcoma

Histological Features

Gross

- Enclosed by a fibrous capsule
- Cut sections show extensions dividing the growth into lobules.
- Neoplastic tissue comprises of bluish white translucent cartilage.

Microscopic Features

- Mature lobules of hyaline cartilage
- Relatively hypercellular
- Mild atypia is present
- Mature cartilage at the centre undergoes degenerative changes like calcification, cystic degeneration and myxomatous changes.
- Nuclei of chondrocyte are small and pyknotic
- Juxtacortical chondroma:
  - Tends to be more cellular than medullary counterpart
  - It may contain occasional plump or double nuclei

Treatment

Solitary Enchondromas

- Observation with serial radiographs
- If the lesion remains radiographically stable and asymptomatic, no further intervention is required
- If a lesion grows, or if it becomes symptomatic, extended curettage is curative.
- Recurrence rates are low.

Multiple Enchondromatosis

- Treatment is more difficult.
- Individual lesions usually are not treated.
- Obvious deformities can be corrected by osteotomy.
- Patients must be monitored indefinitely for malignant change.

Q20. Discuss the clinical features, histopathological, radiological and management of chondrmyxoid fibroma.

Chondromyxoid fibroma (CMF) is a rare, slow-growing bone tumour of cartilaginous origin. Jaffe and Lichtenstein first described the condition in 1943.

Incidence

- Accounts for <0.5% of primary bone tumours.
- Occur at any age, most occur in patients 10–30 years old.
- Males and females are affected equally.
- Genetic predisposition: there occurs clonal rearrangement of chromosome 6. Each of these rearrangements involved band 6q13.

Location

- Metaphyseal region of the long bones.
- Any bone may be involved.
- Proximal tibia is the most common location, followed by the distal femur, pelvis, and foot.
- Flat bone involvement may be seen more often in older patients.

Clinical Features

- Majority of patient have symptoms at the time of diagnosis.
- Pain
- Painless swelling or mass (if the tumour is located in the hands or feet)
- In very rare cases, a limitation of joint motion.

Radiological Features

- Appearance is that of a benign neoplasm.
- It usually is an eccentric well-circumscribed lesion with a rim of sclerosis in the metaphysis of a long bone.
- Medullary margins are scalloped and sclerosed Sometime it may have bubbly appearance mimicking a non-ossifying fibroma.

- In contrast to other cartilaginous lesions, radiographic evidence of intralesional calcification usually is absent (except in the rare cases of a surface lesion in which calcification may be abundant)

Histological Features

Grossly

- Firm, greyish-white masses.
- Lobulated or pseudolobulated

Microscopically

- Lobulated
- Center of the lobules contains loose myxoid tissue, and the periphery contains a more cellular fibrous tissue.
- The background often appears chondroid, although distinct areas of hyaline cartilage are rare. Microscopic calcification may be present.
- The lesion may contain areas with atypical cells.

Treatment

- Resection or extended curettage with bone grafting
- Local recurrence occurs in ~ 20% of patients and is treated with repeat surgery.
- Sarcomatous change or metastasis is rare.

Q21. Discuss the differential diagnosis of cysts and cyst-like lesions of bone.

Simple Bone Cyst

- Most common sites are the proximal humerus and femur (metaphyseal region)
- Elongated
- Needle aspiration reveals straw coloured fluid.

ABC (Aneurysmal Bone Cyst)

- Peak in second decade of life
- Metaphysis of long bones
- Blood-filled reactive lesions of bone (aspiration reveal blood)
- Eccentric, expansile
- Almost spherical

Giant Cell Tumour

- Epiphyseal
- Eccentric
- Cortical penetration and expansion of the cortex

Fibrous Dysplasia

- Usually diaphyseal
- Multiloculated, soap-bubble appearance
- Ground glass appearance

Chondromyxoid Fibroma

- Metaphyseal
- Eccentric
- Cortical expansion

Chondroblastoma

- Located in epiphysis
- Eccentric
- Calcification and trabeculation

Metaphyseal Fibrous Cortical Defect

- Lesion usually situated in the proximal tibia
- Eccentric

Q22. Describe in brief aneurysmal bone cyst.

Aneurysmal bone cysts (ABCs) are locally destructive, blood-filled reactive lesions of bone lined by fibrous septae that include giant cells and areas of osteoid but no true endothelial cells. These are not considered to be true neoplasms.

Incidence

- 85% of patients with ABCs are younger than 20 years old.
- Peak in second decade of life
- Slight female predominance.

Location

- Any bone may be involved but most commonly involve the metaphysis of long bones (including the proximal humerus, distal femur, proximal tibia)
- Posterior elements of the vertebrae (15–20%)
- Also involve the pelvis and scapula

Pathogenesis

- It is uncertain
- It is likely that aneurysmal bone cysts result from local circulatory disturbance leading to raised venous pressure and production of local haemorrhage.

Clinical Features

- Pain (mild to moderate)
- Swelling
- Tenderness on palpation of the involved bone
- Spinal lesions may cause neurological compromise or radicular pain.
- Grow rapidly and frequently cause pathologic fractures.

Radiological Features

- Expansile lytic lesion eccentrically located in the metaphysis
- Lesion remains contained by a thin shell of cortical bone

- "Finger in balloon" sign
- Occasional periosteal new bone formation present
- Well-defined margins or a permeative appearance that mimics a malignancy

Bone Scan

It shows diffuse or peripheral tracer uptake with a central area of decreased uptake.

CT Scan

- Helpful in delineating the cyst in areas of complex anatomy, such as the pelvis or spine.
- In addition, the thin rim of bone surrounding the cyst can be appreciated.

MRI

MRI reveals the multiloculated cavities and fluid levels.

Histological Features

Grossly

- Cavitary lesion with blood-filled septate spaces.
- It is surrounded by a thin layer of bone covered by a raised periosteum

Microscopically

- Hemorrhagic tissue with cavernous spaces separated by a cellular stroma.
- Stroma of spindle cells with giant cells and haemosiderin.
- Cavernous spaces lined by compressed fibroblasts and histiocytes. It usually lacks endothelial lining.
- Haemosiderin-laden macrophages, chronic inflammatory cells, and multinucleated giant cells also are present

Treatment

- Extended curettage and grafting with a bone graft substitute.
- Marginal resection sometimes is indicated for lesions in expendable bones.
- Lesions in the spine or pelvis: can be treated with preoperative embolization to minimize surgical blood loss.
- In locations where curettage would be extremely difficult: Arterial embolization has been used as definitive treatment of aneurysmal bone cysts.
- Low-dose irradiation often associated with rapid ossification; however, it is not used as a routine procedure because of the potential for malignant transformation.

Q23. Discuss the clinical features, histopathological, radiological and management of Simple bone cyst.

Unicameral bone cyst, otherwise known as a *simple bone cyst*, is a *straw coloured* fluid-filled, single chambered thin walled cavity developing most commonly in the *metaphyseal region* of long bone *adjacent to the growth plate*, lined by compressed fibrous tissue (fibroblasts) and single line (usually less than 1 mm thick) of mesothelial cells.

Aetiology

- The exact cause is unknown.
- Theories regarding its origin:
  - Local defect in metaphyseal remodeling blocks interstitial fluid drainage and this increases pressure, which leads to focal bone necrosis and accumulation of fluid (most widely accepted theory).
  - The cysts result from a disorder of the growth plate.
  - Temporary failure of bone formation during skeletal growth.
  - The cysts result from problems with circulation due to developmental anomaly in the veins of the affected bone.
  - Trauma to the growth plate interfering with the enchondral ossification.
  - Synovial 'rest' theory: a 'rest' of synovial tissue during the fetal development, becomes incorporated into the osseous tissue and if this tissue remains or functional, synovial secretion subsequently results in a cyst developing in the bone.

Age

- Predominantly between 5 and 15 years of age.
- Rarely after 20 years of age.
- >80% of the bone cyst occurs in childhood and adolescent.
- Male preponderance (2:1).

Location/Sites

- Metaphyseal in location.
- Proximal humerus (55%) followed by proximal femur (26%).
- Less common site includes ilium, lower humerus and femur, tibia, calcaneus, talus, radius, ulna and ribs.

Clinical Features

- Most lesions are asymptomatic, unless a pathological fracture has occurred.
- The wall of the cyst are very thin, many patient (2/3rd) usually present with a pathological fracture with trivial trauma. A fracture may produce local swelling and tenderness.
- Pathological fracture usually heals spontaneously within few weeks.
- Spontaneous obliteration of cyst occurs following healing of fracture in 15% of cases.
- Non-fractured lesions usually present as an incidental finding on radiographs obtained for other reasons.
- Intermittent limp may be the presenting complaint in case of weight-bearing bone.
- Cyst abutting the growth plate may induce growth disturbances.
- Cyst at the proximal femur may cause coxa vara deformity.
- Occasionally shortening or overgrowth may occur.

Radiograph Findings

- Central and symmetric radiolucent lesion with a well-marginated outline in the metaphyseal lesion.
- Cortices are often thin and expanded.
- It is characteristically equal or slightly greater in diameter to the epiphyseal plate.

- In 20% of cases, *"fallen leaf"* sign present (a fractured fragment falls into distal portion of the cyst confirming its empty cystic nature; pathognomonic of a unicameral bone cyst with a fracture).
- Cyst may expand concentrically, but never penetrates the cortex.
- No periosteal reaction is present, unless there has been a fracture.
- Cysts are classified as active when they are within 1 cm of the physis and latent when they are closer to the diaphysis

Treatment

Conditions/lesion	Treatment
• Small, asymptomatic lesions in the upper extremities	• Observation with serial plain radiographs
• Larger lesions (lesions at risk for pathological fracture)	• Curettage with or without bone grafting or internal fixation
• Symptomatic lesions	• Aspiration and injection (using steroids, bone marrow aspirate, demineralized bone matrix, or other materials)
• Lesions in the lower extremities	
• Pathological fractures in the upper extremity	• Treated conservatively because the fracture may initiate cyst "healing."
• Fractures through cysts in the proximal femur	• Curettage, bone grafting, and internal fixation (usually flexible intramedullary nailing)

Treatment is aimed primarily at preventing recurrent fractures.
- Curettage/bone grafting
- Steroid injection
- Bone marrow injection

After three injections without healing, curettage and bone grafting should be considered.

Prognosis

- Prognosis for a unicameral bone cyst is generally good.
- Most of these cysts do heal with proper treatment and if left alone, most heal spontaneously by the time the skeleton ceases to grow.
- Follow-up care is essential.

Poor prognostic factors (for successful percutaneous treatment):
- Multi-loculated appearance
- Large size
- Radiographically active lesions
- Patient age younger than 10 years

Q24. Write short note on Haemangioma.

Haemangiomas or angiomas of bone are slow growing benign, malformed vascular lesions composed of masses of mature adult blood vessels.

Incidence

- Haemangioma is a common lesion, present in 10–12% of autopsy specimens.
- Overall constituting <1% of all primary bone neoplasms.

Site

- Vertebral body is the most common location, especially in the lumbar and lower thoracic regions.
- Skull (20%) where the lesion usually originates in the meninges and scalp.
- Posterior elements are involved in 10–15% of patients.
- Infrequently the long bones are involved.

Types

Capillary

It comprises of closely packed small blood vessels lined by a single layer of cuboidal endothelial cell.

Cavernous

- More common
- Comprises of large blood filled spaces lined by single layer of endothelial cells

Clinical Features

- Bone hemangiomas are usually asymptomatic lesions discovered incidentally on imaging or postmortem examination
- Patients with symptomatic hemangiomas most commonly have:
  - Pain (60%)
  - Neurological compromise (30%)
  - Symptomatic fracture (10%)

Investigations

- Radiographs detect larger lesions, which have *vertical striations and coarse, thick trabeculae, described as a "corduroy" vertebra.*
- Expansion may be noted in aggressive lesion, with erosion of the vertebral body.
- CT scanning is more sensitive than plain radiography. Vertebral haemangiomas are typified by punctate sclerotic foci representing thickened vertical trabeculae seen in cross-section and giving a *polka-dot appearance.*
- Bone scanning is not particularly helpful because lesions may be either hot or cold.
- MRI has become the standard for diagnosing these lesions. Typical haemangioma is identified by increased intensity on T_1- and T_2-weighted sequences, can be differentiated from Paget's disease because pagetic bone has cortical thickening, and affects the entire vertebral body.
- Angiographic findings confirm the hypervascularity of the lesions. Angiography usually is performed in conjunction with embolization of symptomatic haemangiomas prior to surgery

Treatment

- Most haemangiomas do not require treatment but should be observed by skiagram for any changes in appearance and clinically for developing any neurological deficit.
- *Radiation:* For rare symptomatic lesions, radiation is successful in 50–80%.
- *Embolization:* is useful, especially in patients with progressive neurological deficits, and may provide temporary symptomatic relief.

- *Vertebroplasty*: used successfully for treatment of aggressive haemangiomas by stabilizing pathological bone with an injection of bone cement into the vertebral body.
- *Use of inflatable bone tamps* has had similarly good short-term results.
- *Direct intralesional injection of ethanol*: Effective in obliterating symptomatic vertebral haemangiomas. CT angiography is required before injection to identify functional vascular spaces of the haemangioma and to direct needle placement.
- For progressive neurological deficit, radiation alone may be successful in arresting progression.
- With neurological deficit and fracture: *Surgery* is necessary to remove an aggressive haemangioma, and embolization should be done preoperatively to minimize bleeding intraoperatively.

Q25. Write short note on admantinoma.

Admantinoma is a rare but distinctive low-grade malignant primary bone tumour. The term *Admantinoma* was originally given because histologically it simulates the benign but locally aggressive tumour of the proliferating odontogenic epithelium called *ameloblastoma*.

This low-grade malignant tumour has variety of morphological patterns, most frequently epithelial cell, surrounded by a relatively bland spindle cell osteofibrous component.

Incidence

Rare, <1% of all bone tumours (the number of cases reported is approximately 100).

Age

- It usually occurs in adults.
- Peak incidence seems to be between 10 and 35 years.
- Male preponderance
- Blacks are predisposed.

Site

In the appendicular skeleton *tibia* is the most commonly involved bone.

Clinical Features

- Tumour develops insidiously over a period of many years.
- It may be asymptomatic and discovered incidentally on skiagram or at time, the first indication may be a *pathological fracture*.
- Initial symptoms varies, includes mild-to-moderate *pain, swelling* and *tenderness*.

Radiological Features

- An *eccentrically* sharply defined rarefaction in the medullary location involving the overlying cortex is the characteristic finding.
- With growth of tumour, the cortex becomes thinned-out, attenuated, expanded and often eroded in a characteristic *saw-toothed fashion*.
- *Loculated or Honey-combed* appearance is typical.
- The tumour eventually penetrates the cortex and extends into the contiguous soft tissues.
- Almost no periosteal reaction is noted but following a pathological fracture, extensive periosteal new bone formation produces a large spindle-shaped deformity.

MRI

- Helpful in determining the size of the tumour especially the medullary extension and soft tissue masses associated with it.
- Helpful in recognizing skip lesions.
- Helpful in surgical planning and evaluation of possible recurrence.

CT Scan

- Evaluation of tibial cortical involvement.
- Screening for pulmonary metastases.

Radionuclide Scans

The tumour shows increased uptake both in the vascular phase and in delayed images.

Biopsy

It is necessary for confirmation.

Pathology

Gross

- Tumour is yellowish, greyish white, and firm or fleshy in consistency.
- It may contain cystic space filled with straw-coloured or bloody fluid.

Histology

- Major portion of the tumour is consisting of epithelial cell surrounded by a fibrous stroma.
- Mitotic index is low (0–2 per 10 high-power fields).

Several histologic variant have been describes:

- *Tubular:* With cords of epithelial cells (most typical pattern).
- *Basaloid:* Resembling basal cell carcinoma with palisading of the peripheral layer of cells.
- *Squamous:* Resembling well-differentiated squamous cell carcinoma that may show keratinization.
- *Spindle cell:* That may show a fascicular or storiform pattern.
- *Vascular pattern:* With hyperplastic endothelial vascular channels adjacent to the processes of the tumour cells (angioblastic origin of tumour)

Treatment

- Wide en-bloc excision with substantial margin of normal bone with reconstruction with an allograft or autograft or custom-made prosthesis is the therapy of choice.
- En-bloc excision should always be accompanied by removal of suspiciously involved regional lymph node.
- If excision is followed by recurrence, amputation is indicated.
- Chemotherapy and radiotherapy have not been shown to be effective modalities of treatment.

Prognosis

- It is usually good.
- Local recurrence: 31%
- Metastases with a latency period of 10–20 years: lungs (20%); lymph nodes (6%).

Q26. Discuss in brief chondrosarcoma.

Chondrosarcoma is a malignant, slow growing cartilaginous tumour that arises from a pre-existing cartilage rest or enchondroma; has a longer natural history and better prognosis than osteosarcoma.

Incidence

- It is second most common primary malignant bone tumour.
- It constitutes about 9% of primary malignancies of bone.

Age/Sex

- It Peaks between 40 and 60 years for primary chondrosarcoma and between 25 and 45 years for secondary chondrosarcoma.
- Male preponderance

Locations

- It can occur in any location.
- Majority are located in a proximal location such as the pelvis, proximal femur, and proximal humerus.
- It is extremely rare in hands and feet except in calcaneus.

Types

Primary

Arise de novo from previously normal bone, i.e. tumour has its sarcomatous property from the very beginning

Secondary

- Arise at the site of a preexisting benign cartilage lesion.
- Ollier disease (multiple enchondromas) the incidence is 25% by age 40 years
- Maffucci's syndrome *(multiple enchondromas with soft-tissue haemangiomas)*, the incidence may be even higher

Presentation/Clinical Features

Primary Chondrosarcoma

- Usually asymptomatic
- Most of the time discovered incidentally on a bone scan or radiograph obtained for another reason
- Increasing pain (especially in the presence of pathological fracture)
- Palpable mass

Secondary Chondrosarcoma

Condition associated with the secondary chondrosarcoma:
- Ollier disease (multiple enchondromas)
- Maffucci's syndrome (multiple enchondromas with soft-tissue haemangiomas)
- Synovial chondromatosis

- Chondromyxoid fibroma
- Periosteal chondroma
- Chondroblastoma
- Previous radiation treatment
- Fibrous dysplasia.

Radiological Findings

- Lesion arising in the medullary cavity with irregular matrix calcification
- Pattern of calcification described as "punctate," "fluffy", "popcorn," or "comma-shaped
- Endosteal scalloping may be present; when its depth is more than two-thirds the normal thickness of the cortex, this scalloping is useful in distinguishing chondrosarcoma from enchondroma
- Cortical destruction
- Compare to enchondroma, chondrosarcoma has a more aggressive appearance with cortical erosions, bone destruction, periosteal reaction, and rarely a soft-tissue mass.

CT Scan

- Lucent areas containing chondroid matrix calcification
- Endosteal scalloping and cortical destruction

It can be helpful:
- To show endosteal erosions
- To show other evidence of a destructive lesion
- To differentiate benign from malignant cartilage lesions.

MRI

It is used to assess:
- Soft-tissue extension (extraosseous extension of a chondrosarcoma)
- The intramedullary extent of the tumour
- Thickness of the cartilage cap

Secondary Chondrosarcoma

Size of cartilaginous cap:
- The size of the cartilaginous cap of an osteochondroma, as evaluated with CT or MRI, is important in evaluating the possibility of a secondary chondrosarcoma.
- If the cartilaginous cap is >2 cm in a skeletally mature patient, a secondary chondrosarcoma must be considered.

Histological Finding

- Conventional chondrosarcomas are composed of malignant cells with abundant cartilaginous matrix
- Hypercellularity
- Plump nuclei
- More than occasional binucleate cells
- Permeative pattern
- Entrapment of bony trabeculae

Histological Subtypes

- *Dedifferentiated chondrosarcoma:*
  - High-grade sarcoma
  - On X-rays, it show a more aggressive radiolucent area
- *Clear cell chondrosarcoma:*
  - It consists of round cells with abundant clear cytoplasm
  - distinct cytoplasmic borders with a background of cartilaginous matrix
  - Multinucleated giant cells usually are apparent
- *Mesenchymal chondrosarcoma:*
  - · High-grade tumour
  - · Consisting of small round blue cells with islands of benign-appearing cartilage
  - · Cellular portions often have a haemangiopericytomatous pattern of growth with "staghorn-like" vessels

Treatment

Chemotherapy has no role in the treatment of conventional chondrosarcoma and radiotherapy likewise has a limited role and is indicated only as a palliative measure for surgically inaccessible lesions.

Low-grade Chondrosarcoma

- Controversial
- Extended curettage

High-grade Chondrosarcoma

Wide or radical resection or amputation.

For Lesions in an Expendable Location

Primary wide resection without a biopsy may be indicated to decrease the chance of tumour contamination.

Pulmonary Metastases

It should be treated with surgical resection.

Q27. Write short note on synovial cell sarcoma.

This is a malignant tumour arising from the synovial lining of joints, tendons and bursa, around the second decade of life.

Aetiology

- The origin of synovial cell sarcoma is unclear
- In contrast to its name, synovial cell sarcoma is not associated with synovial joints.
- The term *synovial sarcoma* is a misnomer. The term originates from the histological appearance of the cells, which can resemble synovial cells.
- The tumours do not arise from synovial tissue; however, an intra-articular location or even continuity with the joint capsule is extremely rare
- A neurologic origin has been suggested owing to its histologic resemblance between neural cells of malignant peripherical nerve sheath tumour (MPNST) and synovial cell sarcoma

- Synovial cell sarcoma is characterized by a specific chromosomal translocation t(X;18) (p11;q11) (>90% of cases)

Incidence

- Incidence is 2.75 per 100000.
- Synovial cell sarcoma is the third most common soft tissue tumour in adolescents and young patients.
- Approximately 1 in 3 cases occurring in the first 2 decades of life.
- Mean age of patients at diagnosis is approximately 30 years.
- Females are more commonly affected than males

Presentation

- History of a small nodule that has increased rapidly in size
- The mass often is painful and deep.
- Most commonly, it is situated around the knee, but it also can appear in the hands and feet.

Imaging

Plain X-rays

It typically produces a spotty calcification (snowstorm) within the matrix of the soft tissue tumour

CT Scan

- It is used to confirm the presence of a mass, its size, and its location, but it is non-diagnostic
- May detect secondary bony involvement
- Synovial sarcoma is a malignant disease; therefore, CT scanning of the chest is mandatory to exclude any metastatic disease.

MRI

- It is the investigation of choice for soft tissue sarcomas
- Low signal intensity is observed on T_1-weighted images, and high signal intensity is observed on T_2-weighted images

Cytogenetic Analysis

It aids the physician in detecting the specific chromosomal translocation t(X;18)(p11;q11)

Histological Findings

Macroscopically

- The tumour is a greyish-white and often has a greasy feel.
- Histologic features of synovial sarcoma are identical in children and adults.

Microscopically

The tumours frequently show a biphasic growth pattern with nests of epithelioid cells surrounded by spindle cells.

Three types have been described:

1 *In monophasic type:*
- There is a predominance of spindle cells, mixed with round cells.
- Cells are arranged in fascicles with a poorly defined cytoplasm.
- The monophasic variant does not have glandular areas.

2. *The biphasic type:*
- This type has a layer of columnar epithelium in addition to spindle cells.
- It consists of plump, round cells and spindle-shaped fibroblasts alternating with glandular-like areas that are lined by synovial-like cells and contain mucin.

3. A third type, called poorly differentiated, has numerous mitosis, high cellularity, and tumour necrosis.
- Punctate areas of calcification may be observed

Spread

- Synovial cell sarcoma has the ability to metastasize via the lymphatic system.
- Venous metastasis can occur as well.
- Synovial sarcoma is most likely to invade adjacent bone.

Treatment

Chemotherapy

- Adjuvant chemotherapy and neoadjuvant chemotherapy have been proposed for patients with metastatic soft tissue sarcomas.
- Combinations of doxorubicin ($75\,mg/m^2$ via continuous infusion over 3 days) and bolus ifosfamide ($2.5\,g/m^2$ daily for 4 days, or ifosfamide with liposomal daunorubicin).
- Granulocyte colony-stimulating factor may stimulate the bone marrow.

Surgery

Wide Surgical excision is still the cornerstone of treatment for synovial cell sarcoma. Primary amputation is required in 20% of patients.

Prognostic Factors

Synovial cell sarcoma has survival rates of 50–60% at 5 years and 40–50% at 10 years. Prognostic factors that correlate with a better prognosis include the following:
- Biphasic histologic pattern
- Patients with SYT/SSX2 fusion genes
- Location in the hand or foot
- Size <5 cm
- Female sex
- Age <50 years
- Negative resection margins.

Q28. What is adjuvant and neoadjuvant chemotherapy?

Adjuvant treatment is the administration of additional therapy (*may include chemotherapy, radiation therapy, hormone therapy, targeted therapy, or biological therapy*) *after primary surgery* to kill or inhibit micrometastases. *Neoadjuvant therapy* refers to the administration of therapeutic agents *prior to the main* treatment.

Advantages

- Early treatment of micrometastasis.
- Reduction of tumour size, increasing chance of limb salvage.
- Decreases neovascularity thus helps define tissue planes better during surgery
- Allows time for custom made prosthesis
- Allows direct observation of affect of drugs on tumour.
- Less chance of viable tumour spillage during surgery.

Disadvantages

- High tumour burden.
- More chance of selection of drug resistant cells in main tumour, which may metastasize.
- Psychological trauma of retaining the tumour

Q29. Discuss carcinoma metastasized to bone or secondaries and approach to diagnose these secondaries.

Metastatic carcinoma or secondaries are the most common malignancy treated by orthopaedic surgeons. In any patient >40 years, even without any history of malignancy, a newly diagnosed, aggressive-appearing bone lesion is most likely to be metastatic carcinoma or multiple myeloma.

Incidence

- Metastatic carcinoma are the most common malignant bone tumour
- 50–80% of patients with carcinoma have bone metastases at the time of death.
- Axial skeleton is the third most common site of metastasis after liver and lung.
- The axial skeleton is involved more commonly than appendicular.
- Most common site are spine, pelvis, proximal femur, ribs and skull.

Carcinoma Metastasized to Bone

Most carcinomas metastatic to bone are from the breast and prostate, followed by the lung, kidney, thyroid, and gastrointestinal tract in order of decreasing frequency.

Age

Most patients with skeletal metastases are >40 years.

Sex

In females:
- Breasts and lungs are the most common primary disease sites.
- ~80% of cancers that spread to bone arise in these locations.

In males:
Cancers of the prostate and lungs make up 80% of the carcinomas that metastasize to bone.

In patients of both sexes: The remaining 20% of primary disease sites are the kidney, gut, and thyroid, as well as sites of unknown origin.

Pathophysiology

Following step explains the pathogenesis:

- Release of the neoplastic cell from the primary focus by degradative enzymes such as collageneases, hydrolases, cathepsin D.
- Invasion of vascular channels
- Dissemination of these neoplastic cells to tissues distant from source under the influence of local factors such as integrins, cadherins and laminins.
- Endothelial attachment and invasion of the new host.
- Growth of the original colony into the metastatic foci under the influence of tumour angiogenesis factor inducing neovascularization.

Clinical Features

- Pain (most common)
- 25% are painless and discovered accidently
- Pathological fracture
- Functional impairment

Investigation (Approach to Diagnosis)

Clinical Examination

Complete history and physical examination, including breast or prostate

Basic Laboratory Tests

- Complete blood cell count (CBC) with differential, red blood cell indices, and peripheral smear
- Erythrocyte sedimentation rate (ESR)
- Liver and renal profile
- Alkaline phosphatase (markedly elevated)
- Acidic phosphatase
- Serum protein electrophoresis (SPEP) and urinalysis, urine protein electrophoresis (UPEP)
- Prostate-specific antigen
- Urine: Bence Jones protein
- Serum electrolyte: Sodium, phosphorus, calcium (hypercalcaemia), potassium
- Blood sugar, urea and creatinine.

Imaging

- X-rays: Entire involved bone and a chest radiograph
    - Basic assessment of the degree of cortical erosion and the extent of a tumour
    - Chest radiograph: To rule out primary lung tumour or metastases
    - Skeletal survey in multiple myeloma
    - Lesions may be *lytic, blastic, or mixed.*
        - Breast cancer and prostate cancer typically produce blastic lesions.
        - Kidney cancer and thyroid cancer usually are purely lytic.
        - Lung cancer may produce a mixed appearance

- CT scanning: involved bone and of chest, abdomen, and pelvis
  - Best assessment of the extent of cortical destruction
  - Most sensitive imaging modality to detect bone destruction
- Technetium-99m (^{99m}Tc) bone scanning
  - Very sensitive to detect occult lesions and assess the biologic activity of lesions
  - Helps for an unknown primary site to identify any other lesions and to identify the lesion from which to obtain a biopsy
  - Indirect measure of destruction because it actually reflects the activity of osteoblasts
- Magnetic resonance imaging (MRI):
  - Most sensitive study to assess the anatomic (intramedullary and extra-osseous (extra-compartmental)) extent of a lesion
  - USG: Abdomen, thyroid/parathyroid
  - To assess the primary
- Angiography:
  - Essentially has been supplanted by MRI
  - Useful for the preoperative embolization of vascular lesions, such as renal cell carcinomas, thyroid metastases, and (occasionally) myelomas.

Biopsy

- To know the biological behavior of tumour and establish a firm relationship between the primary carcinoma and the suspected metastasis.
- Histological appearance of metastatic carcinoma usually is similar to the primary lesion

Management

Treatment of carcinoma metastatic to bone is multimodal.

General

- *Nutritional*: A nutritional deficiency may retard wound healing and the potential for rehabilitation. High protein and nutritional diet to improve the general condition of the patient.
- *Opioids/NSAIDs*: to relief pain
- *Haematologic*: haematinics, blood transfusion, transfusion of platelets and other factors especially to patients with myeloma, leucaemia, or metastatic carcinoma who have anaemia, thrombocytopenia, and leucopenia secondary to chronic disease and marrow replacement.
- *Broad-spectrum antibiotics*: to prevent infection in view of neutropenia
- *Proteins and coagulation factors*: in view of coagulopathy (liver disease)
- *Prophylaxis with heparin*: to prevent deep vein thrombosis (DVT) and pulmonary embolism
- *Hypercalcemia* is managed with hydration, bisphosphonates, and Mithramycin.
- *Counseling*: proper counseling of the patient and family members about the prognosis of the lesion. Their support boost the patient to fight against the dreadful pathology.

Specific Medical Care

- Chemotherapy: cytotoxic therapy
- Hormone manipulation may be beneficial for patients with breast or prostate cancer
- Radioactive iodine may be beneficial for some patients with metastatic thyroid cancer

- Bisphosphonates: Preventing new metastatic bone lesions and may slow the growth of existing lesions by inhibiting osteoclast resorption of bone.
- Radiation

Surgery

For impending or actual pathological fractures.

Indication for prophylactic internal fixation:
- Pain that has not responded to radiation treatment
- A lesion >2.5 cm
- A lesion that has destroyed > 50% of the cortex
- An avulsion fracture of the lesser trochanter

Mirels Devised a Scoring System

Evaluates the risk of pathological fracture based on:
- Site nature of the lesion
- Size nature of the lesion
- Lytic or blastic nature of the lesion

Variable	Score		
	1	2	3
Site	Upper limb	Lower limb	Peritrochanter
Pain	Mild	Moderate	Functional
Size	< 1/3	1/3–2/3	> 2/3
Lesion	Blastic	Mixed	Lytic

- Prophylactic internal fixation should be considered for any patient with a score of ≥ 8.

Fixation

- Fixation must be stable enough to allow immediate full weight bearing.
- Cavity can be filled with methacrylate (Bone cement) to augment the fixation.
- Lesions of the femoral neck should be considered for hemiarthroplasty or total hip arthroplasty with cementation.

Advantages of prophylactic fixation (compared to fixation after fracture occurs) follow:
- Decreased morbidity
- Shorter hospital stay
- Easier rehabilitation
- Pain relief
- Faster and less complicated surgery
- Decreased surgical blood loss

18

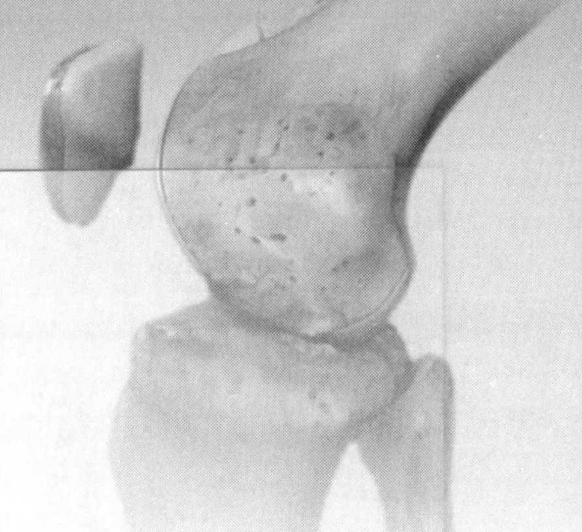

Amputation

Q1. Define amputations. Give indication and important points while doing an amputation.

Surgical removal of part or the whole limb and refashioning the mobile stump with intact sensation, fit for a prosthetic device and subsequent function.

Types

Open or Guillotine Amputation

Guillotine amputation is done in emergency for grossly crushed and infected limbs, all the tissues are cut at the same level and the stump left open with later revision to a more proximal level after the infection is under control and then treated by secondary management.

Closed Amputation

In planned closed amputation, proper flaps are designed and then skin, muscle and fascia followed by bone are cut stepwise and then closed over a drain.

Indications

The only absolute indication for amputation is irreversible ischaemia in a diseased or traumatized limb.

Dead Limb

- Severely crushed and devitalized.
- Irreparable vascular injury in an ischemic limb.

Dying Limb

- Peripheral vascular disease
- Diabetic foot
- Gangrene
- Buerger's disease

Infections

- Gas gangrene
- Madura foot
- Leprosy

Tumours

- Osteogenic sarcoma
- Ewing's sarcoma

Congenital

Deformed and useless limb.

Others

- Thermal or electrical injury to an extremity may necessitate amputation.
- Frostbite

Important Points while Doing an Amputation

Always give a chance of survival, take a second surgical opinion before amputation

While doing any amputation keep in mind the following:

- *Hemostasis:* Except in severely ischaemic limbs, the use of a tourniquet is highly desirable and makes the amputation easier.
- The *level* should be above the safe margin in tumours and vascular lesions, all the same good enough for prosthetic fitting.
- The *suture line* should be anterior or posterior.
- *Flaps* should be kept thick.
- *Unnecessary dissection* should be avoided to prevent further devascularization of already compromised tissues.
- Cut the *bone* and cover it with periosteal sleeve.
- The cut end of the bone should be rasped to form a smooth contour. This is especially important in locations such as the lateral aspect of the femur, anterior aspect of the tibia, and radial styloid.
- *Muscles* usually are divided at least 5 cm distal to the intended bone resection. They may be stabilized by *myodesis* (suturing muscle or tendon to bone) or by *myoplasty* (suturing muscle to periosteum or to fascia of opposing musculature).
- *Nerves* should be isolated, gently pulled distally into the wound, and divided cleanly with a sharp knife so that the cut end retracts well proximal to the level of bone resection (nerves, such as the sciatic nerve, often contain relatively large arteries and should be ligated before cutting.)
- Double ligate the *artery and vein* separately to avoid A-V fistula.
- In potentially *contaminated and crushed limbs*, it is preferable to debride and leave the wound open for secondary closure.
- Remove the *tourniquet* before closure and keep a closed suction drain, apply compression dressing.
- *Mobilize* the stump as early as possible and fit the prosthesis for early ambulation and rehabilitation.

Q2. Enumerate common sites of amputations.

Upper Limb

Fingers and Thumb

All possible lengths should be preserved.

Wrist

- Transcarpal amputation or disarticulation of the wrist is an excellent functional unit and does not require above elbow cuff.
- If done through the transcarpal zone, it provides flexion and extension of the stump.

Forearm

Forearm amputation should always be done at the junction of upper two-thirds and lower one-third, since rotation is preserved and cine plastic procedures can be done.

Krukenberg Operation/Amputation

- It converts the forearm to *forceps* in which the radial ray acts against the ulnar ray.
- It helpful in blind patients with bilateral amputation (provides both prehension and sensibility at the terminal parts of the limb).

Mid Arm

An ideal stump is 2″ proximal to the elbow, to allow the elbow lock mechanism and permit rotation with prosthesis.

Cineplastic Procedure

- This consists of creating a surgical canal through the muscle belly for insertion of a rod, which is connected to a cable.
- Contraction of the muscle belly provides the motor function for the cable attached to the distal part of the prosthesis.

Lower Limb

Amputation through the *toes/metatarsal* gives satisfactory results.

Lisfranc's

- Lisfranc's amputation is at the tarso-metatarsal joints.
- It is unacceptable because of the resulting inversion-equinus deformity.

Chopart's

- Tarsal amputation proximal to insertion of Tibialis anterior
- It results in equino-valgus deformity corrected by TA lengthening.

Syme's

- It consists of a bone section at the distal tibia and fibula 0.6 cm proximal to the periphery of the ankle joint and passing through the dome of the ankle centrally
- The heel flap is brought over the lower end of tibia forming an excellent end-bearing stump, but prosthetic fitting requires a bulk tissue, which is cosmetically not accepted.

Pirogoff Amputation

- Calcaneus is rotated forward to be fused to the tibia after vertical section through its middle
- Arthrodesis between the tibia and part of the calcaneus

- The calcaneus is sectioned vertically, its anterior part is removed, and its remaining posterior part and the heel flap are rotated forward and upward 90° until the raw surface of the calcaneus meets the denuded distal end of the tibia.

Through Leg

This requires about 6 inches or more of the tibia for an adequate prosthetic fit, preferably if the fibula is excised 3 cm proximal to the level of tibial resection. This is an excellent weight bearing stump.

Disarticulation of Knee

This is an excellent end-bearing stump in children as it preserves the growth plate in the distal femur and prosthetic fitting can be made easy by resecting the condylar flare.

Through Thigh

This is done 3 inches proximal to the knee joint and the closure is done either by tendoplasty (the patella is excised and the tendinous part of the quadriceps is sutured across the femoral stump) or myodesis (muscles are attached to the end of the bone providing a dynamic stump). This cylindrical stump is ideal for modern total contact prosthesis.

Hip Disarticulation

This is done in cases of malignant tumours of the bone and is best fitted with Canadian hip disarticulation prosthesis or an ischial weight bearing prosthesis.

> **Q3. What are the traditional sites for an ideal stump and enumerate the complications of amputations.**

The standard amputations are designed to be non-end bearing. The traditional site for ideal stumps is as follows:
- *Above knee*: 11 inches from the top of greater trochanter
- *Below knee*: 5½ inches below the tibial plateau
- *Above elbow*: 8 inches from the tip of acromian process
- *Below elbow*: 7 inches below the tip of olecranon process

Complications

- Infections leading to:
    - Secondary haemorrhage
    - Wound dehiscence
    - Osteomyelitis of the bony stump
    - Stump neuroma
    - Phantom limb
    - Contractures
    - Bony overgrowth in children
- Skin blisters ulceration and dermatitis

19

Imaging in Orthopaedics

Q1. Who Invented MRI?

Raymond Vahan Damadian invented the magnetic resonance imaging (MRI) scanner, which has revolutionized the filed of diagnostic medicine.

Q2. What is the principle of MRI?

MRI is based on the principle of nuclear magnetic resonance (NMR) discovered by Edward M. Purcell and Felix Bloch in 1946.

Mechanism

- Nuclei of elements with odd number of protons or neutrons (especially hydrogen, most prevalent in water molecule) have an intrinsic angular momentum termed as nuclear spin.
- When stimulated in strong magnetic field; causes the hydrogen nuclei to align parallel with the field.
- This alignment is disturbed (causes the hydrogen nuclei to enter in higher energy state) by a pulse of radiofrequency (RF).
- When the RF pulse is switched off, these nuclei gradually return to their original position (lower energy state), releasing small amount of energy in a process called relaxation. This energy is assayed (detected by sensitive MR coils) and converted to images.
- This process of relaxation is described in term of independent constant T_1 and T_2.

Q3. What is Signal Intensity (SE)?

Signal intensity characterize the brightness of tissue on an MR image.

On that basis Tissues may be classified as:
- High-intensity *(bright)*, intermediate-intensity *(grey)* or low intensity *(black)*. or
- *Hyper-intense, iso-intense, or hypo-intense* when signal intensity of tissue of a diseased process is described relative to the normal surrounding tissue.

SE depends on:
- T_1 *(longitudinal relaxation time)* of tissue under evaluation
- T_2 *(horizontal relaxation time)* of tissue under evaluation
- Proton density *(Number of mobile hydrogen ions)* of tissue under evaluation

Q4. Explain the difference between the T_1 and T_2 images?

T_1 *(longitudinal relaxation time)* and T_2 *(Horizontal relaxation time)* are elemental physical properties of tissues and based on response of the *hydrogen nuclei* to the radiofrequency pulse different tissue have different T_1 and T_2 properties.

T_1 and T_2 Images

T_1 Image	T_2 Image
TE (time to echo) 15–30 ms	TE (Time to echo) 60–120 ms
TR (time to repetition) 400–600 ms (<1000)	TR (Time to repetition) 1500–3000 ms (>1000)
Fat appears bright	Water or fluid appear bright (T_2 water white)
Excellent for evaluating structures containing *fat, proteinaceous fluid or haemorrhage*	Excellent for evaluating tissues with *higher water content (CSF, Cysts, Normal intervertebral disc)*
These images demonstrate well defined anatomical structures.	Most useful for contrasting normal and abnormal anatomy (pathological process)

Note:

- **TE: Time of echo**: *Time between the application of radiofrequency pulse and recording of the MR signals.*
- **TR: Time to repetition**: *Time between the RF pulses.*

General Funda

In **T1** water appear **dark**, whereas in T_2 water appears **white** (T_2 Water White)

Q5. Enumerate the uses of an MR image and discuss its advantage and disadvantages?

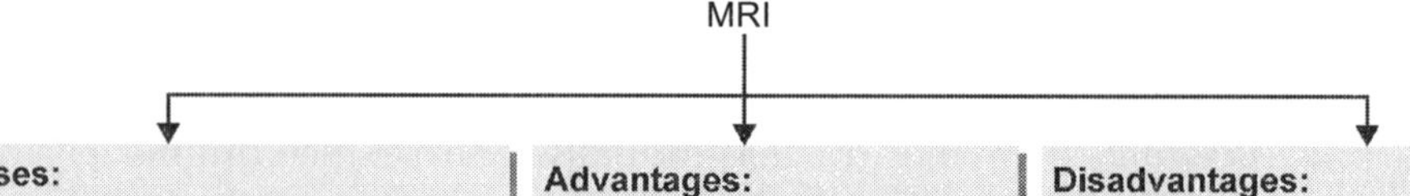

Uses:

For early and accurate diagnosis of:
- Spine and disc related disorders
- Osteonecrosis of femoral head.
- Assessment of tumours.
- Assessment of marrow changes.
- Internal derangement of knee, effusion.
- Articular and peri-articular structure visualization.
- Early detection of bone and joint infections especially in the spine.
- Neural status: spinal cord lesions.

Advantages:
- Non-invasive
- Avoid ionizing radiation (no radiation hazards)
- Multiplanar resolution
- Superior soft tissue contrast resolution.
- High degree of specificity and accuracy.
- Ability to detect disorders of non-osseous structures such as menisci, ligaments, articular cartilage.

Disadvantages:
- Expensive
- Time consuming
- Difficulty in patients suffering from claustrophobia
- Poor cortical outline or delineation
- Require expertise.
- Sophisticated equipment as well as sedation or anaesthesia in the infant or younger child for necessary immobilization.
- Hazards with implants, particularly pacemaker.
- Many life-support systems are incompatible with MRI equipments (difficult to manage the patient in acute trauma)

Q.6: What are the contraindications to obtaining an MR image?

Foreign elements/objects that can be affected by magnetic field constitute a contraindication to MRI.

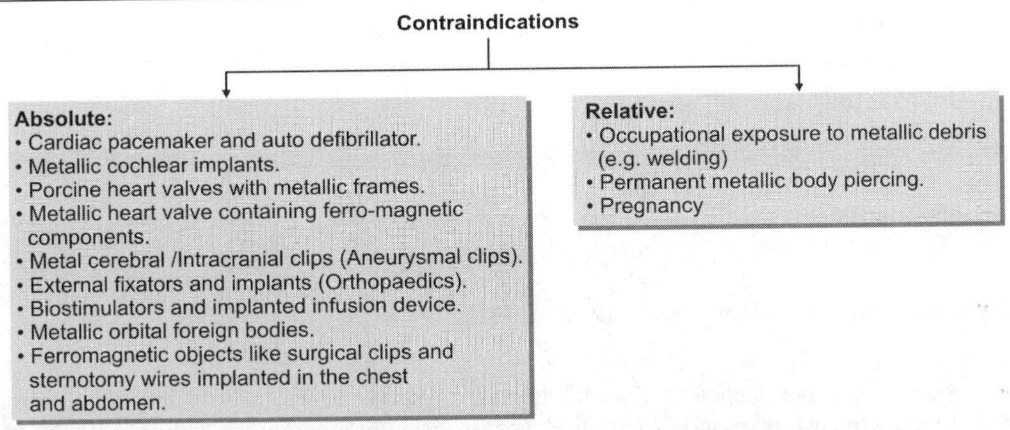

Note: Orthopedic surgeons nowadays favour *titanium implants* as titanium's nonmagnetic properties make it *compatible for use with an MRI* besides their strength and compatibility with body tissues.

Q7. Discuss the uses, advantage, and disadvantage of CT scan.

Invented by Godfrey Hounsfield in 1973.

- Technique of tomography involves moving the X-ray source and receptor around the body in relation to a point in body.
- The resulting film has the image of structures at that point.
- Using a computer, the matrix of data produced can be converted to an image in a plane.
- The clarity of image can be enhanced by using a filter and further by setting a window.
- The thickness of slices produced can be decreased to enhance the clarity.
- The density of a soft tissue mass or bone on a CT scan is called its "attenuation coefficient" and is measured in Hounsfield units (HU).

Uses

- To assess tumour size and spread.
- To diagnose spinal disorders, especially intervertebral disc prolapse, spinal canal stenosis.
- Joint abnormalities
- It is typically the first line of investigation for a pelvic mass.
- To assess intra-articular fractures.
- Assessment of complex fracture and fracture sites not accessible on plain X-ray, e.g. sacroiliac joints, vertebral bodies, carpal bones.
- To assess bone density with contrast media, enhanced and accurate image can be made.

Advantages

- Axial cuts reduce problems of anatomical superimposition.
- Greater radiographic density discrimination.
- 3D images can be built up with the help of advanced software and spiral CT angiography can be done with contrast.
- CT guided biopsies can be done with precision.
- By knowing the Hounsfield unit of a shadow, we may predict the nature of a tissue involved.

Disadvantages

- Radiation is high.
- Cannot do multiplanar imaging.
- Poorer soft tissue contrast.
- Prone for artifact in bony walled areas, e.g. spine.

CT imaging has no absolute contraindications. The relative contraindications are related to the radiation dosage.

Q8. Write short note on *Hounsfield units*.

There is an eventually *linear relationship between voxel signal intensity (image brightness) and X-ray linear attenuation coefficient* μ, which is scaled relative to air and water and converted to an integer. This is expressed in *Hounsfield units (H) with air having a value of* -1000*, water to a value of 0 (zero) and the most soft tissue (except fat) values of about 20–60 H.*

Some of the **more common tissue densities** to be encountered in practices.

On the Hounsfield (HU)

- *Air is* -1000 *and **dense bone** is* $+1000$ *HU.*
- *Normally,* -1000 *HU* is densely **black, while** $+1000$ is densely **white**, when viewed on the cathode ray tube, or film. The **rest** of the densities are seen to be various **shades of grey**.

Tissues	HU	Tissues	HU
Air	−1000	Grey matter (brain)	36–46
Fat	−100 to −50 HU	Clotted blood	60–80 HU
Water	0	Calcification	70–1000
CSF	0–3 HU	Muscle and soft tissue	40
White matter (brain)	22–32	bone	+ 1000

Q9. Discuss the principle uses, and advantage, disadvantage of Ultrasonography.

Principle

In *ultrasonography, the imaging modality is based on the piezoelectric effect.* This effect is based on the fact, that certain substances possess the *quality of conversion of electrical to sound energy, and vice versa.*

Important Features

- The most common substance used in medical ultrasonic is *lead zirconate titanate.*
- A disc of lead zirconate titanate is executed by means of two electrodes, which causes it to resonate the beam of ultrasound, which passes through the tissues.
- High frequency sound waves are produced by a transducer and the reflections from different tissue is recorded as echo.
- *Solids and fat are highly echogenic, while cysts are low echogenic.*

Probes

- The higher frequency probes (5–7.5 mHz) are less penetrating but they provide better resolutions.

- These are mainly used in paediatric scans and scans of small parts or superficial structures.
- For adult scans and for deeper structures the lower frequency probes are preferable (3-5 mHz)

Types

- *Linear*
- *Sector*
- *Arc*
- *Compound*
- *Radial*

Displays

- ***A scan*** *(Amplitude modulation): Vertical deflection*
- ***Beta scans*** *(Brightness modulation): Bright dots*
- *Time position **(M-mode)**: Used in echocardiography*
- *Real-time display:* **Dynamic display**

Uses

- Diagnosis of hip dysplasia in newborn.
- It helps in the accurate deposition of intra-articular injections and can also be used to guide the therapeutic extraction of deposits, e.g. calcium salts at the joints as is commonly seen in the shoulder joint in rotator cuff syndrome.
- Diagnosis of deep seated abscess, cysts and aneurysm.
- Evaluation of tendon and ligament pathologies.
- Quick and non-invasive modality of detecting DVT.
- To evaluate inflammation or inflammatory conditions: In such conditions as osteomyelitis, sub-periosteal inflammatory exudates/collections can be easily detected on ultrasound even before such changes can be appreciated on plain radiographs.
- Used to evaluate:
  - Fracture union and nonunion
  - Infection
  - Ligamentous injury
  - Nerve compression
  - Mechanical impingement caused by hardware.

Advantages

- Non-invasive
- No ionizing radiation
- Cheap
- Portable
- Painless, it does not require sedation

Q10. Write short note on: a. Radionuclide scans (scintigraphy); b. Bone densitometry dual energy X-ray absorptiometry (DEXA); c. Arthroscopy; d. X-rays; e. C-arm.

a. Radionuclide Scans (Scintigraphy)

- This technique based upon the relatively high uptake of the radioisotope in areas of bone with high mineral turnover. It reflects the metabolic process as well as the change in mineralization.
- This positive scan is seen before X-ray changes.
- It can indicate the presence of local infection in the same way as the presence of some metastatic or primary bone tumor.

Procedure

- For a bone scan, the patient is injected intravenously with a small amount of radioactive material such as 5–10 mCi of technetium-99m-MDP (diphosphonate) or HDP (phosphorous). It is then scanned with a gamma camera. The gamma camera detects record and display the activity within its total filed of view (~25 cm in diameter). The increases radioactivity is displayed either as a number of counts on a scale or pictorially as a 'Hot-spot' on a scintiscan (in multiple myeloma three is no hot spots).
- MDP is a phosphate derivative, which can exchange place with bone phosphate in regions of active bone growth, so anchoring the radioisotope to that specific region.

Phases (Triple Phase Bone Scan)

- With Tc99 m-HDP, images are obtained immediately:
    - I: After injection (flow phase)
    - II: At 15 min (blood pooling)
    - III: In 4 hours (bone imaging)
- *Cellulitis* shows up as increased activity in the first 2 phases, and there is little or diffuse increased in activity in the third phase.
- *Osteomyelitis* causes increased uptake in all three phases.

Isotopes

Common Isotopes used in Nuclear Medicine

Many isotopes nowadays used for bone scanning. Among all *Strontium (Sr85)*, which is pure gamma emitter and is taken up by bone in a similar fashion as calcium and more recently *Technetium (Tc99m)* have become popular.

The most commonly used *intravenous radionuclides* are:
- Technetium-99m (technetium-99m)
- Iodine-123 and 131
- Thallium-201
- Gallium-67
- Fluorine-18 Fluorodeoxyglucose
- Indium-111 labeled leukocytes

The most commonly used *gaseous/aerosol radionuclides* are:
- Xenon-133
- Krypton-81m
- Technetium-99m Technegas
- Technetium-99m DTPA

Uses

- Stress fractures
- *Infections:*
  - Osteomyelitis
  - Discitis
- *Tumor:*
  - Spine metastasis
  - Primary bone tumor
  - Skull tumor
- *Disease involving abnormal bone metabolism:*
  - Paget's disease
  - Hyperostosis frontalis interna

b. Bone Densitometry Dual Energy X-ray Absorptiometry (DEXA)

BMD is used to diagnose osteoporosis, and DEXA is the gold standard for screening density. DEXA uses two X-ray beams of different energy levels. The degree of attenuation is measured as the beam passes through the bone. The dual energy beams allow for soft tissue corrections resulting in bone mineral density.

- It can be done at multiple sites, usually two sites, the hip and wrist, are measured in combination for accurate diagnosis.
- It is measured in grams/cm^2.
- BMD is defined by:
  - *T-score*: This signifies patient's level compared to peak bone mass in normal young adults.
  - *Z-score*: This is patient's BMD compared to the peak bone mass in age/sex matched adults.

The WHO criteria define patient's bone density.

T-score: Value 1 is normal. Its value <1 leads to osteopenia. Between −1 and −2.5 is osteoporosis.

Advantages

- Quick
- Simple
- Non-invasive
- Minimal radiation exposure
- Inexpensive

Uses

- This is used for the screening of osteoporosis in-patient with risk factors.
- It is used for prediction of fractures.
- Confirmation of clinical diagnosis of osteoporosis.
- Determination of rate of bone loss for prognostic treatment of osteoporosis.
- For risk assessment of osteoporosis in perimenopausal women who are willing to take HRT.
- For monitoring the response to a particular mode of treatment of osteoporosis

c. Arthroscopy

Arthroscopy is an important tool for use in diagnosis and treatment of joint disorders.
- Arthroscopy offers distinct advantaged over open exploration of joints.
- The entire joint can be visualized and low morbidity of arthroscopy allows rapid rehabilitation.
- Arthroscopy is done for diagnostic examination of joint or for therapeutic surgical interventions.

Joints

- Common joints for arthroscopy are knee, shoulder, elbow, ankle, and wrist joint.
- The knee is the joint in which arthroscopy has its greatest diagnostic and intra-articular surgical application

System

- An arthroscope is an optical instrument.
- Fibre-optic arthroscope consist of a rod lens systems surrounded by multiple light conducting glass fibrils.
- These two systems are enclosed in a metal sheath.
- Lens is angled in the scope, usually with inclination of 25–90°.
- Diameter of arthroscope varies from 1.7 to 7.0 mm one end of the scope has eyepiece for viewing.
- A television camera can be attached to eyepiece for viewing on television set.
- Among the keys to success in arthroscopy are adequate *light, distentions of the joint and precise localization of the portals of entry* for the arthroscope and accessory instruments.

Indications

- Meniscal injuries
- Loose bodies
- Knee instability (cruciate and collateral ligaments)
- Selected tibial plateau fracture
- Patellar chondromalacia or malalignment
- Chronic synovitis
- Recurrent effusions
- Acute haemarthrosis
- Chondral and osteochondral fractures

d. X-rays

Medical X-rays for diagnostic imaging have been used for over a century, soon after the published discovery by *Roentgen* in 1895. These are a form of electromagnetic radiation, similar to visible light. Unlike light, however, X-rays have higher energy and can pass through most objects, including the body.

In a radiographic room there are few basic components to produce X-ray beams includes *tube, tube housing, generator, beam filtration system, and collimator.* The X-ray tube is the source of the X-ray beam.

X-rays are produced by firing electrons at high speed form cathode in an X-ray tube onto a positively charged rotating anode. A uniform X-ray beam incident on the patient interacts with the patient's soft tissues and bones *(depends upon their radiological density),* producing a variable transmitted X-ray flux casting what are effectively *'shadows'* which are displayed as images on an appropriately sensitized plate portions of the beam are attenuated. The more dense and impenetrable the tissue, the greater the X-ray attenuation and therefore the more blank, or white, the image that is captured. Thus, a metal implant appears intensely white, bone less so and soft tissues in varying shades of grey depending on their 'density'.

Uses

- Detects fractures
- Status of joints (arthritis)
- Certain tumors and other abnormal masses
- Calcifications
- Foreign objects (Implants)
- Dental problems

Limitations

- It involves exposure of the patient to ionizing radiation, which under can lead to radiation-induced cancer
- It provides poor soft-tissue contrast: For example, it fails to distinguish between muscles, tendons, ligaments and hyaline cartilage.

e. C-arm (Computer-assisted Radio Monitoring)

The intraoperative use of *C-arm fluoroscopy* in orthopaedics has become an important tool in the most orthopaedic procedures. It is a mobile digital unit to show real-time images (single still images or to continuously capture 25–30 images per second) in orthopaedic procedures. Prior to 1955, X-ray systems were unable to change direction. Philips therefore developed the first *C-arm, an X-ray system in the form of a half moon*. Doctors could now move the X-ray equipment in various directions. Since the C-arm is flexible, diagnoses can be made quicker and procedures can be performed faster, which is more comfortable for patients and surgeons.

The intraoperative use of C-arm uroscopy in orthopaedic surgical practice has become an important arsenal in most orthopaedic procedures. The intraoperative use of C-arm uroscopy in orthopaedic surgical practice has become an important arsenal in most orthopaedic procedure.

The intraoperative use of C-arm uoroscopy in orthopaedic surgical practice has become an important arsenal in most orthopaedic procedure.

Benefits

- Enhances the surgeon's expertise
- Ease of operative procedure
- Minimizes soft tissue trauma/devitalization
- Shortened operative time
- Decreased patient morbidity
- Documentation of intraoperative images
- Improved procedural outcome

Limitations

Radiation hazards to surgical team.

Gait, Orthosis/Prosthesis and Physical Therapy

Gait is rhythmic coordinated movement of the upper and lower limb in cyclic order balancing the pelvis and spine, helping the person in forward propagation.

Strides Characteristics

These are fundamental variables/data needed for gait analysis. Stride characteristics are sensitive indicators of diseases and disorders that primarily affects gait. These include velocity (speed), gait cycle, stride length, step length, single and double limb support, and swing and stance time.

Velocity (Speed)

- It is measure of forward progression of an individual centre of gravity, which is normally located midline and anterior to sacrum.
- It is expressed as meters/min.

Gait Cycle

- It is measured as number of seconds from the point of initial ground contact of one lower extremity to the point at which, same extremity touches the ground again.

Stride

It is the combination of two steps, i.e. right and left step, which is equivalent to one gait cycle.

Step Length

- Step length is the distance between the point of initial contact of one foot (heel strike) and the point of initial contact of the opposite foot (heel strike).
- In normal gait, right and left step lengths are similar.

Stride Length

- Stride length is the distance between successive points of initial contact of the same foot (i.e. heel strike of one foot to heel strike of same foot).
- Right and left stride lengths are normally equal.

Cadence or Walking Rate

- The number of step taken by the patient per unit of time is cadence.
- It is calculated in steps per minute.

Foot Angle or Degree of Toe out

Foot angle or toe out describes an angle between the line of progression and a line drawn between the midpoints of the calcaneus and the second metatarsal head.

Double Support Phase

- It is a phase when both feet are in contact with the ground.
- During normal gait, for a moment, the two lower extremities are in simultaneous contact with the ground. This happens between push off and toe off on one side and between heel strike and foot flat on the contralateral side. During this period, both legs support the body weight and this is known as *'double support'*.

Q2. Discuss gait cycle in brief.

A normal gait must be rhythmic and soundless, having springiness in the feet, which work alternatively in a definite cyclic order.

A normal gait cycle is divisible into two phases for each extremity.
- *Stance phase*, during this phase the foot is on the ground (60%).
- *Swing phase*, when the foot is off the ground (40%).

Classification

The stance and swing phase is divided into its subdivision under following classification:

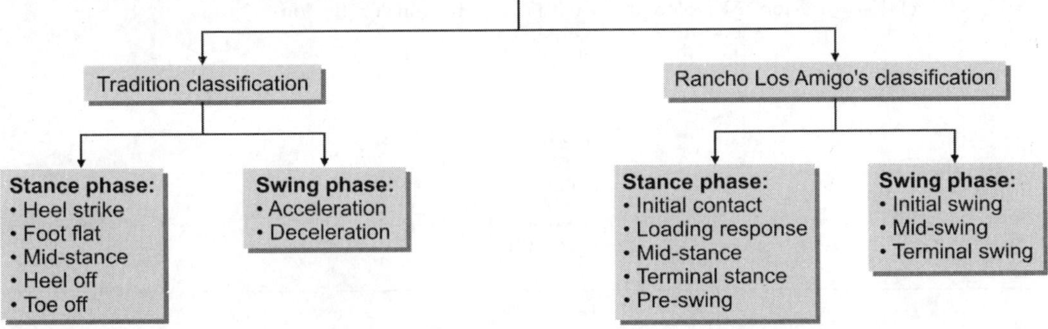

Traditional Classification

Stance Phase

- *Heel strike*: It is initiation of stance phase when heel is in contact with the surface or ground.
- *Foot flat*: When the sole of the foot comes in contact with the ground following heel strike.
- *Mid stance*: It is the point when body weight passes through the reference extremity.
- *Heel off*: In this phase heel of the reference extremity, leave the ground following mid stance.
- *Toe off*: During this phase, the toe of the reference extremity is in contact with the ground.

Swing Phase

- *Acceleration:* following toe off the toe leaves the ground to the point when the reference extremity is below the body.
- *Deceleration:* this is the end of the wing phase when the foot is preparing for heel strike.

Position of Various Joints in a Normal Gait Cycle

| Position of joint | Initial contact (heel strike) | Stance phase (60%) | | | Swing phase (40%) | | | |
		Loading response (flat foot)	Mid stance	Terminal stance (heel off)	Pre-swing (toe off)	Initial swing	Mid-swing	Terminal swing
Trunk	Erect neutral	Erect neutral	Erect neutral	Erect neutral	Erect neutral	Erect neutral	Erect neutral	Erect neutral
Pelvis	Level: maintains forward rotation	Level: less forward rotation	Level: neutral rotation	Level: backward rotation 5°	Level: backward rotation 5°	Level: backward rotation 5°	Level: neutral rotation	Level: forward rotation 5°
Hip	Flexion 30° Neutral rotation Abduction adduction	Rotation 30° Neutral rotation Abduction adduction	Extending to neutral Neutral rotation Abduction adduction	Apparent hyper-extension 10° Neutral rotation Abduction adduction	Neutral extension Neutral rotation Abduction adduction	Flexion 20° Neutral rotation Abduction adduction	Flexion 20–30° Neutral rotation Abduction adduction	Flexion 30° Neutral rotation Abduction adduction
Knee	Full extension	Flexion 15°	Extending to neutral	Full extension	Flexion 35°	Flexion 60°	Flexion 60–30°	Extension to 0°
Ankle	Neutral Heel first	Plantar flexion 15°	From plantar flexion to 10° dorsi flexion	Neutral with tibia stable and heel off prior to initial contact opposite foot	Plantar flexion 20°	Plantar flexion 10°	Neutral	Neutral
Toes	Neutral	Neutral	Neutral	Neutral IP Extended MP	Neutral IP	Neutral	Neutral	Neutral

Q3. Discuss briefly the different type of gait patterns.

There can be several variations in a normal gait depending upon the *weight, posture, the gymnastic activities,* the *shape of the foot* and the *ground over* which the individual walks. Everyone adapts the *least energy consuming* style of walking.

The lay description of abnormal gait can be divided into two patterns—*limping and lurching.*

- In *limping* the patient avoids weight bearing on the affected side as far as possible (diminished stance phase). Limping denotes a painful condition on the affected side.
- In *lurch,* the patient prolongs the stance phase to improve the stability. Lurching denotes variable failure of the abduction mechanism.

Recognized patterns of gait, which occur in particular conditions:

Scissor Gait

- It is due to spasm of adductor muscle spasm of hip joint.
- Here one leg crosses directly over the other with each step, like crossing of the blades of a scissor, e.g. cerebral palsy.

High-steppage Gait or Foot Drop Gait

- It is also known as slapping gait.
- It is due to weakness of dorsi-flexors of ankle joint.
- Here the patient flexes the hip and knee excessively in order to clear the ground, for example, foot drop.

Spastic Gait/Hemiplegic Gait

- Here the patient muscles do not allow the hip and knee to be flexed enough for the foot to clear the ground. Therefore, the patient partially drags his weight on the spastic leg.
- In this attempt, there is some circumduction effect on the lower limb, example hemiplegia for ground clearance.

Lathyric Gait

In this gait, there is a combination of spasticity, hyperabduction and dragging.

Waddling Gait/Duck Gait

There is increased lordosis; the body sways from side to side on a wide base. Therefore, the patient lurches on both sides while walking, e.g. bilateral congenital dislocation of hip, osteomalacia, pregnancy, myopathy.

Trendelenburg Gait

- It is also known as gluteus medius gait.
- It may be unilateral or bilateral.
- Bilateral Trendelenburg gait is almost like the waddling gait.
- When unilateral, the patient lurches on the affected side.
- In stance phase there is *"side ways dipping of shoulder"*.
- Any condition, in which there is *deficit in abduction mechanism* of the hip joint, e.g. CDH, polio paralysis.

Ataxic/Drunkards/Reeling Gait

- Here the patient tends to walk irregularly on a wide base, swinging sideways with tendency of falling with each step
- It is seen in cerebellar incoordination, or in drunkard state.

Festinating /Short Shifting Gait

- It is characterized by shortened stride, increase cadence, lack of heel strike and toe off and decreased arm swing.
- Here the patient with stooping body is propelled forward quickly in succession as if trying to catch up with the centre of gravity, e.g. parkinsonism.
- In a few cases of parkinsonism 'retropulsion' occurs, i.e. if the patient is pushed backwards, he starts walking backward involuntarily.

Antalgic Gait

- Painful gait.
- The patient adopts a lateral trunk displacement towards the involved joint in order to reduce the total joint force through the involved joint.
- Due to pain, the patient avoids weight bearing on the affected limb *(reduced stance phase)*.
- Commonly seen in patients following fracture or injury to lower limb.

Jack Knife Gait

- This is also known as gluteus maximus gait.
- It occurs due to paralysis/weakness of gluteus maximus (chief extensor of hip).
- In order to prevent the trunk from falling forward at the flexion of hip joint, the patient throws his trunk posteriorly at heel strike.

Stamping /Charcot's Gait

- The patient raises his feet abnormally high and jerks them forward to strike the ground with a stamp.
- Occurs in sensory ataxia, e.g. tabes dorsalis.

Knock Knee Gait

The gait here is also a typical one, i.e. *while walking*, the patient flexes the hip slightly, the knees point and oppose each other, the ankles and feet are kept apart with tendency of toe in.

Short Limb Gait

- It is due to limb length discrepancy.
- In stance phase there is vertical dipping of the shoulder (or excessive rise or fall of shoulder in vertical plane)
- Initially the shortening is made up by equinus, with more shortening; the patient dips his pelvis on that side.

Q4. What are characteristic an Ideal orthosis, prosthesis, and what are various steps in providing an orthotic or prosthetic device?

Characteristics of an Ideal Orthosis and Prosthesis

- Function (meets user's need, simple, easily learned)
- Strength
- Stiffness
- Durability (fatigue resistance)
- Density
- Corrosion resistance
- Ease of fabrication (fast, modular, readily widely available and take off, lightweight, adjustable)
- Cost (affordable, cost-effective)
- Availability
- Cosmesis (looks, smell, sound normal, easily cleaned, stain resistant)
- Comfort (fits well, easy to put on and take off, lightweight, adjustable)

Steps in Providing Prosthesis and Orthosis

- Step 1: Evaluation/prescription
- Step 2: Measurement/impression taking (plaster)
- Step 3: Fabrication/bench alignment
- Step 4: Fitting/static alignment
- Step 5: Modification/dynamic alignment
- Step 6: Re-evaluation/follow-up

Q5. Define an orthosis and discuss its uses.

It is an appliance, which is added to the patient, to enable better use to be made of that part of the body to which it is fitted.

It is a mechanical device to promote stability, relieve pain, control deformity and restrict movements, e.g. *axillary crutches, brace, cervical collar, calipers, surgical shoes.*

Functions of an Orthosis

- Provide stability
- Overcome weakness
- Relieve pain
- Controls deformity

Spinal Orthosis

Function

- Supportive and corrective
- To relieve pain
- To support weakened and paralyzed muscles and unstable joints
- To immobilize the spine (vertebral column) in functional position
- To prevent the occurrence of the deformity
- To correct an existing deformity

For cervical spine:
- Thomas collar
- SOMI (sterno-occipital-mandibular-immobilizer)
- Four-poster cervical collar
- Halo-body orthosis

For thoracic and lumbar spine:
- Taylor spinal brace
- Fischer spinal brace
- Thomas spinal brace
- Anterior hyperextension spinal brace (AHS brace)
- Moulded spinal brace

For cervico-thoracic and lumber spine:
- Milwaukee brace
- Boston brace

Lower limb orthosis:
Aim: To enable the patient to walk.

Function:
- Provide stability
- Relieve pain
- Control deformity
- Relieve weight bearing

Calipers

Weight relieving calipers (KAFO): The weight is transmitted from the ischial tuberosity to a padded ring through side metal bars and hence the ground.

Non-weight relieving calipers (KAFO):
- Here the body weight is not supported on a ring as in the weight relieving calipers.
- These types of caliper are mainly used to control deformity or to restrict the movement of the joints of the lower joints.

Hip Weakness

Pelvic band with hip joint: Provides rotational stability with significant mediolateral pelvic stability. This is essential for patients with weak abductors and in obese amputees.

Knee

- Quadriceps weakness-AK with anterior knee stop.
- Hamstrings weakness: AK with posterior knee stop.

Ankle

- Surgical shoes with caliper below knee (BK)
- Equinus: BK caliper with posterior knee stop.
- Calcaneus: BK caliper with anterior knee stop.

Subtalar

- *Valgus heel*: Outside iron with inside T-strap.
- *Varus heel*: Inside iron, outside T-strap.

Foot drop

- Static: Ortholene foot drop splint.
- Dynamic: BK with toe raising device/ spring.

Q6. Write short note on walking aids.

These are mechanical aids to support a weak part of the body to help it to perform its normal function.

Crutches

- This helps by aiding the lower limb during the stance phase of the locomotion by sharing the weight bearing.
- It may be used individually or as a pair.
- It consists of an axillary pad supported by two parallel bars connected by a handgrip and a non-slip rubber tip covering the lower end.

- It is measured from the anterior fold of the axilla to the heel of the foot to which 2 inches is added for the ground clearance or subtract 16 inches (41 cm) from the height of the patient.
- The handgrip should be approximately at the level of a greater trochanter to keep the elbow in 30° of flexion.
- It may be made up of wood, aluminium, or steel.

Elbow Crutch

This is a modified walking stick, which has a handgrip and a forearm cuff support to give it a wider area of contact for weight transmission through the elbow and forearm.

Walking Stick

- It is used for elderly patients and following lower limb injuries for partial weight bearing.
- It is usually bent at the level of the greater trochanter for handgrip. The tip is single, tripod or quadripod to give it a wider base.

Q7. Define prosthesis and mentions its types.

This is an artificial device designed to replace appearance/function of the part of the body, which has been removed, or it is a mechanical device that replaces the missing part of the body.

Types
Upper Limb

Above/below elbow and hand, this may be cosmetic or dynamic.

Lower Limb

I. HKAFO (Hip knee ankle foot prosthesis) for hip disarticulation
II. Above knee, prosthesis has:
- In young patient needs quadrilateral suction socket.
- In old patient: Total contact suction socket for old patients with pelvic band and hip joint. Suction thigh socket, (II) knee hinge, (III) tibial component with a distal, (IV) SACH foot (solid ankle and cushion heel) or a Jaipur foot.

III. *Below knee*, patellar tendon bearing prosthesis has a PTB total contact socket with SACH foot
IV. *Syme's prosthesis*: This is total contact socket to accommodate ankle and heel pad.

Q8. Discuss the comparison between Jaipur foot and SACH (Solid Ankle Cushion Heel) foot.

Characteristic	SACH foot	Jaipur foot (devised by Prof PK Sethi)
Appearance	• SACH foot does not look like a normal foot. • SACH foot requires a closed shoe to protect as well as hide it.	• It looks like a normal foot • There is no such need or requirement with Jaipur foot. But in case someone wants to wear a shoe, he can do it comfortably with a flat heel shoe

(Contd.)

Characteristic	SACH foot	Jaipur foot (devised by Prof PK Sethi)
Movements and activities of daily living	• Wooden Keel is long enough to trict/limit movements in all direc tion and what so ever movements take place, they occur at unnatural sites • Squatting is not possible with SACH foot, as it requires dorsi flexion at ankle joint, which due to its rigid keel is not possible • No cross-leg sitting is possible because it requires adduction at forefoot and transverse rotation of foot in relation to shank. • As there is almost no movement at sub-tarsal joint inversion or eversion is not possible; so SACH Foot is suitable only for walking on level ground walking on uneven grounds and rough terrain is very uncomfortable • Bare-foot walking is not possible • As no transverse rotation of the foot in relation to leg is possible, the amplified uneven ground reaction while walking on uneven ground and rough terrain is transmitted over the stump, so great discomfort is complained by amputees	• Metallic keel (carriage bolt) is confined to ankle only. Therefore, no restriction of movement and all the movements take place at natural sites • Squatting is easily achieved; as a sufficient range of dorsiflexion is attainable comfortably • Cross-legged sitting is possible because sufficient forefoot adduction and transverse rotation of foot in relation to shank is available • As there is adequate inversion and eversion at sub-tarsal level, so walking on uneven ground and rough terrain is very comfortable • Bare-foot walking is possible • As transverse rotation of foot in relation to leg is possible, no complaint of discomfort while walking on uneven ground
Availability of material and cost	• Stern training and skills are required to fabricate SACH foot • Raw material for fabrications is not locally available (in many parts of world) • It is costly and unavailability of the material further adds to the cost	• Requires very little training to fabricate • Raw material for fabrication is locally available • It is very economical
Financial advantage	• 8000 US $	• 35 US $
Fitment time	• 3 months	• 1 hours

It is a temporary prosthesis. A temporary prosthesis consists of the *socket, pylon, and foot.*
• The *pylon* is the component between the socket and foot.
• It provides a central support around which is built up the prosthesis with or without cosmetic cover on pylon.
• An exoskeleton pylon has a rigid exterior, known as a crustacean shank.
• The endoskeletal, modular, pylon have a central support and have shock absorbing mechanism.
• Shock-absorbing pylons compresses to absorbs the vertical shock in early stance phase and in push off phase they rebound to improve propulsion. This provides protection to

the residual limb from injury, particularly if the skin is fragile and the joints are arthritic.

Advantage

- It is used for 3–6 months following the date of amputation.
- Provide morale and psychological support to the patient.
- It allows early ambulation and promotes residual limb shrinkage.
- Its use enables the wearer to weight bear and significantly reduces oedema.
- It may be converted to a definitive or final prosthesis with necessary cosmetics modifications.

Q10. Discuss in brief: a. TENS; b. Short wave diathermy; c. Microwave diathermy; d. Cryotherapy.

a. TENS (Transcutaneous Electrical Nerve Stimulation)

Based on the Gate control theory (Melzack and Wall) of pain, TENS produces pain relief by inhibiting the passage of sensory inflow to the cortex. TENS also decreases pain by endorphin production. The currently proposed mechanisms by which TENS produces neuromodulation include the following:

- Pre-synaptic inhibition in the dorsal horn of the spinal cord
- Endogenous pain control (via endorphins, enkephalins, and dynorphins)
- Direct inhibition of an abnormally excited nerve
- Restoration of afferent input.

Uses

- Peripheral nerve injuries
- Entrapment neuropathy like carpal tunnel syndrome
- RSD (reflex sympathetic dystrophy)
- Phantom pain
- Brachialgia (avulsion injury)
- Postherpetic neuralgia
- Postoperative pain

Contraindications

- Epilepsy
- Anesthetic skin
- Cardiac pacemaker
- First three month of pregnancy
- Haemorrhage
- Cardiac diseases

b. Short Wave Diathermy (SWD):

Principle

The heating effects of diathermy are produced by placing the patient within an electric field created by high frequency AC current having wavelength of 3–30 m, in which the patient forms the part of the secondary circuit of a high frequency generator.

Physiological Effects

SWD produce deep heating directly in the tissues of body. Hyperaemia, sedation, and analgesia are the basic physiologic effects. The reduction in muscle spasm due to muscle relaxation is a result of increased vascular supply to the treated area

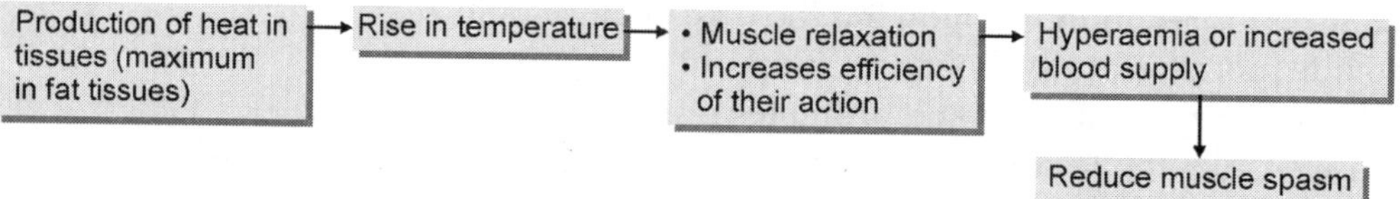

Uses

The following problems can be treated with short-wave diathermy, depending upon the individual condition of each patient and the desired treatment goals:
- Localized musculoskeletal pain
- Inflammation (joint or tissue)
- Pain/spasm
- Sprains/strains
- Tendinitis
- Tenosynovitis
- Bursitis
- Rheumatoid arthritis
- Periostitis
- Capsulitis

Contraindications

Short-wave diathermy (SWD) has the following precautions or contraindications:
- Malignancy
- Sensory loss
- Tuberculosis
- Metallic implants or foreign bodies
- Pregnancy
- Application over moist dressings
- Ischaemic areas or arteriosclerosis
- Thromboangiitis obliterans
- Phlebitis
- Use extreme care with paediatric and geriatric patients
- Cardiac pacemakers
- Contact lenses
- Metal-containing intrauterine contraceptive devices
- Metal in contact with skin (e.g. watches, belt buckles, jewellery)
- Use over epiphyseal areas of developing bone

c. Microwave Diathermy

It has a shorter wavelength than short-wave diathermy. The microwave has an antenna or director, which beams energy that is both absorbed and reflected.

Physiological Effects

- Microwave diathermy, a form of electromagnetic radiation, is another deep heat modality that selectively heats tissues with high water concentration.
- *Hyperaemia, sedation*, and *analgesia* are the physiologic effects, similar to the results of shortwave diathermy.
- Secondary local vascular dilatation results in increased local metabolism.

Frequencies

- The two frequencies designated for microwave diathermy are *2456 MHz* and *915 MHz*, the latter being the most commonly used.
- The lower frequency is preferred because it provides selective heat deep into muscle, and less energy is converted to heat in the subcutaneous fat.

Uses

- More useful in localized conditions.
- Traumatic or inflammatory pain
- Pain/spasm
- Sprains/strains
- Tendinitis
- Tenosynovitis
- Bursitis

Contraindications

- Malignancy
- Sensory loss
- Paralytic patient
- Tuberculosis
- Metallic implants or foreign bodies
- Pregnancy
- Ischemic areas or arteriosclerosis
- Thromboangiitis obliterans
- Phlebitis
- Use extreme care with pediatric and geriatric patients
- Cardiac pacemakers
- Contact lenses
- Metal-containing intrauterine contraceptive devices
- Metal in contact with skin (e.g. watches, belt buckles, jewellery)

d. Cryotherapy

It is application of cold to tissues, resulting in the cooling of the injured part by the transfer of heat energy from the part to the cooling medium.

Method of administration of cryotherapy:

- Ice massage
- Immersion
- Ice packs

- Evaporation cooling
- Application of cooling agents such as ice, gel, chemicals, Freon.

Physiological Effects

- Reduction in swelling and inflammation (due to rapid vasoconstriction → decrease circulation → decrease swelling and inflammation)
- Reduction in pain
- Reduction in spasm due to pain reduction
- Limiting the extent of initial injury.

Therapeutic Uses

- As a first-aid measure to produce vasoconstriction.
- To reduce pain
- To reduce and prevent oedema
- To reduce spasticity
- Soft tissue injures like strain, sprain and contusion
- To produce a temporary anaesthetic effect.

Contraindications

- Circulatory disorders—coronary heart disease
- Allergy to cold
- External haemorrhage.

Q11. Write short note on: a. Ultrasound; b. Interferential therapy; c. infra-red rays.

a. Ultrasound

Principle

Therapeutic ultrasound is a physical agent with its effect being due to heating and mechanical phenomenon within the tissues. Ultrasound energy is generated by the piezoelectric effect; electrical energy is applied to a crystal (lead zinconate titanate), causing it to vibrate at a high frequency and to produce ultrasound.

Frequencies

- Ultrasound is a deep heating modality that uses high-frequency acoustic vibration above the human audible spectrum, defined as frequencies >17,000 Hz.
- Therapeutic ultrasound is in the frequency range of 0.8–1.0 MHz
- Ultrasound is delivered by continuous or pulsed wave (the goal is to produce non-thermal effects such as streaming and cavitation) and provides a high heating.

Biological Effects

Therapeutic ultrasound causes the following biologic effects:
- Temporary analgesia
- Increased peripheral blood flow
- Increased vascularity with associated hyperemia/inflammatory response

- Increased cell membrane permeability
- Peripheral nerve conduction changes (reversible conduction block with high intensity ultrasound exposure)
- Relief of muscle spasms

Uses

- Rheumatology and traumatology
- Chronic indurated oedema
- Capsulitis
- Myalgia
- Epicondylitis
- Sprains
- Tendinitis
- Joint contracture
- Joint adhesions
- Calcific bursitis
- Hematoma resolution
- Radicular neuropathy: lumbago, sciatica
- Ankylosing spondylitis (early stages)

Contraindications

- Sensory loss
- Thrombophlebitis
- Malignancy
- Acute pathology·
- Tuberculosis
- Active infection
- Intra-tissue prosthetic metal implants
- Vascular deficit

b. Interferential Therapy

It is the application of two medium frequency currents to the tissues. The interference produced by two currents in the tissue is called beat frequency and this is the principle of therapy.

It is possible to produce any desired frequency by varying the frequency difference of the carrier current.

Physiological effects

Muscle stimulation $\rightarrow\uparrow$ blood supply $\rightarrow$ reduces swelling, relieve pain! improves cellular functions and induce healing

Advantages

- Localized effect; unnecessary irritation of the skin is avoided
- It can be used for pain relief as well as for muscle stimulation.

Uses

- Arthritis
- Rheumatism

- Postoperative pain conditions (as metal is not the contraindication)
- Sprain
- Sports injury
- Neuralgia
- Neuritis
- Soft tissue injury

Contraindications

- Avoid on infants and children
- Avoid its use over eyes
- Sensory loss

c. Infrared Rays

Infrared rays are electromagnetic waves, the heat energy obtained from the rays are used to relieve pain.

Uses

- Pain
- Muscle strain and pain

Contraindication

- Defective blood supply to the area, e.g. in case of diabetes
- Any blood loss
- Defective skin sensation (nerve damage)

Q12. Write in short: a) Isotonic exercise, b) Isometric exercise.

a. Isotonic Exercise

- These are heavy, slow, concentric and eccentric resistance training
- It is a form of resistance training
- It is performed using free weights to strengthen a specific muscle area
- Static weight is used to maintain muscle tension during the action. This in-turn affects the muscle, expanding the muscle fibres and increasing the pounds of weight that the muscle can lift
- Isotonic contraction: (constant tension in the contraction as the muscle length changes).
- Isotonic contraction broadly classified into two types: *concentric and eccentric.*
- Concentric contractions cause the muscular tension to increase in response to resistance, and then stabilize as the muscle shortens.
- Eccentric contraction causes the muscle to lengthen as the resistance exceeds the force produced by the muscle.
- Isotonic training consists of both eccentric and concentric exercises
- These exercise intended to increase muscle strength and endurance.

b. Isometric Exercises

- Isometric exercise (skeletal muscle contraction without shortening)
- Also known as *static exercises* and are performed by increasing tension in a muscle while keeping its *length constant*

- Isometric muscle contraction: No change in muscle length during contraction
- These exercises do not require any equipment and provides an eccentric stimulus using bodyweight.
- Isometric strengthening is somewhat joint angle specific
- Isometric exercises improve muscle strength at other angles by 10–50% and have the most effect when performed with the muscle in a lengthened rather than a shortened position.
- Isometric training is gentle on the joints, while maintaining and increasing strength
- It is ideal for individuals who require low-impact exercise due to an arthritic condition or injury
- These exercises build muscle mass, strength, and bone density, while reducing cholesterol and improving digestion.

21

Plaster of Paris, Splints and Traction

The name *plaster of Paris* originated from an accident to a house built on deposits of gypsum salt, in Paris. The house burnt down and when rain fell, it was noted that footprint in the mud set rock-hard. This led to the rediscovery of method of heating gypsum salt to make smooth walls. When Hennery III visited Paris, he appreciated the smooth lustrous whiteness of the walls and popularized the use of plaster of Paris in England.

Chemistry

- Plaster of Paris is made from gypsum, a naturally occurring material.
- To make plaster of Paris, gypsum salt is heated to drive off water. When water is added to the resultant form, the original mineral reforms and heat is released.

$$2(CaSO_4 \cdot 2H_2O) + Heat \leftrightarrow 2(CaSO_4 \cdot \tfrac{1}{2}H_2O) + 3H_2O$$

| Calcium sulphate dihydrate | Calcium sulphate semi-hydrate | Water |

POP-bandages

- A Dutch military surgeon Antonius Matthysen from Paris first used these POP-bandages.
- The material used is semi-hydrated calcium sulphate powder finely sprayed over gauze bandages stiffened by starch or dextrose.

Application of POP Bandages

- On immersion in water, it undergoes an exothermic reaction and starts setting into a solid structure.
- The speed of setting depends on the material used, temperature of water and humidity.
- It is always advisable to apply a fair amount of cotton padding and stockinet before applying a cast to avoid compartmental syndrome or skin damage.
- It can be used as a *slab*, which is a support-encircling half or three-fourths of the limb, or as a *cast*, which requires a circumferential application of the bandages around the limb and then shaped and contoured before its sets.

Instructions to the patients after application of cast:

- Elevate the limb
- Encourage active finger/toe movements
- Avoiding wetting of plaster
- Immediately report to the doctor in event of:
  - Excruciating pain in the limb

– Progressive oedema over the finger/ toes
– Numbness, tingling, pale and cyanotic changes in the fingers
– Paralysis or painful finger movements

Q2. What are the advantages and disadvantages of using plaster of Paris bandages.

Plaster of Paris bandages have following advantages and disadvantages:

Advantages

- Easy available
- Durable
- Cheap
- Strong
- Simple to apply
- Radio-translucent
- Non-inflammable
- Material requiring very little apparatus for application
- It can be used anywhere, anytime and in any part of the body

Disadvantages/Complications

- Oedema due to tight plasters and even causing compartmental syndrome
- Circulatory embarrassment (impairment of circulation)
- Pressure sores
- Dermatitis
- Skin blisters
- Nerve palsy
- Deep vein thrombosis
- Stiffness of joints
- Sudeck's atrophy
- Osteoporosis
- Disuse atrophy of muscles

Contraindication

- Anaesthetic limb
- Severe skin dermatitis
- Trophic ulcers
- Circulatory embarrassment
- Non-compliant patient

Q3. What properties should make any casting material an ideal one?

An ideal casting should have the following properties:
- It should be suitable for direct application to the patient.
- Easy to mould
- It should be non-toxic (both to patient and to user)

- It should be unaffected by fluids such as water
- It should be transparent to X-rays
- Easy to setting and be quick setting
- Easy to remove
- It should have Superior mouldability and flexibility
- It should be able to transmit air, odour, water and pus
- It should be strong but light in weight
- It should be non-inflammable
- It should be cheap

Q4. What is traction and countertraction?

When a limb is painful as a result of fracture of bones or any inflammatory pathology of joint, the controlling muscles (*agonist and antagonistic*) go into spasm and more powerful muscle will result in deformity that seriously hampered the function of limb.

Traction

- *Traction* is application of mechanical forces to counteract the deforming forces of an inflamed, injured, diseased or deformed part of the body, against counter-traction
- Traction, when applied to injured limb overcomes the effect of deforming forces (*muscle spasm, gravity*) and by doing this it can relieve pain and allow the patient's limb to be rested in the best possible functional position.
- It allows constant controlled force for initial stabilization of long bone fractures and help in reduction during surgical procedures.
- The option for skin versus skeletal traction is case dependent.

Countertraction

- A traction force applied to the affected part of the limb will overcome muscle spasm only if another force acting in opposite direction. This opposite force is *counter-traction*.
- If countertraction force is not applied, the body will be pulled in the direction of the traction force and as a result, the muscle spasm will not be overcome.

Q5. What is fixed and sliding traction.

- *Fixed traction*: When counter-traction acts through an appliance or fixed point, which obtains a purchase on a part of body, the arrangement is called fixed traction.
- *Sliding traction*: When gravity is utilized to provide counter traction force just by tilting the bed so that the patient tends to slide in the opposite direction to that of the traction force or when the weight of all or part of body, acting under the influence of gravity, is used to provide counter-traction, the arrangement is called sliding traction.

Q6. What is skin traction and discuss its complication.

Traction force is applied over a large area of skin. It is applied through adhesive or non-adhesive plaster bandaged to the part distal to the deformed or injured part. The maximum of 15 pounds (6.7 kg) can be applied.

Type

- Adhesive
- *Non-adhesive*: These are useful on thin or atrophic skin, or when there is sensitivity to adhesive strapping

Contraindications

- Abrasions
- Lacerations
- Impaired circulation (varicose ulcers, impending gangrene)
- Dermatitis
- Marked shortening (weight required will greater than can be applied through the skin)

Complications

- Allergic reaction
- Excoriation of the skin
- Pressure sores around the bony prominence (malleoli) and over the tendocalcenus
- Common Peroneal Nerve palsy

Q7. What is skeletal traction and discuss its application.

Through a metal wire or pin, the traction force is applied directly to the skeleton. It is indicated when heavy traction has to be applied, the skin condition is unhealthy and needs frequent monitoring.

Devices Through which Skeletal Traction Applied

Steinmann Pin

Rigid stainless steel pin of varying length, 4–6 mm in diameter.

Denham Pin

- Similar to Steinmann pin except the raised threaded length in the middle
- Threaded portion engages the bony cortex and reduces the risk of pin sliding.
- Particularly suitable for:
  - Cancellous bone (calcaneus)
  - Osteoporotic bone

K or Kirschner Wire

- Most often used in the upper limb, e.g. olecranon traction.
- These are easy to insert
- Minimize the chance of soft tissue damage or infection.

Uses

- It is used frequently in the management of lower limb fractures.
- It may be employed as a means of reducing or of maintaining the fracture in reduced state.
- It can applied to the conditions where skin traction is contraindicated

Complications

- Introduction of infection into bone.
- Damage to neurovascular structures
- Incorrect placement may causes:
  - Failure of traction system

    – Cut out of bone causing pain
    – Results in uneven pull
    – Make application of splint difficult
    – Control of rotation of limb is difficult
- Distraction at the fracture site leading to non-union.
- Ligamentous damage (if large traction is applied for prolonged time).
- Damage to the epiphyseal growth plate (especially in children).
- Depressed scar.

Q8. Discuss common site of application of skeletal traction.

The common sites of application of skeletal traction are as follows.

Olecranon

- Site: 3 cm distal to the tip of olecranon to avoid the elbow joint
- Direction of pin insertion: medial to lateral to avoid injury to ulnar nerve.

Second and Third Metacarpals

Point of insertion: 2–2.5 cm proximal to the distal end second metacarpal.

Upper End of Femur (Greater Trochanter)

Point of entry: is on lateral surface; 2.5 cm below the most prominent part of greater trochanter, mid-way between the anterior and posterior surface.

Lower End of Femur

- Point of insertion: Just proximal to the upper limit of the lateral condyle about 3 cm proximal to the joint line.
- Direction: Lateral to the medial (or vice versa as in literature)
- Care: Avoid injury to the femoral artery; To avoid entering the knee joint

Disadvantages

Predisposes to knee stiffness so lower femoral pin; must be removed after 2–3 weeks and replaced by one through the proximal tibia.

Upper End of Tibia

- Point of insertion: 2.0 cm behind the crest, just below the level of the tubercle of tibia
- Direction: from lateral to medial side to avoid damage to common peroneal nerve.

Lower End Tibia

Point of insertion: It is 5.0 cm above the level of ankle joint, mid-way between the anterior and posterior borders of tibia.

Calcaneus

Point of insertion: 2.0 cm below and behind the lateral malleolus or 3.0 cm below and behind the medial malleolus.

Q9. Give advantages and disadvantage of using traction.

Goal of applying traction is to relieve the muscle spasm and hence deformity.

Advantages

- It maintains length of a limb, alignment and stability at the fracture site.
- It allows joint movement   and maintains the joint space.
- It can overcome muscle spasm and pain associated with bone or joint disease.
- Oedema is reduced in an extremity by a traction unit that elevates the affected part above the heart.
- Correction of soft tissue contractures by pulling them gradually.
- Correction of deformity.

Disadvantages

- Costly in terms of hospital stay
- Hazards of prolonged bed rest
  - Thromboembolism
  - Decubiti
  - Pneumonia
- Requires meticulous nursing care
- Sometimes it can develop contractures

Q10. Enumerate various types of splint and their uses.

Splints

Name	Use
Thomas splint	Fracture femur
Bohler–Braun splint	Fracture femur
Aluminium splint	Immobilization of fingers
Denis-Browne splint	CTEV
Toe-raising	Foot drop
Volkmann's splint	Volkmann's ischaemic contracture
Aeroplane splint	Brachial plexus injury
Cock-up splint	Radial nerve palsy
Knuckle bender splint	Ulnar nerve palsy
von Rosen splint	CDH

Q11. Write short note on: a. Thomas splint, b. Braun's splint, c. Cramer wire splint, d. Dennis-Browne hip splint.

a. Thomas Splint

Thomas splint was described by Hugh Owen Thomas as a knee appliance which he initially used for ambulant management of subacute or chronic (TB) of knee joint.

Uses

- For all types of injuries involving the lower limb
- Dislocation of hip

- Trochanteric fractures
- Tibial injuries

Components
Thigh Ring

- Oval metal ring to which are attached sidebars.
- The ring is inclined at an angle of 120° to the inside bar

Two Sidebars

- Sidebars are of unequal length
- The outer bar is angled by about two inches (5 cm) for trochanteric clearance.
- These bars joined together at the distal end to form "W"

Measurement

The splint is measured as:
- Ring diameter equaling the thigh girth in line of the inguinal ligament (oblique circumference of thigh just below the gluteal fold and ischial tuberosity) plus two inches added to it for cotton padding/to accommodate swelling.
- The length of the splint is measured from the groin (crotch) to heal and six inches added to it for the traction and spreader kit.

For knee mobilization during traction: Pearson's knee attachment is a modified Thomas splint, which has a knee joint for flexion in traction to mobilize the knee during the period of immobilization.

Advantage

Both skeletal as well as skin traction can be applied through this frame.

b. Braun's Splint

- This is used for injuries involving the femur and tibia including knee and ankle injuries for application of skeletal traction.
- It has a basic frame for support of the thigh and leg with a pulley for traction.
- This is an excellent splint for immobilization, elevation and traction for injuries of the lower limb.
- **Bohler's** modification of Braun's splint has additional overhead three pulleys:
  - For femoral, supracondylar traction
  - For upper tibial pin traction
  - Foot drop support traction
- **Problems:**
  - Makes nursing care difficult
  - It is a heavy cumbersome frame
  - May cause deformity at fracture site (especially in the cases of supracondylar fracture of femur) as: distal fracture fragment and limb is immobile relative to proximal fragment and body of the patient together so always support at the fracture site and not at the knee joint to prevent angulation.

c. Cramer wire splint

Friedrich Cramer (1847–1903) is noted for the development of a malleable wire ladder splint. This is a very light weight, versatile and malleable support and can be used for supporting injured limbs for temporary immobilization during transport of the patient pending final stabilization.

Components

It consists of two thick parallel wires with fine interlacing wires.

Use

Temporary stabilization (temporary immobilizer) of fracture during transportation (especially during emergency situation)

Advantages

- Malleable and fits all sizes and shapes of limbs.
- It can be autoclaved

Disadvantages

- It does not provide rigid immobilization
- It casts radio-opaque shadow on X-rays.

d. Dennis-Browne splint

It is a type of *static splint* and keeps the hips in *abduction and flexion (hip abduction brace)*. It is used in the management of *developmental dysplasia of hip or congenital dislocation of the hip*. If the condition is diagnosed soon after the birth, the splint is retained for about twelve weeks. In cases of older child, it is retained until there is radiological evident of adequate acetabulum development and congruity of femoral epiphysis in the acetabulum.

Components

- Strong metal bar to which two thigh bands are attached and position of these bands can be altered.
- The thigh bands are fastened over the child's thighs either by straps and buckles
- A waterproof pad, on which the child's sacrum rests, is attached to the centre of the bar between the thigh bands.

Advantages

- The splint does not have to be removed to keep the child clean
- Early recognition of unstable hip reduction

Disadvantage

They seem to have a higher rate of complications like avascular necrosis (AVN), femoral nerve palsy

Q12. Write short note on bone cement.

Chemically bone cement is poly methyl methacrylate (PMMA).

This is used as:

- Space filler in bone cavities after curettage of tumours.
- Load transferring when used along with the implants THR, TKR for cementing the implant and greater area contact at the bone-implant interface.

Components

It has two components:

Polymer powder containing:

- PMMA grains 10–150 microns—89%
- Radiopaque barium sulphate—10%
- Polymerization initiator—1% (benzyl peroxide)
- Stabilizer: Hydroquinone, ascorbic acid

Liquid monomer containing:

- Methyl methacrylate
- Activator 3% DMP toluidine

Chemical reaction:

- When these two components are mixed there is an exothermic reaction
- Components mixing occur in three different phases: "Dough time"; "Working time" and "Setting time".
- Within 2–3 minutes, it forms uniform dough (Dough time :uniform dough; does not stick to the non-powered surgical gloves)
- This is then filled (working time: 5–8 minutes) at the desired space (finger packing or Cement gun usage)
- If used with an implant, this is pressed for the next few minutes (setting time: sum of dough and working time; average is 8–10 minutes) till it becomes hard.

Mixed with antibiotics:

- Antibiotics can be added while mixing the two components.
- Antibiotic used: thermostable and well-eluted antibiotic like aminoglycosides, penicillins, cephalosporins, and clindamycin.

Precautions

- It is very important to lavage away all the bony debris and blood by thorough saline irrigation, before putting in the cement and hold the implant steady and well pressed while the cement is setting.
- Watch for hypotension during cement application.

Instruments and Implants

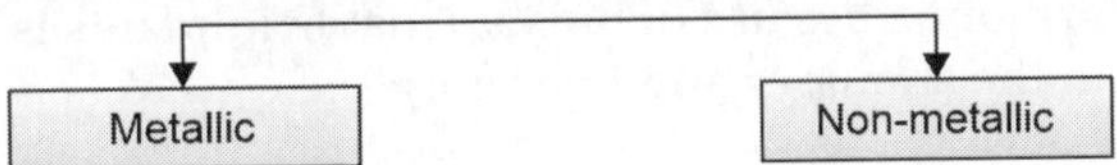

Material used in making implants can be divided into:

```
                    Metallic              Non-metallic
```

Metals

- They are strong, ductile and biocompatible.
- Metals used in making implants are generally alloys of various metals.
- Purpose of using alloys: Carbon decreases corrosion and lowers freezing point.
- Nickel is a stabilizer, chromium increases corrosion resistance, molybdenum being antichloride increases corrosion resistance, iron increases fatigue strength and toughness.
- Common alloys:

Steel	Cobalt based alloys	Titanium Based Alloys
Steel: Steel is iron and carbon. If to this, chromium, nickel and molybdenum are added, it becomes stainless steel. The modulus of elasticity of stainless steel is 12 times that of cortical bone. **Most common alloy:** 316L stainless steel	• Cast vitallium: Co, Cr, Ni, Mo. *Superior corrosion resistance, biocompatible, tough and strong but very expensive.* **Wrought vitallium:** Co, Cr, Ni, and Tungsten • *Extremely strong, can be machined but very expensive and high local disintegration.*	Ti (90%), Al (6%), Vanadium (4%) are excellent corrosion resistant but not so strong. **Disadvantages:** • High coefficient of friction • Low wear resistance makes it a poor material for joint surface. Most common alloy: Ti-6Al-4V

Non-metallic Materials

- *Polymeric materials* can avoid corrosion, but ductility is doubtful.
- *Biodegradable polymeric* materials- avoid removal of implant but tissue clearance is a problem.
- *Ceramic materials, hydroxy apatite and tricalcium phosphate*, gives improvement on bone growth but brittleness and limited strength restricts their use as material for internal fixation.
- *Carbon* used for making artificial ligaments.
- *Silicon* used for making artificial tendons and joint lubricant.

Q2. Write a short note on the Bioabsorbable implants?

The key factors that led to the escalation of research in this regard, were social but also economic, targeting to improve the quality of life, by reducing the use of traditionally permanent metallic implants (cobalt-based alloys, stainless steel, and titanium alloys) which involve the second implant removal surgery and other undesirable effects (stress shielding, metal ion releases and corrosion).

Bioabsorbable Implants

Polyglycolic acid (PGA) was the first totally synthetic bioabsorbable suture and was introduced in 1970 as dexon. This was followed in 1975 by vicryl, a copolymer of 92% PGA and 8% polylactic acid (PLA) and polydioaxanone (PDS) in 1981. PDS was the first bioabsorbable material to be made into screws. Currently, PGA, PDS, polylevolactic acid (PLLA), and racemic poly D, L- lactic acid (PDLLA) are the alpha polyesters used for bioabsorbable materials.

The most common orthopaedics use of bioabsorbable implants is for the attachment of soft tissue to bone, as in the shoulder and knee surgeries.

Advantages

- Gradual load transfer to the healing tissue
- Reduced need for hardware removal, and radiolucency, which facilitates postoperative roentgenographic evaluation.
- Natural biodegradation capacity, excellent biocompatibility.

Disadvantages

- Due to limited mechanical properties they are of interest for implants which must resist only minor loading and where surgical removal is a major undertaking. An ideal sterilization process is not yet available.
- Some cautions is advised in situations susceptible to infection, as degradable material seems to exhibit a reduced resistance to infection if compared to the best metal implants.

Note: *Magnesium-based metal alloys* are presently the new generation of biodegradable metal materials with a good osseointegration property.

Q3. Discuss various instruments and implants.

Orthopedic implants is defined as medical devices used to replace or provide fixation of bone or to replace articulating surfaces of a joint while *Surgical instruments* are tools or devices that perform such functions as cutting, dissecting, grasping, holding, retracting, or suturing during surgical procedures.

ORTHOPAEDICS INSTRUMENTS

1. Periosteal Elevators

Farabeuf Periosteal Elevator

- This has a flat handle, a narrow neck and a wide blade.
- The proximal part of the blade is serrated at the top for the thumb grip, while the tip is straight, bevelled and sharp. Its tip may be straight or curved.

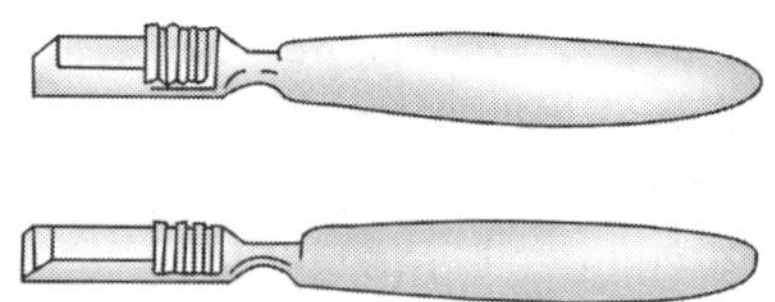

Farabeuf periosteal elevator

Bristow's Periosteal Elevator

- This has small oval fenestrated handle and a long shaft, which is gently curved and sharp at the tip.
- This is used for stripping off the periosteum cum bone lever.

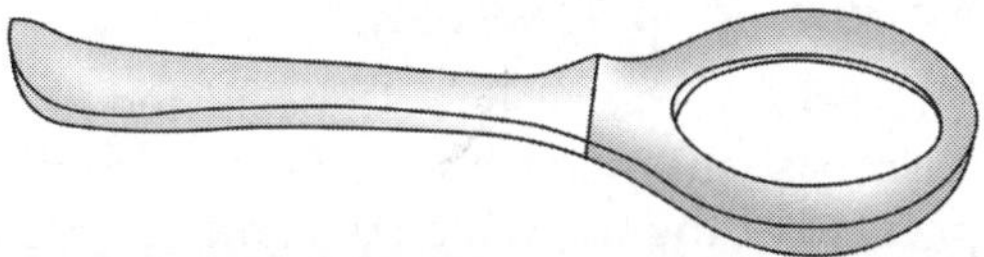

Bristow's periosteal elevator

Mitchell's Periosteal Elevator

This has a round handle for a good grip, elevated and serrated thumb rest and a straight sharp tipped blade.

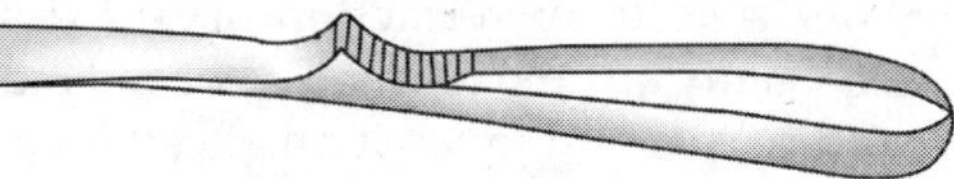

Mitchell's periosteal elevator

Uses

· Stripping off the periosteum before application of bone levers/forceps, to avoid damage to muscles/vessels and nerves overlying the bone.

Doyan's Periosteal Elevator

This has a smooth round handle, a conical shank and a U-curved cutting blade.

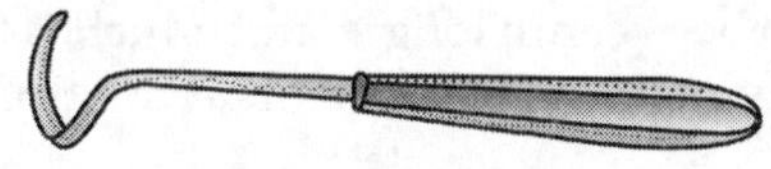

Doyan's periosteal elevator

Uses

t is curved in right and left direction and is exclusively used as a rib raspatory for stripping of the periosteum from the rib, while protecting the intercostal vessel and nerve.

2. Bone Levers

Lane's Bone Lever (Plain)

This has a fenestrated oval handle for a finger grip, a long shank and a narrow blade, which is smooth and conical at the tip, which is gently curved.

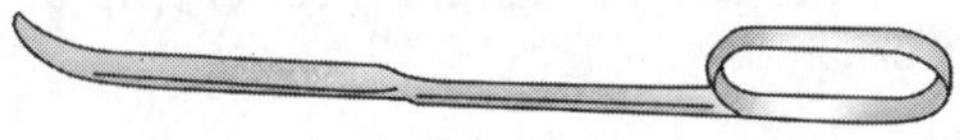

Lane's bone lever (plain)

Use

This is used for long bones of the upper and lower extremities. The periosteum is first stripped from the bone by periosteum elevator and while the periosteum elevator is still in place the lever is introduced so that the soft tissues are separated along with the periosteum from the bone allowing room for the bone forceps to hold the bone.

Lane's Bone Lever (Serrated Tip)

- This has a round thumb grip, a long shank and a serrated curved blade at the terminal end.
- This is used for femur and tibia. The serrated blade prevents it from slipping while the bone is being levered out.

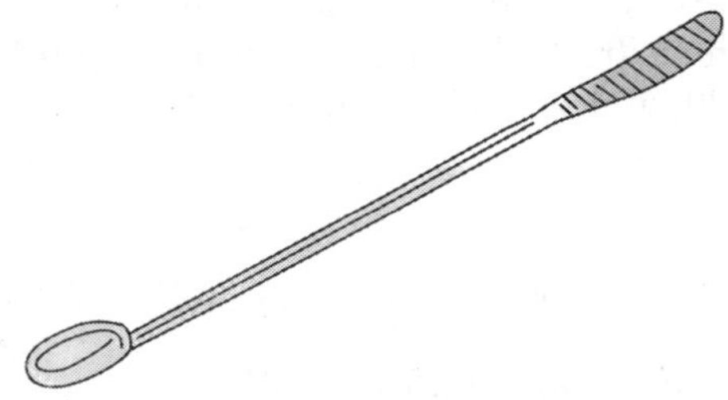

Lane's bone lever (serrated tip)

Narrow Blade Bone Lever

This bone retractor has a fenestrated handle, a narrow shank, and a blade, which is conical and pointed at the tip, which is gently curved

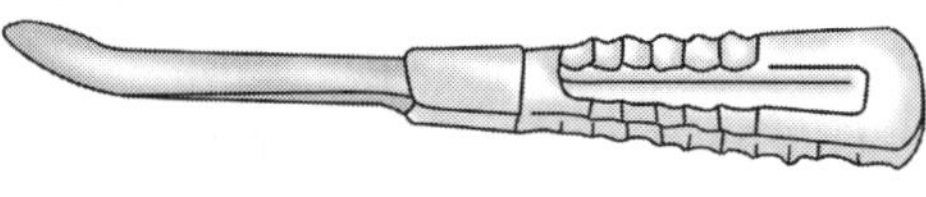

Narrow blade bone lever

Broad Blade Bone Lever (Hohmann's retractor)

· This is used for retraction of soft tissue especially around joints. The broad blade and narrow tip gives it an excellent and minimal engagement on the bone, all the same, a wide area of soft tissue retraction giving freedom of instrumentation. It is available as straight and angled shank.

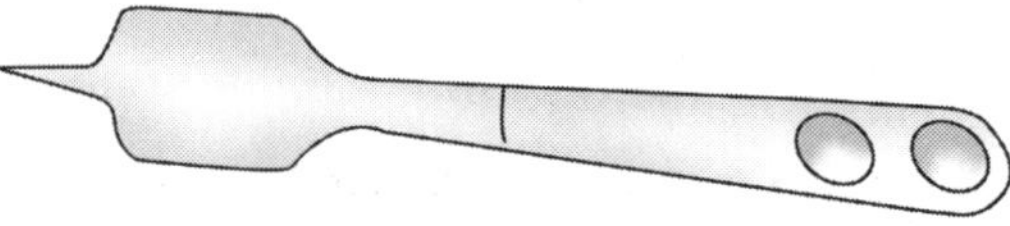

Hohmann's retractor

3. Skin Hooks

Single Hook Skin Retractor

This has a small, thin and flat handle, serrated in between, a long shank which is tapered and shaped into a fine hook at the tip.

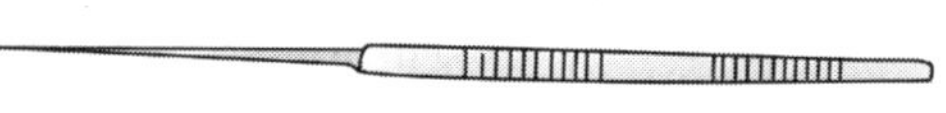

Single hook skin retractor

Uses

- This is used for retraction of soft tissue while doing micro-dissection as in the cases of neonates and neurovascular surgery.
- During preparation of skin graft

Double Hook Skin Retractor

This has two prongs for a better grip in the skin.

Double hook skin retractor

Four Prong Skin Retractor

This is used for paediatric surgery.

Four prong skin retractor

4. Retractors

Paton's Retractor

· This is used for the retraction of sub-cutaneous tissue, muscles and vessels.

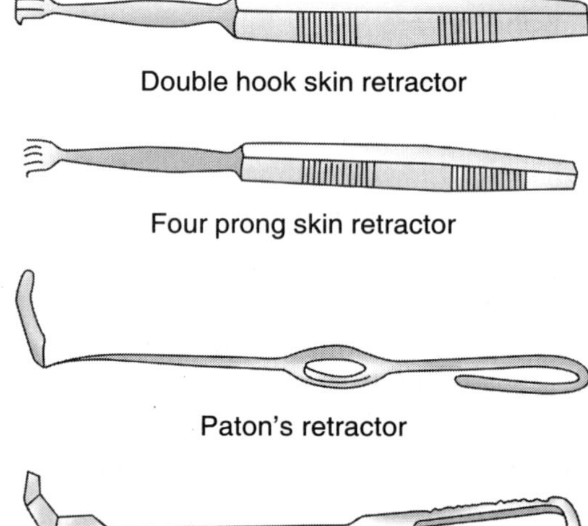

Paton's retractor

Langenbeck Retractor

This has a long shank, serrated triangular, fenestrated handle. The blade is angled at 90° and bent at the tip with long and short lengths.

Langenbeck retractor

Uses

This is very useful for retraction of deep tissues and muscles during surgery.

Volkmann's Retractor

This has a long shank with a triangular serrated fenestrated handle at one end

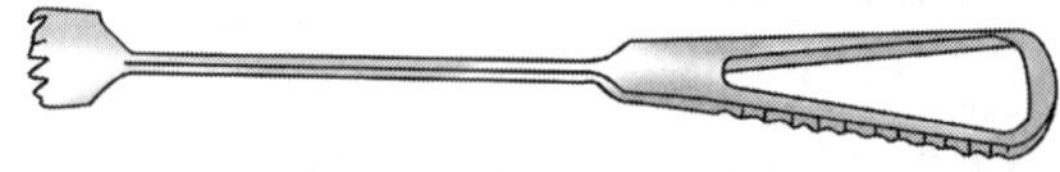

Volkmann's retractor

and four hooked prong sharp retractor at the other. This is also known as *cat's paw retractor*.

Uses

This is an excellent soft tissue retractor as the hooks bite into the subcutaneous tissue and prevents slippage of the skin during surgery

Kocher's Hook Retractor

This has a handle and a long shank that is conical, tapered and the tip is bent to form a hook, which is smooth tipped.

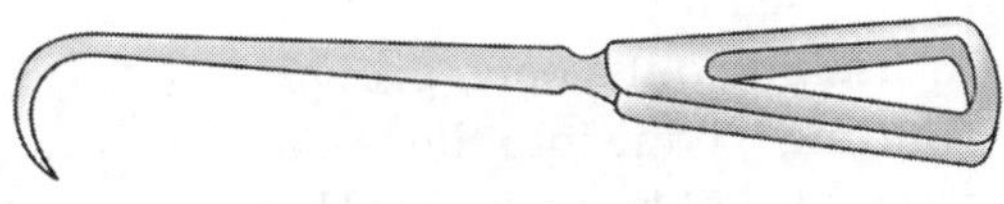

Kocher's hook retractor

Uses

This is used for hooking/retraction of the bone during surgery.

Beckmann–Adson Self-retaining Retractor

This has an outfaced hook multipronged retraction tip, long-curved arms which are hinged to be bent at a suitable angle, a handle with a rachet lock.

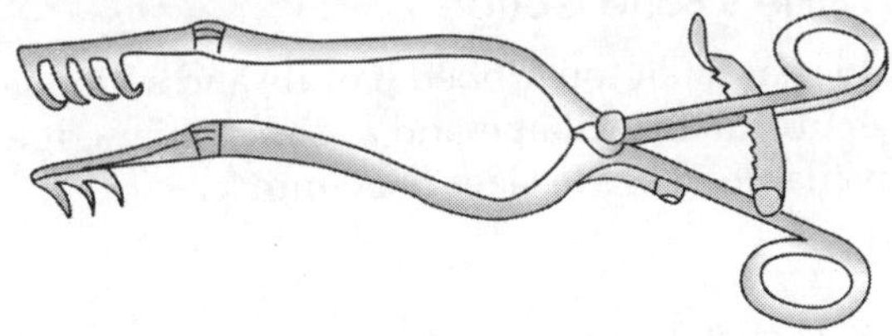

Beckmann-Adson self-retaining retractor

Uses

- Posterior spinal surgery
- This is used for retraction of muscles especially in posterior spinal surgery. The muscles are first retracted by a Langenbeck's retractor on both sides of the spinous process, the prongs are then introduced, the jaws are then opened up and are held automatically at the desired retraction by the rachet lock.
- The blades can be bent at a suitable angle so that deep retraction can be achieved. To release the retraction, the rachet lock is pressed and the jaws close by themselves. Two retractors are invariably used, one for the proximal and other for the distal soft tissue retraction so that the wide area of laminae and spine is visible and does not require help of an assistant to do the same.

5. Osteotome

Smith-Peterson's Osteotomes

This has a smooth, round handle, a narrow neck, a long blade and a flat top for hammering. It is available in blade sizes varying from 5 to 35 mm.

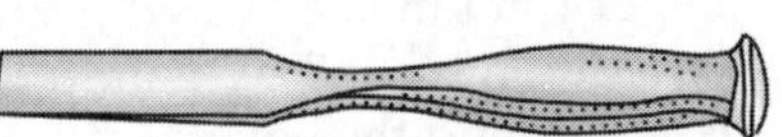

Smith-Peterson's osteotomes

Uses

This is used for:
- Osteotomy
- Cutting the bone for correction of deformities (corrective osteotomy such as French osteotomy, Mcmurays osteotomy)
- Making a window into the bone (saucerization)
- Triple arthrodesis
- During bone grafting
- Excision of exostosis

6. Stille's Chisel

This has a flat top for hammering, a narrow cylindrical handle which is ribbed and a blade which is bevelled at the tip. This is available in blade sizes 5–30 mm.

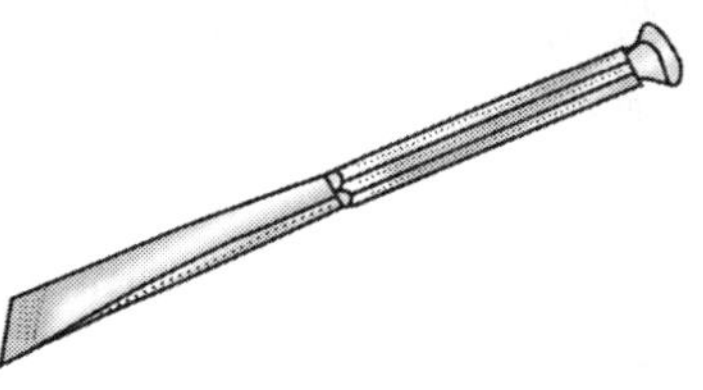

Stille's chisel

Uses

This is used for:

- Chiselling out a bony growth
- Cutting wedge into the bone
- Removal of bone grafts (This is either straight or curved. The latter is more convenient while removing bone grafts from the iliac crest or while cutting through a curved surface.)
- To remove excess callus while operating on hypertrophic non-union or old malunited fractures.

7. Stille's Bone Gouge

This has a flat top, ribbed handle and a blade which is semitubular in shape and has a cutting edge. This is available in blade sizes 5–30 mm.

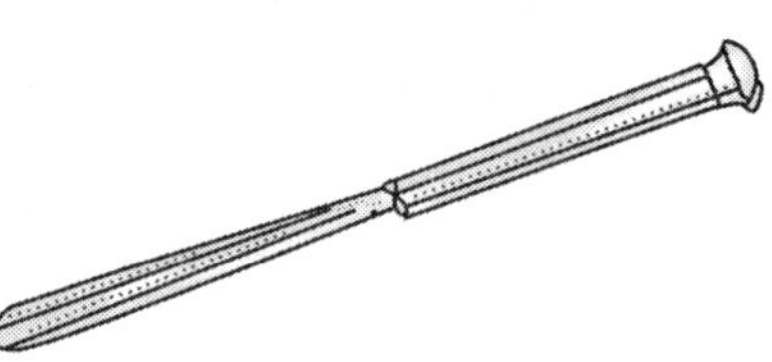

Stille's bone gouge

Uses

This is used:

- To gouge out bone cavities
- Removal of bone grafts
- Lateralization of medullary canal for insertion of prosthesis during hemiarthroplasty. This is necessary for valgus setting of the prosthesis.

8. Gigli's Wire Saw With Hook Handle

This Gigli's wire is a useful device for sawing the bone as in the:

- Cases of amputation
- Correction of deformities

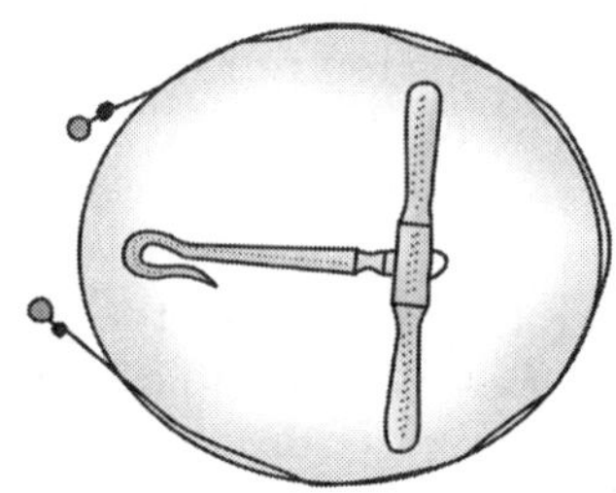

Gigli's wire saw with hook handle

How?

- The periosteum is elevated from all around the bone, the soft tissue retracted by Lane's lever and then the wire is passed around the bone.
- The tips are then held in T-hook handles and by sea-saw movement the bone is cut through by the spiked wire. *One must always take precautions to protect the soft tissues adequately while sawing through the bone.*
- The wire is available in lengths of 30–70 cm

9. Volkmann's Curette

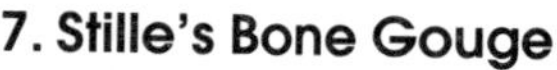

Volkmann's curette

This has a flat handle serrated in between and has two scoops at either end. It is available in cup sizes of 2–12 mm. It usually has a small cup on one side and a large cup on the other.

Uses

This is used for curetting out bone cavities in cases of:
• Bone tumour
• Osteomyelitis (after saucerization)
• Refreshing the fracture ends during ORIF
• Freshening fistula or sinus

10. Mallet

Heath Mallet

This is a stainless steel hammer with serrated handle. It is available in different weights of 1–2 pounds with a standard handle length of 8 inches.

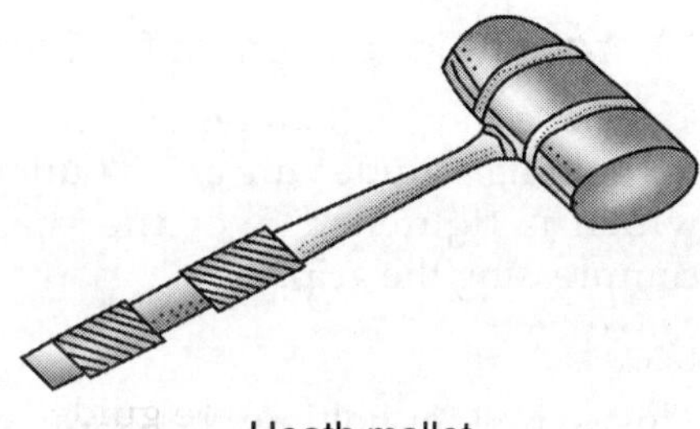

Heath mallet

Uses

This is used for hammering during introduction of nails for intramedullary fixation of fractures, cutting the bone while using a chisel or osteotome. In cases of prosthetic use, one end of the head of the hammer is tufnol tipped to avoid any indentation or damage to the surface of the prostheses.

Fibre Mallet

This is made up of fibre with a tufnol head.

Uses

It has the same strength as that of a brass hammer and has an excellent advantage of not hammering chisel or other cutting tools or the head of prostheses during introduction.

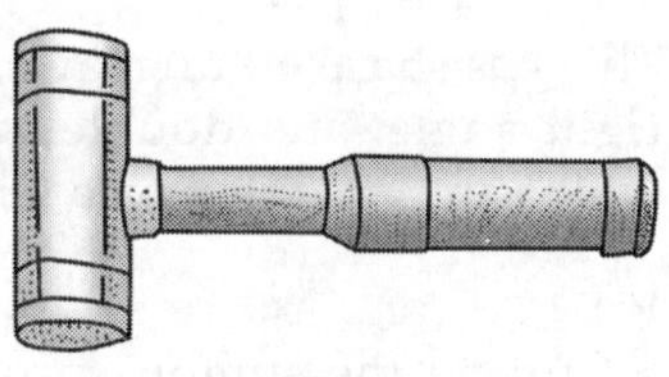

Fibre mallet

This mallet is perfectly balanced, sympathetic to touch, non-spark and can be autoclaved or boiled in a routine way.

11. Universal Bone Drill

This has a manual rotational gear, which is connected to the shaft by cog-wheel. It has a Jacob's chuck for loading K-wire and drill bit which is tightened by a key. The shaft is cannulated for the long K-wire to pass through from front to back.

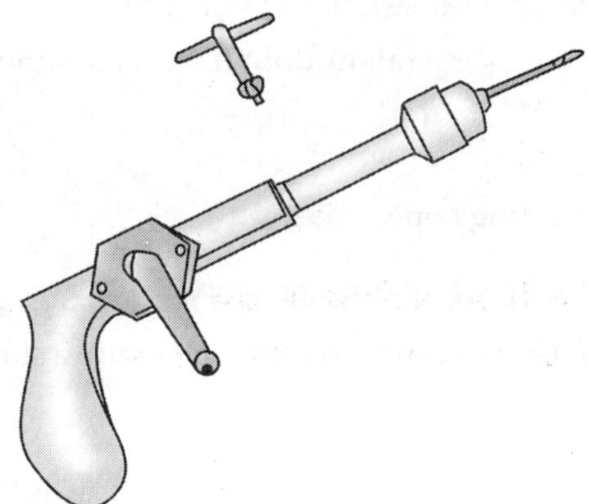

Universal bone drill

Uses

It is very useful instrument for:
• Drilling in K-wire
• Steinmann pin
• Making holes with drill bit for introduction of screws

12. Steinmann Pin Introducer

This has a long T-handle, the shaft of which is cannulated throughout its length with Jacob's chuck at the end.

Uses

This is used for introduction of K-wire, guide wire, Steinmann pin and Shanz pin into the bone. The wire is first introduced into the shaft and while a desired length is allowed to remain outside. The chuck is tightened with the key.

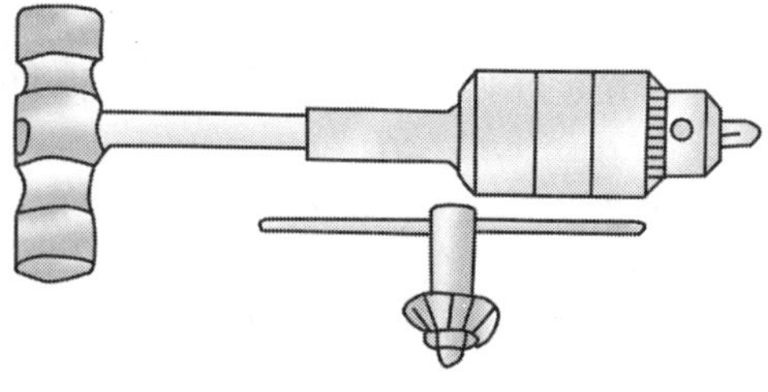

Steinmann pin introducer

13. Watson–Jones Handle for Guide Wire

This has a short 'T' handle, which is cannulated for holding a guide wire and a butterfly sleeve, which is tightened over the shaft thereby compressing the grip.

Uses

This is used for holding the guide wire during introduction into the neck of femur, by gentle oscillating movements.

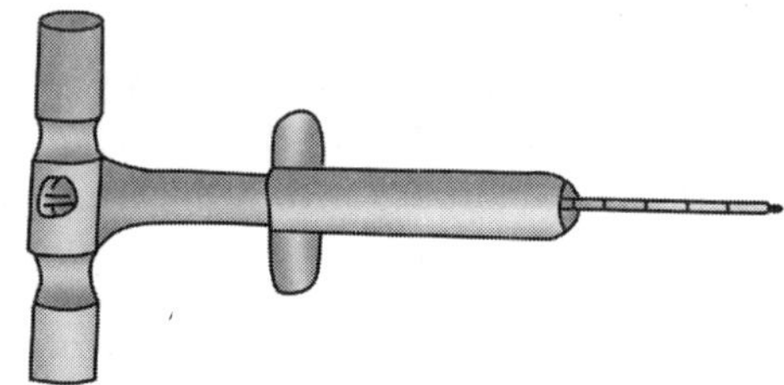

Watson-Jones handle for guide wire

14. Stille Horsley Bone Cutting Forceps

This has sharp cutting jaws, which are bent at right angle, and double-hinged lever arms, which are separated by a tension strip.

Uses

- Cutting the spinous process during laminectomy
- Can also be used to cut bone spikes and edges to give it a uniform edge

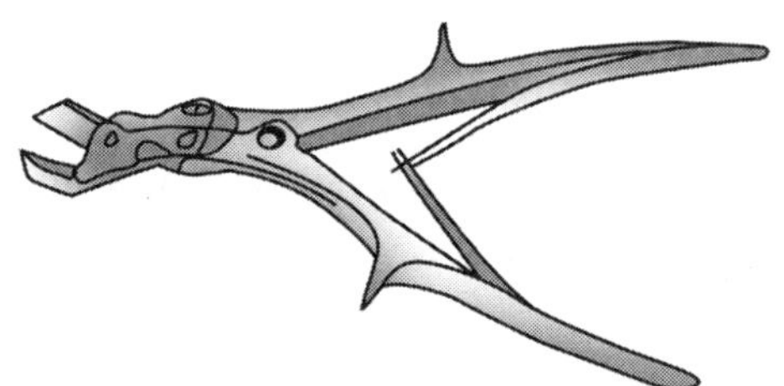

Stille-Horsley bone cutting forceps

Ruskin Bone Cutting Forceps

This is a straight double-hinged bone cutting forceps.

Uses

Cutting bone spikes.

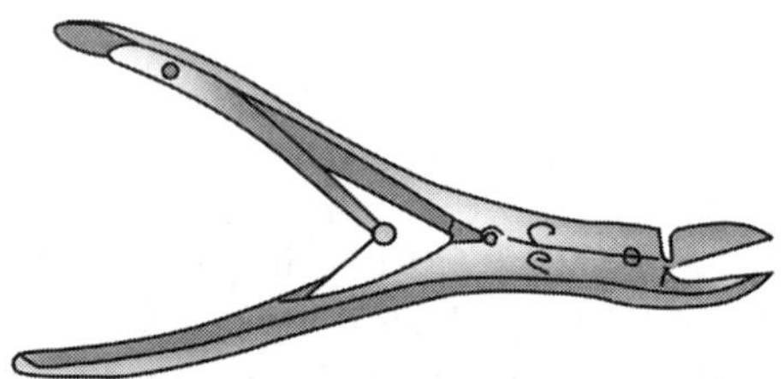

Ruskin bone cutting forceps

15. Bone Nibbler Single Action Straight

This is a straight bone nibbler with a single hinge and a tension strip in between the handles.

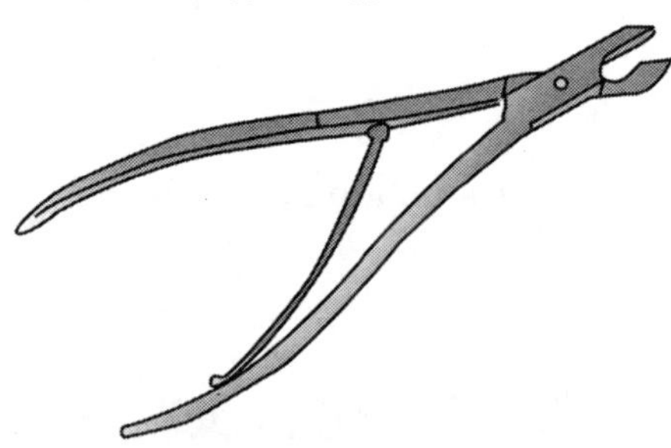

Bone nibber single action straight

Uses

Nibbling away the bone margins in a piece meal style to give it a uniform edge or desired contour

16. Sargent Rongeur

This is a strong double-hinged nibbler with angled jaws.

Uses

This is used for nibbling cortical bone; the angled tip gives it an extra advantage for in depth working and the strong jaws can cut out bone with ease.

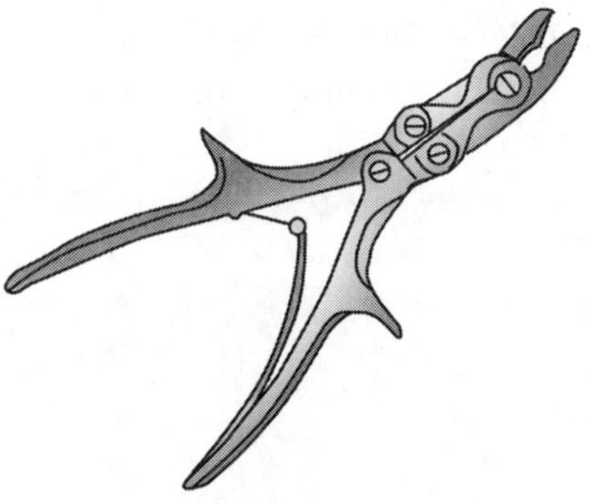

Sargent rongeur

Northfield's Rongeur Heavy Double Action

This is a straight double-hinged bone nibbler.

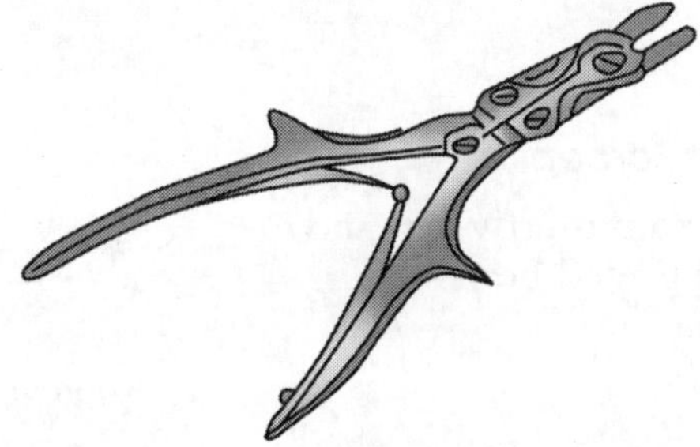

Northfield's rongeur heavy double action

Heyjack Rongeur (Kerrison's Punch)

This has a handle, which on grip closing causes the long twin shafts to slide over one another and close the cutting tips. It is available in up cutting as well as down cutting tips.

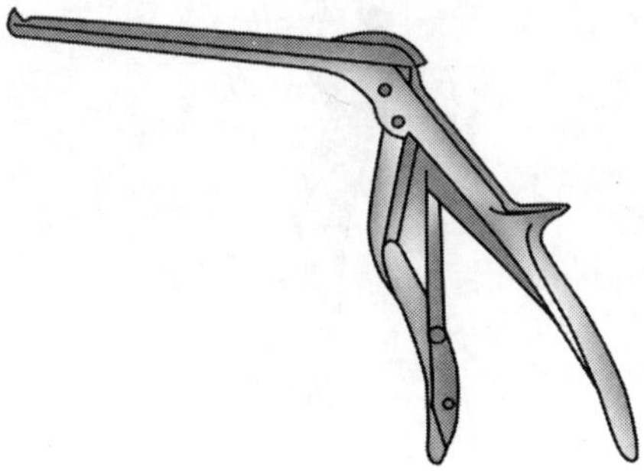

Sargent rongeur

Uses

- This is used for cutting/nibbling the laminae and a pedicle while doing a spinal decompression, the long shaft is a great advantage to cut the deeply placed bone
- It is also used as a sphenoid punch.

17. Straight Disc Punch

This is a scissor type of instrument with a long shaft and small terminal jaws.

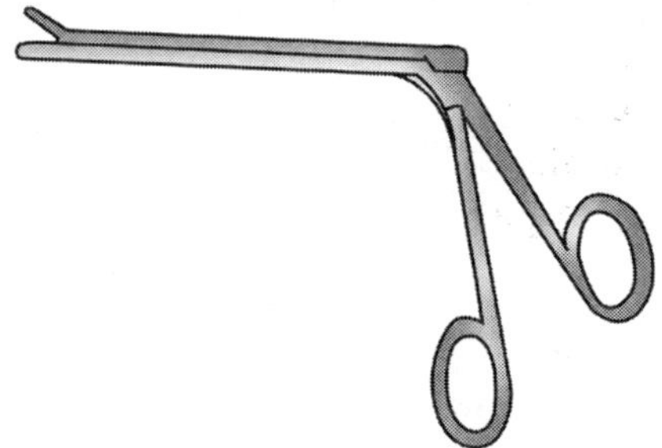

Straight disc punch

Uses

Catching and pulling out disc material in between the vertebral bodies in cases of disc prolapse

18. Bone Holding Forceps

Heygrove's Bone Holding Forceps

This has long handles with a butterfly nut and bolt at the base to lock the griped bone, a long shaft and curved serrated jaws.

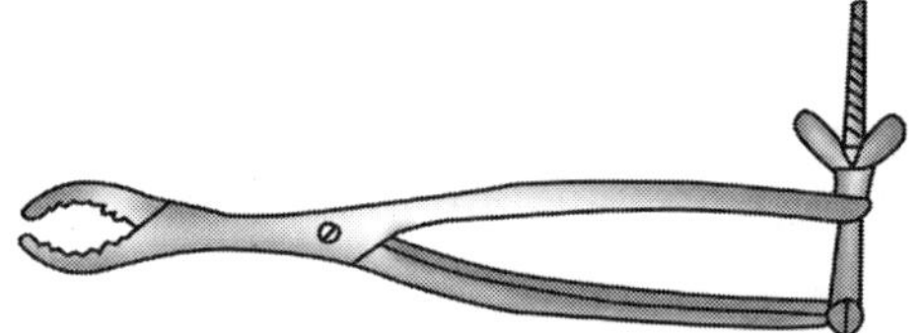

Hegrove's bone holding forceps

Uses

This is used for holding the long bones. The bone is held and the butterfly nut is tightened for a fixed grip to avoid slippage during reduction of fractures.

Burn's Bone Holding Forceps

· This has a rachet lock handle and fenestrated jaws.

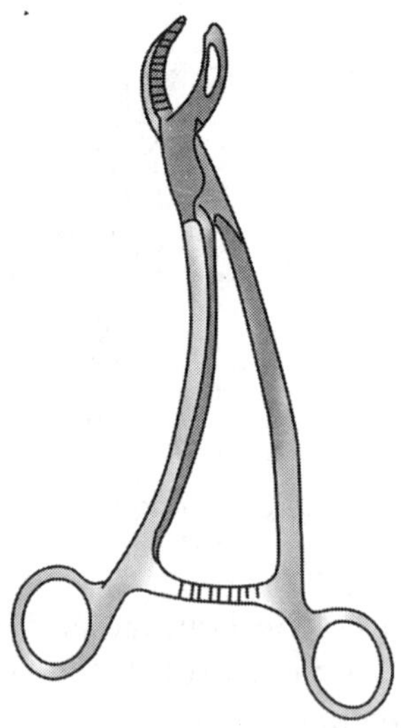

Burn's bone holding forceps

Uses

This is a very useful instrument for holding the forearm bones during reduction and fixation, the fenestrated jaws are a great advantage as it allows to drill and pass a screw through it while holding the plate on the bone.

Lanes Fagg's Bone Holding Forceps

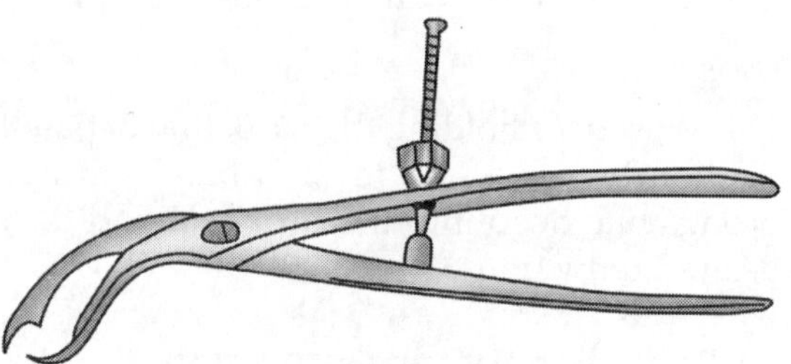

Lanes Fagg's bone holding forceps

- This is a long, large bone holding forceps.
- It has two serrated arms, one of which is curved to avoid slipping of grip while manipulating the bone during reduction of fracture.
- The thick lion toothed jaws give a firm grip on the bone. It is about 12 inches long.

Uses

- This is used for holding the femur and tibia during ORIF.
- It should be used with caution in osteoporotic bones for the fear of crushing the bones

Self-centering Bone Holding Forceps

- This forcep has a beaked jaw, the grip of which is variable by the use of eccentric hinge in the shank.
- The handle has a butterfly-nut to fix the grip on the bone.
- It is available in sizes varying from 150 mm for small bones to 280 mm for femur and tibia.

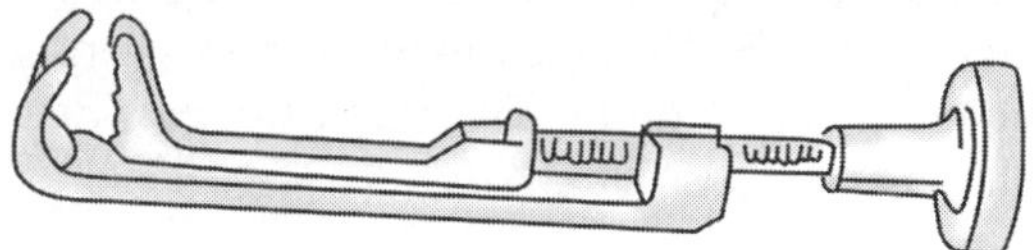

Self-centering bone holding forceps

Uses

- This instrument is used for holding the bone of variable dimension. The conical beaked tips hold the bone with minimal stripping of periosteum and the grip is self-adjusting because of its peculiar hinge.
- It can also be used for holding the plate after reduction of fracture. Once the plate and the bone are firmly gripped, the handles are locked using the nut and bolt. This ensures that the forceps will not allow the bone or the plate to slip off during reduction and fixation.

19. Lowman's Bone Holding Clamp

- This has two inter-sliding jaws, which are serrated and controlled by a chuck nut.
- It is available in sizes varying from 4–8 inches.

Lowman's bone holding clamp

Uses

This is a useful instrument for holding the plate on the bone while it is being fixed by screws.

20. Reduction Forceps

- This has a sharp serrated pointed jaw, and handles with a locking device.
- It is available in sizes varying from 140 to 170 mm in length.

Uses

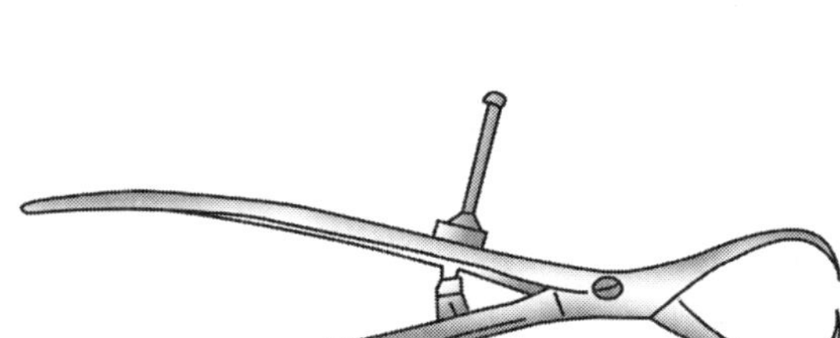

Reduction forceps

- This is used for holding long bones during manipulation and reduction of fractures. The sharp teeth give it a firm bite in the bone and prevent the slipping of forceps.
- This should be used with caution in osteoporotic bones since it may cause crushing of the bones.

21. Patella Forceps

- This is shaped like a large towel clip with sharp pointed prongs and a bolt lock in the handle.
- It is available in single and double prongs in each jaw and is about 175 mm.

Uses

This is used for holding the reduction of patellar fragments during fixation by screws or tension band wiring. The sharp pointed prongs bite deep into the proximal and distal fragments to give desired reduction.

Patella forceps

22. Reduction Forceps with Points

- This is a modified towel clip with bolt lock in the handles.
- It is available in sizes 130–200 mm.

Uses

This is used for reduction of small fragments like medial malleolus, olecranon butterfly fragments, etc. and the spiked jaws bite into the bone and give it a good grip.

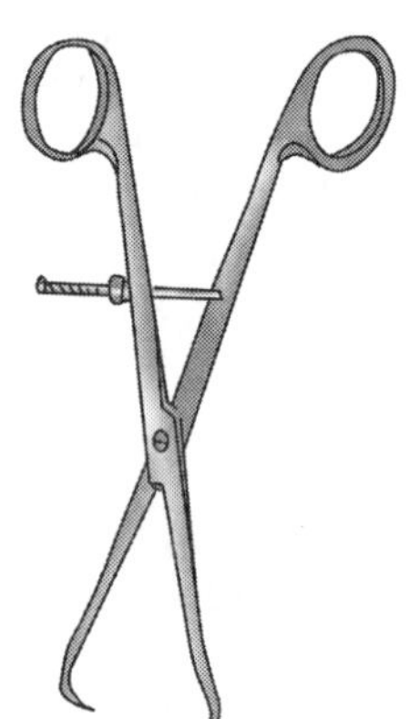

Reduction forceps with points

23. Charnley's Compression Clamp

This has a self-collapsing shaft with two pairs of clamps to hold the Steinmann pin. The clamps are loaded over a butterfly nut bolt.

Uses

- This is used extensively for arthrodesis of the knee and ankle. It can also be used for controlling and compressing osteo-tomies around the knee.

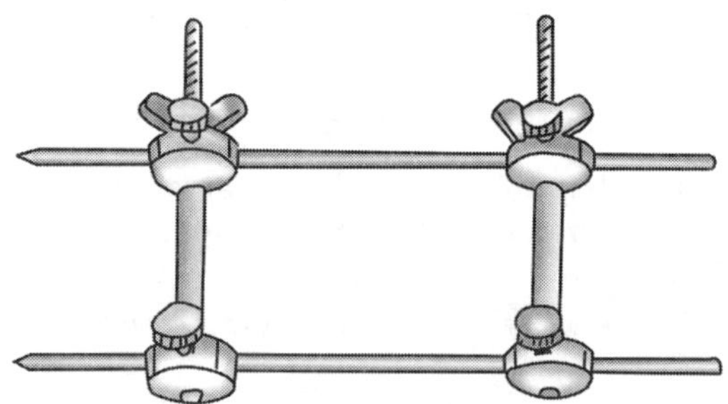

Charnley's compression clamp

- First, the joint is excised and Steinmann pin are passed in each fragment.

- The Steinmann pins are then passed through the hole in the clamp on each side of the joint.
- The butterfly-nut on tightening causes compression of the joint thereby causing an early bony ankylosis. These clamps are available in single and double pin option.

24. K-Nail Extractor with Two Hooks

- This has a long smooth shaft threaded at both ends.
- The proximal end is for the hook extractor and the distal end is for fixing the handle.
- A sledge-hammer freely moves along the shaft. All the components can be dismantled. The sledge hammer weighs 1–3 pounds.

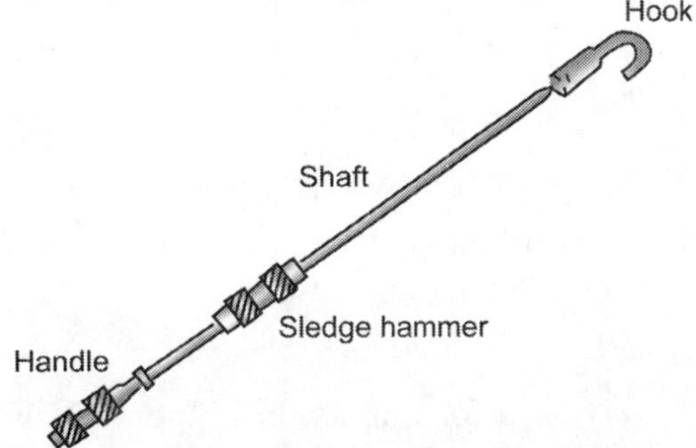

K-nail extractor with two hooks

Uses

This is a very useful instrument required for the extraction of intramedullary ordinary nails (K. nail and V. nail).

How?

- The hook is first passed through the eye of the nail and then the shaft is threaded into it.
- The sledge hammer is then loaded onto the shaft after which the handle is tightened into the tail end. Once this unit is assembled, the sledge hammer is moved to and fro, hammering onto the handle.
- This gives pulling force in the axis of the shaft, thereby extracting the nail.
- This is available with a set of three hooks which are sharp, round and acute tipped.
- One must always keep spare hooks whenever extraction of the femoral nail has been planned.

25. Kuntscher's Diamond Pointed Awl

· This has a U-shaped handle, an angled shaft and a diamond pointed tip.

Uses

- This is used for making an opening hole (entry portal) in the trochanter and tibial condyles for introduction of intramedullary nails. The starting hole is made along the medial surface of the greater trochanter preferably the piriform fossa for a femoral nail or the proximal end of the tibial tuberosity of tibia.

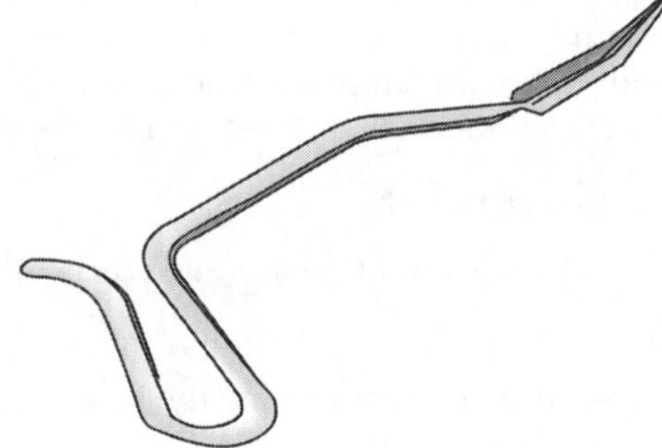
Kuntscher's diamond pointed awl

- The sharp point is thrust into the bone and then subsequently directed into the line of the medullary canal by twisting movements.
- Always direct the awl in the long axis of the bone to prevent perforation of the posterior cortex.

26. Bone Awl with Eye

This has a smooth and oval-shaped handle, a narrow straight shaft, and diamond tipped cutting edge with a small eye.

Uses

- This is a useful instrument for making entry holes in the radius and ulna for intramedullary nailing.
- The eye in the tip can be used to pull out stainless steel wire or suture material through the bone.

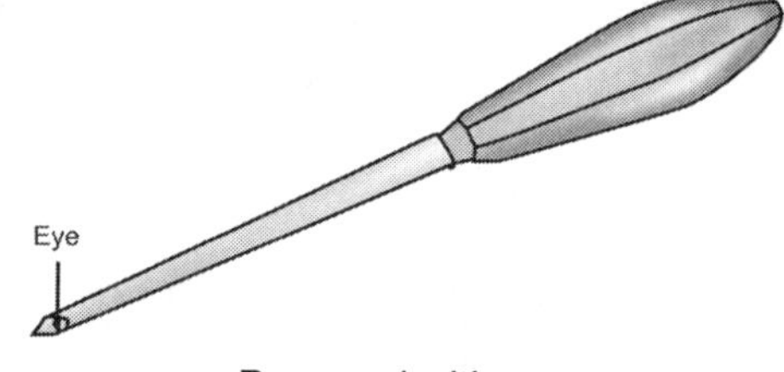

Bone awl with eye

27. Smith-Peterson Impactor

This has a bell-shaped tip, a hollow shaft and a top for hammering.

Uses

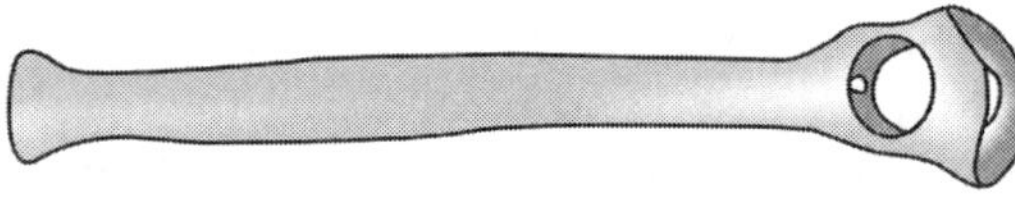

Smith-Peterson impactor

This is used for impaction of the neck of femur following fixation by SP-nail or parallel pins. The Impactor is placed on the lateral surface of the greater trochanter and hammered in the axis of the neck of femur. The hollow bell-shaped tip gives room for the protruding tip of the implant.

28. Cannulated Sterling Holder Punch

To hammer the bone after the pins have been passed through the fracture site.

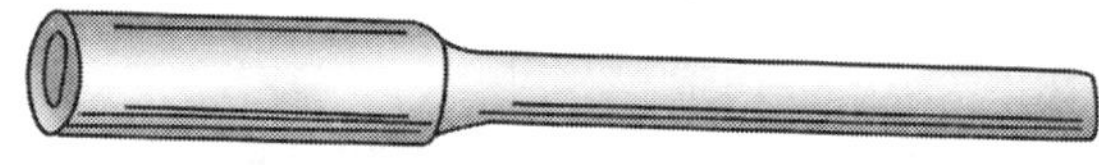

Cannulated sterling holder punch

29. Kuntscher's Nail Driver

- This is a solid rod with a hollow tip, which is slotted.
- The grip is serrated.

Uses

This is used for impaction of K-nail into the femur. The hollow tip allows the eye of the nail to remain out of the trochanteric bone so

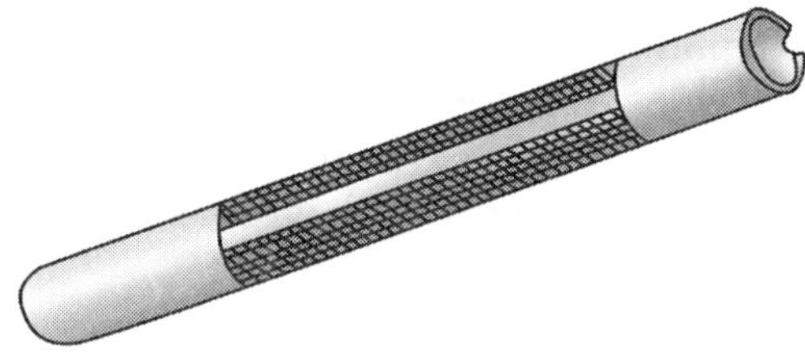

Kuntscher's nail driver

that the hook can be fitted into it whenever it is necessary to extract the nail.

30. K-Nail Punch

This is a solid rod with a small stud at the tip.

Uses

This is used for hammering the K-nail into the femur. The stud enters into the hollow of the nail and hence does not allow the punch to wander during hammering, and keeps the eye of nail out of the bone for easy extraction.

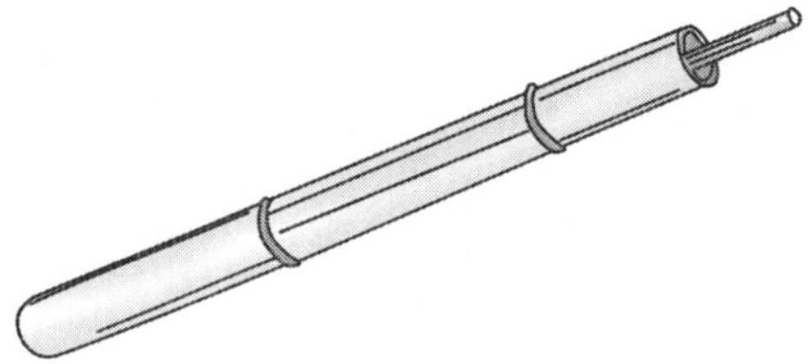

K-nail punch

31. Intramedullary Reamer

- This is a long T-shaped instrument with a spiral-cutting flute.
- It is available in sizes varying from 1.5 to 15 mm and can be used for practically all long bones requiring intramedullary fixation.

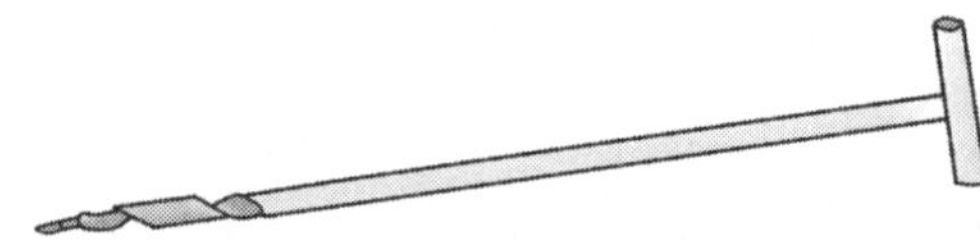

Intramedullary reamer

- The modified reamers are now available which can be motor driven and are flexible in cases of closed interlocking nail fixation of long bones.

Uses

This is used for reaming of the medullary cavity so as to make a uniform canal for the intramedullary nail. The reamer is introduced into the bone after making an entry hole by an awl or directly through the fracture site while doing open reduction, the self-cutting and reaming tip makes a bore along the medullary canal so that the nail is not jammed at the isthmus of the bone.

32. Plate Bender Pair

This has a long-tempered shaft with oval terminal ends, which are slotted to accommodate the plate.

Uses

This is used for bending of plates, both narrow as well as broad. The plate is held
in between two bending irons at the desired junction and while one bender holds the plate the other bender contours it.

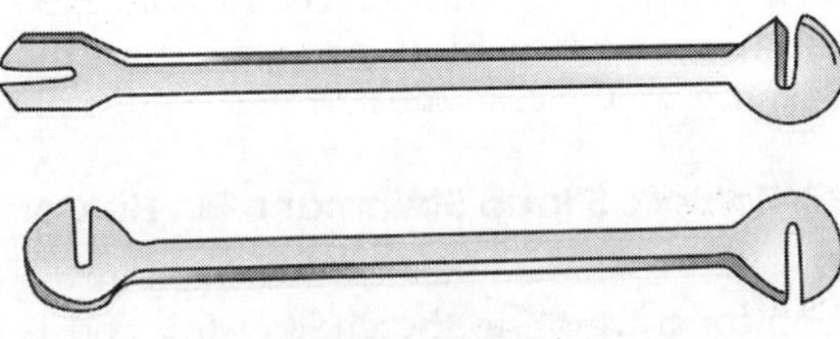

Plate bender pair

33. Flat-nosed Parallel Plier

This is used for twisting the circlage wire and holding K-wires during extraction. This is available in sizes varying from 4 to 12 inches.

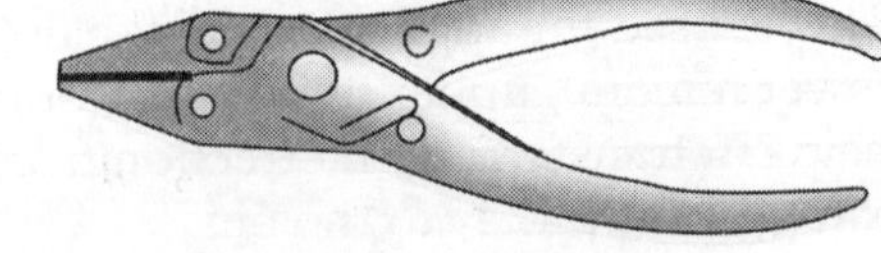

Flat-nosed parallel plier

34. Plaster Saw with Aluminium Handle

This has an aluminium handle with a semilunar stainless steel cutting blade attached to it.

Uses

This is used to saw the plaster for removal or to make a window into the POP cast for inspection of wounds.

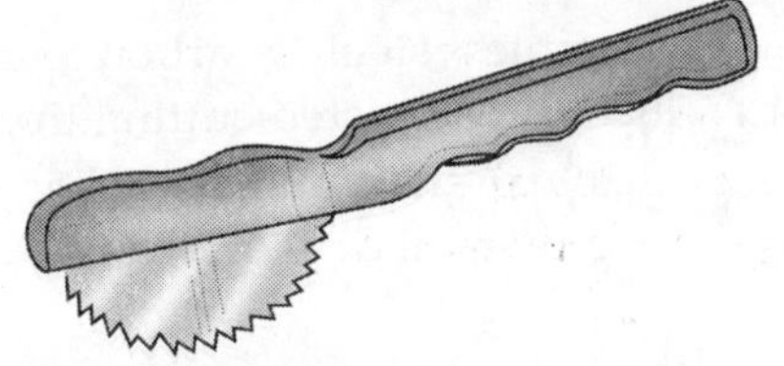

Plaster saw with aluminium handle

35. Bohler's Plaster Cutting Scissor

This is a strong large scissor with the upper blade a little shorter than the lower, which is extended blunt tipped.

Uses

- This is used for cutting the plaster casts, cotton and bandage.
- The lower blade is introduced inside the cast; the blunt tip protects the skin. While cutting, the scissor cuts through the hard POP material and avoids any entrapment of the soft tissue.

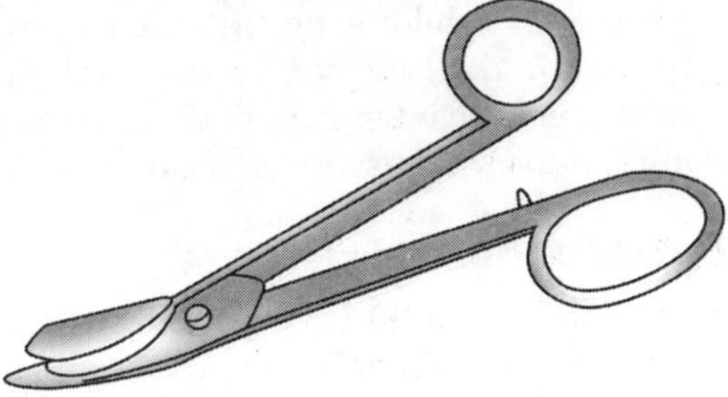

Bohler's plaster cutting scissor

36. Henning's Plaster Cast Spreader

This has two long handles, a narrow hinged shank and wide blades which are serrated on the outer side.

Uses

This has a peculiar function, i.e. on closing the handles the blades open out. The plaster cast is first cut, opened by saw or shear and then the spreader is introduced into the gap, the handles are then pressed thereby opening up the cast, the serrated blades prevent the slippage of the spreader.

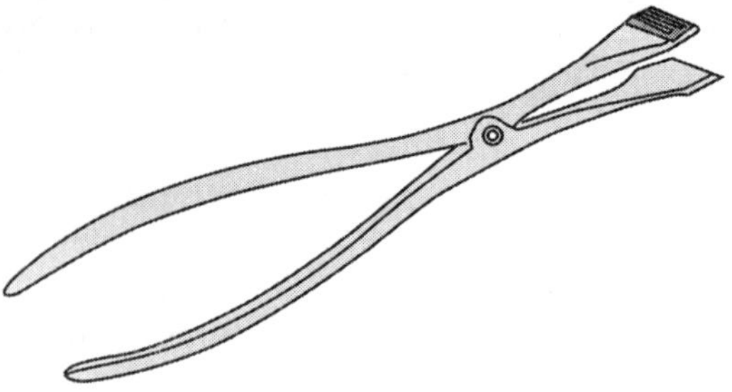

Henning's plaster cast spreader

37. Bohler's Stirrup Steinmann Pin Holder

This is a U-shaped steel rod twisted at the base to form a loop for traction, to the ends of this rod is attached small clamps to hold a Steinmann pin which can be tightened by the help of small bolts.

Uses

This is used for application of skeletal traction through the lower femoral, upper tibial or lower tibial sites. The stirrup helps in transferring the traction from the weights hanged through the pulley to the pin.

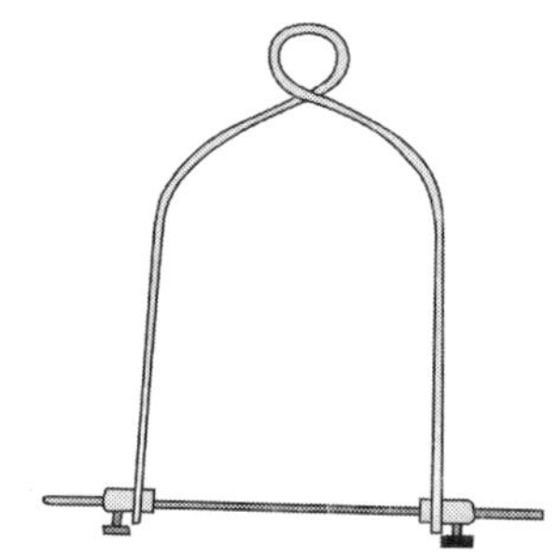

Bohler's stirrup Steinmann pin holder

38. Drill Bit

- This is a stainless steel or carbon tempered rod, which has a twisted cutting tip.

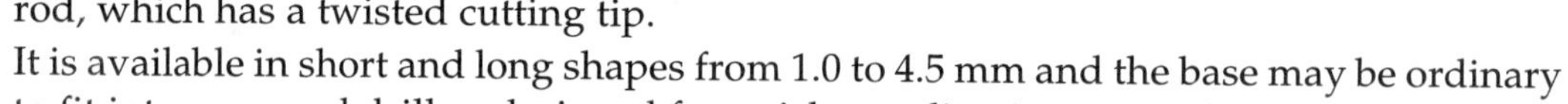

Drill bit

- It is available in short and long shapes from 1.0 to 4.5 mm and the base may be ordinary to fit into a manual drill or designed for quick coupling in powered instruments.

Uses

- This is used for drilling holes in the bone for introduction of screws, pins and nails.
- It is important to protect the soft tissues adequately while using the drill bit, by using the drill sleeve, as its rotatory movement can entangle soft tissue fascia, muscle and vital tissues extensively.

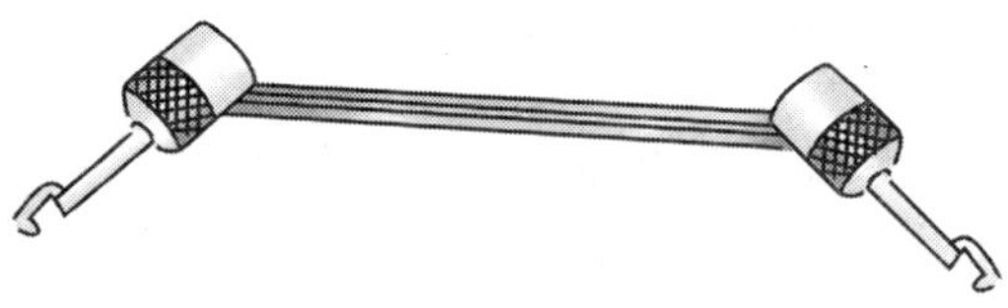

39. Twin DCP Drill Guide

- This has a handle with eccentric drill guide on one end and neutral on the other.
- The guide on one side has a central/neutral hole while the other has an eccentric/loaded hole for compression screw.
- They are used for 2.0 mm as well as 3.2 mm drill bits.

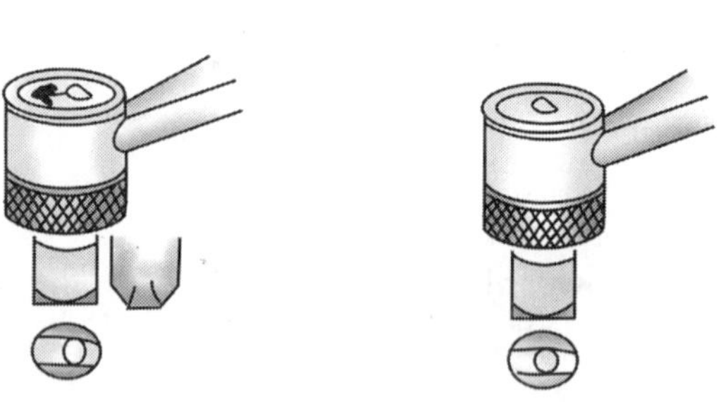

Twin DCP drill guide

Uses

- This is used for drilling holes in the bone for cortical screws.
- The dynamic compression plate is fixed on the bone and the hole drilled with neutral guide on the one side, and eccentric (with arrow towards fracture) on the other side of the fracture. For compression greater than 1 mm at the fracture site, the holes on both the sides of the fracture can be drilled using an eccentric drill guide. The tip of the guide is flattened on the sides to exactly fit into the plate holes down to the bone. The guides are mounted on the rings of the handle end so that they can be conveniently rotated.

40. Mini Drill Sleeve (3.5/2 mm)

This has a small handle with two sleeves attached on each handle.

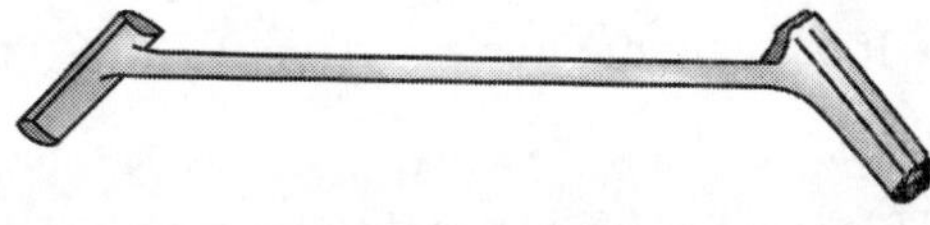

Mini-drill sleeve

Uses

The sleeves are to accommodate drill bits inside and prevent the entanglement of soft tissues while the drill is being rotated.

41. Countersink

This is a T-handle with a small cutting tip of 4.5 mm.

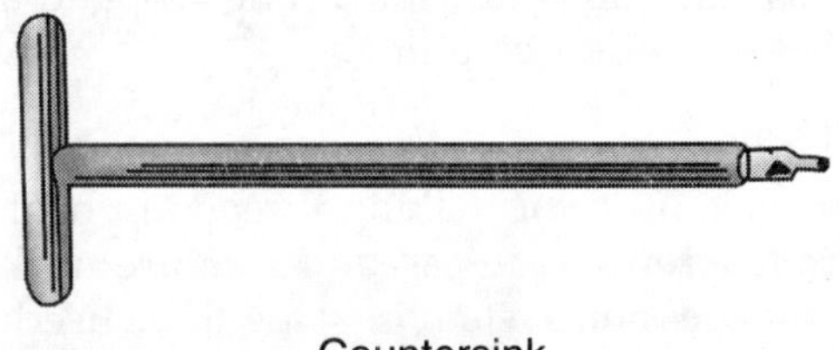

Countersink

Uses

This is used for making room for the head of the screw in the proximal cortex, when used as a lag screw, so that the head sinks into the bone and does not protrude out especially if the screw is introduced along the subcutaneous surface of the bone.

42. Depth Gauge

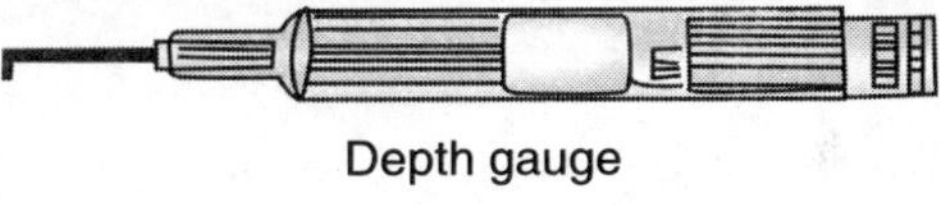

Depth gauge

- This has a flat scale to which is attached measuring rod, which is bent at the tip. It moves inside a tubular sleeve.
- Separate depth gauges are available for 2.5 mm, 3.5 mm and 4.5 mm screws.

Uses

- This is used for measuring the depth of the hole in the bone for selecting appropriate length of the screw to be used. The hole is first drilled by a twist drill bit and then the rod of depth gauge is passed through the plate hole and the bone bypassing the opposite cortex.
- The outer sleeve is fixed to the plate, while the rod tipped scale is pulled up, the bent end of the rod engages the outer cortex at the far end. The depth of the hole is then read directly looking at the scale.

43. Tap

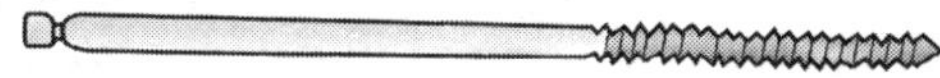

Tap

- This is a quick coupling tap for making threads in the holes drilled in the bone for introduction of screws.
- It is available in sizes varying from 2.7 to 6.5 mm.
- It is used in power driven instruments.

Uses

This is used for making threads for non-self tapping cortical screws, cancellous screws and malleolar screws.

44. Tap with Fixed Handle

- This is a T-shaped tempered rod with cutting threads and flutes. The flutes allow the bone debris to come out while the hole is being tapped.
- It is available in sizes from 2.7 to 6.5 mm.

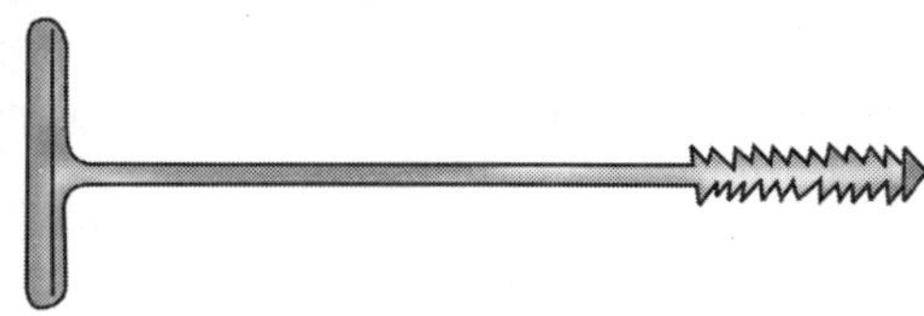

Tap with fixed handle

Uses

This is used for manual threading of holes in cortico-cancellous bone for screws.

45. Cancellous Tap (6.5 mm)

This has a smooth cannulated shaft, which has cancellous threads at one end and a flat base for quick coupling.

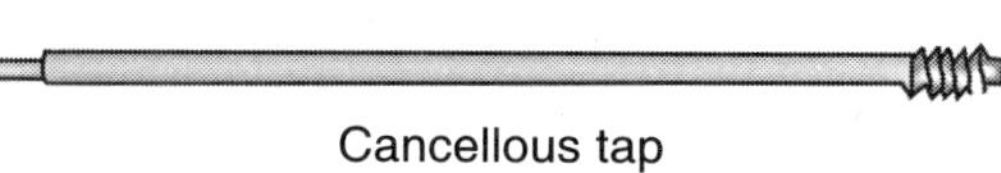

Cancellous tap

Uses

This is used for making threads in healthy adult cancellous bone for introduction of 6.5 mm screws as in cases of fracture neck of femur or condylar fractures where dynamic compression system is going to be used. It is used with power instruments.

46. Screwdriver

This is an ordinary screwdriver, flat tipped with a fibre handle.

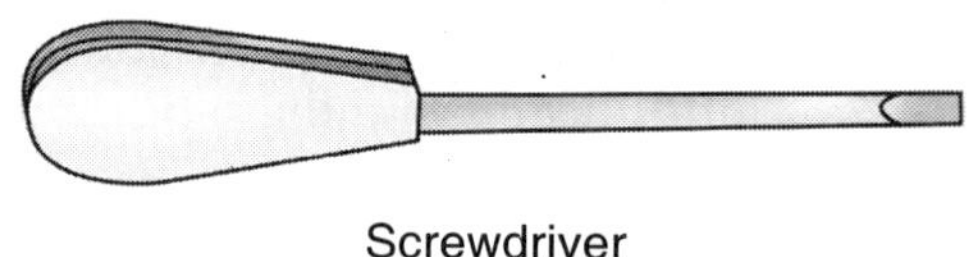

Screwdriver

Uses

This is used for screws with ordinary heads, which are now obsolete.

47. Hexagonal Screwdriver with Fibre Blade

- This has a flat fibre handle and a smooth shaft which has a high tempered hexagonal shaft at the tip (as shown in insert).
- The flat handle is a great advantage during tightening of the screw and the hexagonal tip gives it a mechanical grip on the head of the screw, which does not require the need of applying vertical pressure during rotational tightening.
- It is available in 3.5 and 4.5 mm. The latter can also be used for malleolar as well as 6.5 mm cancellous screws.

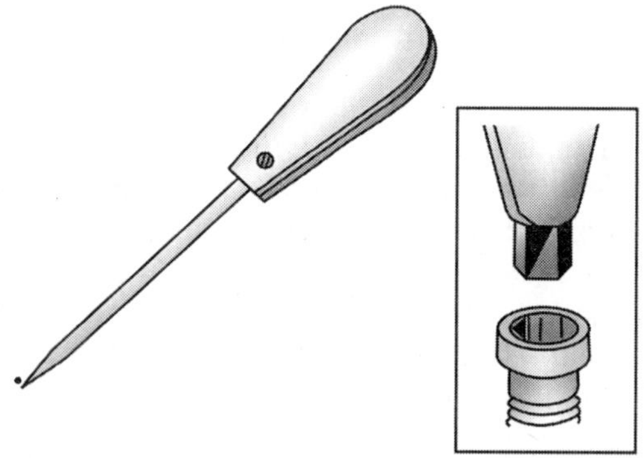

Hexagonal screwdriver with fibre blade

Uses

This is used for introduction of dynamic compression screws for plate fixation and directly on the bone also.

48. Guide Wire

- This is a tempered stainless steel wire with alternate dark and light marks along its smooth round shaft, which is pointed at one end and blunt at the other
- It is available in a standard 9 inches length and 2.5 mm diameter.

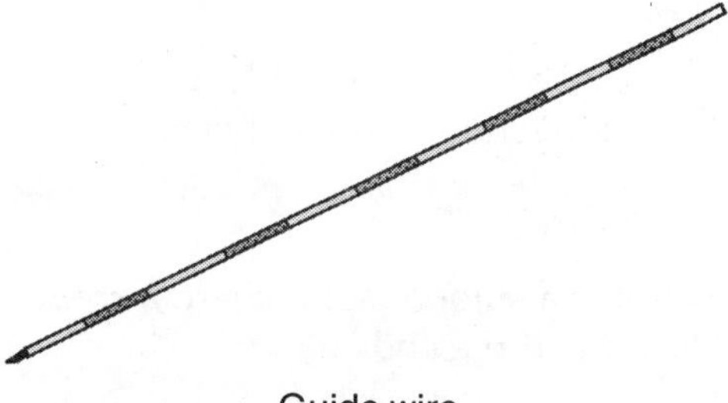

Guide wire

Uses

This is used for deciding the length of the implant (SP-nail, cancellous screw, etc.) in cases of fracture neck of femur. After reduction of the fracture, the guide wire is passed using an angle guide so that the wire enters at an appropriate depth and at a desired angle. The position is further checked by X-ray. The part of the wire, which remains outside the bone, is deducted from the total length thereby giving an exact intramedullary distance.

49. Angle Guide (Fixed)

- This is a T-shaped instrument with a fenestrated tube connecting the horizontal with the vertical bar.
- It is available in a wide range of angles of 120°–170° and allows a guide wire of 2.5 mm to pass through.
- Adjustable angle guides are also available

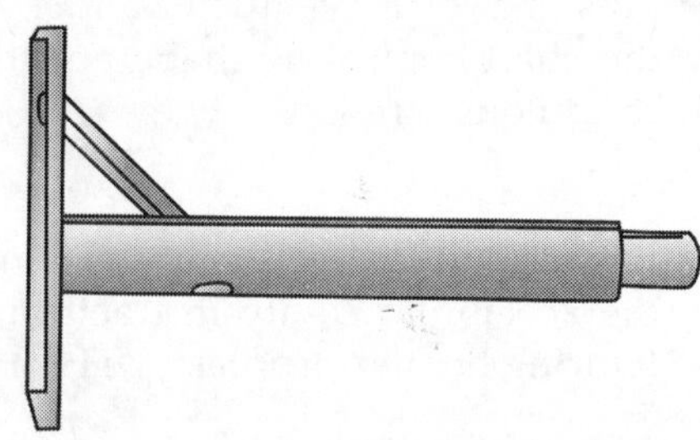

Angle guide (fixed)

Uses

This is used as a fixed angle guide for introduction of the guide wire in the neck of femur.

50. Triple Reamer

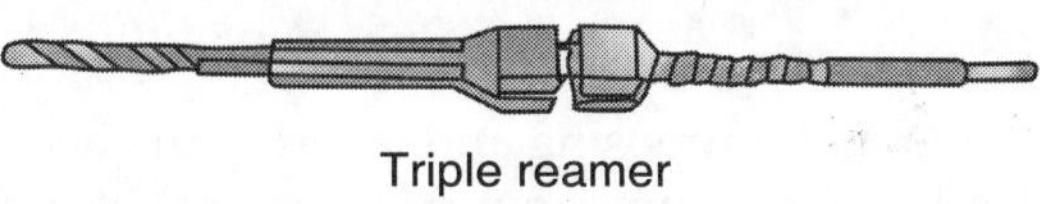

Triple reamer

- This has a cannulated drill bit combined with a slotted shank for the screw and a tapering collar for the barrel of the plate.
- This is used for 3-in-1 functions, i.e. to make a drill hole along the guide wire for the shaft of the screw as well as a larger hole in the proximal cortex for the barrel of the DHS to fit in. The length of the drill bit and the collar shaft can be conveniently adjusted. This is used with powered instrumentation.

Uses

It is used for fracture neck of femur, trochanteric fracture in the proximal end of femur and also intercondylar/ supracondylar fracture at the distal end of femur

51. CHS Wrench (Cannulated Hip Screw)

- This is a T-handle with a hollow tip for introduction of cannulated hip screw in cases of fracture neck of femur.
- It has a vertical plate in the tip to fit into the slot of cancellous screw.
- A guide wire is first passed, the hole is then drilled and tapped. An adequately sized screw is loaded into the wrench and then tightened.

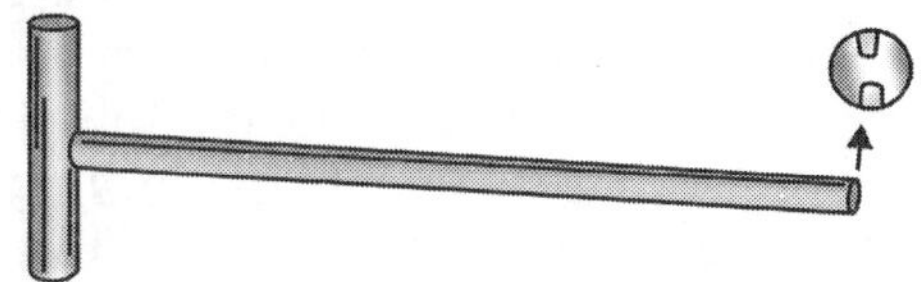

CHS wrench (cannulated hip screw)

Uses

This is used for the introduction and extraction of 6.5 mm compression hip screws in the neck of femur and condyles.

52. Impactor

This has a smooth solid shaft, a round head and a blunt tip at the end.

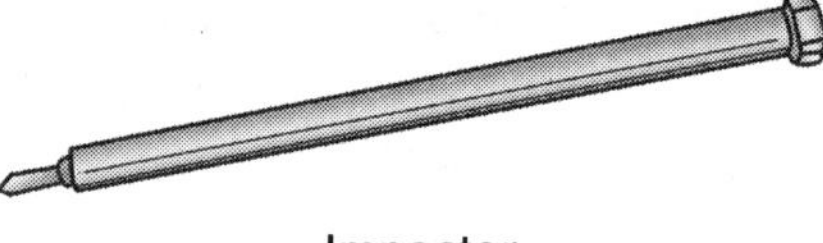

Impactor

Uses

- This is used for impaction of the plate barrel assembly onto the compression screw in the trochanteric area
- It can also be used for impaction of bipolar prosthesis in cases of fracture neck of femur.

53. Judet Femoral Head Extractor

- This is a long T-shaped handle, with the tip of the shaft conical in shape and threaded like a cancellous screw.

Uses

- It is used for extraction of the femoral head from the acetabular cavity in fracture neck of femur (During hemiarthroplasty/THR).

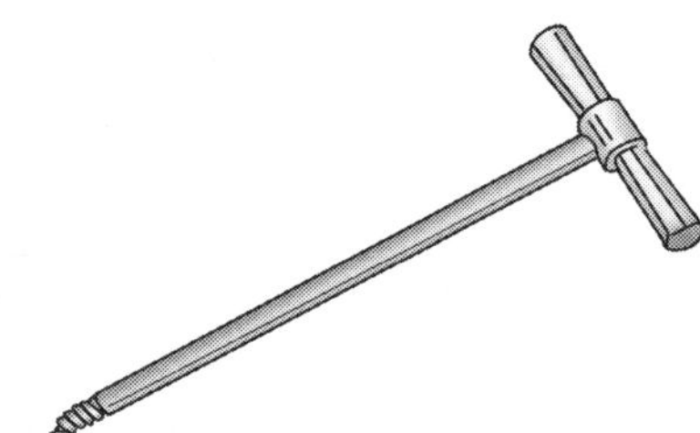

Judet femoral head extractor

54. Murphy's Skid

This has a wide and narrow spoon-shaped ends, smooth on one side and serrated on the other side.

Uses

It is used for reposing and levering the head of the femoral component of the prosthesis into the acetabulum during replacement surgery.

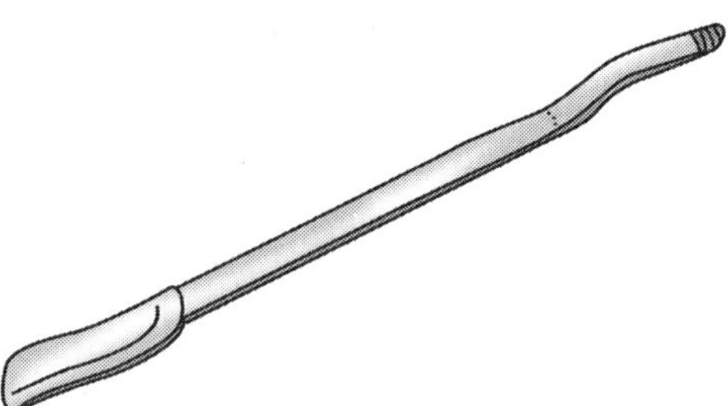

Murphy's skid

55. Austin Moore's Rasp

This has a long curved shaft with serrated tapering tip, a fenestrated handle, square top and a tommy bar.

Uses

This is passed into the medullary canal of the neck of femur after accurate positioning which is helped by the tommy bar and is hammered into the shaft to make room for the stem of the prosthesis. The tommy bar helps in guiding the rotational adjustment of the rasp and in extraction too.

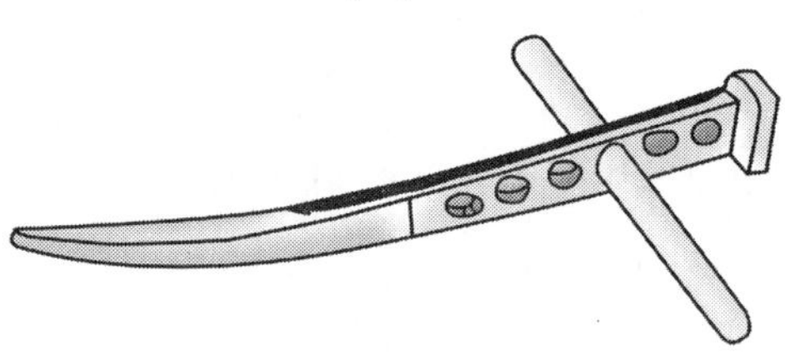

Austin Moore's rasp

56. Prosthesis Impactor/Punch

This is made of aluminium or steel handle and has Teflon tip on one end.

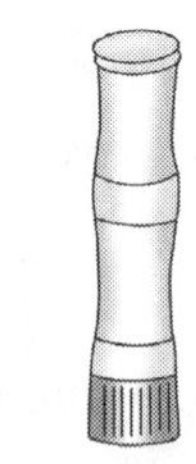

Prosthesis impactor/punch

Teflon Tip

Orthopaedic Implants

1. Smith-Petersen Nail

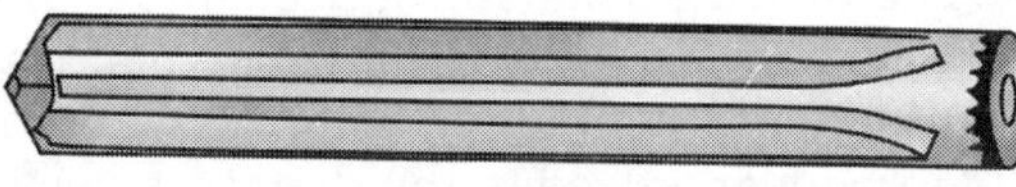

Smith-Petersen nail

- This is a triflanged nail, the shaft is cannulated, the core is threaded with serrated base and sharp pointed tip.
- It is available in a wide range of length of 2.5–5".

Uses

- This triflanged cannulated nail is used for fracture neck of femur (not used these days) and as a part of McLaughlin plate for cervico-trochanteric fractures. It has a cannulated core for the insertion.
- First, a guide wire is introduced into the neck of femur and after satisfactory localization, the length of SP nail is decided and the nail is hammered into the neck of femur over the guide wire. It has a threaded, serrated base for fixation of introducer and extractor.
- It can be fixed to the McLaughlin plate with a bolt in case of cervico-trochanteric fractures. It also has a triflanged shaft, for three-point fixation in the neck of femur, which prevents rotation, and sharp pointed tip for easy penetration.

2. McLaughlin Plate with Washer and Bolt

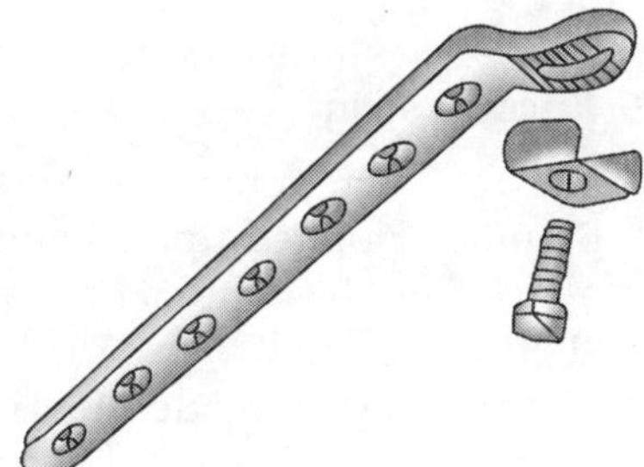

McLaughlin plate with washer and bole

- This has three components a plate, washer and bolt.
- The plate is rigid with 3–8 holes with the proximal end contoured like a spoon to adapt to the base of the SP nail and is serrated both on the medial and lateral surface to provide better fixation.
- It has a washer and bolt, which helps to fix the SP nail to the plate.
- The disadvantage of this device is its inherent weakness of the junction of nail, plate and the bolt which invariably gives away and is an insecure fixation.

Uses

- This is used in combination with SP nail for fixation of cervico-trochanteric fractures and has the advantage of fixation that can be done at a wide range of neck shaft angle.
- The SP nail is introduced into the neck of femur and then the plate is fixed to the shaft of femur to stabilize the neck shaft angle.

3. Jewett Nail Plate

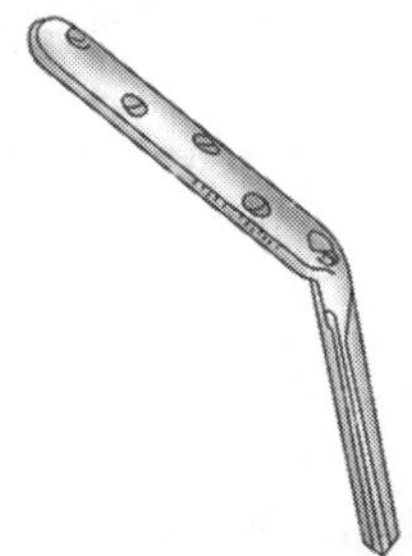

Jewett nail plate

- The components are triflanged cannulated nail in the proximal end and a plate in the distal end.
- This is a rigid nail plate fixation implant with fixed nail plate angle available with 130–145° angle.
- It has 6–8 hole plate, a rigid SP nail fixed to it as a single unit and scores over McLaughlin plate because of its fixed nail plate angle, which gives it the advantage of a strong cervico-trochanteric stabilization system.

Uses

- Cervico-trochanteric fractures stabilization
- A guide wire is first introduced into the neck and after deciding the exact length and the neck shaft angle, an appropriate nail plate is selected. The triflanged proximal end is guided and hammered into the neck threaded over the guide wire and the plate is subsequently fixed to the shaft by screws.

4. Austin Moore's Pin

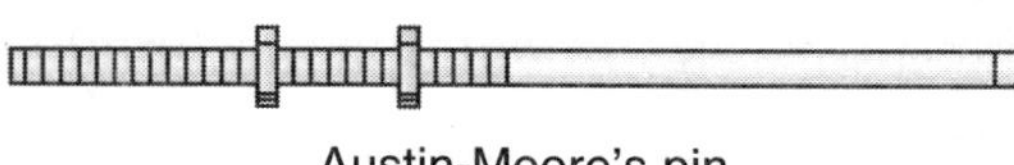

Austin-Moore's pin

- This has a smooth shaft with diamond pointed tip and a threaded base with 2 nuts.
- It is available in a wide range of sizes varying from 2.5" to 7".
- The disadvantage of this pin is frequent loosening of the nuts, proximal migration of the pin and bending.

Uses

- This is used for fixation of fracture neck of femur in children.
- After reduction of the fracture 3 to 4 parallel pins are introduced into the neck and 2 nuts are threaded over the base of the pin and are interlocked to prevent proximal migration of the pin.

5. Knowle's Pin

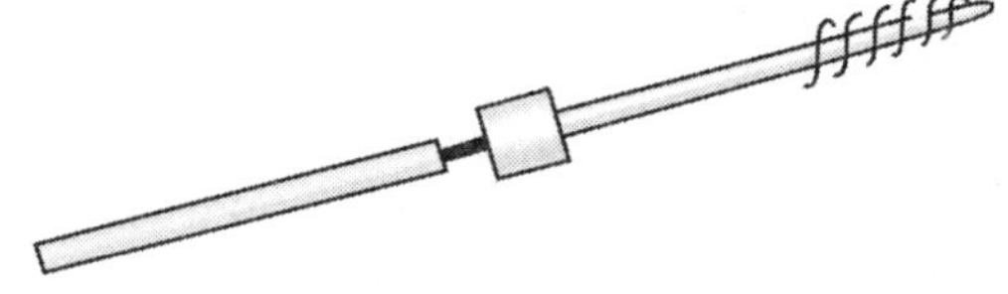

Knowle's pin

- This is a tempered pin with a threaded diamond pointed tip, a smooth shaft with a broad nut base and a breakable proximal shaft.
- Because of its threaded tip, it has a secure fixation in the head of femur which prevents its proximal migration which is further aided by the nut-shaped base.
- Because of its tempered steel, the chances of bending are less. After introduction of the pin, the tail end of the nail is broken off.
- It is available in 4 mm diameter ranging from 2" to 5" in length.

Uses

This is used for fixation of neck of femur in children and adults

6. Cannulated Bolts

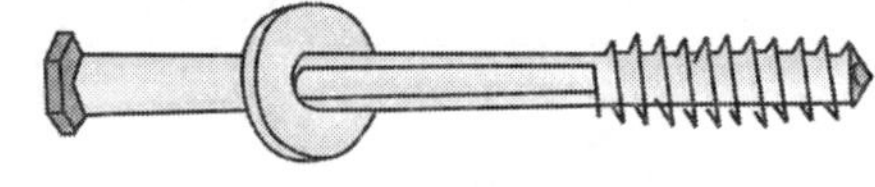

Cannulated bolts

- This has a cannulated shaft with cancellous thread at the tip, a washer over the shaft and base is nut shaped.
- A guide wire is passed after reduction of the fracture and the bolt is tightened over it, the washer prevents the sinking in of the bolt.

Uses

This is used for fixation of:
- Fracture neck of femur in adults
- Intercondylar fractures of femur and tibia

7. Thompson's Hip Prosthesis

- This has a smooth polished head, neck and shaft.
- The neck of this prosthesis compensates for the absorbed neck of femur. After extraction of the head and shaping the remaining neck, the medullary canal is rasped.
- The size of the prosthesis is selected depending on the head of the femur, which is extracted, and measured by a gauge.
- The prosthesis is then hammered into the medullary cavity.
- if necessary in osteoporotic patients Bone cement may be used.
- The bevelled tip of the shaft prevents perforation of the lateral cortex during introduction of the prosthesis. It is available in a wide range of sizes from 35 to 55 mm of head size.

Uses

This is used for replacement of the head of femur following fracture neck in elderly patients where the calcar is less than 2.5 cm.

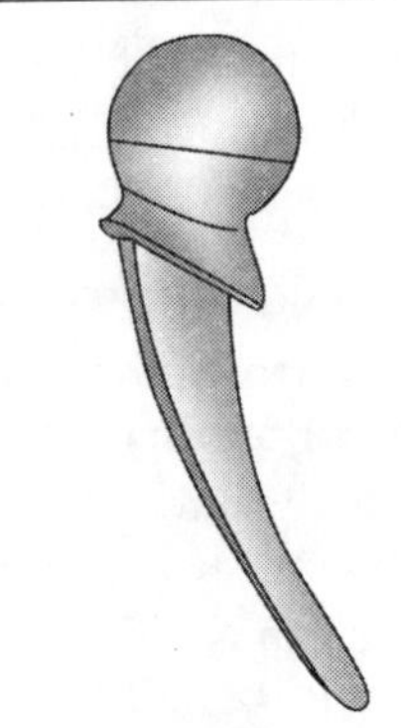

Thompson's hip prosthesis

8. Austin Moore's Prosthesis

- This has a smooth polished head, short neck with hole for extraction, shank with sharp lateral ridge and fenestrated shaft with bevelled tip.
- The fenestrations in the shaft make it light and give room for introduction of bone grafts
- The rigid shank gives a good hold in the trochanter
- The bevelled tip prevents lateral perforation during introduction.
- Bone cement can be used where there is a risk of loosening in osteoporotic patients .
- It is available in size 39–55 mm.

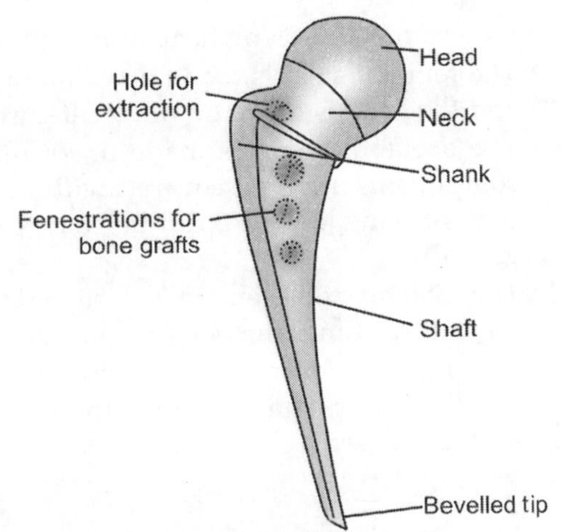

Austin-Moore's prosthesis

Uses

This is used for replacement of head and neck (hemiarthroplasty) of femur in patients with fracture neck of femur, beyond the age of 60, with a calcar of at least 2.5 cm and has a good articular cartilage lining, the acetabular cavity.

9. Bipolar Hip Prosthesis

- The components are an acetabular cup with an outer polished surface and an inner polyethylene core, the metallic stem with a small head, which fits into this cup.
- The modern bipolar prosthesis has two articulations (Bipolar), both of which contribute to total hip motion.

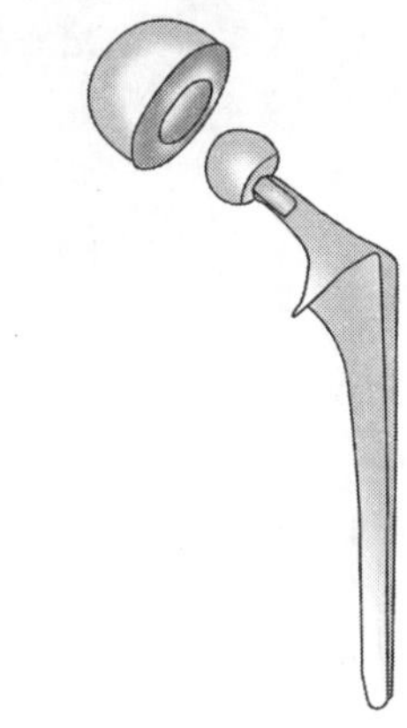

Bipolar hip prosthesis

- The outer joint, the large bipolar head against the acetabular cartilage
- The inner articulation is formed by the small femoral head that fits into the large head cup.

Uses

- Hemiarthroplasty (head and neck (hemiarthroplasty) of femur in patients with fracture neck of femur)
- It is indicated when degeneration is limited to the femoral side of the hip joint as in cases of osteonecrosis, tumour invasion or displaced fracture neck of femur in elderly patients.
- The stem is either press fit inserted into the medullary canal or in elderly patients bone cement is used.
- In younger patients, revision is very easy and in old patient's conversion to total hip can be conveniently done by changing the acetabular cup. This hemiarthroplasty is more conservative than total hip replacement since the articular cartilage is not removed.
- It is not indicated in patients who have developed advanced osteoarthritis of the hip with acetabular erosion. Modular porous are now available with variable head and neck lengths.

10. Total Hip Prosthesis (Father of modern THR: Sir John Charnley)

- It has a metallic stem, head and high-density polyethylene cup.
- The femoral stem is made up of titanium alloy, which has high stress transfer quality, and the head is made up of cobalt-chrome alloy which has superior wear resistance.
- The acetabular cup is made up of ultra high-molecular weight polyethylene, many components are now covered with metal shell to improve stress transfer to underline cement bone junction, can be coated with hydroxyapatite which encourages bone in growth.
- The total hip replacement is designed to enable the implant to support the loads, which reach three times the body weight during walking.
- Femoral components with large cross section are stronger, proper neck length selection helps in restoration of the hip motion, accurate femoral offset decrease the bending stress with each step.

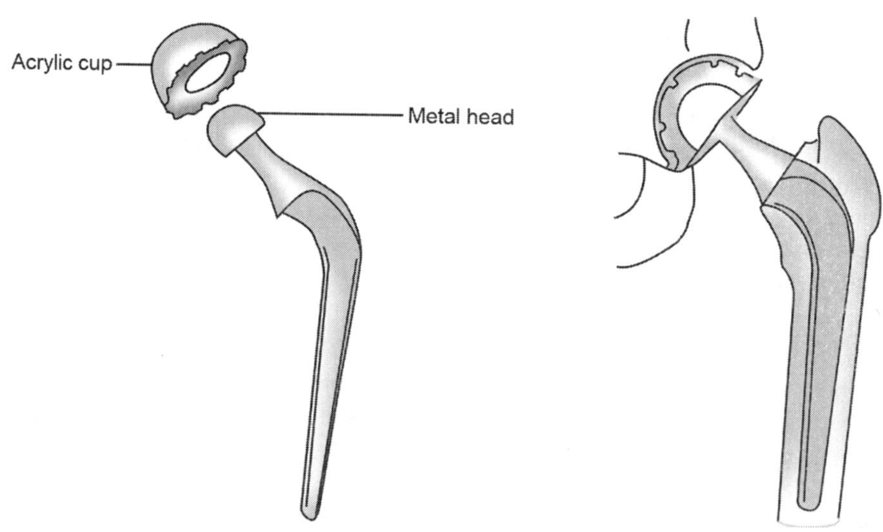

Total hip prosthesis

- The femoral component is either press fit in young patients or cemented in elderly.
- The acetabular cup is used with cement or screw fixed. Occasionally bone grafts are packed in the acetabular floor if it is deficient.
- Modular variety is also available with different sizes of head, neck length and shaft diameter.

Uses

Indications for *total hip replacement (THR)* are:

- Primary/secondary osteoarthritis
- Inflammatory diseases
- Avascular necrosis
- Displaced fracture neck of femur and non-union in elderly
- Bone tumours
- Metabolic and dysplastic involvement of hip
- Rheumatoid arthritis
- Ankylosing spondylitis
- Gout
- Congenital dislocation of hip
- Perthes' disease
- Slipped capital femoral epiphysis

11. Total Knee Prosthesis

Femoral and tibial component is made up of cobalt and chromium alloy, the tibial insert and patellar component is made up of UHDMP. Both are cemented onto the prepared precut bone surface.

Indications

- Advanced osteoarthritis of the knee
- Rheumatoid arthritis
- Ankylosed knee following trauma or infection

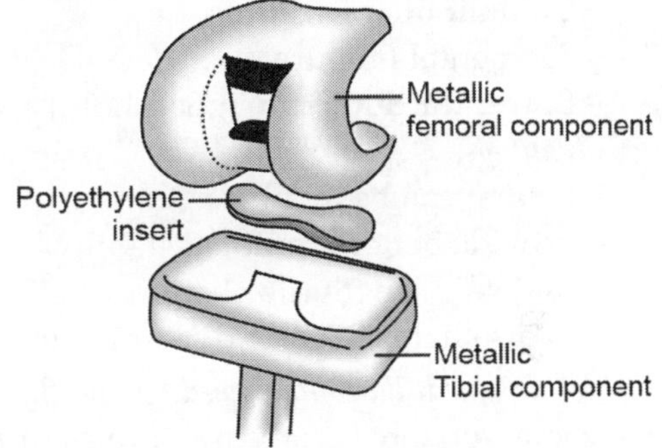

Total knee prosthesis

12. Femoral Intramedullary Nails

Kuntscher's clover leaf nail for femur:

- This is a long sheet moulded into cloverleaf shape as seen in cross-section.
- There are two eyes at each end for extraction of the nail.
- The shape gives it the strength to resist bending force.
- The straight nail inside a twin curved medullary canal gives it a three-point fixation.

Procedure

- After exposure of the fracture site, the length of the nail and diameter is assessed by reaming the canal to

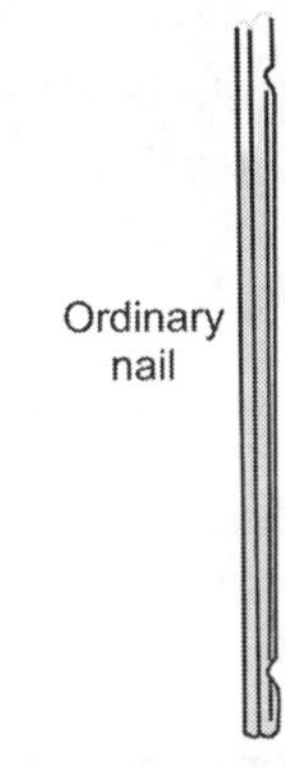

Femoral intramedullary nails

the maximum diameter and then using a guide wire, adding at least 2" to the intramedullary length for the nail eye to protrude above the tip of the trochanter for easy extraction

- This can be inserted *prograde,* i.e. from the piriform fossa in the distal direction entering the proximal fragment first and then across the fracture site into the distal fragment as is done in closed intramedullary nailing.
- It can also be introduced *retrograde* by first exposing the fracture site, introducing the nail in the proximal fragment out through the trochanter and then back into the distal fragment after reduction of the fracture, the nail is in this case hammered over the punch from the greater trochanter.

Use

It is used for intramedullary fixation of the upper two-thirds of femur shaft.

Disadvantage of intramedullary nailing

- Disrupts the medullary vessel network
- Because of the wide medullary canal it is not suitable for the lower third femoral shaft fractures

Newer nails

Interlocking nails (two screw holes in the proximal and distal ends)
- *Indicated in:*
  - Comminuted fracture
  - Segmental fracture
  - Lower third fracture (good hold)
- *Advantages:*
  - Patient can be mobilized early
  - Provide better rotational stability
  - Maintain length (no chances of collapse as seen with the K-nail)
  - It also helps in early dynamization of fracture

Other intramedullary nails used for specific fracture configuration:
- Reconstruction nail: for fracture shaft femur with ipsilateral fracture neck femur
- Proximal femoral nail (PFN): Subtrochanteric fracture femur
- Intertrochanteric nail (IT): Intertrochanteric fracture
- Enders nail: Shaft fracture humerus, fracture shaft tibia and fracture shaft femur in children
- Sofield's telescoping rods: Use in cases of osteogenesis imperfecta
- Peter William's rods: Pseudo-arthrosis of tibia

13: Rush Nail

- This is a malleable nail.
- One end is hook-shaped while the other is bevelled.
- The hooked tip prevents sinking in of the nail and helps during extraction.

Uses

It is used for intramedullary fixation of:
- Fracture shaft humerus

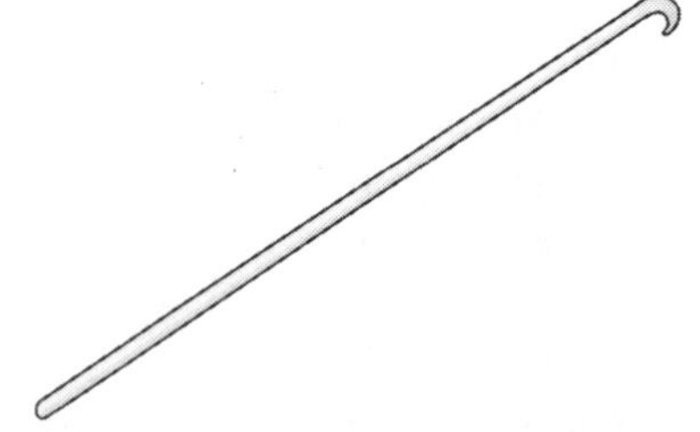

Rush nail

- Fracture of long bones in children as it can be bent to a desirable shape, the bevelled tip prevents penetration of the cortex.

14. Kuntscher's "V" Straight Nail For Humerus

- This is a straight nail with an eye at one end for extraction; the tip is pointed and bevelled
- The nail has a triangular cross section, which gives it three-point fixation, but the disadvantage is that it cannot provide compression at the fracture site and hence distraction often occurs.
- It has now been modified and has a hole above and below for transfixation screws so that the nail can be interlocked for early mobilization of the elbow.
- It is available in 5–8 mm diameter and 20 to 30 cm in length.

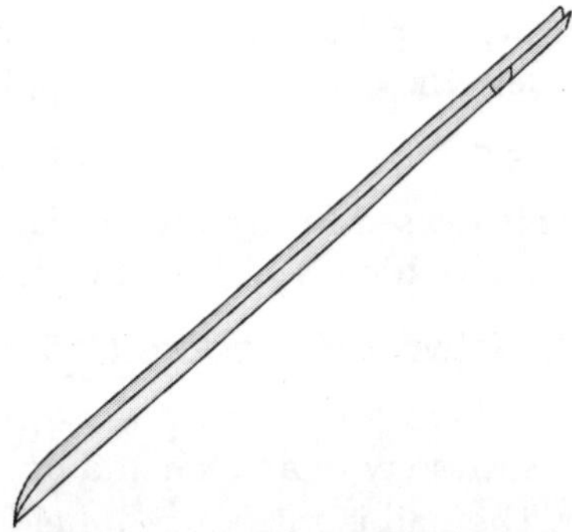

Kuntscher's "V" straight nail for humerus

Uses

- This is used for intramedullary fixation of humerus (fracture shaft humerus), the nail is inserted from the greater tuberosity across the fracture site into the distal fragment and the bevelled tip prevents the perforation of the cortex during insertion.
- It can be introduced in the retrograde direction through the roof of the olecranon fossa.

15. Kuntscher's "V" Angled Nail for Tibia

- This is a proximally angled at the junction of upper one-fourth and lower three-fourths, has an eye in the proximal end, the tip is pointed and bevelled.
- It is inserted in prograde direction medial to the tibial tuberosity or from above it. Because of wide medullary cavity in the upper part of the tibia it has a poor hold. It has now been modified with two screw holes above and below for interlocking and can be used for a large variety of fracture of the tibia.
- The angulation in the upper one-third, helps it for a better localization in the medullary canal and is an advantage during extraction.
- It is available in 6–11 mm diameter and 20–36 cm in length.
- For early mobilization, *modified interlocked nails* (Herzog bend: located at the junction of upper 1/3 and lower 2/3 length) have holes in the proximal as well as distal ends for interlocking screws, using Cotter pins.

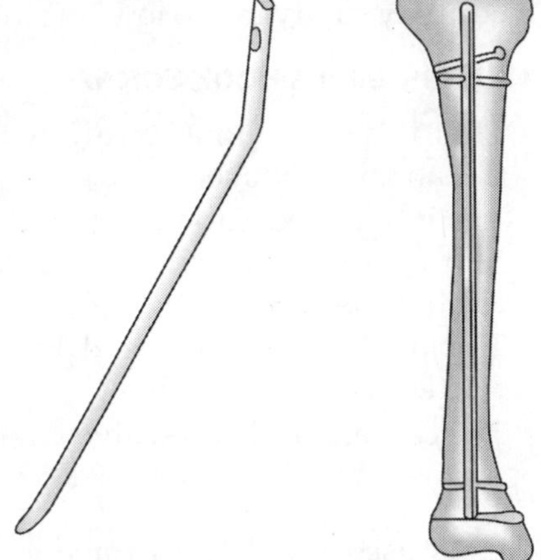

Kuntscher's "V" angled nail for tibia

Uses

This is used for intramedullary fixation of lower two-thirds of fracture tibia.

16. Talwalkar's Square Nail for Ulna

- This is straight nail square in cross-section with a pointed tip and a threaded base.
- It is introduced through the tip of the olecranon into the proximal fragment through the fracture site into the distal fragment.

- Due to its square cross section, it has a multi-point fixation here.

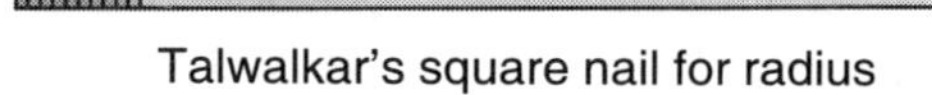

Talwalkar's square nail for ulna

- The threads in the base are used for attachment of the extractor device. It is available in 2–4 mm diameter and 17–30 cm in length.

Uses

This is used for intramedullary fixation of the lower half of ulna, because the medullary canal of ulna is wide in the proximal third, this is unsuitable for fixation here.

17. Talwalkar's Square Nail for Radius

Talwalkar's square nail for radius

- This is a straight nail, square in cross section with a notch and bevelled tip. The tail end is threaded.
- The nail is introduced, held in a T-handle and the point of entry is either the styloid process or lateral to the Lister's tubercle into the distal fragment across the fracture site into the proximal fragment up to the head of radius.
- The bevelled tip prevents perforation of cortex while negotiating the curved medullary canal.
- The threads in the base are used for attachment of the extractor device.
- It is available in 2–4 mm diameter and 17–30 cm in length.

Uses

This is a nail used for intramedullary fixation of upper half of radius, because of wide medullary cavity in the lower third, it is unsuitable for fixation.

18. Cancellous Hook Screw

- This is a cancellous screw with a long thread and a hooked head.
- It is introduced into the head and neck of femur through the trochanter for application of traction.
- The hooked head is used for applying traction through weights

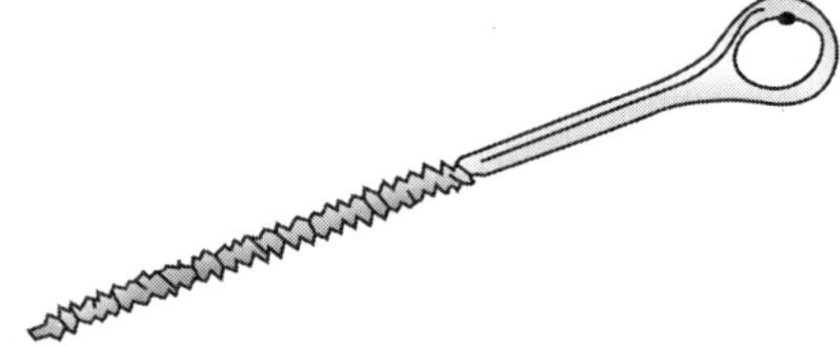

Cancellous hook screw

- The cancellous threads give an excellent purchase in the head and neck of femur.

Uses

This is used for skeletal traction in cases of central fracture dislocation of hip and pelvic injuries.

19. Cortical Screw (4.5 mm)

- It has spherical head of 8 mm diameter and hexagonal socket for screwdriver with asymmetric full-length threads and a non-tapping tip.
- The thread diameter is 4.5 mm the core diameter is 3 mm and requires a drill bit of 3.2 mm for the threaded hole and of 4.5 mm for gliding hole and a tap of 4.5 mm diameter.
- The spherical head gives it a maximum contact with the plate even if it is introduced at an angle.

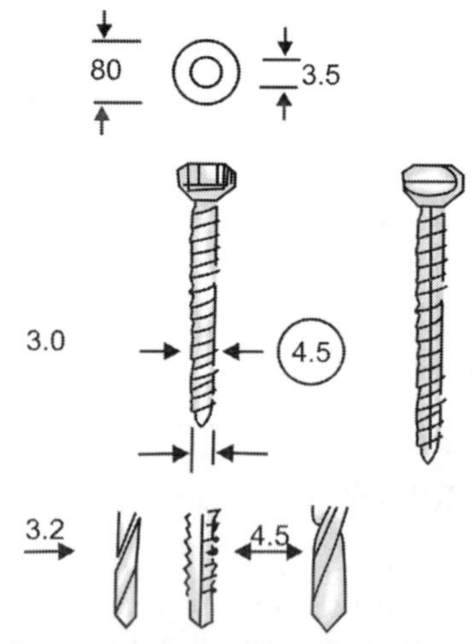

Cortical screw (4.5 mm)

- The hexagonal socket gives it an advantage over an ordinary screw head and does not require axial pressure during introduction or extraction.
- The thread profile is suitable for hard cortical bones and requires predrilled hole in which the threads are precut by a tap.
- Asymmetric thread gives an excellent bone contact.
- It is available in a wide range of length from 12 to 70 mm.
- Smaller screws with 1.5–3.5 mm diameters are also available for use in thin and small bones like radius, ulna and metacarpals.

Uses

- This is used for diaphyseal fractures and plate screw fixation of femur, tibia and humerus
- It can be used as a bicortical fixation alone or with a plate and can also be used as a lag screw if the near hole is over drilled by a 4.5 mm drill bit.

20. Cancellous Screw (6.5 mm)

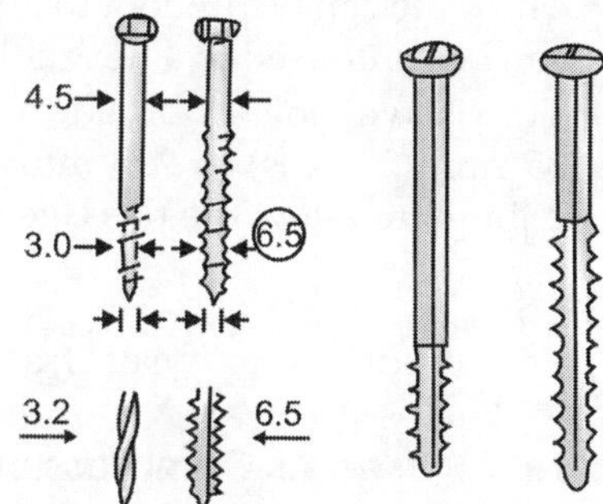

- This has a partial or full-threaded shaft, spherical head with hexagonal socket and has a self-tapping tip. The thread dimension is 6.5 mm; shaft is 4.5 mm, while the core is 3 mm.
- The deep threads and coarse pitch ensures a good hold in the compressed cancellous trabeculae.
- After the hole is predrilled only the cortex needs to be tapped, the screw tip is capable of cutting its own path through the cancellous bone.
- It is available in a wide range of length from 25 to 110 mm.
- Smaller cancellous screws of 4.5 mm and 4 mm diameters and lengths ranging from 10 to 70 mm are also available.

Cancellous screw (6.5 mm)

Uses

- This is used in epiphyseal and metaphyseal injuries for intercondylar and supracondylar fractures.
- It can be used alone or at the end hole of a plate in cancellous area.

21. Malleolar Screw

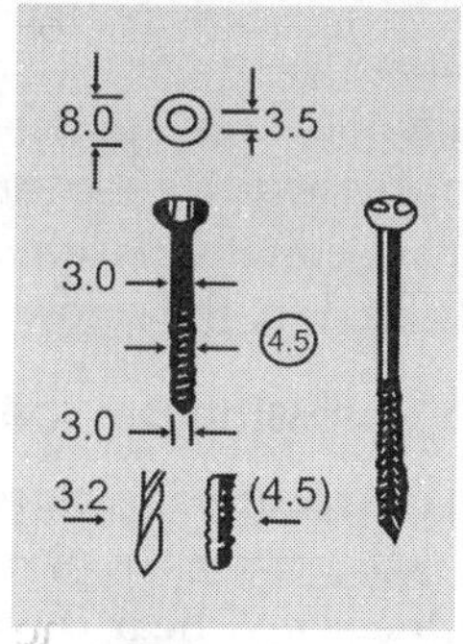

- This has a spherical head, a smooth shaft, and cortical threads in the distal half.
- The thread profile is like a cortical screw and the tip can cut its own thread, hence tapping is seldom necessary, the thread diameter is 4.5 mm, while the core and shaft diameter is 3 mm and requires a 3.2 mm drill bit to make a hole.
- It is available in lengths of 25–70 mm

Malleolar screw

Uses

These screws are used as lag screw for fixation of epiphyseal and metaphyseal injuries, e.g. fracture of medial malleolus.

22. Dynamic Compression Plate

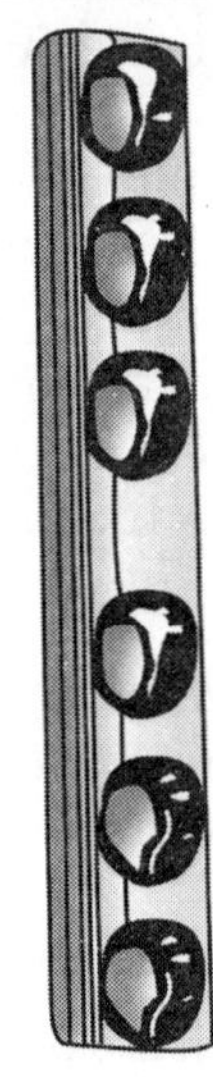

- This is a flat rigid plate with multiple spherical gliding holes on each side the middle zone.
- It is an improvement over traditional round hole plates with several additional advantages due to its special hole geometry.
- When the screw is inserted through these holes, it moves in a downward and horizontal direction because of its slanting cylindrical shape of the hole which causes the underlying bone to move horizontally thereby creating interfragmentary compression.
- The oval screw holes allow screws to be inserted at an angle to the plate. An eccentrically loaded screw can cause compression of 1 mm at the fracture site on either side even in segmental fractures, thereby eliminating the use of compression device.
- The plate can be prebent to give compression at the far cortex and can be contoured to a desirable shape to suit the underlying bone.
- This is available as broad, narrow, and mini sizes varying from 39 mm (2 holes) to 295 mm (18 holes). The end holes are large enough to allow the passage of 6.5 mm cancellous screws.

Dynamic compression plate

Uses

This is used for diaphyseal fracture stabilization of long bones.

23. DCP Used As Compression Device

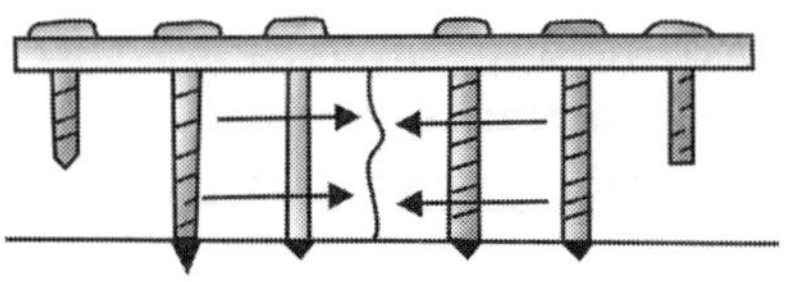

If the holes on either side of the fracture site are eccentrically drilled then a compression of 2 mm can be achieved at the fracture site.

DCP used as compression device

24. Lag Screw through DCP

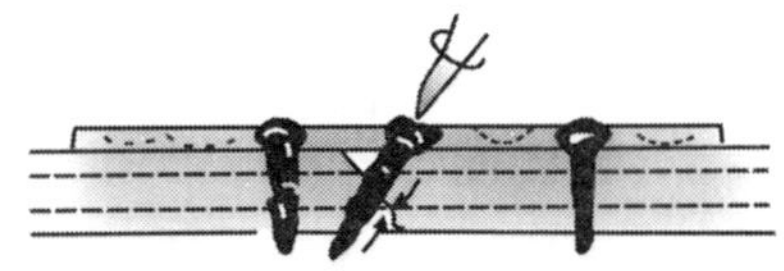

- In dealing with oblique fractures, an oblique lag screw is a great advantage (while using a DCP). All the screws are inserted as usual, the inter fragmentary screw hole is first drilled using a 3.2 mm drill bit, the screw length gauged and the hole tapped with 4.5 mm tap.

Lag screw through DCP

- The near hole is then over drilled with 4.5 mm drill and then the appropriate screw is tightened to get compression at the fracture site.
- The screw is placed perpendicular to the fracture line. In such situations, it is mandatory to first fix the screw on the obtuse angle side.

Compression Device

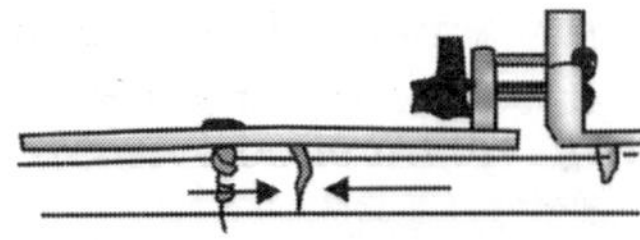

- The fracture is reduced and appropriate sized, contoured and prebent plate is placed across the fracture site.
- One screw near the fracture is inserted and the hook of the compression device is attached to the slot in the last hole of the DCP.

Compression device

- The device is fixed to the bone with a screw inserted in only one cortex, the compression bolt is then tightened to achieve the desired compression and the screw in the near hole is fixed.

25: Limited Contact DCP (LC-DCP)

- The newly designed LC-DCP stands for a new approach to plate fixation:
- Reduced trauma to bone
- Preservation of blood supply
- Avoidance of producing stress risers at implant removal
- The contact of the plate with the bone is limited and the plate-induced remodelling is small.
- Grooves on the under surface (as shown by an arrow)of the LCDCP improve blood circulation, allow for a small bone bridge beneath the plate at a place which is otherwise weak, result in more evenly distribution of stiffness of the plate than in conventional plate

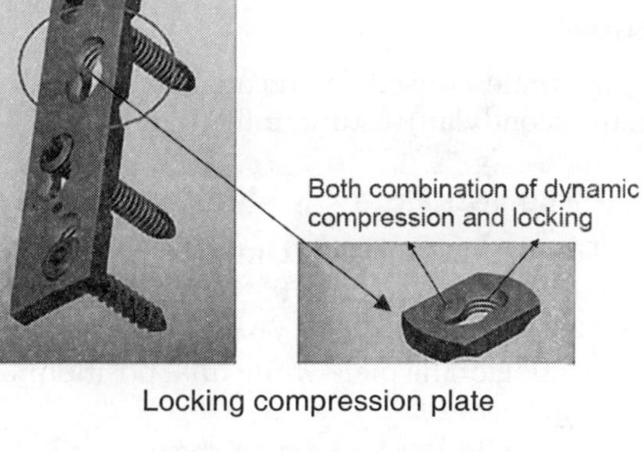

Limited contact DCP (LC-DCP)

26. Locking Compression Plate

- The newly designed Locking Compression-DCP stands for a new approach to plate fixation: providing both dynamic compression and locking.
- The screw head and the hole in the plate are both threaded to snuggly fit into each other for a better stable screw head and plate hole stability thereby preventing any toggle of the screw in osteoporotic bones.

Uses

Locking plates are ideal for fractures in osteoporotic bone.

Both combination of dynamic compression and locking

Locking compression plate

27. Reconstruction Plates

- This plate has lateral notches making it possible to bend the plate in three dimensions.
- The oval holes permit self-compression.
- The screws used are of size 3.5 mm.
- It is available in 5 holes (58 mm) to 12 holes (142 mm).

Uses

This is used for:
- Mandibular fixation and reconstruction
- Pelvic injuries (acetabular/rim fracture)
- Distal humeral fracture with intercondylar component

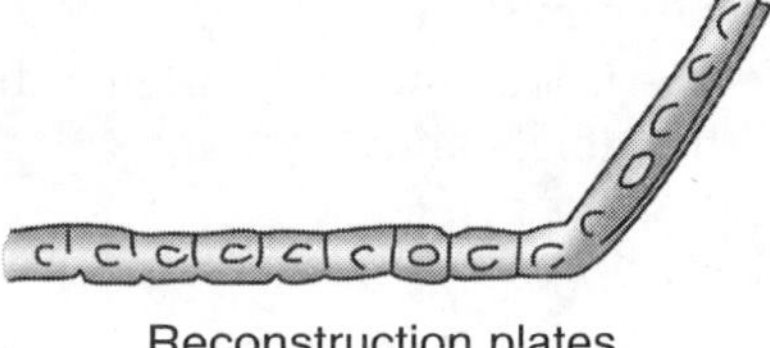

Reconstruction plates

28. T-mini Plate

- These small 2 mm buttress plates are available in various shapes.

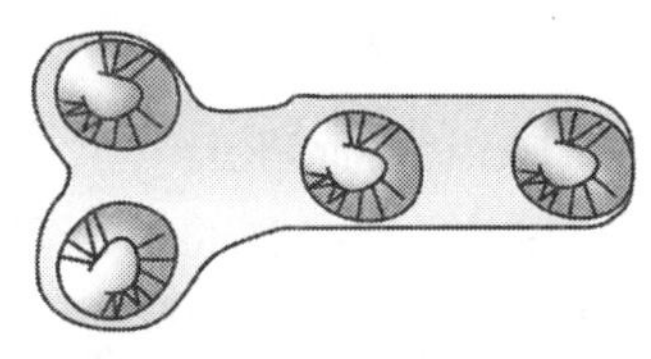

Mini plates

- 2 mm drill bit and 2.7 mm tap is used for insertion of 2.7 mm mini screws, which have a spherical head and hexagonal socket.
- These have 3–6 holes.
- Smaller plates (mini) for 2 and 1.5 mm cortical screws are also available.

Uses

It is used for fixation of small bones of the hand and feet.

29. Y-Reconstruction Plate

- Because of its peculiar shape, it can be moulded in three dimensions, which can be contoured to suit the distal flare of the humerus.
- The arms of this plate can support the medial and lateral pillars of the supracondylar area and can be bent and cut short using pliers, stem of the Y-segment of the plate is screwed onto the shaft of the humerus by 3.5 mm screw.
- It is available in a standard 10 mm size.

Uses

This plate is used for reconstruction of inter- and supracondylar fracture of the humerus.

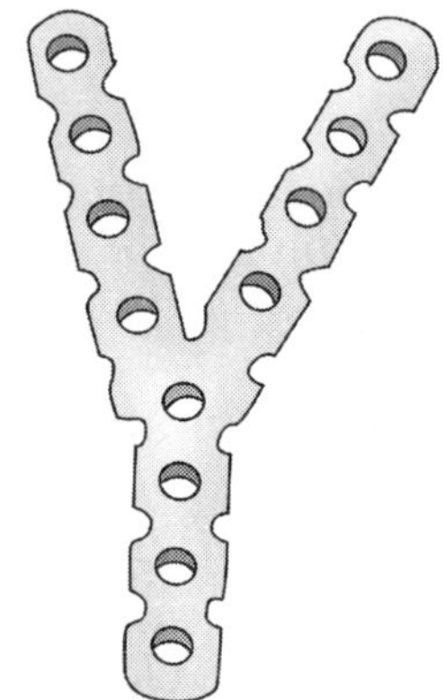

Y-reconstruction plates

30. T-Buttress Plate

- This is T-shaped with 2 holes in the upper part and several compression holes in the vertical part.
- The oval middle hole meant for temporary cortical screw fixation of the plate while final positioning and compression is done
- It also allows a lag screw to be inserted at a wide range of angle.
- It is available in the sizes ranging from 84 mm (4 holes) to 116 mm (6 holes).
- The upper end of the plate is bent to adjust to the flare of the tibial condyles.

Uses

- This is used for stabilization of metaphyseal fractures as in intercondylar fractures of the tibia and prevents the collapse of fracture fragments held by screws.
- It is also used for the fractures of the upper end of the humerus.

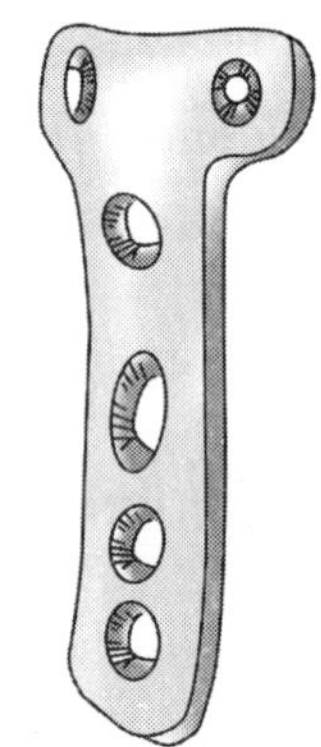

T-buttress plate

31. Condylar Plate

- This has a blade, which is U-shaped in cross-section, giving it high strength with minimal bone displacement, fixed at an angle of 95–130° with the plate

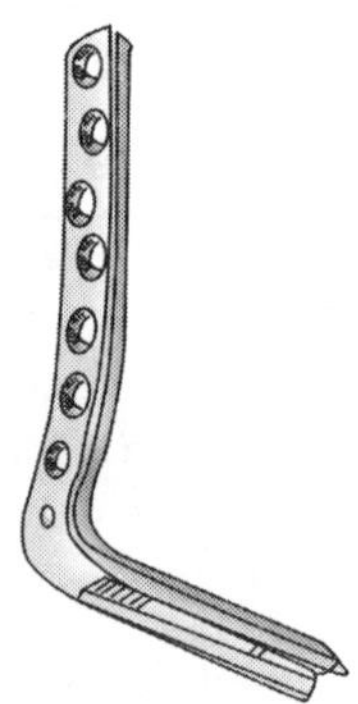

Condylar plate

- The upper two holes in this plate can take cancellous screws of 6.5 mm, while the other holes take cortical screws at various angles.
- It is available in a wide range of sizes, the blade is 50 to 80 mm in length and 6.5 mm thick
- Plate has 5–10 holes and is 92–204 mm in length.

Uses

This is used for proximal and distal femoral fractures.

32. Richard's Compression Hip Assembly

Compression Hip Screw:

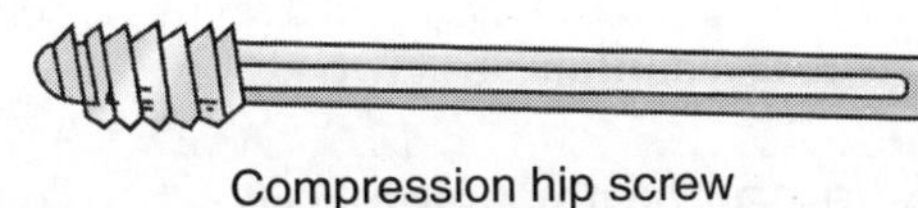

Compression hip screw

- This has a rectangular cannulated shaft, slotted at one end for the wrench for introduction and extraction, the tip has 6.5 mm cancellous threads.
- The cannulation is meant for the guide wire.
- The guide wire is first passed into the anteroinferior quadrant of the head and neck of femur over which the hole is drilled and tapped by a triple reamer.
- The screw length is gauged and then an adequate sized screw is loaded on the T-wrench and then introduced into the head.
- Following which the guide wire is withdrawn and the barrel plate is then loaded over the slotted end of the screw.
- It is available in sizes ranging from 50 to 115 mm.

Uses

This is used as a part of the dynamic compression hip system as a lag screw, in cases of fracture neck of femur and trochanteric fractures.

Compressing Screw or Top Screw:

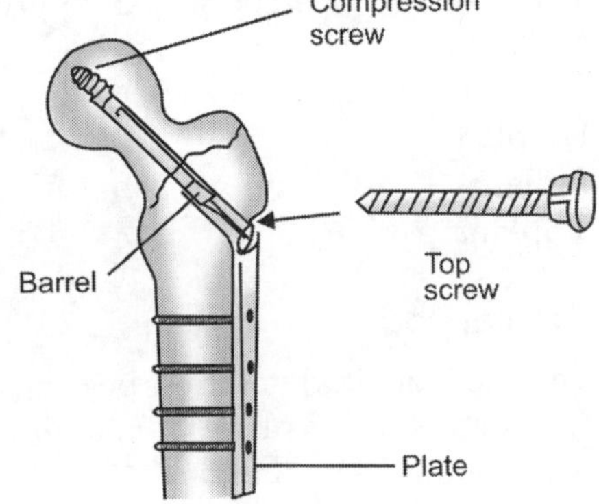

Compression screw or top screw

- This is a screw with hexagonal head and machine threads, it is basically a bolt.
- This is part of the DHS assembly.
- After insertion of the cancellous screw and loading the barrel plate over it, this screw is passed through the barrel into the threaded, slotted distal end of the cancellous hip screw.
- On tightening, it causes compression between the cancellous screw, which grips the head on one side, and the barrel plate, which holds the shaft of femur on the other.

Uses

This is used for compression of fracture neck of femur and trochanteric fractures.

Barrel Plate

- This has a short barrel circular in shape and the inner core rectangular in cross-section to match the shaft of the cancellous screw inclined at and angle of 130–150° to the plate, which has 4–6 compression holes for cortical screws.

- The barrel slides over the compression hip screw and then the plate is fixed to the shaft of femur by cortical screws.
- The first hole is meant for the cancellous screw and the compressing screw is finally tightened through this hole, thereby creating compression at the fracture site.
- The last hole is slotted for attachment of compression device.
- It is available in barrel size of 38 mm in an angle of 130°–150° and the plate of 4–6 holes.

Uses

- This is used for fracture neck, cervicotrochanteric and subtrochanteric fractures.

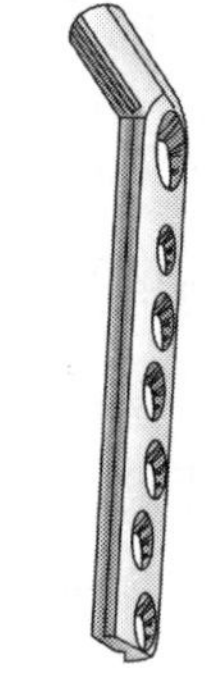
Barrel plate

External Fixator Assembly

This is an AO type of external fixator system used for temporary stabilization of:
- Open or compound fractures
- Load bearing splints
- Interfragmental compression
- Arthrodesis
- Corrective osteotomies
- Stabilization of pelvic fractures

The *components* are the basic frame made up of:
- Tubular rods
- The Schanz's pins hold the bone.
- The clamps connect the Schanz's pins to the tubular rods.
- The rods are interconnected to give three-point stability.

The *assembly* can be:
- Uniplanar
- Biplanar
- Triplanar

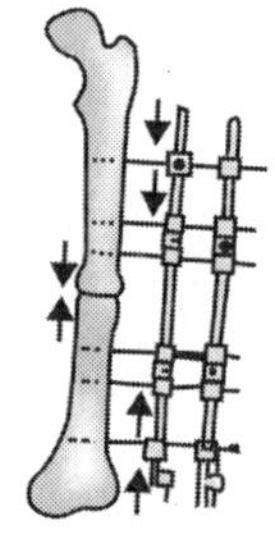
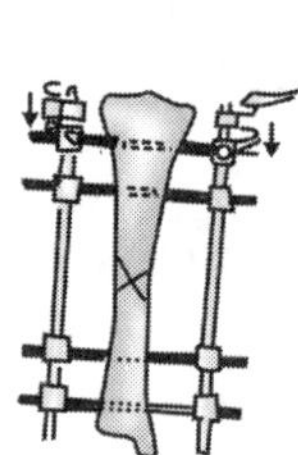
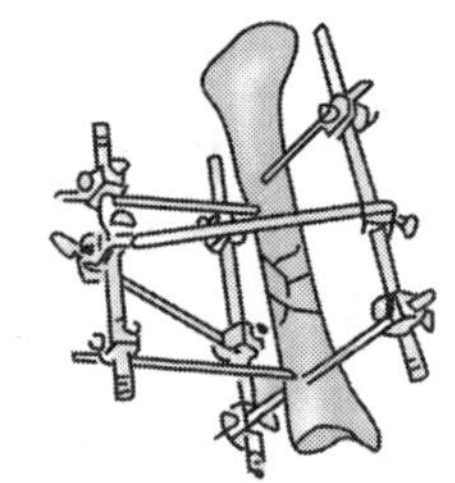
External fixator assembly

1. Tubular Rod

- These are longitudinal stress bearing hollow, tubular rods used as columns in 1–3 planes for stabilizing the skeletal system
- It is available in standard 11 mm and 8 mm diameter and lengths varying from 10 to 45 cm.

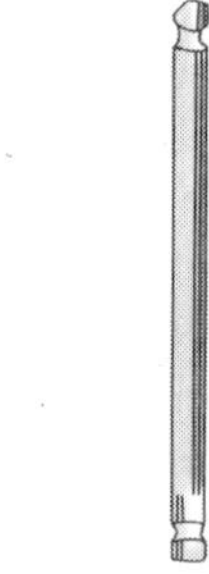
Tubular rod

2. Standard Adjustable Clamp

- This is a versatile device, which connects the Schanz's pins, holding the bone to the tubular rods. It permits over 15° adjustments in the frontal plane.
- It has a 5 mm space for the Schanz's pin on one side and 11 mm on the other side for the

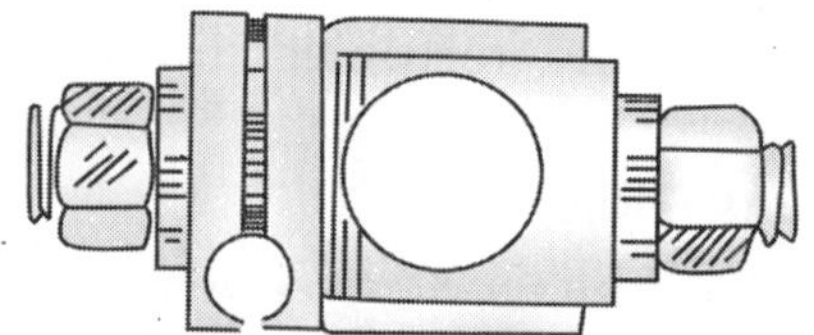
Standard adjustable clamp

tubular rod. Nuts on the either side can compress both of these holes by an 11 mm spanner.

- Specially designed clamps for holding 2 parallel Schanz's pins are also available.

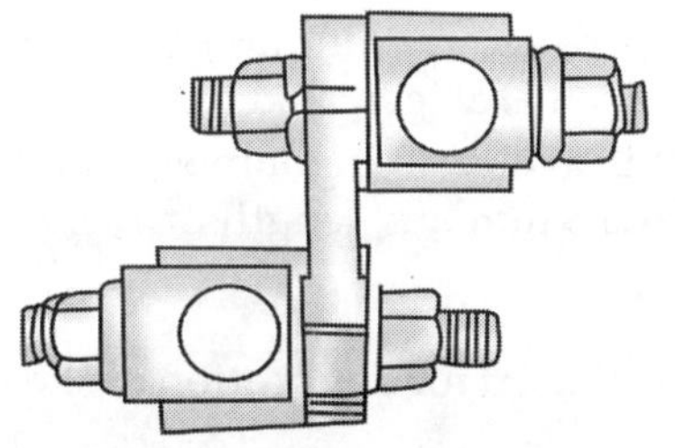
Universal joint for two tubes

3. Universal Joint for Two Tubes

- This is a coupled AO clamp hinged together for holding and stabilizing two rods together.
- •The hinge allows adjustment in one plane.

4. Transverse Pin Adjusting Clamps

- This is a long plate with a central hole for fixation of the tube and two side rectangular sockets for pin holding clamps. This is used for the stabilization of condylar fractures of the tibia.

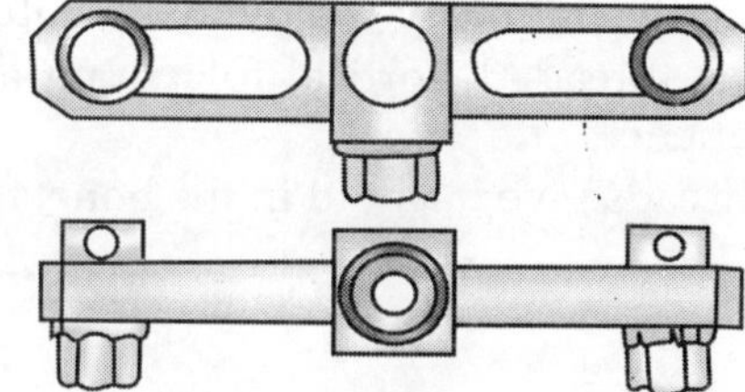
Transverse pin adjusting clamps

5. Schanz's Pin

- This is a modified Steinmann pin with a smooth shaft having cortico/cancellous threads at the tip, which is self-cutting.

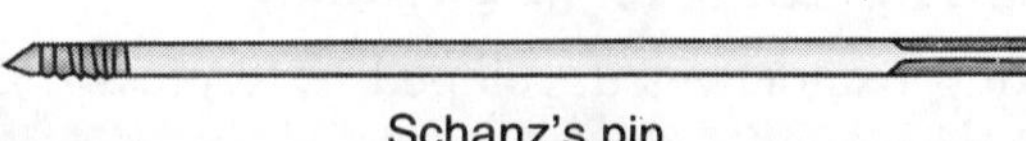
Schanz's pin

- The tail end is triangular for holding in a T-handle or drill. It is available in a wide range of diameter of 1.8–6.5 mm and 10–25 cm in length.
- The threads at the tip may be short or long.

Uses

Cortical threads are used for fixation in diaphyseal part of the bone, while cancellous long threads are used for condylar fixation and the neck of femur.

6. Asculab Clamp

- This is a modified clamp in which Schanz's pin can be placed at a variable rotational position connected with two parallel 8 mm rods.
- A single nut fixes both the components.
- It is ideal for fixation of humerus and forearm bones.

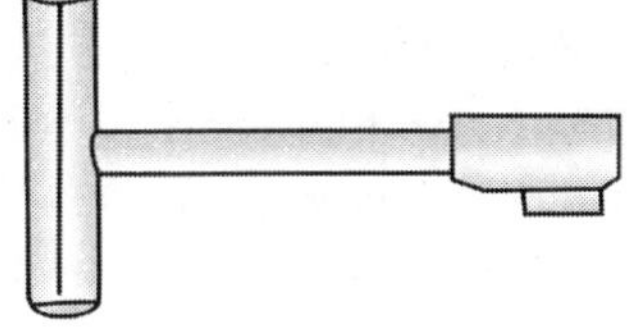
Asculab clamp

7. 'T' Handle

This 'T' shaped handle has a triangular socket for holding and quick coupling of Steinmann/Schanz's pin for introduction in the bone.

'T' handle

8. Steinmann' Pin

- This is the most commonly used implant in the wards.
- It has a smooth shaft with a diamond pointed tip and a triangular tail end.
- The diamond pointed tip makes it easy for the pin to enter the hard cortical bone, while the triangular base gives it a three-point grip and prevents slipping during introduction using a drill.

- There are certain modifications of this pin, which are described as under.
- It is available in diameter ranging from 1.8 to 6.5 mm and length of 12.5–30 cm.

Uses

This is used for application of skeletal traction.

9. Denham's Pin

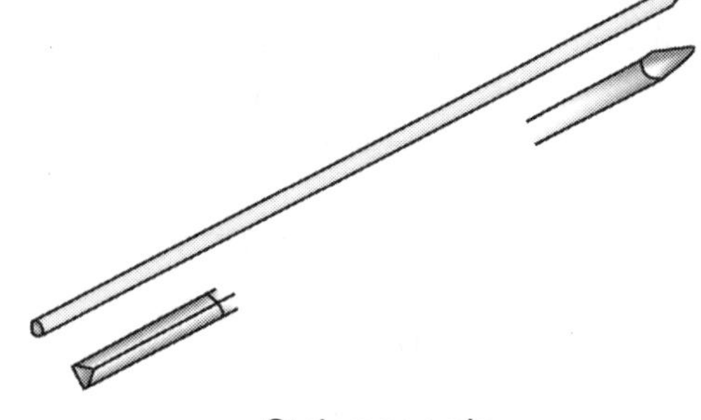

Steinmann pin

- This is a modified Steinmann pin in the sense that the middle of the pin has a cutting flute.
- It is threaded, cortical for young adults and cancellous threads for osteoporotic old patients.
- Threads give it a hold in the bone, thereby preventing its migration or slipping.

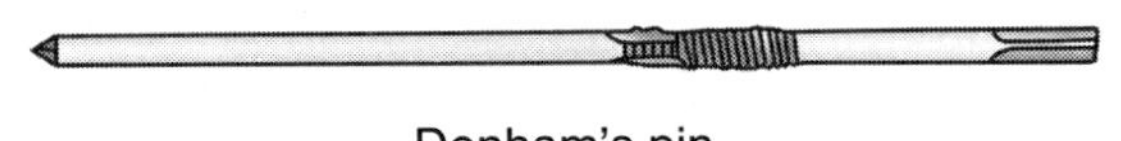

Denham's pin

Ilizarov Fixator (or Ring Fixator)

Ring fixator was developed by Professor Garvil A Ilizarov (Magician of Kurgan).

- Illizarov ring system is a highly versatile simple assembly made up of an external skeleton comprising of rings.
- These rings are interconnected by several long-threaded rods spanning the length of the limb, this is then connected to the bone through fine wires which pass through the bone and are tightened to the rings with the help of small wire fixation bolts.

Uses

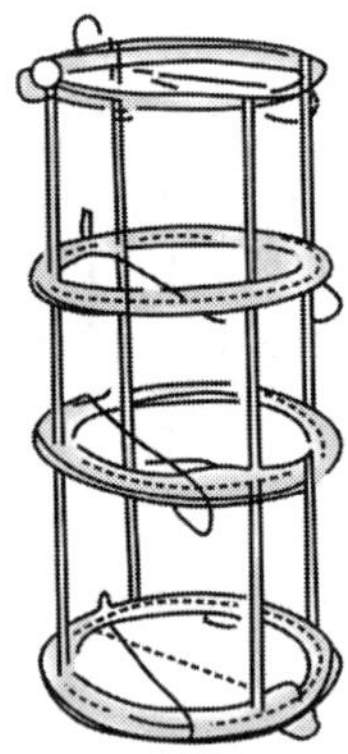

Ilizarov fixator

This can be used for a wide range of conditions varying from:
- Stabilization of fractures
- Correction of deformities
- Limb lengthening
- Management of non-union
- Malunion
- Arthrodesis

The components are as follows:

Primary components:
- Half rings
- Threaded rods
- K-wires
- Fixation bolts

Secondary components:
Used to construct the frame of apparatus e.g. bolts, nuts, rancho cubes.

1. Rings

- This contains two and a half rings in sizes varying from 80 to 240 mm in diameter with 18–28 holes for introduction of bolts or threaded rods
- Each hole is 8 mm in diameter and spaced 4 mm from the next hole
- The two and a half rings are connected to each other by small bolts converting into a full-ring.
- These rings are made of stainless steel.
- The newer ones are made up of carbon, which is light and radiolucent, but very expensive.

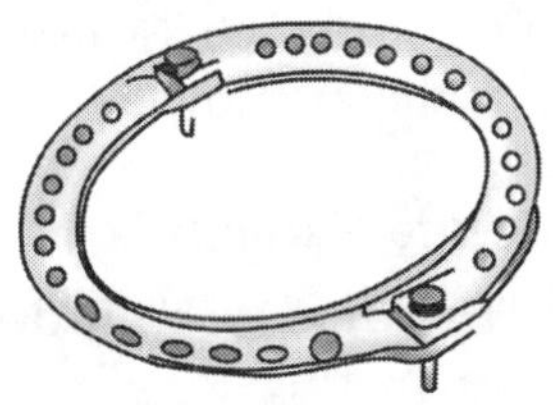

Rings

2. Threaded Rod

- These are stainless steel threaded rods 6 mm in diameter and is used for connecting the rings together to form the external frame and is available in 60 to 400 mm in length.
- The distance between two threads (pitch) is precisely 1 mm so that the compression or distraction can be accurately done everyday.
- It is preferable to do 0.25 mm eight hourly. This is controlled by twisting of the nut at a desired rate.
- One full circle of which moves the thread by 1 mm usually about 4 rods at equidistance are used for connecting the rings.
- Telescoping rods are available which give an automatic shift of 1 mm everyday

Threaded rod

3. K-wires

- These are specially tempered K-wires of 1.5 mm for children and 1.8 mm for adults.
- The tip of these wires may be: (i) trocar for cancellous bone; (ii) bayonet for hard cortical bone; (iii) olive wires are used as stoppers and available in lengths of 300–400 mm.
- The wires are passed through the bone using a drill keeping in mind the safe corridor and are then transfixed to the rings by bolts.
- These wires, are tensioned after introduction to increase its strength.
- The olive wires are used to act as stopper for controlling transverse traction in a butterfly fragment or for side-to-side translation.

On basis of tip:
- Trocar tip
- Bayonet tip
- Olive wire

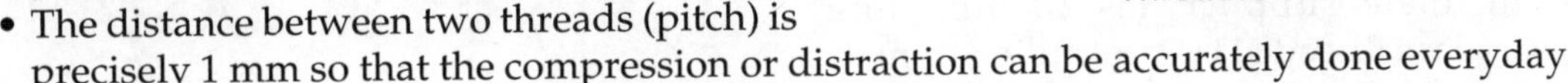

Different tips

4. Dynamometric Wire Tensioner

- The wire is first firmly fixed to the ring by bolts at one end while the other end is tensioned using a dynamometer so as to create a strength of 50–120 kg, which increases the strength of K-wires enabling them to withstand enormous loading forces.

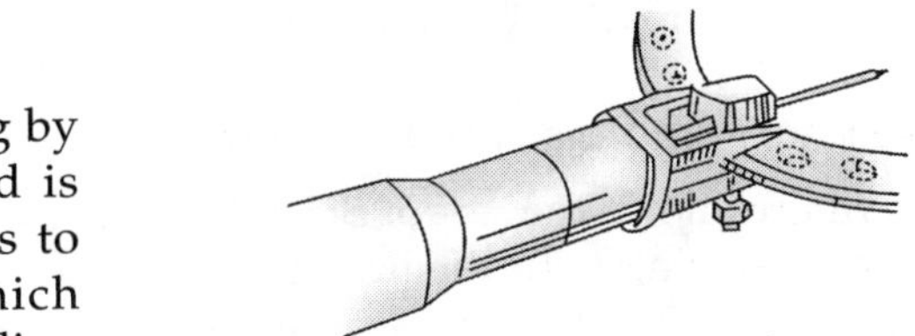

Dynamometric wire tensioner

- Once the wire is tensioned, it is fixed to the ring with the help of bolt and the tensioner is then removed.

5. Wire Fixation Bolts

- These are specially designed to fasten the K-wires to the rings.
- They are:
  - Slotted, so that the wire passes from the groove under the head of the bolt
  - Cannulated, in which there is a 2 mm hole in the middle of the neck of the bolt through which the wire passes.
- These bolts have heads with 6 mm diameter and a 3 mm smooth neck which sinks into the ring holes.

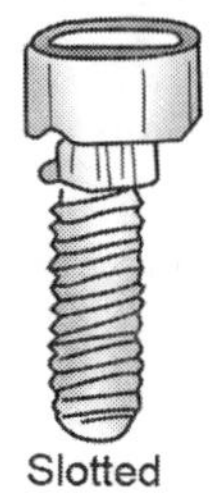
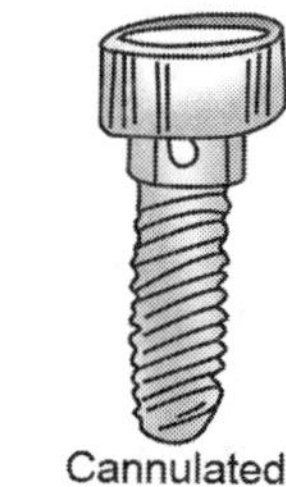

Wire fixation bolts

6. Male and Female Posts

- The male support has 13 mm long, standard threaded leg protruding from the butt end.
- The female post has no protruding rod, but 10 mm deep threaded hole at the butt end.
- This hole serves to connect bolts or rods.
- Their main advantages are that they can be placed virtually at any location, they can be turned 360° around their axis and they can be fixed in desirable position.
- They can be further modified, coupled together and converted into hinges as shown in the diagram.

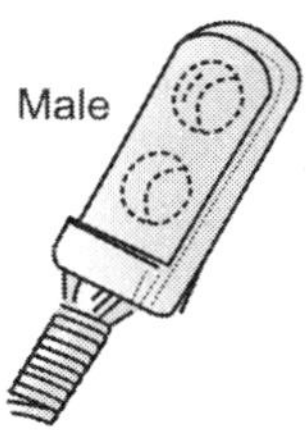

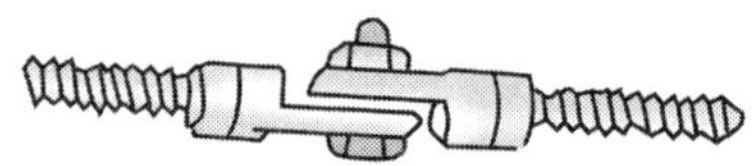

Male and female posts

7. 90° Femoral Arch (Italian Arch)

- This is exclusively used for proximal femoral fixation. Schanz's pin can be fixed to this arch, with the help of bolts and posts, which is subsequently connected to the rings below by three-threaded rods, one at each end and other in the middle.
- Larger ones of 120° are also available.

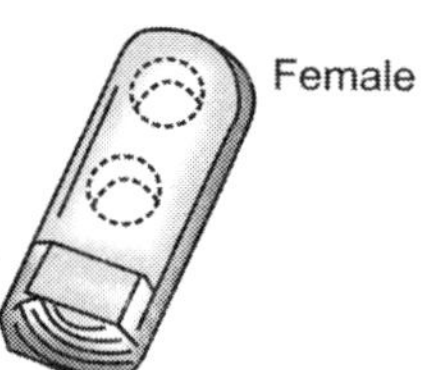

90° femoral arch (Italian arch)

8. Oblique Support Connector

This helps in connecting the proximal and distal arches in the upper femoral fixation assembly.

1. Proximal Femoral Fixation Assembly

- The figure shows the use of Schanz's pins connected to the 90° half ring with the help of posts and the second half ring of 120°, which are interconnected by oblique connectors.

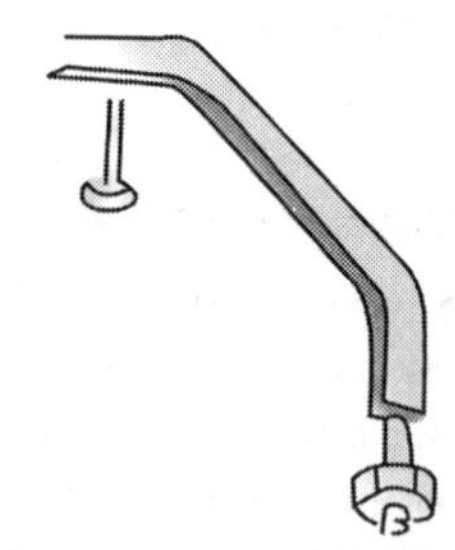

Oblique support connector

* This is an excellent assembly for the fixation of the upper third of the femur, i.e. the head, neck and subtrochanteric zone, which can be further connected down with the standard ring fixator.
* The above assembly circumvents the need to pass wires through the limb avoiding injury to important neurovascular structures.

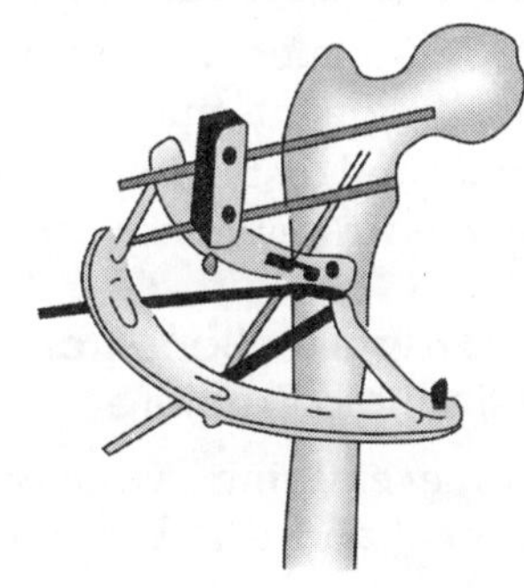

Proximal femoral fixation assembly

2. Assembly Frame to Show Stabilization of Subtrochanteric and Shaft of Femur Fractures

Several half rings are used in the proximal part through which Shanz pins and K-wires are passed and subsequently connected to full rings below.

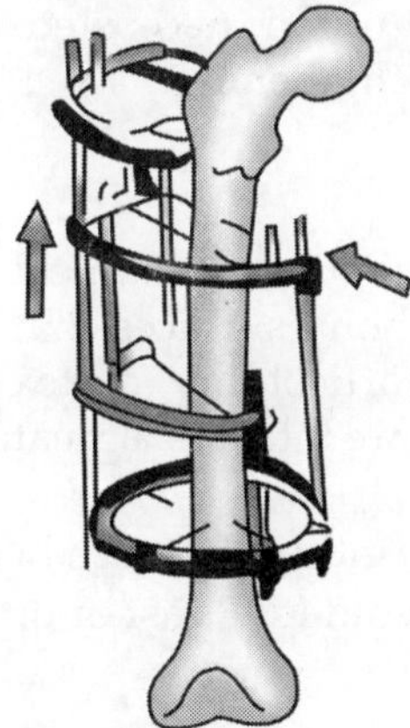

Assembly frame to show stabilization of subtrochanteric and shaft of femus fractures

3. Assembly for Communited Fracture of Tibia

* This shows the utilization of several rings, at least two in the proximal and two in the distal fragment stabilizing the main fragments

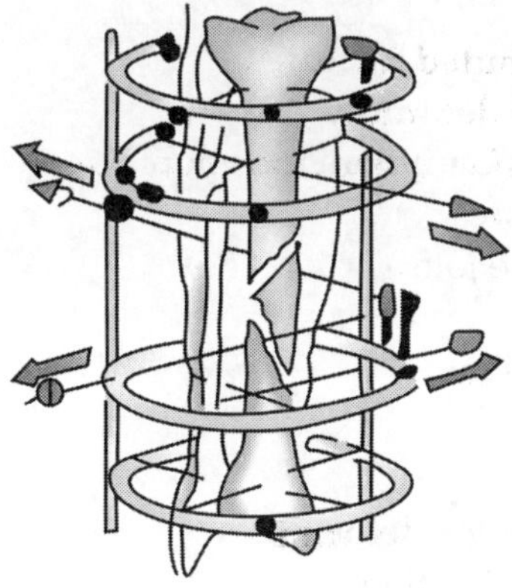

Assembly for communited fracture of tibia

- The butterfly fragment is fixed and compressed utilizing olive wires, which are passed through the fragments and fixed to the frame with the help of posts.
- The proximal and distal rings exert a vertical compression while the olive wires provide transverse interfragmentary compression.

4. Assembly Frame for Bone Transportation for Non-union of Distal Tibia Fracture

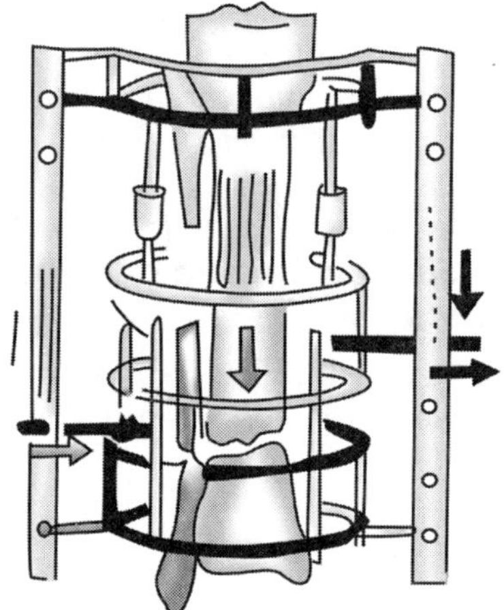

- This shows several rings, which are stabilized, in the main proximal and distal fragments by connecting long plate.
- A corticotomy is done in the proximal tibia and distraction between the second and third ring to produce neo-osteogenesis, while there is simultaneous compression between the fourth and fifth ring thereby managing the fracture non-union.
- This versatile frame can manage union, neo-osteogenesis as well as provides limb lengthening.

Assembly frame for bone transportation for non-union of distal tibia fracture

Principle

- *Distraction neo-osteogenesis* which is mechanical induction of new bone between bony surfaces that are gradually pulled apart after corticotomy (cortex is cut, but medulla and its vessels are intact to a greater extent) as regenerate (new bone) forms.
- *Compression* to destroy infection, induce fracture healing in delayed and non-union.
- Stabilization of fracture so as to avoid POP cast or open reduction and internal fixation.

Distraction Osteogenesis

- Fibrovascular network forms in first 2 week.
- Mineralization in next 2 week.
- Bone with haversian system-4 month
- Distraction should be done at a rate of 1 mm/day (0.25 mm/6 hours)

Indications

- Reduction of displaced, comminuted fractures
- Limb lengthening, correction of deformity
- Bone transport in bone loss for non-union, infection
- Intra-articular, malunited fractures
- Arthrodiastasis (stretching of the joint)
- Arthrodesis by compression
- Congenital pseudoarthrosis of tibia

Advantages

- Simultaneous correction of complex deformities
- Early ambulation and joint mobilization
- Light-weight, high strength, radiolucent rings

- Minimal surgical intervention
- Secure and rigid fixation of fractures

Disadvantages

· Cumbersome and heavy (new low weight carbon rings are available but very expensive).
· Time consuming
· Difficult to arrange rings
· Soft tissue management impossible

Sterilization, Autoclaving and Suture Materials

Microorganisms are ubiquitous. Since they cause contamination, infection and decay, it becomes necessary to remove or destroy them from materials or from areas. This is the object of sterilization.

- *Sterilization* is defined as the process by which an article, surface or medium is freed of all living microorganisms either in vegetative or spore state.
- *Disinfection* means the destruction or removal of all pathogenic organism, or organism capable of giving rise to infection.

Various agent used in sterilization can be classified as follows:

Physical

- Sunlight
- Drying
- Dry heat: Flaming, incineration, hot air
- Moist heat: Pasteurization, boiling, steam under normal pressure, steam under pressure
- Filtration: Candle, asbestos pads, membranes
- Radiation: Ionizing (X-rays, gamma rays and cosmic rays); Non-ionizing (infrared, ultraviolet radiation)
- Ultrasonic and sonic vibrations

Chemical

- Alcohols: Ethyl, isopropyl, trichlorobutanol
- Aldehydes: formaldehyde, glutaraldehyde
- Dyes
- Halogens
- Phenols
- Surface active agents
- Metallic salts
- Gases: Ethylene oxide, formaldehyde gas

Autoclaving

- The commonest mode, which we across in OT is autoclaving.
- The principle of autoclave or steam sterilizer is that water boils when its vapor pressure equals that of the surrounding atmosphere. Hence, when pressure inside a closed vessel increases, the temperature at which water boils also increases.

Recommended temperature and duration for heat sterilization

Method	Temperature (°C)	Holding time (in min)
Autoclaving	121	15
	126	10
	134	3

Remember: Different method of sterilization for article used in day-to-day procedures in OT:

Material	Method
Skin	Tincture iodine
OT	Formaldehyde gas
Orthopaedics implants	Autoclaving
Suture material except catgut	Autoclaving
Catgut	Ionizing radiation (dose of 2.5 M rad)
Surgical instrument except sharp instrument	Autoclaving
Sharp instrument	5% cresol
Endoscope	Glutaraldehyde (cidex 2%) or ethylene oxide
Glass syringes	Hot air oven (180°C× 1 hour)
Disposable syringes	Ionizing radiation
Gloves, catheters	Autoclaving

Other Sterilization Procedures

- Prosthesis and bone cement are presterilized and comes in sealed packages.
- Prostheses are sterilized using *Ethylene Oxide gas or Gamma rays* and are supplied sterile for single use only.
- Formalin tablets, kept in closed chamber (air-tight) especially for arthroscopic instruments and electric drills.

Q2. What are the characteristic of ideal sutures?

Suture Materials

The characteristic of an ideal suture:
- It should be *non-electrolytic, non-capillary, non-allergenic* and *non-carcinogenic.*
- It would consist of material which permits its use in any operation.
- It should handle comfortably and naturally to the surgeon.
- Tissue reaction stimulated should be minimal
- It should not create a situation favorably to bacterial growth
- The breaking strength should be high in small caliber.
- A knot should hold securely without fraying or cutting.

Q3. Comment on Size and Tensile Strength of suture?

Size denote the diameter of the material, stated numerically, *the more zeros (0) in the number, the smaller the size* of the strand. As the number of 0's decreases, the size of strand increases. The 0's are designated as 5–0 for example, meaning 00000 which is smaller than a size 4–0.

The *smaller the size, the less tensile strength* the strand will have. Tensile strength of a suture is the measured force in pounds that the strands will withstand before it breaks when knotted.

Q4. Discuss in brief the types of sutures and mention suture materials commonly used in surgery?

Suture can be conviently be divided into two broad groups: absorbable and nonabsorbable. Absorbable sutures can be associated as temporary, most nonabsorbable are permanent. Regardless of its nature, suture material is a foreign body to the human tissues in which it is implanted.

Types of Suture

- All suture material which is digested by body enzymes or hydrolyzed by tissue fluids is called *absorbable*.
- Tissue enzymes cannot dissolve some suture materials. These are called *non-absorbable*.

Monofilament

- It is made of a single strand
- It resists harboring microorganisms
- It ties down smoothly

Multifilament

- It consist of several filaments twisted or braided together
- This gives good handing and typing qualities

Suture Materials Commonly Used in Surgery

Suture	Types	Raw Material	Absorption rate	Contraindication	Uses
Surgical gut	Plain Plain	Collagen derived from healthy mammals	Digested by body enzymes within 70 days	Should not be used in tissues that heal slowly and require support	Ligate superficial vessels; Sutures subcutaneous and other tissues that heal rapidly. Sometime used in presence of infection; Ophthalmology
	Chronic	Collagen derived from healthy mammals Treated to resist digestion by body tissues	Digested by body enzymes within 90 days	Being absorbable should not be used where prolonged approximation of tissue under stress is required	May be used in presence of infection; Used in tissues that heals relatively slowly but intended for used as absorbable suture or ligature. Ophthalmology
Coated vicryl	Braided	Copolymer of lactide and glycolide coated with polyglactin-370 and calcium stearate	Minimal until about 40th day. Essentially complete between 60–90 days. Absorbed by slow hydrolysis	Being absorbable should not be used where prolonged approximation of tissue under stress is required	Ligate or suture tissues where an absorbable suture is desirable except where approximation under stress is required

(Contd.)

Suture	Types	Raw Material	Absorption rate	Contraindication	Uses
PDS	Mono-filament	Polyester polymer	Minimal until about 90th day. Essentially complete within 210 days absorbed by slow hydrolysis	Being absorbable should not be used where prolonged approximation of tissue under stress is required	Abdominal and thoracic closure. Subcutaneous tissue, colon and rectal surgery, can we in presence of infection, Orthopaedic; plastic
Surgical silk	Braided	Natural protein fibres of raw silk spun by silk worm	Usually cannot to found after two years	Should not be used for placement of vascular prosthesis and artificial heart valve	Most body tissues for ligating and suturing. General surgery, ophthalmology and plastic surgery
Ethilon nylon	Mono-filament	Polyamide polymer	Degrades at a rate of about 15–20% per year	None	Skin closure, retention, plastic surgery, ophthalmology and micro-surgery
Mersi-lene	Braided	Polyester polyethylene terephthalate	Nonabsorbable: remains encapsulated in body tissues	None	Cardiovascular general and plastic surgery, retention, ophthalmology
Prolene	Mono-filament	Polymer of propylene	Nonabsorbable: remains encapsulated in body tissues	None	General, plastic, cardiovascular surgery and skin closure; ophthalmology

Q5. Write short note on surgical staples?

In 1978, Ethicon, INC introduced the world's first reassembled disposable staging instrument. The staples are gently placed across the junction of the skin edges so they informally span the incision line. Approximately of the skin edges by stapling minimizes tissue compression. Skin staples are flexible in terms of their application.

Uses

They can be used virtually anywhere, regardless of the contour of the body they may be employed for routine skin closure in a wide variety operative procedure, to severe skin greater on burn patients, and for lacerations closed in the emergency department. These are quicker and easier than sutures.

Disadvantage

- There is a significantly higher risk of developing a wound infection when the wound is closed with staples especially during hip surgery.
- More expensive and require a special instrument (specific staple remover) for the removal.

Contraindications

When it is not possible to maintain at least 5 mm from the stapled skin to underlying bones, vessels, internal organs, the use of staples for skin closure is contraindicated.

Q6. Discuss in short about Tourniquet?

Tourniquet use is a common practice in operative procedure especially orthopedic and plastic surgeries. They are compressive devices that occlude arterial flow distal to the device to control extremity bleeding and provide a clearer surgical field and decrease the perioperative blood loss.

Application

Pneumatic tourniquet with a hand pump and an accurate pressure gauge is probably the safest, but a constantly regulated pressure tourniquet is quite satisfactory if it is properly maintained and checked. A tourniquet should be applied by an experienced person.

Several sizes of pneumatic tourniquets are available for the upper and lower extremities. The upper arm or the thigh is wrapped with several thicknesses of smoothly applied cotton cast padding. An assistant manually grasps the flesh of the extremity just distal to the level of tourniquet application and firmly pulls this loose tissue distally before the cast padding is placed. Traction on the soft tissue is maintained while the padding and tourniquet are applied and the latter is secured. The assistant's grasp is then released, resulting in a greater proportion of the subcutaneous tissue remaining distal to the tourniquet. This bulky tissue tends to support the tourniquet and push it into an even more proximal position. All air is expressed from the sphygmomanometer or pneumatic tourniquet before application.

When a sphygmomanometer cuff is used, it should be wrapped with a gauze bandage to prevent its slipping during inflation. Every effort is made to decrease tourniquet time; the extremity often is prepared and ready before the tourniquet is inflated. The extremity is then elevated for 2 minutes, or the blood is expressed by a sterile sheet rubber bandage or a cotton elastic bandage. Beginning at the fingertips or toes, the extremity is wrapped proximally to within 2.5–5.0 cm of the tourniquet. If a Martin sheet rubber bandage or an elastic bandage is applied up to the level of the tourniquet, the latter will tend to slip distally at the time of inflation. The tourniquet should be inflated quickly to prevent filling of the superficial veins before the arterial blood flow has been occluded.

Tourniquet cuff pressure: When applied *at the thigh*, the minimum effective tourniquet pressure is *90–100 mm Hg above systolic BP*, and in a normotensive, non-obese patient, pressure of *250 mm Hg* is sufficient. Similarly, an *arm* tourniquet pressure of *200 mm Hg* is recommended.

Complications

- *Tourniquet paralysis* can result from (1) excessive pressure, (2) insufficient pressure, resulting in passive congestion of the part, with haemorrhagic infiltration of the nerve, (3) keeping the tourniquet on too long, or (4) application without consideration of the local anatomy. This complication is thought to be related to the duration of ischaemia and not to the mechanical effect of the tourniquet.
- *Post-tourniquet syndrome* is a common reaction to prolonged ischaemia and is characterized by edema, pallor, joint stiffness, motor weakness, and subjective numbness. Spontaneous resolution usually occurs within 1 week.
- *Compartment syndrome*, rhabdomyolysis, and pulmonary emboli are rare complications of tourniquet use.
- *Vascular complications* can occur in patients with severe arteriosclerosis or prosthetic grafts. A tourniquet should not be applied over a vascular graft.

24

Eponymic (Named) Fractures/Attitudes

Q1. Enumerate important Eponymic fractures.

Eponymic (Named) Fractures

Barton's Fracture

Fracture of the distal end of the radius stable, oblique intra-articular fracture of the dorsal or ventral surface of the distal radius.

Bennett's Fracture

Fracture of the base of the first metacarpal, running into the carpo-metacarpal joint and complicated by subluxation.

Cotton's Fracture

Also called a tri-malleolar fracture. It refers to a combination of fractures involving medial malleolus, lateral malleolus and posterior lip of tibia.

Dupuytren's Fracture

Rupture of the deltoid ligament, fracture of medial malleolus, lateral subluxation of the talus and disruption of the distal tibiofibular syndesmosis with fracture of the distal fibula.

Essex-Lopresti Fracture

Comminuted, impacted fracture of the radial head and neck with associated distal radio-ulnar joint dislocation.

Hutchinson's Fracture

Also called the Chauffeur's fracture, a sagittally oriented, intra-articular fracture of the distal radial styloid.

Jefferson's Fracture

A burst fracture (compression) involving both anterior and posterior arches of the atlas.

Jone's Fracture

Proximal diaphyseal fracture of the fifth metatarsal.

Lisfranc's Fracture

Fracture dislocation of the tarso-metatarsal joints (Lisfranc's joint).

Maisonnneuve's Fracture

Rupture of the deltoid ligament, lateral subluxation of the talus and disruption of the distal tibiofibular syndesmosis with fracture of the proximal fibula.

Malgaigne's Fracture

A supra-malleolar transverse, oblique or comminuted fracture of the distal tibia. Also refers to fracture of the anterior and posterior pelvic arches on the same side.

Moore's Fracture

Fracture of distal radius with ulnar head dislocation and entrapment of the ulnar styloid beneath the annular ligament.

Pott's Fracture

It is a bimalleolar fracture with subluxation of talus.

Boxer's Fracture

A transverse fracture through the metacarpal neck, resulting in volar angulation of the head. The fracture name is derived from the common mechanism of injury, punching a solid object with a bare fist.

Bucket-handle Fracture

Fracture of the anterior and posterior pelvic arches on the opposite sides.

Bumper Fracture

Fracture of one or both legs caused by the impact of an automobile bumper, often occurs just below the knees and involves the tibial plateau.

Buttonhole Fracture

Perforation of the bone by a missile (bullet or other small, rapidly moving object).

Chance Fracture

Thoracolumbar distraction injury involving transverse fracture through the posterior elements, which may extend into the postero-superior or postero-inferior portion of the vertebral body.

Clay-Shoveler's Fracture

Avulsion fracture of a spinous process, most often of the C_7 vertebra.

Fulcrum Fracture

Thoracolumbar distraction injury involving transverse fracture through the posterior elements and transverse fracture of the vertebral body.

Hangman's Fracture

Bilateral avulsion fractures through the pedicles of the axis C_2 with or without subluxation of the C_2 vertebra on the third.

Nutcracker Fracture

Crushing of the cuboid between the 4th and 5th metatarsal and the anterior calcaneus during lateral subluxation of the midtarsal joint (Chopart's joint).

Paratrooper Fracture

Fracture of the posterior articular margin of the tibia and/or of the medial/lateral.

Pilon Fracture

A comminuted fracture of the tibia involving the medial malleolus, lateral malleolus, anterior tibial lip and the distal tibia proximal to the articular surface. Its results from impact of the talus against the plafond. A hallmark of the pilon fracture is an anteriorly displaced fracture of the anterior tibial lip, often maintained in association with the talus.

Sprinter's Fracture

Avulsion fracture of the antero-superior or antero-inferior iliac spine, caused by violent muscular action.

Straddle Fracture

Bilateral fracture of both pubic rami.

Chauffer's Fracture

Fracture of radial styloid process.

deQuervain's Fracture/Dislocation

Anterior dislocation of lunate, along with the proximal fragment of a fractured scaphoid.

Fischer's Fracture

Dorsal avulsion of the triquetrum.

Colles' Fracture

Fracture of distal radius within 20–30 mm of the joint (cortico-cancellous junction) and dorsal angulation of the distal fragment.

Smith Fracture

Fracture of distal radius within 20-30mm of the joint (cortico-cancellous junction) and volar angulation of the distal fragment.

Bar-room fracture

4th or 5th metacarpal neck fracture with anterior displacement of the head.

Gamekeeper's Fracture

Disruption of the ulnar collateral ligament at the first metacarpophalangeal joint.

Sideswipe or Baby Car or Traffic Fracture

Fracture of the distal humerus, proximal radius, and ulna when an elbow protruding from a car/buss window is struck by an object.

Chisel Fracture

Vertical fracture of the radial head extending 10 mm from the anterior surface.

Galeazzi's or Piedmont's Fracture

Fracture of the junction of the distal and middle third of the radial shaft and dislocation of the inferior radio-ulnar joint.

Kocher's Fracture

Osteochondral fracture of the capitellum.

Little Leaguer's Elbow

Avulsion of the medial epicondyle

Monteggia Fracture

Fracture of the proximal ulnar shaft with dislocation of radial head.

Nightstick or Parry Fracture

Fracture of the ulna shaft when the arm is raised to protect the head from a blow.

Aviator's or Aviator's Astragalus Fracture

Fracture through the neck of the talus.

Beak Fracture

Avulsion of the posterior calcaneal tubercle.

March fracture

Stress fracture of the 2nd or 3rd metatarsal.

Flake Fracture

Osteochondral fragment separated from the medial facet of the femoral surface of the patella after dislocation.

Segond's Fracture

Avulsion of the lateral tibia at the insertion of the tensor fascia lata.

Q2. List important attitudes that help in making diagnosis in Orthopaedics.

Important Attitudes Following an Injury or Disease or Deformity

Injury	Attitude
Claw hand	Hyper-extension of the metacarpophalangeal joint Flexion of the interphalangeal joint
Erb's palsy	Arm: adduction and internal rotation Forearm: extension and pronation
Perthes disease	Flexion adduction, external rotation and shortening

(Contd.)

Injury	Attitude
Slipped capital femoral epiphysis	Adduction, external rotation and shortening
OA of hip	Flexion, adduction, external rotation shortening
Central dislocation of hip	Abduction, flexion, shortening
Anterior dislocation of hip	Flexion, abduction and external rotation
Posterior dislocation of hip	Flexion, adduction and internal rotation
Intracapsular fracture neck femur	External rotation, shortening
Extra-capsular fracture neck femur or intertrochanteric fracture	External rotation, lateral surface of the foot touching the couch, shortening
Anterior dislocation of the shoulder	Arm: Abducted and externally rotated. Forearm and elbow supported by other hand.
Posterior dislocation of shoulder joint	Classical sling position" of shoulder internal rotation and adduction
Inferior dislocation of shoulder joint	Upper limb in fixed abduction with the hand raised and inability to bring the elbow back to the body.
Supracondylar fracture of humerus	
Extension type (most common)	Distal fragment with elbow displaced posteriorly, laterally, shifted proximally and gets pronated
Flexion type (less common)	Distal fragment with elbow displaced proximally, anteriorly, laterally and supinated
Posterior dislocation of elbow	Posterior prominence of olecranon elbow flexed at 130°
Colles fracture	Impaction, Dorsal tilt and shift, Lateral tilt and shift, Supination (6 D or 6 displacement fracture)
Smith's fracture	Reverse of colles (with volar angulation)

Q3. List important osteotomies in Orthopaedics.

Important osteotomies in Orthopaedics

Osteotomy	Pathology/deformity
French (lateral closed wedge osteotomy)	Cubitus varus deformity
King's (medial open wedge osteotomy)	Cubitus varus deformity
Fernandez (dorsal wedge osteotomy)	Colles fracture
Campbell (lateral wedge osteotomy)	Colles fracture
McMurrays (oblique, intertrochanteric, displacement osteotomy based on biomechanical principles) Shanz Pauwel's	For non-union fracture neck femur
Salter Pemberton Steel Chiari Derotation	CDH
Innominate osteotomy	Perthes diseases
High tibial osteotomy	Genu varum in OA
Dwyer (lateral closed osteotomy)	Varus deformity of foot
Japa's "V" osteotomy	Cavus foot
Keller's	Hallux valgus deformity

Multiple Choice Questions

Bone Fracture

1. **Commonest fracture in childhood is:**
   - a. Femur
   - b. Distal humerus
   - c. Clavicle
   - d. Radius
   - **Ans:** b, i.e. Distal humerus

2. **Patients comes with fracture femur in an acute accident, the first thing to do is:**
   - a. Secure airway and treat the shock
   - b. Splinting
   - c. Physical examination
   - d. X-ray
   - **Ans:** a, i.e. Secure airway and treat the shock

3. **Most sensitive structure in a joints is:**
   - a. Articular cartilage
   - b. Synovium
   - c. Fibrous capsule
   - d. Bone
   - **Ans:** c, i.e. Fibrous capsule

4. **Chemical synovectomy is done by:**
   - a. Osmic acid
   - b. Chymopapain
   - c. Chymotrypsin
   - d. Trypsin
   - **Ans:** a, i.e. Osmic acid

5. **Fat embolism is associated with:**
   - a. Petechial haemorrhages
   - b. Haemarthrosis
   - c. Haematuria
   - d. Bruise below the line of lesion
   - **Ans:** a, i.e. Petechial haemorrhages

6. **Maximum weight used for skin traction is**
   - a. 5 kg
   - b. 7 kg
   - c. 10 kg
   - d. 15 kg
   - **Ans:** a, i.e. 5 kg

7. **K-wire is used in:**
   - a. Circalage
   - b. Fixing forearm bones
   - c. Prior to plating
   - d. All of the above
   - **Ans:** d, i.e. All of the above

8. **The term orthopaedics was coined by:**
   - a. Nicholas Andrey
   - b. Hugh Owen Thomas
   - c. Thoma Bryant
   - d. Sir Rober Jones
   - **Ans:** a, i.e. Nicholas Andrey

9. **Avascular necrosis of bone is most common is:**
   - a. Scapula
   - b. Scaphoid
   - c. Calcaneus
   - d. Cervical spine
   - **Ans:** b, i.e. Scaphoid

10. **Which is not a principle of compound fracture treatment:**
    a. No tendon repair
    b. Aggressive antibiotics cover
    c. Wound debridement
    d. Immediate wound closure
    Ans. d, i.e. Immediate wound closure
11. **The structure responsible for longitudinal growth is:**
    a. Epiphysis
    b. Epiphyseal plate
    c. Metaphysis
    d. Diaphysis
    Ans: b, i.e. Epiphyseal plate
12. **The precartilaginous analogue to bone arises from:**
    a. Ectoderm
    b. Endoderm
    c. Mesenchyme
    d. None of the above
    Ans: 'c' i.e. Mesenchyme
13. **Fabella is:**
    a. Same as fibula
    b. An accessory projection from fibula
    c. A seasamoid bone
    d. None of the above
    Ans: c, i.e. A seasamoid bone
14. **The last step in the healing of a fracture is:**
    a. Hematoma formation
    b. Consolidation
    c. Remodeling
    d. Callus formation
    e. Demineralization of bones
    Ans: c, i.e. Remodeling
15. **Arthroplasty means:**
    a. The joint is made of plastic material
    b. The articulating parts of bones forming the joint are excised and made to fuse together
    c. The joint is excised and bones are so kept as to avoid fusion
    d. Any of the above
    Ans: c, i.e. The joint is excised and bones are so kept as to avoid fusion
16. **The characteristic of collagen is presence of:**
    a. Glycine
    b. Methionine
    c. Hydroxyproline
    d. None of the above
    Ans: c, i.e. Hydroxyproline
17. **Bone graft with maximum osteogenic potential is:**
    a. Fresh autograft
    b. Fresh cortical autograft
    c. Osteoperiosteal graft
    d. Vascular bone graft
    Ans: a, i.e. Fresh autograft
18. **Distal femoral epiphysis is seen at the age of:**
    a. Just after birth
    b. 10 weeks
    c. 20 weeks
    d. 34 weeks
    Ans. d, i.e. 34 weeks
19. **Osteoblasts produce:**
    a. Collagen
    b. Calcium
    c. Pyrophosphate
    d. Monosodium urate
    Ans: a, i.e. Collagen
20. **Stress fracture are known to occur in the:**
    a. Metatarsals
    b. Tibia
    c. Femur
    d. Pelvis
    e. Radius and ulna
    Ans. Four options, i.e. 'a, b, c, and d' are correct

21. **The most important factor in fracture healing is:**
    a. Good alignment
    b. Accurate reduction and 100% apposition of fractured fragments
    c. Immobilization
    d. Adequate calcium intake
    Ans. b, i.e. Accurate reduction and 100% apposition of fractured fragments
22. **Spontaneous rupture of the Achilles tendon in an 18-year-old make it most likely to be due to excess stress beyond:**
    a. Tendon strength
    b. Bone strength
    c. Muscle strength
    d. Musculo-tendinous junction strength
    Ans: a, i.e. Tendon strength
23. **Which of the following muscles are stance phase muscles:**
    a. Quadriceps
    b. Hamstring muscles
    c. Anterior tibial
    d. Peroneus longus
    e. Soleus-gastrocnemius
    Ans. All options are correct
24. **Mc Murray's osteotomy operation is based on the following principle:**
    a. Mechanical
    b. Biological
    c. Bio-mechanical
    d. None
    Ans: c, i.e. Bio-mechanical
25. **Intramedullary nailing is contraindicated in fracture shaft femur if:**
    a. The fracture is compound
    b. The fracture is near the knee joint
    c. The epiphysis have not fused
    d. Any of the above is present
    e. None of the above
    Ans: 'e', i.e. None of the above
26. **The type of displacement of fractured fragment in which bone is not remodelled:**
    a. Anterior angulation
    b. Posterior angulation
    c. Lateral angulation
    d. Rotation
    Ans: d, i.e. Rotation
27. **Most common cause of pathological fracture in a child is:**
    a. Malignancy
    b. Bone cyst
    c. Fibrous dysplasia
    d. Paget's disease
    Ans: b, i.e. Bone cyst
28. **Normal bone remodelling in response to stress was described by:**
    a. Kuntscher
    b. Wolf
    c. Pauwels
    d. Hugh Owen Thomas
    Ans: b, i.e. Wolf
29. **Cock-up splint is used in management of:**
    a. Ulnar nerve palsy
    b. Brachial plexus palsy
    c. Radial nerve palsy
    d. Combined ulnar and median nerve palsy
    Ans: c, i.e. Radial nerve palsy
30. **Most common bone fracture in body is:**
    a. Radius
    b. Clavicle
    c. Femur
    d. Vertebra
    e. Pelvis
    Ans: b, i.e. Clavicle

31. **Fracture which most often requires open reduction and internal fixation:**
    a. Lateral condyle of humerus
    b. Femoral condyle
    c. Distal tibial epipyseal separation
    d. Fracture both bones forearm
    Ans: a, i.e. Lateral condyle of humerus

32. **Which of the following is best related to fat embolism:**
    a. 20% of polytrauma
    b. 40% of bilateral fracture femur
    c. 90% of trauma
    d. Only 15%
    Ans: b, i.e. 40% of bilateral fracture femur

33. **Longitudinal bone growth is dependent on:**
    a. Metaphysis
    b. Diaphysis
    c. Epiphysis
    d. None
    Ans: c, i.e. Epiphysis

34. **Ideal site for bone graft harvesting:**
    a. Iliac crest
    b. Skull bones
    c. Femur cortex
    d. Tibial cortex
    Ans: a, i.e. Iliac crest

35. **Pathognomic sign of traumatic fracture:**
    a. Swelling
    b. Tenderness
    c. Redness
    d. Crepitus
    Ans: d, i.e. Crepitus

36. **Most common joint where arthroscopy is performed is:**
    a. Hip
    b. Knee
    c. Ankle
    d. Shoulder
    e. Elbow
    Ans: b, i.e. Knee

37. **Most common bone fracture during birth:**
    a. Scapula
    b. Humerus
    c. Clavicle
    d. Radius
    e. **Ans:** c, i.e. Clavicle

38. **Avascular necrosis occurs due to fracture of:**
    a. Medial femoral epicondyle
    b. Olecranon
    c. Talus
    d. Fibula
    Ans: c, i.e. Talus

39. **Common injury to baby is:**
    a. Fracture humerus
    b. Fracture clavicle
    c. Fracture radius – ulna
    d. Fracture femur
    Ans: b, i.e. Fracture clavicle

40. **Most common joint to undergo dislocation is:**
    a. Shoulder
    b. Radio-ulnar
    c. Hip
    d. Patello-femoral
    Ans: a, i.e. Shoulder

41. **Avascular necrosis is commonest one of the following fractures:**
    a. Garden 1 and 2 fracture of femoral neck
    b. Garden 3 and 4 fracture of femoral neck
    c. Sub-trochanteric fracture of femoral neck
    d. Baso-trochanteric fracture
    Ans: b, i.e. Garden 3 and 4 fracture of femoral neck

42. **A man was diagnosed to have myositis ossificans progressive at the age of 20 years. He died 5 years. later. What is the most probable cause of death:**
    a. Starvation and chest infection
    b. Myocarditis
    c. Hypercalcaemia
    d. Hyperphosphataemia
    Ans: a, i.e. Starvation and chest infection

43. **Myositis ossificans is commonly seen at the ... joint**
    a. Knee
    b. Elbow
    c. Shoulder
    d. Hip
    Ans: b, i.e. Elbow

44. **Most common cause of pressure sore in the foot in India is:**
    a. Diabetes
    b. Syringomelia
    c. Leprosy
    d. Thorn prick
    Ans: c, i.e. Leprosy

45. **Phalen's test is positive in:**
    a. Tennis elbow
    b. deQuervain's disease
    c. Carpal tunnel syndrome
    d. Ulnar bursitis
    Ans: c, i.e. Carpal tunnel syndrome

46. **Which of the following causes acute compartment syndrome most frequently?**
    a. Fractures
    b. Post ischemic swelling
    c. Exercise initiated syndrome
    d. Soft tissue injury
    Ans: a, i.e. Fractures

47. **Pointing index is due to:**
    a. Ulnar nerve injury
    b. Radial nerve injury
    c. Medial nerve injury
    d. Injury to flexor digitorum profundus tendon
    Ans: c, i.e. Medial nerve injury

48. **15 years old lady sustained a lacerated wound on the back of right thigh by the horn of a bull. The wound was sutured. Two months later she developed foot drop. The most likely diagnosis is:**
    a. Chronic ischaemic to limbs due to popliteal artery injury
    b. Partial injury to sciatic nerve
    c. Complete division of sciatic nerve
    d. Injury to hamstring muscles
    Ans: c, i.e. Complete division of sciatic nerve

49. **Diabetic Charcot's joint affects most commonly:**
    a. Knee
    b. Ankle
    c. Hip
    d. Foot joint
    Ans: d, i.e. Foot joint

50. **Which among the following benefits from cervical sympathectomy?**
    a. Sudeck's dystrophy
    b. Compound palmar ganglion
    c. Osteoarthritis of first MCP joint
    d. deQuervain's tenosynovitis
    Ans: a, i.e. Sudeck's dystrophy

51. **Commonest type of shoulder dislocation:**
    a. Subcoracoid
    b. Subglenoid
    c. Posterior
    d. Subclavicular
    Ans: a, i.e. Subcoracoid

52. **Fracture surgical neck of humerus results in:**
    a. Wrist drop
    b. Loss of sensations over forearm
    c. Loss of roundness of shoulder
    d. Claw hand
    Ans: c, i.e. Loss of roundness of shoulder

53. **Treatment of fracture clavicle in an infant is best treated by:**
    a. Cuff and sling
    b. Figure of 8 bandage
    c. Open reduction
    d. Shoulder cast
    Ans: b, i.e. Figure of 8 bandage

54. **Anterior dislocation of shoulder causes all *except*:**
    a. Circumflex artery injury
    b. Avascular necrosis head of humerus
    c. Brachial plexus injury
    d. Chip fracture scapula
    Ans: b, i.e. Avascular necrosis head of humerus

55. **Nerve most commonly involved in fracture of surgical neck of humerus:**
    a. Radial N
    b. Axillary N
    c. Ulnar N
    d. Median N
    Ans: b, i.e. Axillary N

56. **Hill Sach's lesions is:**
    a. Avulsion of glenoid labrum
    b. Rupture of capsule near scapula
    c. Bony defect in humeral head
    d. Rupture of capsule near humerus
    Ans: c, i.e. Bony defect in humeral head

57. **Commonest cause for recurrent shoulder dislocation is:**
    a. Shallow glenoid labrum
    b. Bankart's lesion
    c. Weakness of subscapularis muscle
    d. Injury to humeral head
    Ans: 'b' and d, i.e. Bankart's lesion, Injury to humeral head

58. **Treatment of choice for fracture neck of humerus in a 70-year-old male:**
    a. Analgesic with arm sling
    b. U-slap
    c. Arthroplasty
    d. Open reduction-internal fixation
    Ans: a, i.e. Analgesic with arm sling

59. **All are components of Rotator cuff *except*:**
    a. Supraspinatus
    b. Infraspinatus
    c. Subscapularis
    d. Teres major
    Ans: d, i.e. Teres major

60. **Most commonly injured nerve in anterior dislocation shoulder is:**
    a. Nerve of Bell
    b. Axillary nerve
    c. Radial nerve
    d. Median nerve
    Ans: b, i.e. Axillary nerve

61. **Treatment of anterior dislocation of shoulder is by:**
    a. Kocher's manoeuvre
    b. Denis Browne splint
    c. Barlows manoeuvre
    d. Surgery
    Ans: a, i.e. Kocher's manoeuvre

62. **Most common nerve damage in shoulder dislocation is:**
    a. Radial nerve
    b. Axillary nerve
    c. Ulnar
    d. Median
    Ans: b, i.e. Axillary nerve

63. **Commonest recurrent dislocation is seen with:**
    a. Shoulder
    b. Patella
    c. Elbow
    d. Hip
    Ans: a, i.e. Shoulder

64. Luxatio erecta:
a. Tear of the glenoidal labium
b. Inferior dislocation of shoulder
c. Anterior dislocation of shoulder
d. Defect in humeral head
Ans: b, i.e. Inferior dislocation of shoulder

65. Most common complication of clavicle fracture is:
a. Non union
b. Stiffness of finger
c. Vascular injury
d. Sudeks dystrophy
Ans: 'None'

66. Ideal treatment with fracture neck of humerus in a old lady will be:
a. Triangular sling
b. Hemiarthroplasty
c. Chest arm bandage
d. Internal fixation
Ans: a, i.e. Triangular sling

67. Bankert's lesions involves:
a. Anterior aspect of the head of humerus
b. Anterior aspect of glenoid labrum
c. Posterior aspect of glenoid labrum
d. Posterior aspect of head of humerus
Ans: b, i.e. Anterior aspect of glenoid labrum

68. A patient with recurrent dislocation of shoulder presents to the hospital. The doctor tries to abduct his arm and to extend the elbow and external rotation, but the patient does not allow to do so. This test is called.
a. Duga's test
b. Hamilton's test
c. Callway's test
d. Apprehension test
Ans: d, i.e. Apprehension test

69. If the greater tuberosity of the humerus is lost, which of the following movements will be affected?
a. Adduction and flexion
b. Abduction and lateral rotation
c. Medial rotation and adduction
d. Flexion and medial rotation
Ans: b, i.e. Abduction and lateral rotation

70. All are related to recurrent shoulder dislocation *except*:
a. Hill-Sachs defect
b. Bankart lesion
c. Lax capsule
d. Rotator cuff injury
Ans: d, i.e. Rotator cuff injury

71. Treatment of fracture head of radius in young patients:
a. Excision of head of radius
b. Immobilization in cast
c. Late excision after trial immobilization
d. None of the above
Ans. Two options are correct, i.e. 'a and b'

72. In supracondylar fracture, the segment is often displaced:
a. Laterally
b. Medially
c. Anteriorly
d. Posteriorly
Ans: d, i.e. Posteriorly

73. Tardy ulnar nerve palsy is due to:
a. Cubitus valgus
b. Fixation of nerve in the groove by osteoarthritis
c. Excision of elbow joint
d. Fracture of internal condyle
Ans: a, i.e. Cubitus valgus

74. **Tardy ulnar nerve palsy is seen in:**
    a. Cubitus valgus
    b. Dislocation of elbow
    c. Fracture scaphoid
    d. Supracondylar fracture of humerus
    Ans: a, i.e. Cubitus valgus
75. **In Volkmann's ischaemia, surgery should be done:**
    a. Immediately
    b. After 6 hours
    c. 24 hours
    d. 72 hours
    Ans: a, i.e. Immediately
76. **Which fracture in children requires operative reduction?**
    a. Epiphyseal separation
    b. Both upper limb bones
    c. Dislocation of elbow
    d. Fracture humerus
    Ans: d, i.e. Fracture humerus
77. **Muscles involved in Volkmann's ischaemic contracture:**
    a. Flexor policis longus
    b. Flexor digitorum profundus
    c. Flexor sublimes
    d. All
    Ans. Two option are correct, i.e. 'a and b'
78. **The cause of gun stock deformity is:**
    a. Supracondylar fracture
    b. Fracture both bones forearm
    c. Fracture surgical head of humerus
    d. Fracture fibula
    Ans: a, i.e. Supracondylar fracture
79. **True flexors of the elbow joint are:**
    a. Biceps
    b. Brachialis
    c. Brachioradialis
    d. Teres minor
    Ans. Three options are correct, i.e. 'a, b and c'
80. **Myositis ossificans is most common around the ... joint:**
    a. Knee
    b. Elbow
    c. Wrist
    d. Hip
    Ans: b, i.e. Elbow
81. **The most important sign in Volkmann's ischaemic contracture:**
    a. Pain
    b. Pallor
    c. Numbness
    d. Obliteration of radial pulse
    Ans: a, i.e. Pain
82. **Open reduction in children is done for:**
    a. Supracondylar fracture
    b. Forearm both bone fracture
    c. Femoral condyle fracture
    d. Lateral condyle of humerus fracture
    Ans: d, i.e. Lateral condyle of humerus fracture
83. **Triangular relation of elbow is maintained in:**
    a. Fracture ulna
    b. Anterior dislocation of Elbow
    c. Posterior dislocation of Elbow
    d. Supracondylar fracture
    Ans: d, i.e. Supracondylar fracture
84. **Treatment of acute myositis ossificans is:**
    a. Active mobilization
    b. Passive mobilization
    c. Infra red therapy
    d. Immobilization
    Ans: 'd' i.e, Immobilization
85. **Which fracture in children requires open reduction**
    a. Fracture tibial epiphysis
    b. Fracture shaft of femur
    c. Fracture both bones forearm
    d. Fracture femoral condyle
    Ans: 'a' i.e, Fracture tibial epiphysis

86. Tardy ulnar nerve palsy is seen with:
a. Lateral humeral condyle fracture
b. Supracondylar fracture
c. Medial humeral condyle fracture
d. Fracture Capitellum
Ans: 'a' i.e, Lateral humeral condyle fracture

87. Volkmann's ischaemic contracture mostly involves:
a. Flexor digitorum superficialis
b. Pronators teres
c. Flexor digitorum profundus
d. Flexor carpi radialis longus
Ans: c, i.e. Flexor digitorum profundus

88. Pulled elbow is:
a. Disarticulation of elbow
b. Subluxation of distal radio-ulnar joint
c. Subluxation of proximal radio-ulnar joint
d. None of the above
Ans: c, i.e. Subluxation of proximal radio-ulnar joint

89. Open reduction for supracondylar fracture in a child is *not* preferred because of the fear of:
a. Injury to nerve and vessels in that region
b. Myositis ossificans traumatica
c. Permanent stiffness of the elbow
d. Infection
Ans: c, i.e. Permanent stiffness of the elbow

90. Earliest sign of Volkmann's ischaemic contracture is:
a. Pain during passive extension
b. Pulselessness
c. Necrosis of muscles
d. Loss of adduction
Ans: a, i.e. Pain during passive extension

91. Treatment after removal of plaster for supracondylar fracture of humerus is:
a. Active mobilization at elbow joint
b. Massage
c. No treatment
d. Passive movements at elbow joint
Ans: a, i.e. Active mobilization at elbow joint

92. Most common type of supracondylar fracture is:
a. Extension type
b. Flexion type
c. Abduction type
d. Adduction type
Ans: a, i.e. Extension type

93. Excision of fractured fragment is practiced in all fractures *except*:
a. Patella
b. Olecranon
c. Head of radius
d. Lateral condyle humerus
Ans: d, i.e. Lateral condyle humerus

94. Pulled elbow is due to:
a. Fracture of radius
b. Fracture of ulna
c. Supracondylar fracture humerus
d. Subluxation of radial head
Ans: d, i.e. Subluxation of radial head

95. All the following requires open reduction and internal fixation almost always *except*:
a. Lateral condyle of humerus
b. Olecranon
c. Patella
d. Volar Barton's fracture
Ans. Three options are correct, i.e. 'b, c and d'

96. Suspected medial epicondylar fracture of humerus in a 4-year-old child requires:
a. X-ray both arms with elbow for comparison
b. X-ray same limb only
c. Examination under general anaesthesia
d. POP in full flexed position
Ans: a, i.e. X-ray both arms with elbow for comparison

97. **A young adult presenting with oblique, displaced fracture olecranon treatment of choice:**
    a. Plaster cast
    b. Percutaneous wiring
    c. Tension ban wiring
    d. Removal of displaced piece with triceps repair
    Ans: c, i.e. Tension ban wiring

98. **Earliest sign of Volkmann ischaemic contracture is:**
    a. On passive extension there is pain
    b. Obliteration of radial pulse
    c. Pale and cold hand
    d. Warm and red hand
    Ans: a, i.e. On passive extension there is pain

99. **Carrying angle is decreased in:**
    a. Cubitus varus
    b. Cubitus valgus
    c. Genu valgum
    d. Genu varum
    Ans: a, i.e. Cubitus varus

100. **Treatment in the early stage of myositis ossificans is:**
    a. Immobilization
    b. Massage
    c. Excision of the bone
    d. Active joint movements
    Ans: a, i.e. Immobilization

101. **Volkmann's ischaemic contracture the muscle commonly involved is:**
    a. Palmaris longus
    b. Flexor indicis
    c. Flexor digitorum profundus
    d. Flexor pollicis longus
    Ans. Two options are correct, i.e. 'c and d'

102. **osteotomy bone for malunited supracondylar fracture is:**
    a. French
    b. Shan's
    c. McMurray's
    d. McAllister
    Ans: a, i.e. French

103. **Earliest sign of Volkmann's ischaemic contracture is:**
    a. Pain
    b. Numbness
    c. Paraesthesia
    d. Pallor
    Ans: a, i.e. Pain

104. **The best radiological view for fracture scaphoid is:**
    a. AP
    b. PA
    c. Lateral
    d. Oblique
    Ans: d, i.e. Oblique

105. **Carpal bone fracture is commonly of:**
    a. Scaphoid
    b. Lunate
    c. Hammate
    d. Pisiform
    Ans: a, i.e. Scaphoid

106. **Complication of fracture scaphoid is:**
    a. Injury to radial artery
    b. Avascular necrosis of proximal part
    c. Avascular necrosis of distal part
    d. Injury to radial nerve
    Ans: b, i.e. Avascular necrosis of proximal part

107. **Dislocation of which one of the following carpal bones can present as median nerve palsy?**
    a. Scaphoid
    b. Hamate
    c. Lunate
    d. Trapezium
    Ans: c, i.e. Lunate

108. The complication not common in Colles' fracture is:
a. Malunion
b. Nonunion
c. Sudeck's atrophy
d. Stiffness of wrist
Ans: b, i.e. Non union

109. Oblique view is required to diagnose fracture of:
a. Capitate
b. Scaphoid
c. Navicular
d. Hamate
Ans: b, i.e. Scaphoid

110. Commonest site of fracture scaphoid:
a. Waist
b. Proximal third
c. Distal third
d. Tuberculosis
Ans: a, i.e. Waist

111. In Colles' fracture not seen is:
a. Proximal impaction
b. Lateral rotation
c. Dorsal angulation
d. Medial rotation
Ans: d, i.e. Medial rotation

112. Least common complication of Colles fracture is:
a. Malunion
b. Nonunion
c. Stiffness of fingers
d. Sudeks dystrophy
Ans: b, i.e. Nonunion

113. Most common complication of Colles fracture is:
a. Nonunion
b. Stiffness of fingers
c. Vascular injury
d. Sudek's dystrophy
Ans: b, i.e. Stiffness of fingers

114. Position of immobilization in fracture both bones of forearm in an adult male:
a. Prone
b. Mid-prone
c. Supine
d. $10°$ supine
Ans: b, i.e. Mid-prone

115. A lady presents with a history of fracture radius which was put on plaster of Paris cast for 4 weeks. After that she developed swelling of hands with shiny skin. What is the most likely diagnosis
a. Rupture of extensor pollicis longus tendon
b. Myositis ossificans
c. Reflex sympathetic dystrophy
d. Malunion
Ans: c, i.e. Reflex sympathetic dystrophy

116. Which one of the following statements is *not* correct regarding fracture of the scaphoid?
a. It is the most commonly fracture carpal bone
b. Persistent tenderness in the anatomical snuffbox is highly suggestive of fracture
c. Immediate X-ray of hand may not reveal fracture line
d. Malunion is a frequent complication
Ans. d, i.e. Malunion is a frequent complication

117. Reduction of Bennet's fracture is difficult to keep in position due to the pull of:
a. Abductor pollicis brevis
b. Abductor pollicis longus
c. Flexor pollicis longus
d. Flexor pollicis brevis
Ans: b, i.e. Abductor pollicis longus

118. **In treatment of hand injuries, the greatest priority is:**
     a. Repair of tendons
     b. Restoration of skin cover
     c. Repair of nerves
     d. Repair of blood vessels
     Ans: b, i.e. Restoration of skin cover

119. **A Bennet's fracture is difficult to maintain in reduced position because of the pull of:**
     a. Extensor pollicis longus
     b. Extensor pollicis brevis
     c. Abductor pollicis longus
     d. Abductor pollicis brevis
     Ans: c, i.e. Abductor pollicis longus

120. **Commonest complication of extracapsular fracture of neck of femur is:**
     a. Nonunion
     b. Ischaemic necrosis
     c. Malunion
     d. Pulmonary complications
     Ans: c, i.e. Malunion

121. **Which fracture neck of femur has a poor prognosis?**
     a. Intracapsular
     b. Extracapsular
     c. Both
     d. None
     Ans: a, i.e. Intracapsular

122. **Histology of myositis ossificans mimics:**
     a. Osteosarcoma
     b. Osteochondroma
     c. GCT
     d. Ewing's tumour
     Ans: a, i.e. Osteosarcoma

123. **Avascular necrosis of head of femur can occur in:**
     a. Sickle cell anaemia
     b. Caisson's disease
     c. Intracapsular fracture neck
     d. Trochanteric fracture
     Ans: 'a,b,c', i.e. Sickle cell anaemia, Caisson's disease, Intracapsular fracture neck

124. **Commonest complication of intracapsular fracture neck of femur is:**
     a. Osteoarthritis
     b. Shortening
     c. Malunion
     d. Nonunion
     Ans: d, i.e. Nonunion

125. **Avascular necrosis of the head of femur is not seen in:**
     a. Subcapital fracture
     b. Intertrochanteric fracture
     c. Transcervical fracture
     d. Central dislocation of hip
     Ans: 'b,d', i.e. Intertrochanteric fracture, Central dislocation of hip

126. **In fracture neck of femur in a 64 years old lady the treatment of choice is:**
     a. Prosthetic replacement of head of femur
     b. Conservative
     c. Austin Moores' pin
     d. SP nailing
     Ans: a, i.e. Prosthetic replacement of head of femur

127. **Fracture neck of femur in old persons is best treated by:**
     a. Replacement arthroplasty
     b. Thomas's splint support
     c. No treatment
     d. Internal fixation with SP nail
     Ans: a, i.e. Replacement arthroplasty

128. **In 65-year-old male with history of fracture neck of femur 6 weeks old treatment of choice:**
     a. SP nailing
     b. Mc Murray's osteotomy
     c. Hemiarthroplasty
     d. None
     Ans: c, i.e. Hemiarthroplasty

129. **The most preferred treatment of fracture of neck of femur in young person is:**
    a. Hemiarthroplasty
    b. Total Hip replacement
    c. Conservative treatment
    d. Closed reduction and internal fixation
    Ans: d, i.e. Closed reduction and internal fixation

130. **Bryant's triangle is useful in diagnosis of following *except*:**
    a. Supratrochanteric shortening
    b. Infractrochanteric shortening
    c. Anterior dislocation hip
    d. Posterior dislocation hip
    Ans: b, i.e. Infractrochanteric shortening

131. **The treatment of choice for non-union of intracapsular fracture neck femur is:**
    a. Hip spica
    b. Intramedullary nailing
    c. Internal fixation
    d. Compression plating
    Ans: c, i.e. Internal fixation

132. **Late complication of acetabular fracture is:**
    a. Avascular necrosis of head of femur
    b. Avascular necrosis of iliac crest
    c. Fixed deformity of the hip joint
    d. Secondary osteoarthritis of hip joint
    Ans: 'a,d', i.e. Avascular necrosis of head of femur, Secondary osteoarthritis of hip joint

133. **In the case of 65-year-old person with fracture neck of femur the treatment of choice is:**
    a. Close reduction
    b. Close reduction with internal fixation
    c. Open reduction
    d. Replacement of head and neck of the femur with a prosthesis
    Ans: d, i.e. Replacement of head and neck of the femur with a prosthesis

134. **Commonest type of dislocation of the hip is:**
    a. Anterior
    b. Posterior
    c. Central
    d. Dislocation with fracture of the shaft
    Ans: b, i.e. Posterior

135. **Commonest dislocation of the hip is:**
    a. Posterior
    b. Anterior
    c. Central
    d. None
    Ans: a, i.e. Posterior

136. **The following is true in the treatment of posterior dislocation:**
    a. Closed reduction under anaesthesia
    b. Open reduction
    c. Skeletal traction
    d. Soft tissue release and then internal reduction in 2nd stage
    Ans: a, i.e. Closed reduction under anaesthesia

137. **Flexion, adduction and internal rotation are characteristic posture in:**
    a. Anterior dislocation of hip joint
    b. Posterior dislocation of hip joint
    c. Fracture of femoral head
    d. Fracture shaft of femur
    Ans: b, i.e. Posterior dislocation of hip joint

138. **Dashboard injury cases:**
    a. Anterior dislocation of the hip
    b. Posterior dislocation of the hip
    c. Central dislocation of hip
    d. Fracture neck femur
    Ans: b, i.e. Posterior dislocation of the hip

139. **Dislocation of hip joint palpable on per rectal examination**
    a. Congenital dislocation of hip
    b. Posterior dislocation of hip
    c. Fracture neck of femur
    d. Anterior dislocation of hip
    Ans: b, i.e. Posterior dislocation of hip

140. **The pubic arch in females is above:**
    a. 60–70
    b. 70–75
    c. 100
    d. 130
    Ans: c, i.e. 100

141. **In comminuted fracture of the patella in an old lady the treatment is:**
    a. Excision of a small fragment
    b. Wire fixation
    c. Plaster cylinder
    d. Patellectomy
    Ans: d, i.e. Patellectomy

142. **Which of the following is correct in medial meniscus tear?**
    a. Rotation of femur on tibia
    b. Menisci do not heal
    c. Locking and unlocking episodes
    d. Menisci should be excised
    e. All of the above are correct
    Ans: 'a,c,d', i.e. Rotation of femur on tibia, Locking and unlocking episodes, Menisci should be excised

143. **Fracture femur in infants is best treated by:**
    a. Open reduction
    b. Closed reduction
    c. IM nailing
    d. Gallow's splinting
    Ans. d, i.e. Gallow's splinting

144. **Comminuted fracture of patella is treated by:**
    a. Tension wire bandage
    b. Surgery and immobilization
    c. Conservative
    d. Patellectomy
    Ans: d, i.e. Patellectomy

145. **Medial meniscus tear is more common than lateral meniscus because of its decreased:**
    a. Nerve supply
    b. Vascularity
    c. Mobility
    d. Fibroelasticity
    Ans: c, i.e. Mobility

146. **Medial meniscus is more vulnerable to injury because of:**
    a. Its fixity to tibial collateral ligaments
    b. Its semicircular shape
    c. Action of adductor magnus
    d. Its attachment to fibrous capsule
    Ans: a, i.e. Its fixity to tibial collateral ligaments

147. **Injury to the popliteal artery in fracture lower end of femur is often due to:**
    a. Distal fragment pressing the artery
    b. Proximal fragment pressing the artery
    c. Tight plaster
    d. Hematoma
    Ans: a, i.e. Distal fragment pressing the artery

148. **Recurrent dislocation of patella in an adolescent could be treated by:**
    a. Patellectomy
    b. Excision arthroplasty
    c. Puttipatt operation
    d. Lateral release
    Ans: d, i.e. Lateral release

149. **Recurrent dislocation of patella is most often associated with:**
    a. Abnormally high patella
    b. Abnormally low patella
    c. Bow leg
    d. Quadriceps contracture
    Ans: a, i.e. abnormally high patella

150. Drawer's sign is diagnostic for injuries of:
a. Neck femur
b. Shaft femur
c. Collateral ligaments of knee
d. Cruciate ligaments of knee
Ans: d, i.e. Cruciate ligaments of knee

151. Treatment of choice for old non-united fracture of shaft of femur:
a. Compression plating
b. Bone grafting
c. Nailing
d. Compression plating with bone grafting
Ans: d, i.e. Compression plating with bone grafting

152. Stiffness in knee is maximum when traction is at:
a. Skin
b. Lower end femur
c. Upper end tibia
d. Calcaneum
Ans: c, i.e. Upper end tibia

153. Most common cause of hemarthrosis knee joint is:
a. Hemophilia
b. Anterior cruciate ligament tear
c. Medial meniscus tear
d. Lateral meniscus tear
Ans: c, i.e. Medial meniscus tear

154. A positive pivot shift test in the right knee joint of an athlete is suggestive of injury to:
a. Lateral meniscus injury
b. Medial meniscus injury
c. Injury to anterior cruciate ligament
d. Injury to posterior cruciate ligament
Ans: c, i.e. Injury to anterior cruciate ligament

155. A football player while playing twists his knee over the ankle. He still continues to play. After 2 days he noticed painful swelling of the knee joint. The diagnosis is:
a. Medial meniscus tear
b. Anterior cruciate ligament tear
c. Medial collateral ligament injury
d. Posterior cruciate ligament injury
Ans: a, i.e. Medial meniscus tear

156. Medial meniscus is more prone for injury because:
a. It is semilunar in shape
b. Medial portion is thicker
c. Medial collateral ligaments is attached to it
d. Avascular
Ans: c, i.e. Medial collateral ligaments is attached to it

157. Best diagnostic procedure for anterior cruciate ligament injury is:
a. Lachman's test
b. Pivot shift test
c. Anterior Drawer test
d. Mc Murray's test
Ans: a, i.e. Lachman's test

158. Infarction of the distal epiphyses of the second metatarsal bone is:
a. Kienbock's disease
b. Kohler's disease
c. Freiburg's disease
d. Perthes' disease
Ans: c, i.e. Freiburg's disease

159. Which joint is not fused in triple arthrodesis?
a. Tibiotalar
b. Calcaneocuboid
c. Talanavicular
d. Talocalcaneal
Ans: a, i.e. Tibiotalar

160. **Fall on heel with fracture os calcis is associated with commonly:**
    a. Fracture clavicle
    b. Fracture vertebra
    c. Fracture femur
    d. Any of the above
    Ans: b, i.e. Fracture vertebra

161. **The most common cause of a sprained ankle is injury of:**
    a. Deltoid ligament
    b. Lateral ligament
    c. Inferior tibiofibular ligament
    d. Anterior talofibular ligament
    Ans: d, i.e. Anterior talofibular ligament

162. **Transverse fracture of medial malleolus is caused by:**
    a. Abduction
    b. Adduction
    c. Rotation of foot
    d. Dorsiflexion of foot
    Ans: c, i.e. Rotation of foot

163. **After a fall from a height calcaneal fracture is associated with fracture of:**
    a. Tibia
    b. Vertebra
    c. Pelvis
    d. Femur
    Ans: b, i.e. Vertebra

164. **Most common ligament injured in ankle sprain:**
    a. Anterior talofibular
    b. Posterior talofibular
    c. Deltoid
    d. Spring ligament
    Ans: a, i.e. Anterior talofibular

165. **A segmental compound fracture tibia with 1 cm skin wound is classified as:**
    a. Type I
    b. Type II
    c. Type III A
    d. Type III B
    Ans: a, i.e. Type I

166. **Traction injury to epiphyses of the vertebra is known as:**
    a. Osgood Schlatter's disease
    b. Sinding Larsen disease
    c. Scheurmann's disease
    d. Severe's disease
    Ans: c, i.e. Scheurmann's disease

167. **Commonest cause of paraplegia is:**
    a. Tuberculosis
    b. Trauma
    c. Secondaries
    d. Trasverse myelitis
    Ans: b, i.e. Trauma

168. **Commonest intramedullary spinal tumours is:**
    a. Secondaries
    b. Neurofibroma
    c. Ependymoma
    d. None of the above
    Ans: c, i.e. Ependymoma

169. **Commonest site of prolapse is:**
    a. C_5–C_6
    b. T_8–T_9
    c. L_4–L_5
    d. L_5–S_1
    Ans: 'a,c', i.e. C_5–C_6, L_4–L_5

170. **The following is true of spondylolisthesis:**
    a. Slipping of SI over L5
    b. Posterior arch defect
    c. Congenital defect
    d. More in pregnancy
    Ans: b, c, i.e. Posterior arch defect, Congenital defect

171. **Intervertebral disc prolapse is treated chemically by:**
    a. Hyalse
    b. Chymotrypain
    c. Chymopapain
    d. Elastase
    Ans: c, i.e. Chymopapain

172. Vertebra plana occurs in:
a. TB spine
b. Secondaries in spine
c. Pyogenic osteomyelitis
d. Eosinophilic granulomas
Ans: d, i.e. Eosinophilic granulomas

173. Vertebra plana is caused by:
a. Malignancy
b. Tuberculosis
c. Syphilis
d. Eosinophilic granuloma
Ans: d, i.e. Eosinophilic granulomas

174. When a person reports with vertebral fracture hemiplegia and urinary retention the acute measure to be taken is:
a. Suprapubic cystostomy
b. Catheterization
c. Hot fomentation
d. Condom drainage
Ans: b, i.e. Catheterization

175. Local application of the following drug is used for eradication of *Pseudomonas* infection from the wound:
a. Acriflavine solution
b. Eusol paraffin
c. Acetic acid
d. Tincture iodine
Ans: c, i.e. Acetic acid

176. Tetanus is noticed usually in:
a. Burn cases
b. Wounds contaminated with faecal matter
c. Open fractures
d. Gunshot wounds
e. All of the above
Ans: e, i.e. All of the above

177. Organism causing osteomyelitis in sickle cell anemia:
a. *Salmonella*
b. *Staphylococcus*
c. *Pneumococcus*
d. *Streptococcus*
Ans. Two options are correct, i.e. 'a and b'

178. Tuberculosis of the spine is known as:
a. Pott's disease
b. Scheurmann's disease
c. Perthes' disease
d. Frieberg disease
Ans: a, i.e. Pott's disease

179. Tuberculous arthritis in advanced cases lead to:
a. Bony ankylosis
b. Fibrous ankylosis
c. Loose joint
d. Charcot's joints
Ans. Two options are correct, i.e. 'a and b'

180. Tuberculosis of the spine starts in:
a. Vertebral body
b. Nucleous pulposus
c. Annulus
d. Fibrosis
e. Paravertebral fascia
Ans: a, i.e. Vertebral body

181. Treatment of triple deformity is:
a. ATT
b. ATT + immobilization
c. ATT + immobilization + debridement
d. None
Ans: d, i.e. None

182. The 1st sign of TB is:
   a. Narrowing of intervertebral space
   b. Rarefaction of vertebral bodies
   c. Destruction of laminae
   d. Fusion of spinous processes
   Ans: a, i.e. Narrowing of intervertebral space

183. The ideal surgical treatment for Pott's paraplegia is:
   a. Laminectomy and decompression
   b. Anterior decompression
   c. Anterolateral decompression
   d. Costotransversectomy
   Ans: c, i.e. Anterolateral decompression

184. Earliest fracture of TB vertebra:
   a. Decreased joint space
   b. Soft tissue swelling
   c. Decreased movements
   d. Pain
   Ans: d, i.e. Pain

185. Most important pathology in clubfoot is:
   a. Congenital talonavicular dislocation
   b. Tightening of tendo Achilles
   c. Calcaneal fracture
   d. Lateral derangement
   Ans: a, i.e. Congenital talonavicular dislocation

186. Treatment of clubfoot should begin:
   a. As soon as possible after birth
   b. 1 month after birth
   c. 1 year after birth
   d. None of the above
   Ans: a, i.e. As soon as possible after birth

187. Treatment of CTEV should start at the age of:
   a. 2 weeks
   b. 1 month
   c. Soon after birth
   d. 9 months
   Ans: c, i.e. Soon after birth

188. In congenital dislocation of knee deformity seen is:
   a. Varus
   b. Valgus
   c. Flexion
   d. Extension
   Ans: d, i.e. Extension

189. Commonest deformity in congenital dislocation of hip:
   a. Small head of femur
   b. Angle of torsion
   c. Decreased neck shaft angle
   d. Shallow acetabulum
   Ans: d, i.e. Shallow acetabulum

190. Osteoblastic bone secondary is usually from:
   a. Ovary
   b. Kidney
   c. Breast
   d. Prostate
   Ans. Two options are correct, i.e. ' c and d'

191. Most radiosensitive bone tumour is:
   a. Chondrosarcoma
   b. Osteoclastoma
   c. Ewing sarcoma
   d. Osteosarcoma
   Ans: c, i.e. Ewing sarcoma

192. Commonest benign bone tumour is:
   a. Osteochondroma
   b. Chondrosarcoma
   c. Osteoid osteoma
   d. Osteosarcoma
   Ans: a, i.e. Osteochondroma

193. Commonest benign bone tumour is:
   a. Bone cyst
   b. Chondroma
   c. Chordoma
   d. Osteoma
   Ans: b, i.e. Chondroma

194. Which of the following is a true tumor:
a. Bone cyst
b. Fibrous dysplasia
c. Osteochondroma
d. Brodies tumour
Ans: None

195. Which tumour does not arise from cartilage:
a. Osteoblastoma
b. Osteochondroma
c. Chondrosarcoma
d. Enchondroma
Ans: a, i.e. Osteoblastoma

196. Malignant growth involving the vault of the skull includes:
a. Osteitis fibrosa cystica
b. Osteoclastoma
c. Myeloid epulis
d. Adamantinoma
e. Nephroblastoma
Ans. Two options are correct, i.e. 'b and e'

197. Physalipharous cells (large vacuolated cells) on histopathology are characteristic of:
a. Osteosarcoma
b. Osteoclastoma
c. Liposarcoma
d. Chondrosarcoma
e. Chordoma
Ans: 'e', i.e. Chordoma

198. Osteoclastoma is common in age group of:
a. Below 10 years
b. 10–20 years
c. 20–40 years
d. All age groups
Ans: c, i.e. 20-40 years

199. Which is the most common site of osteoclastoma:
a. Lower end of femur
b. Upper end of tibia
c. Lower humerus
d. Upper radius
Ans: a, i.e. Lower end of femur

200. True statement regarding osteogenic sarcoma is:
a. Affects middle aged people
b. X-ray shows honey combing
c. Can be a complication of Paget's disease of bone
d. All of the above
Ans: c, i.e. Can be a complication of Paget's disease of bone

201. Commonest benign tumour under 21 years of age:
a. Aneurysmal bone ctst
b. Osteochondroma
c. Giant cell tumour
d. Osteoid talus
Ans: d, i.e. Osteoid talus

202. Multiple exostosis usually presents at:
a. Birth
b. Puberty
c. After 21 years
d. At 5 years of age
Ans: d, i.e. At 5 years of age

203. Densely calcified metastatic shadows are found in:
a. Synovial cell carcinoma
b. Osteosarcoma
c. Chondrosarcoma
d. Chondroblastoma
Ans: b, i.e. Osteosarcoma

204. Most common mode of metastasis in osteogenic sarcoma:
 a. Subperiosteal spread
 b. Hematogenous
 c. Lymphatic
 d. Transcortical
 Ans: b, i.e. Hematogenous

205. In a 8 years old child the least common cause of lytic bone lesion in proximal femur:
 a. Plasmacytoma
 b. Histiocytoma
 c. Metastasis
 d. Brown tumour
 Ans: a, i.e. Plasmacytoma

206. Aneurysmal bone cysts:
 a. Are true aneurysms of nutrient arteries
 b. Occur only in flat bones
 c. Are the same as osseous haemangiomas
 d. Manifest as osteolytic lesions in long bones
 Ans: d, i.e. Manifest as osteolytic lesions in long bones

207. Most common site of Eosinophilic granuloma:
 a. Radius
 b. Femur
 c. Skull
 d. Lumber vertebrae
 Ans: c, i.e. Skull

208. Bone dysplasia is due to:
 a. Faulty nutrition
 b. Faulty development
 c. Vitamin deficiency
 d. Hormonal imbalance
 Ans: b, i.e. Faulty development

209. Rare site of metastasis in bone:
 a. Skull
 b. Spine
 c. Upper end of humerus
 d. Below elbow and knee
 Ans: d, i.e. Below elbow and knee

210. Most reliable method for detecting bony metastases is:
 a. MRI
 b. CT scan
 c. Radiography
 d. SPECT
 Ans: None

211. A 50 years old patient presents with a lesions in the midline involving the sacrum which is sclerotic what is the likely diagnosis:
 a. Osteosarcoma
 b. Chordoma
 c. Metastasis
 d. Osteoclastoma
 Ans: c, i.e. Metastasis

212. A 70 years old lady presented with mild low back pain and tenderness in L3 vertebra. On examination Hb 8 g ESR 110 mm/1 hr, A/G ratio of 2:4 likely diagnosis is:
 a. Waldenstorms
 b. Multiple myeloma
 c. Bone Secondaries
 d. None
 Ans: b, i.e. Multiple myeloma

213. Bamboo spine is seen in:
 a. Ankylosing spondylitis
 b. Rheumatoid arthritis
 c. Scheurmann's disease
 d. Pott's spine
 Ans: a, i.e. Ankylosing spondylitis

214. The cause of Rheumatoid arthritis is:
a. Familial
b. Immunological
c. Infective
d. Traumatic
Ans. Three options, i.e. 'a, b and c' are correct

215. Joint that least affected by neuropathy:
a. Shoulder
b. Hip
c. Wrist
d. Elbow
Ans: None

216. Epiphyseal widening may be seen in:
a. Rheumatoid arthritis
b. Juvenile rheumatoid arthritis
c. Osteoarthritis
d. Gouty arthritis
Ans: b, i.e. Juvenile rheumatoid arthritis

217. Therapeutic programme for gout could include administration of:
a. Heavy dose of vitamin C
b. Phenyl butazone
c. Furadatin
d. Gold therapy
Ans: b, i.e. Phenyl butazone

218. Commonest degenerative joint disease in:
a. Gout
b. Osteoporosis
c. Rheumatoid arthritis
d. Osteo arthritis
Ans: d, i.e. Osteoarthritis

219. In rheumatoid arthritis, the pathology starts in:
a. Articular cartilage
b. Synovium
c. Capsule
d. Muscles
Ans: b, i.e. Synovium

220. Para-articular erosions are most commonly seen in:
a. Osteoarthritis
b. Rheumatoid arthritis
c. Gout
d. Acute suppurative arthritis
Ans: b, i.e. Rheumatoid arthritis

221. In osteoarthritis, following is not a predisposing factor:
a. Diabetes mellitus
b. Defective joint position
c. Weight-bearing joints
d. Incongruity of articular surfaces
e. Old age
Ans: None

222. Treatment of osteoarthritis include all except:
a. Graded muscle exercises
b. Replacement of articular surfaces
c. Correction of deformities
d. Increase the weight-bearing by the affected joint
e. Rest to the joint in acute phase
Ans: d, i.e. Increase the weight bearing by the affected joint

223. Treatment of rheumatoid arthritis include all *except*:
a. Give rest to the joint
b. Correction of deformities
c. Synovectomy
d. Exercises
e. Immunosuppressive drugs
Ans: a, i.e. Give rest to the joint

224. **Osteoarthritis involves all *except*:**
    a. Hip joint
    b. Knee joint
    c. Distal interphalangeal joint
    d. Metacarpophalangial joint of thumb
    Ans: d, i.e. Metacarpophalangial joint of thumb

225. **Calcification of menisci is seen in:**
    a. Hyperparathyroidism
    b. Pseudogout
    c. Renal osteodystrophy
    d. Acromegaly
    Ans: b, i.e. Pseudogout

226. **Osteitis fibrosa cystica is seen in:**
    a. Hyperparathyroidism
    b. Hypoparathyroidism
    c. Hypothroidism
    d. Hyperthyroidism
    Ans: a, i.e. Hyperparathyroidism

227. **Menisci calcification is a feature of:**
    a. Gout
    b. Hyperparathyroidism
    c. Pseudogout
    d. Ankylosing spondylitis
    Ans: c, i.e. Pseudogout

228. **Absence of lamina dura in alveolus occurs in:**
    a. Rickets
    b. Osteomalacia
    c. Deficiency of vitamin C
    d. Hyperparathyroidism
    Ans: d, i.e. Hyperparathyroidism

229. **A finding of phosphoethanolamine in the urine is highly suggestive of:**
    a. Renal osteodystrophy
    b. Hypophosphatasia
    c. Urinary phosphate excretion
    d. Serum calcium level
    Ans: d, i.e. Serum calcium level

230. **Not a complication of menopause:**
    a. Fracture spine
    b. Colles' fracture
    c. Fracture neck of femur
    d. Supracondylar fracture humerus
    Ans: d, i.e. Supracondylar fracture humerus

231. **Soft tissue calcification occurs in all *except*:**
    a. Hyperparathyroidism
    b. Scleroderma
    c. Hyperthyroidism
    d. Hypervitaminosis
    Ans: c, i.e. Hyperthyroidism

232. **Treatment of hypercalcaemia is all *except*:**
    a. Rizdol
    b. Plicamycin
    c. Ritodrinate
    d. Gallium nitrate
    Ans: a, i.e. Rizdol

233. **Calcium content of bone is increased in:**
    a. Prolonged immobilization
    b. Glucocorticoids administration
    c. Hyperparathyroidism
    d. Estrogen supplementation in post-menopausal women
    Ans: d, i.e. Estrogen supplementation in post-menopausal women

234. **What is the diagnostic radiological inding skeletal flurosis**
    a. Sclerosis of sacroiliac joint
    b. Interosseous membrane ossification
    c. Osteosclerosis of vertebral body
    d. Ossification of ligaments of knee joint
    Ans: b, i.e. Interosseous membrane ossification

235. Rocker bottom foot results from:
a. Congenital vertical talus
b. Poliomyelitis
c. Club foot over correction
d. Spina bifida
Ans. Two options are correct, i.e. 'a and c'

236. Sclerotic lesions in the bone is seen in all *except*:
a. Osteitis fibrosa
b. Osteopetrosis
c. Melorheostosis
d. Caffey's disease
Ans: a, i.e. Osteitis fibrosa

237. Recurrent clubfoot is due to failure of development of:
a. Tendocalcaneus
b. Peroneal muscles
c. Plantar fascia
d. Tibialis anterior
Ans: b, i.e. Peroneal muscles

238. Housemaids knee is inflammation of bursa:
a. Subpatellar
b. Suprapatellar
c. Infrapatellar
d. Prepatellar
Ans: d, i.e. Pre patellar

239. Arthrodesis of which is not done to correct flat foot:
a. Talus
b. Cuboid
c. Navicular
d. Calcaneum
Ans: b, i.e. Cuboid

240. Weaver's bottom is:
a. Eczematous lesions over buttocks of weavers due to their sedentary position
b. Ischiogluteal bursitis
c. Coccydynia
d. None of the above
Ans: b, i.e. Ischiogluteal bursitis

241. Trigger finger is most likely to be associated with:
a. Diabetes
b. Trauma
c. Gout
d. Rheumatoid arthritis
Ans: d, i.e. Rheumatoid arthritis

242. All of following may be cause of flexible flat foot *except*:
a. In elderly
b. In children
c. In obese
d. In congenital vertical talus
Ans: d, i.e. In congenital vertical talus

243. In hallux valgus surgery, the patients who are likely to be most satisfied are:
a. Those with pain
b. Those with hammer toe
c. Those with metatarsus primus varus
d. Young age
Ans: d, i.e. Young age

244. The long flexor tendon of the thumb can be advanced for more than 1 cm for repair in Zone 1 because:
a. Paratendinous adhesions are fewer following advancement than following free tendon graft
b. Only two annular pulleys bind the tendon to bone
c. Vascularity of the tendon is not compromised because vinculum is absent
d. The tendon is long enough to allow easy advancement
Ans. Two options are correct, i.e. 'a and c'

245. **Earliest changes in Perthes' disease is seen in:**
    a. X-ray
    b. CT
    c. MRI
    d. US
    e. Nuclear scan
    Ans: 'e', i.e. Nuclear scan

246. **Accessory navicular is called:**
    a. Os trigonum
    b. Os tibiale Internum
    c. Os tibiale externum
    d. Os navicular
    Ans: c, i.e. Os tibiale externum

247. **Sever's disease refers to:**
    a. Calcaneum
    b. Radius
    c. Talus
    d. Capitulum
    Ans: a, i.e. Calcaneum

248. **Dysplasia epiphysis hemimelica is:**
    a. Trevor's disease
    b. Blount's disease
    c. Streeter's dysplasia
    d. Leri's disease
    Ans: a, i.e. Trevor's disease

249. **Adventitious bursa is:**
    a. Found normally over any joint
    b. Due to degeneration of connective tissue over a joint
    c. Found over bony prominences
    d. Can turn into malignancy
    Ans: c, i.e. Found over bony prominences

250. **Osteochondritis dissecans occurs at:**
    a. Lateral surface lateral condyle
    b. Medial surface of lateral condyle
    c. Medial surface medial condyle
    d. Lateral surface medial condyle
    Ans: d, i.e. Lateral surface medial condyle

251. **Engelmann's disease is:**
    a. Multiple epiphyseal dysplasia
    b. Infantile cortical hyperostosis
    c. Cleidocranial dysplasia
    d. Progressive diaphyseal dysplasia
    Ans: d, i.e. Progressive diaphyseal dysplasia

252. **Sprengel's shoulder is due to deformity of:**
    a. Scapula
    b. Humerus
    c. Clavicle
    d. Vertebra
    Ans: a, i.e. Scapula

253. **Subperiosteal new bone formation is seen in all *except*:**
    a. Scurvy
    b. Osteosarcoma
    c. Osteomyelitis
    d. Eosinophilic granuloma
    Ans: d, i.e. Eosinophilic granuloma

254. **Commonest cause of loose bodies in joints in adults:**
    a. Tuberculous tenosynovitis
    b. Rheumatoid arthritis
    c. Osteoarthritis
    d. Osteochondritis dissecans
    Ans: c, i.e. Osteoarthritis

255. **Trouser leg appearance on an ascending myelogram suggestive of tumour:**
    a. Extradural
    b. Extramedullary
    c. Intramedullary
    d. None of the above
    Ans: c, i.e. Intramedullary

256. Myositis ossificans is commonly seen at the ... joint:
   a. Knee
   b. Elbow
   c. Shoulder
   d. Hip
   Ans: b, i.e. Elbow

257. Pectus excavatum is seen in:
   a. Cretinism
   b. Senile osteoporosis
   c. Osteogenesis imperfecta
   d. Chronic asthma
   Ans: d, i.e. Chronic asthma

258. Tissue most sensitive to radiation is:
   a. Osteoblast
   b. Cartilage
   c. Epiphysis
   d. Metaphysis
   Ans: c, i.e. Epiphysis

259. The cause of short fourth metacarpal bone is:
   a. Down syndrome
   b. Edward syndrome
   c. Turner's syndrome
   d. Pseudohypo-parathyroidism
   Ans. Two options are correct, i.e. 'c and d'

260. Increased density of skull vault is seen in:
   a. Hyperparathyroidism
   b. Multiple myeloma
   c. Fluorosis
   d. Renal osteodystrophy
   Ans. Two options are correct, i.e. 'c and d'

261. Soft tissue calcification around the knee is seen in:
   a. Scurvy
   b. Scleroderma
   c. Hyperparathyroidism
   d. Pseudogout
   Ans. Three options are correct, i.e. 'b, c and d'

262. Increased density in metaphysis is seen in:
   a. Hypervitaminosis
   b. Healed rickets
   c. Congenital syphilis
   d. Perthes' disease
   Ans: a, i.e. Hypervitaminosis

263. Meyer's operation is done for:
   a. Dislocation of patella
   b. Fracture neck of femur
   c. Dislocation of shoulder
   d. Fracture fibula
   Ans: b, i.e. Fracture neck of femur

264. Bleeding into joint cavities is *not* common in:
   a. Hemophilia
   b. ITP
   c. Christmas disease
   d. None of the above
   Ans: b, i.e. ITP

265. Battle's sign is seen in:
   a. Fracture middle cranial fossa
   b. Fracture base of skull
   c. Fracture anterior cranial fossa
   d. All of the above
   Ans. Two options are correct, i.e. 'a and b'

266. Duga's test is helpful in:
   a. Dislocation of hip
   b. Scaphoid fracture
   c. Fracture neck of femur
   d. Anterior dislocation of shoulder
   Ans: d, i.e. Anterior dislocation of shoulder

267. **Trendelenburg sign is *not* seen in:**
    a. Tuberculous arthritis
    b. Rheumatoid arthritis
    c. Posterior dislocation Hip
    d. Tom Smith arthritis
    Ans: d, i.e. Tom Smith arthritis

268. **Gaenslen's test is positive in:**
    a. Tennis elbow
    b. deQuervain's disease
    c. Carpal tunnel syndrome
    d. Ulnar bursitis
    Ans: 'None'

269. **Bone growth is influenced maximally by:**
    a. Estrogen
    b. Thyroxin
    c. Growth hormone
    d. Testosterone
    Ans: c, i.e. Growth hormone

270. **Cartilage is quite vascular in:**
    a. Embryonic life
    b. Early childhood
    c. Early adulthood
    d. Old age
    Ans: a, i.e. Embryonic life

271. **A recessive form of osteogenesis imperfecta may closely resemble:**
    a. Alkaptonuria
    b. Cretinism
    c. Hypophosphatasia
    d. Homocystinuria
    Ans: c, i.e. Hypophosphatasia

272. **Who is acclaimed world wide for total joint replacement:**
    a. Paul Brand
    b. John Charnley
    c. Paul Harrington
    d. Huckstep
    Ans: b, i.e. John Charnley

273. **Ossification in foetus starts in:**
    a. 1st week of intrauterine life
    b. 2nd week of intrauterine life
    c. 5th week of intrauterine life
    d. 5th month of intrauterine life
    Ans: c, i.e. 5th week of intrauterine life

274. **During the surgical procedure:**
    a. Tendons should be repaired before nerve
    b. Nerve should be repaired before tendons
    c. Tendons should not be repaired at the same time
    d. None is true
    Ans: b, i.e. Nerve should be repaired before tendons

275. **Which of the following is NOT true regarding synovial fluid:**
    a. Contains HCO_3 and CI ions more than plasma
    b. Contains minerals ions less than plasma
    c. Contains uric acid more than plasma
    d. Contains fibrinolysin
    Ans: c, i.e. Contains uric acid more than plasma

276. **Which of the following is NOT found normally in synovial membrane:**
    a. Two layers of lymphatics
    b. Paccinian corpuscles
    c. Basement membrane
    d. A fibrocollagenous layer
    Ans: c, i.e. Basement membrane

277. **Bilateral symmetrical idiopathic fractures are most commonly seen in:**
    a. Osteoporosis
    b. Osteogenesis imperfecta
    c. Polytrauma
    d. Stress fracture
    Ans: b, i.e. Osteogenesis imperfecta

278. Synovial tissue is seen earliest in a developing point at the age of:
a. 8th week of intrauterine life
b. 12th week of intrauterine life
c. 15th week of intrauterine life
d. 28th week of intrauterine life
Ans: b, i.e. 12th week of intrauterine life

279. Adult bone trabeculae are differentiated from foetal bone trabeculae histologically by the presence of:
a. Haversian system
b. Lamellar structure
c. Certain special staining characteristics
d. Different type of bone cells in each
Ans: b, i.e. Lamellar structure

280. The tensions resistance of normal fascia per square inch, such as the fascia lata, has been determined to be:
a. 550 pounds
b. 1000 pounds
c. 2000 pounds
d. 5000 pounds
e. 7000 pounds
Ans: 'e', i.e. 7000 pounds

281. Macewen's osteotomy is performed in cases of:
a. Coxa vara
b. Tibia vara
c. Genu valgum
d. Tom Smith disease
Ans: c, i.e. Genu valgum

282. Infection in ring finger in acute tenosynovitis is most likely to spread to:
a. Dorsum of hand
b. Thenar space
c. Parona's space
d. Mid palmar space
Ans: d, i.e. Mid palmar space

283. Sclerosis of bone is seen in all *except*:
a. Fluorosis
b. Osteopetrosis
c. Secondries from prostate
d. Hyperparathyroidism
Ans: d, i.e. Hyperparathyroidism

284. Triple deformity of knee is seen in:
a. Polio
b. Tuberculosis
c. Villonodular synovits
d. Rheumatoid arthritis
Ans. Three options are correct, i.e. 'a, b and d'

285. Cause of painful limb are all *except*:
a. Perthes' disease
b. Congenital coax vara
c. Slipped femoral epiphysis
d. TB hip
Ans: b, i.e. Congenital coax vara

286. Phocomelia is best described in:
a. Defect in development of long bones
b. Defect in development of flat bones
c. Defect of intramembranous ossification
d. Defect of cartilage replacement by bone
Ans: a, i.e. Defect in development of long bones

287. Pseudoarthrosis of tibia is best treated by:
a. Internal fixation
b. Internal fixation and bone grafting

   c. Above knee POP cast
   d. Below knee POP cast
   Ans: b, i.e. Internal fixation and bone grafting

288. **Viscosity of synovial fluid depends on:**
   a. Chondroitin sulphate
   b. Keratosulphate
   c. Hyaluronic acid
   d. Heparin sulphate
   Ans: c, i.e. Hyaluronic acid

289. **Triple deformity is a complication of:**
   a. Rheumatoid arthritis
   b. Tuberculosis
   c. Osteoarthritis
   d. Septic arthritis
   Ans. Two options are correct, i.e. 'a and b'

290. **Epiphyseal enlargement is a manifestation of:**
   a. Rickets
   b. Ankylosing spondylitis
   c. Spondylo-epiphyseal dysgenesis
   d. Scurvy
   Ans: a, i.e. Rickets

291. **Limb salvage primarily depends on:**
   a. Vascular injury
   b. Skin cover
   c. Bone injury
   d. Nerve injury
   Ans: a, i.e. Vascular injury

292. **Maximal shortening of lower limb is with:**
   a. Posterior dislocation
   b. Central dislocation
   c. Fracture neck of femurs
   d. Trochanteric fracture
   Ans: a, i.e. Posterior dislocation

293. **One of the following fracture requires plaster of Paris cast with equines position:**
   a. Distal fracture both bones leg
   b. Distal fracture fibula
   c. Bimalleolar
   d. Fracture talus
   Ans: d, i.e. Fracture talus

294. **Pathological changes in Caison's disease is due to:**
   a. N_2
   b. O_2
   c. CO_2
   d. CO
   Ans: a, i.e. N_2

295. **Treatment based on "Gate theory' is:**
   a. Short wave diatherapy
   b. Ultrasound
   c. Electrical nerve stimulation
   d. Infrared therapy
   Ans: c, i.e. Electrical nerve stimulation

296. **Osteophytes developing at the joint at Luschka characteristically compresses spinal nerve at:**
   a. Intervertebral foramen
   b. Anterior part of body
   c. Posterior part of body
   d. Paradural areas
   Ans: a, i.e. Intervertebral foramen

297. **Schmorl node is:**
   a. Radiological findings protruded nucleus pulposus into the vertebral body
   b. Soft tissue tumour in relation to the vertebral body
   c. A tumour in the intervertebral disc
   d. None of the above
   Ans: a, i.e. Radiological findings protruded nucleus pulposus into the vertebral body

298. Osteosclerotic rim is seen in:
   a. Growing epiphysis
   b. Giant cell tumor
   c. Enchondroma
   d. Old people
   Ans: a, i.e. Growing epiphysis

299. Least correction in remodelling of bone in children is seen in:
   a. Fracture shaft of humerus
   b. Fracture shaft of femur
   c. Subtrochanteric fracture
   Ans: a, i.e. Fracture shaft of humerus

300. Steinman pin is used for all *except*:
   a. Joint dislocation
   b. Ligament laxity
   c. Osteoporosis
   d. Blue sclera
   Ans: d, i.e. Blue sclera

301. Ortolani test is done for:
   a. Congenital dislocation of hip
   b. Congenital dislocation of knee
   c. Acquired dislocation of hip
   d. Acquired dislocation of knee
   Ans: a, i.e. Congenital dislocation of hip

302. On measurement, the base of Bryant's triangle on the left side is found to the short by 2 cm as compared to the right side. This indicates:
   a. Fracture of the neck of the femur
   b. Fracture of the shaft of the femur
   c. Osteoarthritis of hip joint
   d. Rheumatoid arthritis of the hip joint
   Ans: a, i.e. Fracture of the neck of the femur

303. Actinomycosis is commonly seen in:
   a. Tibia
   b. Mandible
   c. Scapula
   d. Femur
   Ans: b, i.e. Mandible

304. Meyer's operation is done for:
   a. Recurrent dislocation of patella
   b. Dislocation of shoulder joint
   c. Dislocation of hip joint
   d. # Scaphoid
   Ans: 'None'

305. Resorption of the terminal phalanx is not seen in:
   a. Hyperparathyroidism
   b. Reiter's syndrome
   c. Scleroderma
   d. Psoriasis
   Ans: b, i.e. Reiter's syndrome

306. Short wave diathermy is used for all of the following *except*:
   a. Back pain
   b. Haemophiliac joint
   c. Osteoarthritis
   d. Sprain
   Ans: b, i.e. Haemophiliac joint

307. Fracture blisters commonly appear on how many days:
   a. 1–3 days
   b. 3–5 days
   c. 5–7 days
   d. 5–9 days
   Ans: a, i.e. 1-3 days

308. Champagne glass pelvis on X-ray is seen in:
   a. Achondroplasia
   b. Congenital dislocation hip
   c. Strongyloid infection
   d. Rickets
   Ans: a, i.e. Achondroplasia

309. Minimal intra-discal pressure in vertebral column is seen when a person is:
   a. Standing
   b. Sitting
   c. Lying flat
   d. Lying on one side
   Ans: c, i.e. Lying flat

310. **A 3-year-old child falls from 2 metres height. On X-ray no abnormality of lower leg was seen. After 2 years, the child presents with calcaneal valgus. Probable cause is:**
   a. Undiagnosed
   b. Tibial epiphyseal plate injury
   c. Vascular necrosis of talus
   d. Rocker bottom foot
   Ans: b, i.e. Tibial epiphyseal plate injury

311. **Young man with # tibia of left side 2 months ago, is having popliteal cast. Now needs mobilization with single crutch. Which will be the preferred site:**
   a. Left sided crutch
   b. Right sided
   c. Any side
   d. Both sides
   Ans: b, i.e. Right sided

Bone Infection

1. **Bony ankylosis result from:**
   a. Pyogenic arthritis
   b. TB arthritis
   c. Osteoarthritis
   d. Rheumatic arthritis
   Ans. Two options are correct, i.e. 'a and b'

2. **The joint commonly involved in syphilitic arthritis is:**
   a. Hip
   b. Shoulder
   c. Wrist
   d. Knee
   Ans: d, i.e. Knee

3. **Commonest organism causing osteomyelitis in children under 3 years is:**
   a. *Haemophilus*
   b. Staphylococcal
   c. Streptococcal
   d. *Salmonella*
   Ans: b, i.e. Staphylococcal

4. **Commonest site for acute osteomyelitis in infant is:**
   a. Hip joint
   b. Tibia
   c. Femur
   d. Radial
   Ans: b, i.e. Tibia

5. **Osteomyelitis of the spine is mostly caused by:**
   a. *Salmonella*
   b. *Pneumococcus*
   c. Tubercle bacilli
   d. *Staphylococcus*
   Ans: c, i.e. Tubercle bacilli

6. **Osteomyelitis in a cases of sickle cell anaemia is caused by:**
   a. *Salmonella*
   b. *Pneumococcus*
   c. *Streptococcus*
   d. *Haemophilus*
   Ans: a, i.e. Salmonella

7. **Acute hematogenous osteomyelitis is treated with all *except*:**
   a. Antibiotics
   b. Splinting
   c. Analgesics
   d. Surgery
   Ans: 'None'

8. **Which is true regarding acute osteomyelitis:**
   a. *Staphylococcus* is the usual organism
   b. Rest and elevation relieves pain
   c. Parental antibiotics are given
   d. Surgery is the only treatment
   Ans. Three options are correct, i.e. 'a, b and c'

9. **What is Brodie's abscess:**
   a. Long standing localized pyogenic abscess in the bone
   b. Cold abscess

   c. Subperiosteal abscess
   d. Soft tissue abscess
   Ans: a, i.e. Long standing localized pyogenic abscess in the bone

10. **Brodie's abscess usually involves:**
   a. Long bones
   b. Short bones
   c. Pelvic bones
   d. Flat bones
   Ans: a, i.e. Long bones

11. **Viral osteomyelitis seen usually is due to vaccination for:**
   a. Smallpox virus infection
   b. Influenza virus infection
   c. Coxsackie virus infection
   d. Dengue fever
   Ans: a, i.e. Smallpox virus infection

12. **When osteomyelitis disseminates by hematogenous way the most affected part bone is:**
   a. Metaphyses
   b. Epiphyses
   c. Diaphysis
   d. Any of the above
   Ans: a, i.e. Metaphyses

13. **Tom Smith arthritis manifest as:**
   a. Increase hip mobility and instability
   b. Hip stiffness
   c. A + b
   d. Shortening of limb
   Ans. Two options are correct, i.e. 'a and d'

14. **Commonest cause of hematogenous osteomyelitis:**
   a. *Streptococcus*
   b. *Staph. aureus*
   c. *Salmonella*
   d. *H. influenza*
   Ans: b, i.e. *Staph. aureus*

15. **Actinomycosis is commonly seen in:**
   a. Tibia
   b. Mandible
   c. Scapula
   d. Femur
   Ans: b, i.e. Mandible

16. **All are seen in chronic osteomyelitis *except*:**
   a. Sequestrum
   b. Amyloidosis
   c. Myositis ossificans
   d. Metastatic abscess
   Ans: c, i.e. Myositis ossificans

17. **Acute osteomyelitis can best be distinguished from soft tissue infection by:**
   a. Clinical examination
   b. X-ray
   c. CT scan
   d. MRI
   Ans: a, i.e. Clinical examination

18. **Commonest site of skeletal tuberculosis is:**
   a. Tibia
   b. Radius
   c. Humerus
   d. Vertebrate
   Ans: d, i.e. Vertebrate

19. **Earliest manifestation of spinal TB is:**
   a. Cold abscess formation
   b. Paraplegia
   c. Gibbus
   d. Muscle spasm
   Ans: d, i.e. Muscle spasm

20. **Commonest site of TB spine is:**
   a. C8-T2
   b. T2-T6
   c. T10-L1
   d. L1-L4
   Ans: c, i.e. T10-L1

21. **Earliest sign in X-ray in TB spine:**
    a. Paravertebral shadow
    b. Narrowing of disc space
    c. Gibbus
    d. Straightening of the spinal curves
    Ans: b, i.e. Narrowing of disc space
22. **The early feature of Pott's paraplegia is:**
    a. Flexor spas,
    b. Increased tendon jerk
    c. Ankle clonus
    d. Sensory loss
    Ans: c, i.e. Ankle clonus
23. **Recovery in TB spine is delayed in children because of:**
    a. Inadequate rest
    b. Fragile bone
    c. More cartilage
    d. Increased vascularity
    Ans: a, i.e. Inadequate rest
24. **Commonest site of TB spine:**
    a. Dorsolumbar
    b. Lumbar
    c. Sacral
    d. Cervical
    Ans: a, i.e. Dorsolumbar

Metabolic Bone Disease

1. **Triradiate pelvis is seen in:**
    a. Paget's disease
    b. Rickets
    c. Osteomalacia
    d. Chondroma
    Ans: c, i.e. Osteomalacia

2. **Pseudofracture or looser's zone is seen in:**
    a. Osteoporosis
    b. Osteomalacia
    c. Hypoparathyroidism
    d. Pseudohypoparathyroidism
    Ans is b, i.e. Osteomalacia

3. **In Burton's disease there is:**
    a. Scurvy and rickets
    b. Scurvy and syphilis
    c. Syphilis and rickets
    d. Scurvy and pellagra
    Ans: a, i.e. Scurvy and rickets

4. **Senile osteoporosis is radiologically manifest only when ..... of skeleton has been lost:**
    a. 20%
    b. 30%
    c. 40%
    d. 80%
    Ans: c, i.e. 40%

5. **Fish-head appearance of the vertebral bodies is seen in:**
    a. Paget's disease
    b. Rickets
    c. Osteomalacia
    d. Osteoporosis
    Ans: d, i.e. Osteoporosis

6. **Increased bone density occurs in:**
    a. Cushing syndrome
    b. Hypoparathyrodism
    c. Fluorosis
    d. Hyperthyroidism
    Ans: c, i.e. Fluorosis

7. **Commonest site of fracture in senile osteoporosis is:**
    a. Neck of femur
    b. Shaft of femur
    c. Radius
    d. Vertebra
    Ans: d, i.e. Vertebra

8. Drug of choice for senile osteoporosis is:
- a. Oestrogens
- b. Androgens
- c. Calcitonin
- d. Ethidronate

Ans: d, i.e. Ethidronate

9. Metaphyseal fracture is commonly seen in:
- a. Osteogenesis imperfecta
- b. Scurvy
- c. Rickets
- d. None

Ans: b, i.e. Scurvy

10. In long-term therapy in vitamin-D-resistant rickets, the best guide to safe treatment is:
- a. Urinary phosphate excretion
- b. Urinary calcium excretion
- c. Serum alkaline phosphatase
- d. Serum phosphate level
- e. Serum calcium level

Ans: d, i.e. Serum phosphate level

11. All of following conditions may be responsible for osteoporosis *except*:
- a. Steroid therapy
- b. Prolonged weightlessness in spaceship
- c. Hyperparathyroidism
- d. Hypoparathyroidism

Ans: d, i.e. Hypoparathyroidism

12. Marker for bone formation:
- a. Osteocalcin
- b. TRAP
- c. 5 mucleotidase
- d. Parathormone

Ans: a, i.e. Osteocalcin

13. Most common site of fracture in osteoporosis:
- a. Fracture neck femur
- b. Vertebra
- c. Hip bone
- d. Humerus

Ans: b, i.e. Vertebra

Congenital Anomalies

1. Clubfoot seen in a 15-year-old could be treated successfully by:
- a. Appropriate foot wear
- b. Soft tissue operation
- c. Triple arthrodesis
- d. Quardriple fusion

Ans: c, i.e. Triple arthrodesis

2. Clubfoot in a newborn is treated by:
- a. Surgery
- b. Manipulation by the mother
- c. Dennis-Brown splint
- d. Strapping

Ans: b, i.e. Manipulation by the mother

3. Treatment of CTEV should begin:
- a. Soon after birth
- b. After discharge from hospital
- c. After one month
- d. At 2 years

Ans: a, i.e. Soon after birth

4. Clubfoot (CTEV) should be treated at the age of:
- a. 10–12 years of age of child
- b. From the day of birth
- c. 2-3 years of age of child
- d. After epiphyseal fusion

Ans: b, i.e. From the day of birth

5. Treatment of chronic cases of clubfoot is:
   a. Triple arthrodesis
   b. Dorsomedial release
   c. Amputation
   d. None
   Ans: a, i.e. Triple arthrodesis

6. In correction of clubfoot by manipulation, which deformity should be corrected first:
   a. Forefoot adduction
   b. Varus
   c. Equines
   d. Internal tibial torsion
   Ans: a, i.e. Forefoot adduction

7. Child aged 3¼ years is treated for CTEV by:
   a. Triple arthrodesis
   b. Posteromedial soft tissue release
   c. Lateral wedge resection
   d. Tendo Achilles lengthening and posterior capsulotomy
   Ans: b, i.e. Posteromedial soft tissue release

8. Which of the following is seen in bilateral congenital dislocation of hip:
   a. Waddling gait
   b. Shenton's line is broken
   c. Trendelenburg test positive
   d. Telescopy not positive
   Ans. Two options are correct, i.e. 'a and b'

9. In a newborn child abduction and internal rotation produces a click sound. It is known as:
   a. Ortolani's sign
   b. Telescoping sign
   c. Mc Murray's sign
   d. Lachman's sign
   Ans: a, i.e. Ortolani's sign

10. Sprengel's deformity of scapula is:
   a. Undescended/elevated scapula
   b. Undescended neck of scapula
   c. Exostosis scapula
   d. None of the above
   Ans: a, i.e. Undescended/elevated scapula

11. Cleidocranial dysostosis may show:
   a. Wide foramen magnum
   b. Absence of clavicles
   c. Coax vara
   d. All of the above
   Ans: b, i.e. Absence of clavicles

12. Phocomelia is caused by ingestion of … during pregnancy:
   a. Steroids
   b. Tetracycline
   c. Thalidomide
   d. Barbiturates
   Ans: c, i.e. Thalidomide

Developmental Disorder

1. The following is *false* of achondroplasia:
   a. Autosomal dominant
   b. Mental retardation
   c. Due to gene mutation
   d. Shortening of limbs present
   Ans: b, i.e. Mental retardation

2. Shepherd Crooke's deformity is seen in:
   a. Achondroplasia
   b. Gaucher's disease
   c. Hypothroidism
   d. Fibrous dysplasia
   Ans: d, i.e. Fibrous dysplasia

3. **Trident hand is seen in:**
   a. Achondroplasia
   b. Scurvy
   c. Mucopolysaccharidosis
   d. None
   Ans: a, i.e. Achondroplasia
4. **All are seen in osteogenesis imperfecta *except*:**
   a. Joint dislocation
   b. Ligament laxity
   c. Osteoporosis
   d. Blue sclera
   Ans: c, i.e. Osteoporosis
5. **Not associated with osteogenesis imperfecta is:**
   a. Blue sclera
   b. Cataract
   c. Deafness
   d. Fractures
   Ans: b, i.e. Cataract
6. **Marble bone disease is also known as:**
   a. Osteogenesis imperfecta
   b. Osteopetrosis
   c. Perthes' disease
   d. Ochronosis
   Ans: b, i.e. Osteopetrosis
7. **Multiple bone fracture in a newborn is seen in:**
   a. Scurvy
   b. Syphilis
   c. Osteogenesis imperfecta
   d. Morquio syndrome
   Ans: c, i.e. Osteogenesis imperfecta
8. **Musculoskeletal abnormalities in neurofibromatosis is:**
   a. Hypertrophy of limb
   b. Scoliosis
   c. Pseudo arthrosis
   d. All
   Ans: d, i.e. All
9. **Bilateral symmetrical idiopathic fractures are most commonly seen in:**
   a. Osteogenesis imperfecta
   b. Stress fracture
   c. Polytrauma
   d. Osteoporosis
   Ans: a, i.e. Osteogenesis imperfecta

Disease of Joints

1. **Herbeden nodules are seen in:**
   a. Osteoarthritis
   b. Rheumatoid arthritis
   c. Rheumatic arthritis
   d. Psoriatic arthritis
   Ans: a, i.e. Osteoarthritis
2. **HLA B27 is associated with:**
   a. Rheumatoid arthritis
   b. Ankylosing spondylitis
   c. Rheumatic arthritis
   d. Gouty arthritis
   Ans: b, i.e. Ankylosing spondylitis
3. **Bamboo spine is seen in:**
   a. Tuberculosis
   b. Rheumatoid arthritis
   c. Ochronosis
   d. Ankylosing spondylitis
   Ans: d, i.e. Ankylosing spondylitis
4. **The following is involved in rheumatoid arthritis:**
   a. Synovial fluid
   b. Synovial membrane
   c. Cartilage
   d. Subchondral bone
   Ans: b, i.e. Synovial membrane

5. Gaensien's operation is done for:
a. Cervical spondylosis
b. Recurrent shoulder dislocation
c. TB arthritis of knee joint
d. Sacroilliac subluxation
Ans: d, i.e. Sacroilliac subluxation

6. Bouchards nodes are seen in:
a. Proximal IP joints
b. Distal IP joints
c. Sterno-clavicular joints
d. Knee joints
Ans: a, i.e. Proximal IP joints

7. Most common cause of neuropathic joints:
a. Diabetes
b. Leprosy
c. Syphilis
d. Rheumatoid arthritis
Ans: a, i.e. Diabetes

8. Osteo-arthritis does *not* affect:
a. Knee joint
b. Hip joint
c. Interphalangeal joint
d. Metacarpophalangeal joint
e. Shoulder joint
Ans: d, i.e. Metacarpophalangeal joint

9. Positivity of HLA B27 in ankylosing spondylitis:
a. 10%
b. 90%
c. 78%
d. 100%
Ans: b, i.e. 90%

10. Earliest visible change in osteoarthritis is:
a. Loss of water
b. Fibrillation
c. Decreased collagen content
d. Decreased hyaluronic acid level
Ans: b, i.e. Fibrillation

11. Distal interphalangeal joint is *not* involved in:
a. Rheumatoid arthritis
b. Osteoarthritis
c. Psoriatic arthropathy
d. Multiple histocytosis
Ans: a, i.e. Rheumatoid arthritis

12. Disease where distal interphalangeal joint is:
a. Psoriatic arthritis
b. Rheumatoid
c. SLE
d. Gout
Ans: a, i.e. Psoriatic arthritis

13. The factor/ responsible for viscosity of synovial fluid:
a. Chondritin sulfate
b. Hyaluronic acid
c. Heparin sulfate
d. All of the above
Ans: b, i.e. Hyaluronic acid

14. In hemophilia pseudotumor is found in:
a. Gastrocnemius
b. Quadriceps
c. Ilio psoas
d. Semimembranous
Ans: c, i.e. Ilio psoas

Orthopaedics Neurology

1. Claw hand is seen in:
a. Ulnar nerve injury
b. Carpal tunnel syndrome
c. Syringomyelia
d. Cervical rib
Ans. Three options are correct, i.e. 'a, c and d'

2. **Pointing index sign is seen in ... nerve palsy:**
   a. Ulnar
   b. Radial
   c. Median
   d. Axillary
   Ans: c, i.e. Median

3. **Nerve abscess is seen in the ... nerve:**
   a. Median
   b. Ulnar
   c. Lateral fibular
   d. Sciatic
   Ans: b, i.e. Ulnar

4. **Commonest cause of wrist drop is:**
   a. Intramuscular injection
   b. Fracture humerus
   c. Dislocation of elbow
   d. Dislocation of shoulder
   Ans: b, i.e. Fracture humerus

5. **The lesion of Klumpke's paralysis is in:**
   a. Cervical plexus
   b. Lower brachial
   c. Upper brachial
   d. Sacral plexus
   Ans: b, i.e. Lower brachial

6. **Dorsum of middle finger is supplied by:**
   a. Radial nerve
   b. Median nerve
   c. Ulnar nerve
   d. a and b
   Ans. Three option are correct, i.e. 'a, b and c'

7. **Sensory supply of the tip of the ring finger is:**
   a. Radial nerve
   b. Median nerve
   c. Ulnar nerve
   d. Posterior interosseous nerve
   Ans. Two option are correct, i.e. 'b and c'

8. **Which nerve repair has worst prognosis:**
   a. Ulnar
   b. Radial
   c. Median
   d. Lateral popliteal
   Ans: a, i.e. Ulnar

9. **A patient presented with claw hand after a supracondylar fracture was reduced and plaster applied. The diagnosis is:**
   a. Median nerve injury
   b. Volkmann's ischaemic contracture
   c. Ulnar nerve injury
   d. Dupuytren's contracture
   Ans: Two options are correct, i.e. 'b and c'

10. **Phalen's test is positive in:**
    a. Ulnar bursitis
    b. Tennis elbow
    c. Carpal tunnel syndrome
    d. deQuervain's disease
    Ans: c, i.e. Carpal tunnel syndrome

11. **Total claw hand is caused by injury to:**
    a. Radial nerve
    b. Ulnar and radial nerve
    c. Ulnar and medial nerve
    d. Radian and median nerve
    Ans: c, i.e. Ulnar and medial nerve

12. **Radial nerve injury above elbow lead to:**
    a. Ape thumb
    b. Trigger finger
    c. Wrist drop
    d. Claw hand
    Ans: c, i.e. Wrist drop

13. **Peripheral nerves can withstand ischaemia up to:**
    a. 30 minutes
    b. 1 hour
    c. 2 hours
    d. 4 hours
    Ans: 'None', correct ans is 8 hours.

14. **Axillary nerve injury at its origin leads to paralysis of:**
    a. Deltoid and teres minor
    b. Deltoid
    c. Deltoid and teres major
    d. Latissmus dorsi and deltoid
    Ans: a, i.e. Deltoid and teres minor

15. **Radial nerve injury of the type recovers with conservative management:**
    a. Neurotmesis
    b. Crush injury
    c. Neuropraxia
    d. Chemical injury
    Ans: c, i.e. Neuropraxia

16. **Polio paralysis differs from paralysis due to other causes:**
    a. Weakness
    b. Deformity of limbs
    c. No sensory loss
    d. Full recovery is possible
    Ans: c, i.e. No sensory loss

17. **Tendon transfer in polio is done at age of:**
    a. Less than 6 months
    b. 5 months to 1 year
    c. 2 years
    d. 5 years
    Ans: d, i.e. 5 years

18. **The 'Card test' tests the function of:**
    a. Median nerve
    b. Ulnar nerve
    c. Axillary nerve
    d. Radial nerve
    Ans: b, i.e. Ulnar nerve

19. **Injury of median nerve at wrist is best detected by:**
    a. Action of abductor pollicis brevis
    b. Action of flexor pollicis brevis
    c. Loss of sensation of radial half of palm
    d. Loss of sensation of tip of ring finger
    Ans: a, i.e. Action of abductor pollicis brevis

20. **Weber-Fechnar law is:**
    a. Magnitude of sensation is proportional to number of receptor stimulated
    b. Magnitude of sensation is proportional amplitude of action potential or receptor
    c. Magnitude of sensation is proportional to logarithm of intensity of stimulus
    d. Intensity of frequency of stimulus
    Ans: c, i.e. Magnitude of sensation is proportional to logarithm of intensity of stimulus

21. **Brachialis is supplied by:**
    a. Radial and ulnar nerve
    b. Median and musculocutaneous nerve
    c. Radial and musculocutaneous nerve
    d. Radial and median nerve
    Ans: c, i.e. Radial and musculocutaneous nerve

22. **Nerve which responds best to repair is:**
    a. Median
    b. Ulnar
    c. Sciatic
    d. Radial
    Ans: d, i.e. Radial

23. **Extension of the metacarpophalangeal joint is lost injury to:**
    a. Radial nerve
    b. Ulnar nerve
    c. Median nerve
    d. Posterior interosseous nerve
    Ans. Two option are correct i.e, 'a and d'

24. Clumsiness of the hand in case of leprosy is due to involvement of:
a. Interosseous muscle
b. Abductor pollicis longus
c. Extensor carpi ulnaris
d. Flexor carpi ulnaris
Ans: a, i.e. Interosseous muscle

Miscellaneous

1. Pain in Pagets' disease is relieved best by:
a. Simple analgesic
b. Narcotic analgesics
c. Radiation
d. Calcitonin
Ans: d, i.e. Calcitonin

2. The complications of Paget's disease is:
a. Osteogenic sarcoma
b. Deafness
c. Heart failure
d. All of the above
Ans: d, i.e. All of the above

3. Deafness in cases of Paget's disease is due to:
a. Thickened cranium
b. Narrowing of foramina of skull
c. Brain compression
d. Otosclerosis
Ans: d, i.e. Otosclerosis

4. The following are radiological sign's of Paget's disease of bone *except*:
a. "Cotton wool" appearance
b. "Picture window frame" appearance
c. "Hair-on-end" appearance
d. "Blade of grass" appearance
Ans: c, i.e. "Hair-on-end" appearance

5. Following are features of Paget's disease *except*:
a. Deformity of bones
b. Secondary osteosarcoma
c. Lowered serum alkaline phosphatase
d. Increased urinary excretion of hydroxyproline
Ans: c, i.e. Lowered serum alkaline phosphatase

6. Drug therapy of Paget's disease (osteitis deformans):
a. Alendronate
b. Etidronate
c. Calcitonin
d. Plicamycin
Ans: d, i.e. Plicamycin

7. Caffey's disease occurs in infant ages:
a. Below 6 months
b. Above 5 years
c. Above 10–20 years
d. 20–40 years
Ans: a, i.e. Below 6 months

8. Treatment of choice for Caffey's disease:
a. Multiple drilling
b. Tetracycline
c. Penicillin
d. Curettage
Ans: c, i.e. Penicillin

9. In Hand-Schuller-Christian disease, which is correct:
a. Proliferation of reticulo endothelial cells
b. Foam cells seen
c. Punched out lesions in X-ray
d. Diabetes insipidus and Exophthalmoses present
e. All are correct
Ans: e, i.e. All are correct

10. **Osteomyelitis of jaw is seen in:**
    a. Osteomalacia
    b. Osteopoikilosis
    c. Osteoporosis
    d. Caffey's disease
    Ans: d, i.e. Caffey's disease

Regional Orthopaedics

1. **Most common cause of scoliosis in children is:**
   a. Unequal limb length
   b. Post poliomyelitis
   c. Hemivertebrae
   d. Marfans' syndrome
   Ans: b, i.e. Post poliomyelitis
2. **Fracture dislocation injury of the spine is caused by:**
   a. Flexion only
   b. Rotation
   c. Extension
   d. Flexion and rotation
   Ans: d, i.e. Flexion and rotation
3. **Slipped femoral epiphysis is commonly seen in the:**
   a. 1st decade
   b. 2nd decade
   c. 3rd decade
   d. 4th decade
   Ans: b, i.e. 2nd decade
4. **Pes cavus is caused by:**
   a. Weakness of intrinsic muscles of the foot
   b. Excessive tone of intrinsic muscles
   c. Collapse of the arch
   d. Fracture of calcaneum
   Ans: a, i.e. Weakness of intrinsic muscles of the foot
5. **Coxa vara is found in:**
   a. Perthes' disease
   b. Tuberculosis
   c. Rickets
   d. Rheumatoid arthritis
   Ans: a and c, i.e. Perthes' disease and Rickets
6. **Painful are syndrome is due to:**
   a. Chronic supraspinatus tendonitis
   b. Sub-acromial bursitis
   c. Fracture greater tubercle
   d. All of the above
   Ans: d, i.e. All of the above
7. **Which is true about Perthes' disease?**
   a. Not painful
   b. It manifests at puberty
   c. Involves head of femur
   d. Viral aetiology
   Ans: c, i.e. Involves head of femur
8. **Earliest changes in Perthes' disease is seen by:**
   a. X-ray
   b. CT
   c. MRI
   d. US
   e. Nuclear scan
   Ans: 'e', i.e. Nuclear scan
9. **Mallet finger is:**
   a. Avulsion fracture of extensor tendon of distal phalanx
   b. Fracture of distal phalanx
   c. Fracture of middle phalanx
   d. Fracture of proximal phalanx
   Ans: a, i.e. Avulsion fracture of extensor tendon of distal phalanx

10. Dupuytren's contracture is:
   a. Thickening of palmar fascia
   b. Base of little finger involved first
   c. Seen in cirrhotic
   d. Seen in epileptics on hydantoin
   e. All of the above
   Ans: a, c and d, i.e. Thickening of palmar fascia, Seen in cirrhotic and Seen in epileptics on hydantoin

11. Dupuytren's contracture is fibrosis of:
   a. Palmar fascia
   b. Forearm muscles
   c. Sartorius fascia
   d. None
   Ans: a, i.e. Palmar fascia

12. Beheaded Scottish terrier sign is seen in:
   a. Disc prolapse
   b. Sacarlisation of L5
   c. Spondylosis
   d. Spondylolisthesis
   Ans: d, i.e. Spondylolisthesis

Bone Tumour

1. Ivory osteoma commonly arises in the:
   a. Skull
   b. Ribs
   c. Pelvis
   d. Vertebra
   Ans: a, i.e. Skull

2. Commonest site of multiple myeloma:
   a. Skull
   b. Ribs
   c. Vertebra
   d. Long bones
   e. Pelvis
   Ans: c, i.e. Vertebra

3. Commonest site of chondroblastoma:
   a. Epiphysis
   b. Diaphysis
   c. Metaphysis
   d. Soft tissues
   e. Periosteum
   Ans: a, i.e. Epiphysis

4. Osteoblastic secondaries can arise from:
   a. Carcinoma prostate
   b. Thyroid carcinoma
   c. Renal carcinoma
   d. Breast carcinoma
   Ans. Two options are correct, i.e. 'a and d'

5. Commonest benign tumour of the bone is:
   a. Osteoma
   b. Osteochondroma
   c. Osteoid osteoma
   d. Chondroma
   Ans: b, i.e. Osteochondroma

6. Sunray appearance is seen in:
   a. Osteogenic sarcoma
   b. Ewings sarcoma
   c. Multiple myeloma
   d. Osteoclastoma
   Ans: a, i.e. Osteogenic sarcoma

7. Tumour arising from diaphysis:
   a. Osteogenic sarcoma
   b. Ewing's sarcoma
   c. Multiple myeloma
   d. Osteoclastoma
   Ans: b, i.e. Ewing's sarcoma

8. **Tumour most sensitive to radiotheraphy is:**
   a. Osteogenic sarcoma
   b. Ewing's sarcoma
   c. Multiple myeloma
   d. Osteoclastoma
   Ans: b, i.e. Ewing's sarcoma

9. **Enchondroma commonly arises from:**
   a. Ribs
   b. Vertebra
   c. Tibia
   d. Phalanges
   Ans: d, i.e. Phalanges

10. **Osteogenic sarcoma can develop in:**
    a. Osteoblastoma
    b. Paget's disease
    c. Osteoid osteoma
    d. All of the above
    Ans: b, i.e. Paget's disease

11. **The treatment of enchodroma is:**
    a. Amputation
    b. Irradiation
    c. Local excision
    d. Curettage and bone chip filling
    Ans: d, i.e. Curettage and bone chip filling

12. **Onion peel appearance in X-ray suggests:**
    a. Osteogenic sarcoma
    b. Ewing's sarcoma
    c. Osteoclastoma
    d. Chondrosarcoma
    Ans: b, i.e. Ewing's sarcoma

13. **Soap bubble appearance in X-ray suggests:**
    a. Osteogenic sarcoma
    b. Ewing's sarcoma
    c. Osteoclastoma
    d. Chondrosarcoma
    Ans: c, i.e. Osteoclastoma

14. **Involvement of regional lymph nodes is seen in:**
    a. Osteogenic sarcoma
    b. Synovial sarcoma
    c. Osteoclastoma
    d. Fibrosarcoma
    Ans: b, i.e. Synovial sarcoma

15. **Pain in osteoid osteoma is specifically relieved by:**
    a. Salicylates
    b. Narcotic analgesics
    c. Radiation
    d. Splinting
    Ans: a, i.e. Salicylates

16. **Osteogenic sarcoma metastasizes to ... commonly:**
    a. Liver
    b. Lung
    c. Brain
    d. Regional lymph nodes
    Ans: b, i.e. Lung

17. **The commonest bone tumour is:**
    a. Osteosarcoma
    b. Osteoclastoma
    c. Secondaries
    d. Multiple myeloma
    Ans: c, i.e. Secondaries

18. **Osteosarcoma have a very poor prognosis because:**
    a. Highly malignant
    b. Resistant to radiotherapy
    c. Inoperable
    d. Spreads to lung very fast
    Ans: d, i.e. Spreads to lung very fast

19. **In carcinoma prostate with metastasis which is raised:**
    a. ESR
    b. Alkaline phosphatase
    c. Acid phosphatase
    d. Billirubine
    Ans: c, i.e. Acid phosphatase

20. Which of the following arises from epiphysis?
   a. Osteogenic sarcoma
   b. Ewings sarcoma
   c. Osteoclastoma
   d. Multiple Myeloma
   Ans: c, i.e. Osteoclastoma

21. Multiple myeloma is most frequently encountered in the ... decade:
   a. Third
   b. Fourth
   c. Fifth
   d. Seventh
   Ans: d, i.e. Seventh

22. Commonest site of bone cyst:
   a. Upper end of humerus
   b. Lower end of tibia
   c. Lower end of femur
   d. Upper end of femur
   Ans: a, i.e. Upper end of humerus

23. Commonest site for osteogenic sarcoma is:
   a. Upper end of femur
   b. Lower end of femur
   c. Upper end of tibia
   d. Lower end of tibia
   Ans: b, i.e. Lower end of femur

24. Commonest site of osteoclastoma is:
   a. Upper end of femur
   b. Lower end of femur
   c. Upper end of tibia
   d. Lower end of tibia
   Ans: b, i.e. Lower end of femur

25. In multiple myeloma which of the following is seen?
   a. Raised serum calcium
   b. Raised alkaline phosphatase
   c. Raised acid phosphatase
   d. All
   Ans: 'a', i.e. Raised serum calcium

26. Commonest tumour arising from the metaphysis is:
   a. Osteoclastoma
   b. Osteosarcoma
   c. Ewing's sarcoma
   d. Synovial sarcoma
   Ans: b, i.e. Osteosarcoma

27. Treatment of solitary bone cyst is:
   a. Curettage
   b. Excision
   c. Curettage and bone grafting
   d. Irradiation
   Ans: c, i.e. Curettage and bone grafting

28. Age group of osteogenic sarcoma is:
   a. 1–10
   b. 10–20
   c. 20–30
   d. 30–40
   Ans: b, i.e. 10-20

29. The lytic lesion in the epiphysis in children is seen:
   a. Osteogenic sarcoma
   b. Osteoclastoma
   c. Aneurysmal bone cyst
   d. Chondroblastoma
   Ans: d, i.e. Chondroblastoma

30. In which of the following tumour of the extremity of limb is excision of regional lymph node done?
   a. Adamantinoma
   b. Osteoclastoma
   c. Ewing's sarcoma
   d. Synovial cell sarcoma
   Ans: d, i.e. Synovial cell sarcoma

31. Bone cysts most commonly occur in:
   a. Spine
   b. Humerus
   c. Femur
   d. Tibia
   Ans: b, i.e. Humerus

32. **Most common site of ivory osteoma:**
    a. Orbit
    b. Maxilla
    c. Frontal sinus
    d. Mandible
    Ans: c, i.e. Frontal sinus

33. **Fibrous dysplasia of bone with precocious puberty and pigmentation is seen in:**
    a. Adrenal hypoplasia
    b. Achondroplasia
    c. Albright's syndrome
    d. Gardner's syndrome
    Ans: c, i.e. Albright's syndrome

34. **Most common site of aneurysmal bone cyst is:**
    a. Lower end of humerus
    b. Pelvic bones
    c. Radius
    d. Upper end of tibia
    Ans: d, i.e. Upper end of tibia

35. **The most confirmatory test for myeloma is:**
    a. Aspiration of the lesion and histology
    b. Bence-Jones protein in urine
    c. Serum electrophoresis
    d. Technitium 99 radionuclide bone scan
    Ans: c, i.e. Serum electrophoresis

36. **Pain in thigh more at night relieved by aspirin is:**
    a. Osteosarcoma
    b. Osteoclastoma
    c. Ewing's tumour
    d. Osteoid osteoma
    Ans: d, i.e. Osteoid osteoma

37. **Bone tumour metastasizing to bone is:**
    a. Giant cell tumour
    b. Ewing's sarcoma
    c. Chondrosarcoma
    d. Osteosarcoma
    Ans: b, i.e. Ewing's sarcoma

38. **Vertical striations on vertebral bodies are seen in:**
    a. Haemangioma
    b. Paget's disease
    c. Vertebral metastasis
    d. Osteoporosis
    Ans: a, i.e. Haemangioma

39. **Most reliable method for detecting bone metastases:**
    a. MRI
    b. CT scan
    c. Radiography
    d. SPECT
    Ans: 'None'

40. **A boy presenting with swelling at lower end of femur with calcified nodular shadow in lung has:**
    a. Osteosarcoma
    b. Osteochondroma
    c. Tuberculosis femur lower end
    d. Osteomyelitis
    Ans: a, i.e. Osteosarcoma

41. **Ewing's tumour arises from:**
    a. Mesothelial cell
    b. Endothelial cell
    c. Squamous cell
    d. None of the above
    Ans: d, i.e. None of the above

42. **Most common lesion of hand is:**
    a. Enchondroma
    b. Synovioma
    c. Exostosis
    d. Osteoclastoma
    Ans: a, i.e. Enchondroma

43. **A child with upper leg swelling with pulmonary nodule most probable diagnosis is:**
    a. Osteoclastoma
    b. Chondrosarcoma
    c. Osteosarcoma
    d. Chondroblastoma
    Ans: c, i.e. Osteosarcoma

44. **An 8 years old child has a swelling in diaphysis of femur. Histology reveals small clear round symmetrical cells minimum cytoplasm, necrotic areas, minimum osteoid and chondroid material cells. Most likely, it contains:**
    - a. Mucin
    - b. Lipid
    - c. Iron
    - d. Glycogen

    Ans: d Glycogen

45. **Kachrumal, a 46 years old man has expensive growth metaphysis with endosteal scalloping and dense punctate calcification. Most likely bone tumour is:**
    - a. Osteosarcoma
    - b. Chondrosarcoma
    - c. Osteoclastoma
    - d. Osteoid osteoma

    Ans: b, i.e. Chondrosarcoma

46. **Most common site of tumours of bone is –**
    - a. Femur
    - b. Tibia
    - c. Humerus
    - d. Vertebral column

    Ans: a, i.e. Femur

Amputation

1. **Distance from elbow in forearm amputation … inches:**
   - a. 5
   - b. 7
   - c. 8
   - d. 9

   Ans: b, i.e. 7

2. **Distance from the acromian in arm amputation is … inches:**
   - a. 5
   - b. 7
   - c. 8
   - d. 9

   Ans: c, i.e. 8

3. **Distance from the lip of greater trochanter in thigh amputation is … inches:**
   - a. 5
   - b. 7
   - c. 9
   - d. 11

   Ans: d, i.e. 11

4. **Distance from the knee joint in below knee amputation is … inches:**
   - a. 4
   - b. 5.5
   - c. 6
   - d. 7

   Ans: b, i.e. 5.5

5. **Complications of an amputation stump may be:**
   - a. Phantom limb
   - b. Stump neuroma
   - c. Ring sequestrum
   - d. All the above

   Ans: d, i.e. All the above

6. **Symes amputation is contra indicated in:**
   - a. Malignancy of big toe
   - b. Diabetic foot
   - c. Madura mycosis foot
   - d. Crush injury

   Ans: 'None'

Splints

1. **Nondynamic splint is:**
   - a. Banjo
   - b. Opponons
   - c. Cock-up
   - d. Brand

   Ans: c, i.e. Cock-up

2. Aeroplane splint is used for:
   a. Brachial plexus palsy
   b. Volkmann's ischaemic contracture
   c. Myositis ossificans
   d. Fracture talus
   Ans: a, i.e. Brachial plexus palsy

3. von Rosen splint is used in:
   a. CTEV
   b. CDH
   c. Fracture shaft of femur
   d. Fracture tibia
   Ans: b, i.e. CDH

4. Milwaukee brace is used in:
   a. Scoliosis
   b. Fracture skull
   c. Fracture tibia
   d. CTEV
   Ans: a, i.e. Scoliosis

Eponymous Fracture

1. Shoveller's fracture is:
   a. Stress fracture of spinous processes
   b. Fracture of forearm bones
   c. Fracture of the body of atlas
   d. Fracture dislocation of axis vertebrae
   Ans: a, i.e. Stress fracture of spinous processes

2. March fracture affects:
   a. Neck of 2nd metatarsal
   b. Body of 2nd metatarsal
   c. Neck of 1st metatarsal
   d. Fracture of lower end of tibia
   e. Fracture of lower end of fibula
   Ans: a, i.e. Neck of 2nd metatarsal

3. March fracture is:
   a. Stress fracture of neck of second metatarsal
   b. Stress fracture of neck of talus
   c. Compression fracture of calcaneum
   d. Fracture lower end of fibula
   Ans: a, i.e. Stress fracture of neck of second metatarsal

4. Jefferson fracture occurs at:
   a. C1
   b. C2
   c. C1, C2
   d. C2, C3
   Ans: a, i.e. C1

5. Lisfranc dislocation is
   a. Tarsometatarsal dislocation
   b. Lunate dislocation
   c. Scaphoid dislocation
   d. Posterior dislocation of elbow
   Ans: a, i.e. Tarsometatarsal dislocation

6. Bennett's fracture is fracture dislocation of base of ... metacarpal
   a. 4th
   b. 3rd
   c. 2nd
   d. 1st
   Ans: d, i.e. 1st

Index

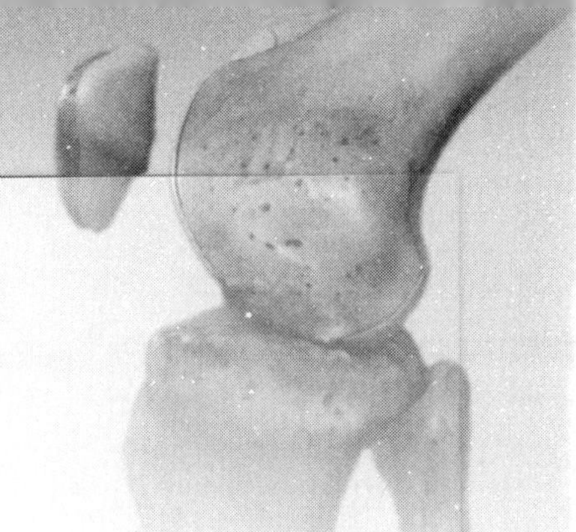